PRINCIPLES IN CONTEMPORARY ORTHODONTICS

Edited by **Silvano Naretto**

INTECHOPEN.COM

Principles in Contemporary Orthodontics
Edited by Silvano Naretto

Published by InTech

Janeza Trdine 9, 51000 Rijeka, Croatia

Edition 2014

Publishing Process Manager Martina Blecic

Technical Editor Teodora Smiljanic

Cover Designer InTech Design Team

Image Copyright Anna Omelchenko, 2011. Used under license from Shutterstock.com

Additional hard copies can be obtained from orders@intechopen.com

Principles in Contemporary Orthodontics, Edited by Silvano Naretto
p. cm.
ISBN 978-953-307-687-4

INTECH

open science | open minds

Contents

Preface IX

Part 1 Technology 1

Chapter 1 **Self-Ligating Brackets: An Overview 3**
Maen Zreaqat and Rozita Hassan

Chapter 2 **Considerations in Orthodontic Bracket Adhesion to Hypomineralized Enamel 31**
Shabtai Sapir

Chapter 3 **External Apical Root Resorption in Patients Treated with Passive Self-Ligating System 43**
Masaru Yamaguchi and Yasuhiro Tanimoto

Part 2 Technique 53

Chapter 4 **Treatment of Class II Deep Overbite with Multiloop Edgewise Arch-Wire (MEAW) Therapy 55**
Paulo Beltrão

Chapter 5 **Sagittal Skeletal and Occlusal Changes of Class II, Division 1 Postadolescent Cases in the Herbst and Activator Therapy 79**
Nenad Nedeljkovic

Chapter 6 **Sterilization and Disinfection in Orthodontics 113**
Alev Aksoy, Gulcın Kılıç, Emad Hussein and Darleen Aboukhalil

Chapter 7 **Laser in Orthodontics 129**
Fekrazad Reza, Kalhori A.M. Katayoun, Ahrari Farzaneh and Tadayon Nikoo

Chapter 8 **Modern Etching and Bonding Materials in Orthodontics 181**
Güvenç Başaran and İlknur Veli

Part 3 Methodology 213

Chapter 9 **An Overview of Selected Orthodontic Treatment Need Indices 215**
Ali Borzabadi-Farahani

Chapter 10 **Orthodontic Retreatment: Dental Trauma and Root Resorption 237**
Pedro Marcelo Tondelli, Fabiana Akemy Kay, Osmar Aparecido Cuoghi and Marcos Rogério de Mendonça

Chapter 11 **Early Treatments in Orthodontics 251**
Ousehal Lahcen and Lazrak Laila

Chapter 12 **Maxillary Lateral Incisor Agenesis (MLIA) 277**
Teresa Pinho

Chapter 13 **Orthodontics and Caries 309**
Farid Bourzgui, Mourad Sebbar and Mouna Hamza

Chapter 14 **New Strategies for Class II Fixed Functional Orthodontics, Including MRI Diagnostics, Manual Functional Analysis and Physiotherapy 327**
Douglas Edward Toll, Nenad Popović and Nicole Drinkuth

Chapter 15 **Treatment and Long Term Follow-Up of a Patient with an Impacted Transmigrant Canine 337**
Neslihan Üçüncü, Belma Işık Aslan and H. Tuğçe Oğuz Türel

Part 4 Orthognathic Surgery 353

Chapter 16 **Orthodontic Contribution to Orthognathic Surgery Cases 355**
Nikolaos Topouzelis

Chapter 17 **Long-Term Outcome of Orthognathic Surgery 381**
Lisen Espeland and Arild Stenvik

Chapter 18 **Orthodontic-Surgical Treatment: Electromyographic and Electrognatographic Evaluation with Three Electromyographic Instruments 397**
Giampietro Farronato, Cinzia Maspero, Lucia Giannini and Guido Galbiati

Chapter 19 **Surgical Orthodontic Treatment of Class III Malocclusions 417**
Paolo Ronchi and Alberto Guariglia

Part 5 Research 445

Chapter 20 **Does Comtemporary Orthodontics Comply with Universal Logic? 447**
Hicham Khayat

Chapter 21 **The Artificial Intelligence Approach for Diagnosis, Treatment and Modelling in Orthodontic 451**
Kazem Bahaa, Garma Noor and Yousif Yousif

Chapter 22 **Biomechanics of Tooth-Movement: Current Look at Orthodontic Fundamental 493**
Joanna Antoszewska and Nazan Küçükkeleş

Chapter 23 **Neural Modulation of Orthodontic Tooth Movement 527**
John K. Neubert, Robert M. Caudle, Calogero Dolce, Edgardo J. Toro, Yvonne Bokrand-Donatelli and L. Shannon Holliday

Chapter 24 **Clinical Application of Three-Dimensional Reverse Engineering Technology in Orthodontic Diagnosis 545**
Bong-Kuen Cha

Chapter 25 **Recent Advances in the Genetics of Orthodontics 569**
Yoko Tomoyasu, Tetsutaro Yamaguchi and Koutaro Maki

Preface

Is there a need for another Orthodontic textbook? Science is a continuum developing of curiosity and mistakes of trail and errors and concepts.

Knowledge presents different areas of inquiry: origin of knowledge, varieties of knowledge, possibility and limit of knowledge, structure of knowledge and methodology of knowledge.

Methodology: not to be mistaken for technology or technique. It refers to the analysis of conceptual, observational and experimental principles and methods that guide a scientific, biomedical and clinical inquiry.

Clinical observations are interpretations in the light of theories and for this reason they are apt to seem to support those theories, and theories or concepts in orthodontics are conjectural and based on a paradigm, a model. Any refutation-corroboration process in medicine and orthodontics is not a cognitive act but a decision making procedure.

In dentofacial orthopedics the process of decision making is based on scientific knowledge and empirical clinical evidence.The distinction between the normal and abnormal is an operation of decision rather than a cognitive act. A discontinuity may be detectable during transition phases but is not necessarily the threshold for the abnormal. Orthodontists are interested in forecasting that if the appropriate requirements are fulfilled, the anticipated event will occur. Clinicians must account for the individual variability, uncontrolled or unknown disturbing factors and unexpected secondary effects.

Written words will last forever, pronounced words will be lost. But the original meaning of this sentence was exactly the opposite. In ancient time until the Middle Age words were written to be pronounced aloud by the few that were able to read them for the people not able to do so, so that "verba volant" words would have been divulged.

Because books were read aloud, it was not necessary to separate letters in phonetic units so writing was a long uninterrupted sequence of letters without capitals letters nor punctuation and was the capability of the reader to give the sense and the interpretation of the written text.

Depending on the place and time these letters in long sequence were from left to right, right to left, from up to down or in two columns or alternatively one line from right and one from left or others zig-zag on the page. Also Marcus Tullius Cicero needed plenty of training before giving a good lecture on the written text and with the correct interpretation.

Julius Caesar was the first one who requested the division of the continuous text in pages to be sent as messages to his troops. In the IV century written text started to be divided "per cola et commata" in lines with a finished meaning. But only between the VII and IX century we can define the beginning of the "silent reading" the method that today seems so natural to the private reader, reading in silence, needed a long time to mature in the present way as pages, paragraphs, lines and punctuations. Books! Books as papyrus scroll rolls were found in Egypt more than 4000 years ago and until Johannes Gutenberg (XV century) was written by hand. And what is next? Would like to report some thoughts:

"Electronic reading has become progressively easier as computer screens have improved and readers have grown accustomed to using them. Still, people read more slowly on

screen, by as much as 20–30%. Fifteen or 20 years ago, electronic reading also impaired comprehension compared to paper, but those differences have faded in recent studies." (Sandra Aamodt is a former editor in chief of Nature Neuroscience)

"Initially, any new information medium seems to degrade reading because it disturbs the balance between focal and peripheral attention. This was true as early as the invention of writing, which Plato complained hollowed out focal memory. Similarly, William Wordsworth's sister complained that he wasted his mind in the newspapers of the day. It takes time and adaptation before a balance can be restored." (Alan Liu is chairman and professor of English at the University of California, Santa Barbara)

"The tools (as usual) are neutral. It's up to us to insist that onscreen reading enhance, not replace, traditional book reading. It's up to us to remember that the medium is not the message; that the meaning and music of the words is what matters, not the glitzy vehicle they arrive in." (David Gelernter, a professor of computer science at Yale University)

In conclusion, whatever the future of writing and reading will be, on paper or on screen, the contents and the thoughts of the authors is the real treasure we have to appreciate and keep as a precious gift.

My acknowledgment goes to all the scientists and clinicians giving their personal effort to contribute to the understanding and developing of our profession.

My acknowledgment goes also to my teachers, mentors and authors for their contribution with their concepts to my personal knowledge in the field of orthodontics.

Silvano Naretto MD, DDS, MSc
Department of Int. Dentistry and Technology
Danube University Krems,
Austria

Part 1

Technology

1

Self-Ligating Brackets: An Overview

Maen Zreaqat and Rozita Hassan
School of Dental Sciences, Universiti Sains Malaysia, Kelantan, Malaysia

1. Introduction

The specialty of orthodontics has continued to evolve since its advent in the early 20th century. Changes in treatment philosophy, mechanics, and appliances have helped shape our understanding of orthodontic tooth movement. In the 1890's, Edward H. Angle published his classification of malocclusion based on the occlusal relationships of the first molars. This was a major step toward the development of orthodontics because his classification defined normal occlusion. Angle then helped to pioneer the means to treat malocclusions by developing new orthodontic appliances. He believed that if all of the teeth were properly aligned, then no deviation from an ideal occlusion would exist. Angle and his followers strongly believed in non-extraction treatment. His appliance, (Fig. 1), consisted of a tube on each tooth to provide a horizontally positioned rectangular slot. Angle's edgewise appliance received its name because the archwire was inserted at a 90-degree angle to the plane of insertion. The rectangular wire was tied into a rectangular slot with steel ligatures (Proffit, 2000). A later shift in thought occurred when one of his pupils, Charles Tweed, observed that some of the patients formerly treated by Angle exhibited a noticeable amount of relapse. Tweed then re-treated a number of these cases by extracting four bicuspids to resolve the crowding and in turn, developed his own treatment mechanics. Another shift in orthodontics occurred when Larry Andrews introduced the straight wire appliance. Instead of bending wires to place teeth in the proper orientation with an edgewise bracket, Andrews' appliance had the angulation and torque values built into the brackets commonly known as the appliance prescription. In theory, these pre-adjusted brackets eliminated the need to repeatedly bend first, second, and third order bends each time the patient progressed to the next wire. The straight wire appliance revolutionized orthodontics by making the bracket much more efficient. Since then, many orthodontic companies have developed their own bracket systems with specific prescriptions, treatment philosophies, and mechanics. However, they all shared one common characteristic - ligatures must be placed around tie wings on brackets to hold arch wires in the bracket slot.

2. Ligatures and ligation properties

Different types of ligatures have been used to hold the archwire in the bracket slot. Steel or elastomeric ligatures have been used mainly. The steel ligatures are made of chrome-alloy stainless steel with dimensions vary from .009" to .012" Inch in diameter and twisted with a hand instrument. In some cases, these ligatures are coated with tooth-colored material such as teflon for aesthetic reasons. Steel ligatures produce a variable effect on the bracket/archwire junction depending on their tightness. The advantages with the steel ligatures are that they do not deteriorate in the oral environment and they retain their shape and strength. They also provide less retention of bacterial plaque and are easier to clean than the elastomeric ligatures (Ridley et al., 1979). The drawbacks with steel ligatures are that they are time-consuming and tiresome on the hand of operator (Maijer & Smith, 1990; Shivapuja & Berger, 1994). Harradine, (2003), found that the use of wire ligatures added almost 12 minutes to the time needed to remove and replace two archwires. They also require careful tucking in of the ends to avoid soft tissue trauma and even then can occasionally be displaced between appointments and cause discomfort (Schumacher et al., 1990; Bendar & Gruendeman, 1993).

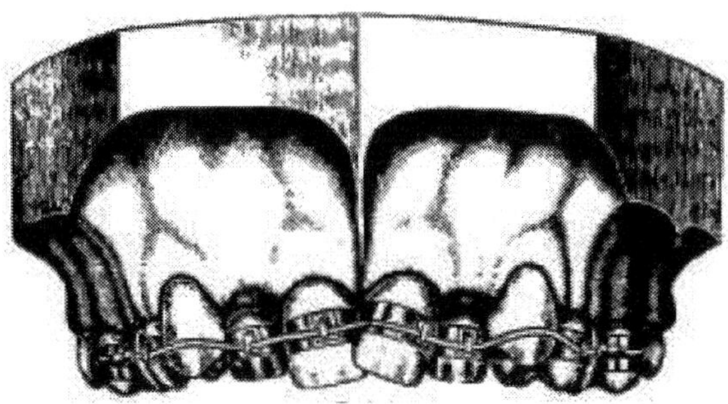

Fig. 1. Early edgewise appliance.

The introduction of elastomeric ligatures in the 1970s is also another milestone in orthodontics which largely replaced steel ligatures. These are quicker and easier to place, and they can be used in chains to close spaces within the arch or prevent spaces from opening. However, conventional ligation with elastomerics fails to provide and maintain full archwire engagement. In addition, they potentially impede good oral hygiene which is a novel situation in orthodontics. Moreover, the physical properties of elastomeric ligatures are imperfect. Elastic ligatures undergo permanent deformation in shape and thus force decays with time. The force decay under constant force application to elastomeric material showed that the greatest amount of force decay occurred during the few hours (Wong, 1976). In addition, they stain permanently shortly after being placed in the oral cavity. More important, elastomeric ligatures have been shown to increase friction in the sliding mechanic systems (Sims et al., 1993; Thomas et al., 1998), and increase the resistance to movement in bracket/archwire systems by 50-175g (Echols, 1975).

2.1 Properties of an Ideal orthodontic ligation system

Regardless of the type of bracket and ligation used, there are several desirable properties for an ideal orthodontic ligation system.

1. Secure and robust ligation

Secure , full archwire engagement maximizes the potential long range of action of modern low modulus wires and minimizes the need to regain control of teeth where full engagement is lost during treatment. Once a wire is ligated, it is desirable that it is resistant to inadvertent loss of ligation. Wire ligatures are good in this respect while elastic ligatures are more easily lost. Elastic ligatures also experience significant force decay over time (Taloumis et al., 1997).

2. Full bracket engagement

Full archwire engagement into the bracket slot is desirable to attain full expression of torque particularly at finishing stages of treatment. Wire ligation can maintain adequate archwire engagement between office visits. On the other hand, elastic ligatures frequently exert insufficient force even on fairly flexible wires.

3. Quick and easy ligation

Wire ligation is a lengthy procedure and this is the main reason they are not frequently used. Elastic ligatures are much faster to remove and replace (Türkkahraman et al., 2005)

4. Low friction

For sliding mechanics, brackets that experience low friction are the most desirable. Low friction is important during the leveling and aligning stages of orthodontic treatment. It will allow a more efficient force delivery, less force dissipation and thus a faster expression of the wire. Low friction is efficient during space closure as well. Wire ligatures are superior to brackets ligated by elastic ligatures in this respect and shown to produce only 30-50% of the frictional forces produced by elastomerics (Shivapuja et al., 1994). Still, forces may reach undesirable levels relative to levels considered ideal for tooth movement (Khambay et al., 2004).

5. Improves patient comfort and hygiene

Wire ligatures can cause tissue laceration if the cut ends are exposed but they are very hygienic. Elastic ligatures are more comfortable than wire ligatures but have the side effect of being less hygienic.

Sliding mechanics in conventional brackets rely on filling the slot with the largest wire possible to provide a certain degree of force control (direction and magnitude) needed to move teeth. With enough force, teeth eventually move to the desired position. Because archwires are held into place with either metal or elastic ligature ties, heavy forces must be introduced into the system in order to overcome the friction created at the bracket/archwire interface before tooth movement can occur. However, some argue that the heavy forces generated by large sized wires and traditional ligation methods are not physiologic because they create force systems high enough to overpower the lip, tongue, and cheek muscular. Clinicians and manufacturers alike sought to develop a product that could replicate the time saving properties of elastomeric modules while lessening or eliminating the friction they caused. This eventually led to the development and popularization of selfligating brackets because they satisfy both criteria and offer a philosophy of orthodontic treatment that greatly differs from this classical school of thought.

3. Self-ligating brackets

3.1 Definition

Self-ligating brackets are ligatureless bracket systems that have a mechanical device built into the bracket to close off the edgewise slot. The cap holds the archwire in the bracket slot and replaces the steel/elastomeric ligature. With the self-ligating brackets, the moveable fourth wall of the bracket is used to convert the slot into a tube.

3.2 Philosophy of self-ligating bracket proponents

Light forces are the key to self-ligation. Proponents suggest that low force, low-friction systems allow teeth to travel to their physiologic position because they do not overpower the musculature or compromise the periodontal tissues. Ischemia is not induced in the surrounding periodontal tissues because the forces generated by the small dimension, high-tech archwires are too low to completely occlude the periodontal vascular supply. Heavy forces on teeth cause hyalinization in the periodontal ligament space which brings tooth movement to a halt. Self-ligating brackets place enough force on the teeth to stimulate tooth movement without completely disrupting the vascular supply and therefore, tooth movement is more effective and physiologic. The final position of the teeth after treatment with the self-ligating bracket systems is determined by the balanced interplay between the oral musculature and periodontal tissues and not by heavy orthodontic forces. Moreover, the design in passive self-ligating bracket also enables teeth to move in the path of least resistance. When the gate is in its closed position, the bracket essentially becomes a tube in which the flexible nickel-titanium archwire can move freely. By greatly reducing the amount of friction with passive self-ligating brackets, low force archwires can work to peak expression and stimulate teeth to move in a more biologically compatible method (Fig. 2). Teeth movement is also more efficient when they are allowed to move individually, and passive self-ligating brackets offer more freedom for teeth to move to their natural position even though they are still interconnected because the archwire is never tightly engaged with the bracket slot (Damon, 1998).

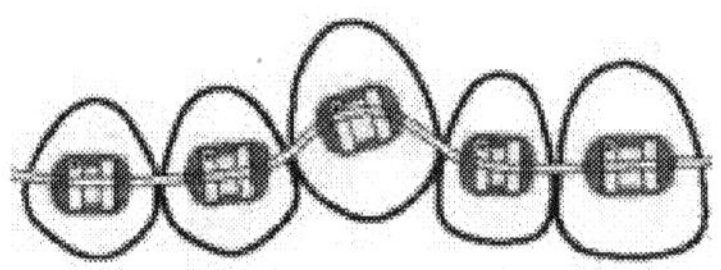

Elastic ligatures create friction and require more force and more frequent adjustments

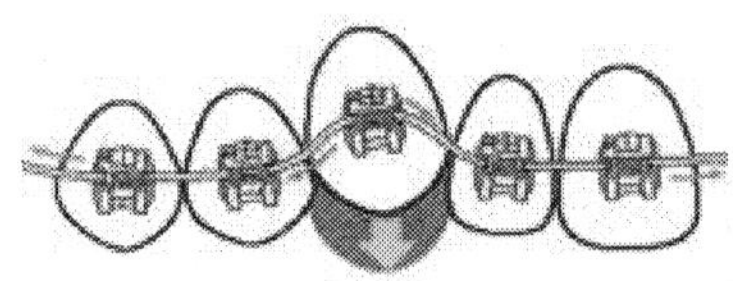

Self-ligating brackets allow freedom of movement, resulting in faster treatment with gentler forces

Fig. 2. Traditional archwire ligation vs. self-ligating brackets.

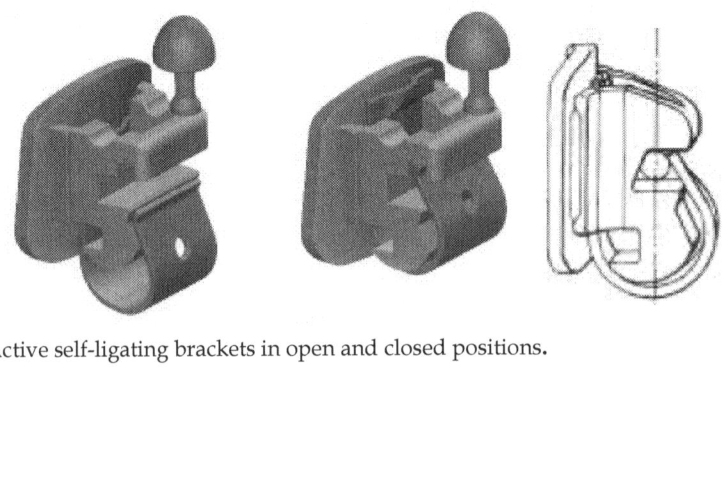

Fig. 3. Active self-ligating brackets in open and closed positions.

3.3 Classification

Two types of self-ligating brackets have been developed, active and passive. These terms refer to the mode in which they interact with the archwire. The active type (Fig. 3) has a spring clip that encroaches on the slot from the labial/buccal aspect and presses against the archwire providing an active seating force on the archwire and ensuring engagement such as In-Ovation (GAC International, Bohemia, NY, USA), SPEED (Strite Industries, Cambridge, Ontario, Canada), and Time brackets (Adenta, Gilching/Munich, Germany).
In the passive type (Fig. 4), the clip does not press against the archwire. Instead, these brackets use a rigid door or latch to entrap the archwire providing more room for the archwire such as Damon (Ormco/"A"Company), SmartClip™ (3M Unitek, USA), and Oyster ESL (Gestenco International, Gothenburg, Sweden).

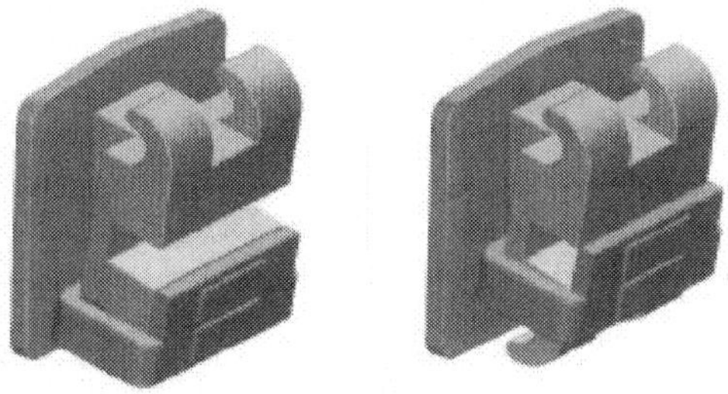

Fig. 4. Passive self-ligating brackets in open and closed positions.

3.4 History and development of self-ligating brackets

Self-ligating brackets were first introduced in the mid-1930s in the form of the Russell attachment by Stolzenberg (Fig. 5). The bracket had a flat-head screw seated snugly in a circular, threaded opening in the face of the bracket that allows for quick and simple archwire changes. Loosening the screw made the system passive and allowed bodily translation on a round wire while tightening it made it active and provided root torquing on a square or a rectangular wire. The bracket system was more comfortable for the patient and resulted in shorter office visits as well. Unfortunately, the Russell attachment did not gain much popularity and virtually disappeared from the market.

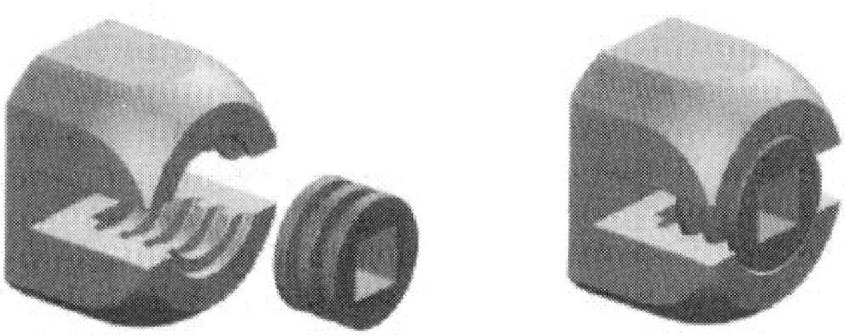

Fig. 5. Russell attachment in open and closed positions

The first modern passive self-ligating bracket (Edgelok- Ormco Corporation, Glendora, CA) was introduced in the early 1970s. The bracket had a round body with a rigid labial sliding cap (Fig.6). Because of its passive nature, orthodontists found precise control of tooth movement to be a challenge. Although many design refinements have been introduced since, the basic design has remained unchanged.

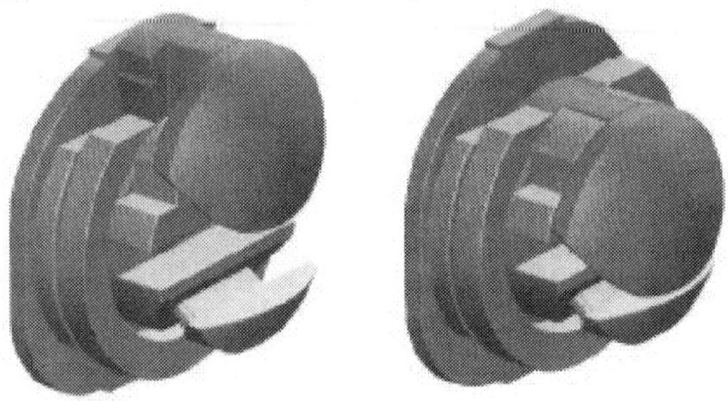

Fig. 6. Edgelok bracket in open and closed positions.

The prototypes of the first active self-ligating bracket (SPEED, Spring-loaded, Delivery) were introduced into the market in 1980. The bracket features a curved, flexible super-elastic nickel-titanium spring clip that embraces the bracket body and passes through the archwire slot.

In 1986, the self-ligating Activa bracket offered another alternative. The Activa bracket had an inflexible, curved arm that rotated occlusogingivally around the cylindrical bracket body (Fig. 7). The arm could be moved into a slot-open or slot-close position with finger pressure alone. Once closed, the rigid outer wall of the movable arm converted the bracket slot into a tube. Another self-ligating bracket model, Time entered the marketplace in 1995. The Time bracket (Fig. 8) features a rigid, curved arm that wraps occlusogingivally around the labial aspect of the bracket body. The stiffness of the bracket arm prevents any substantial interaction with the archwire, thereby rendering Time a passive bracket (Berger & Byloff, 2001).)

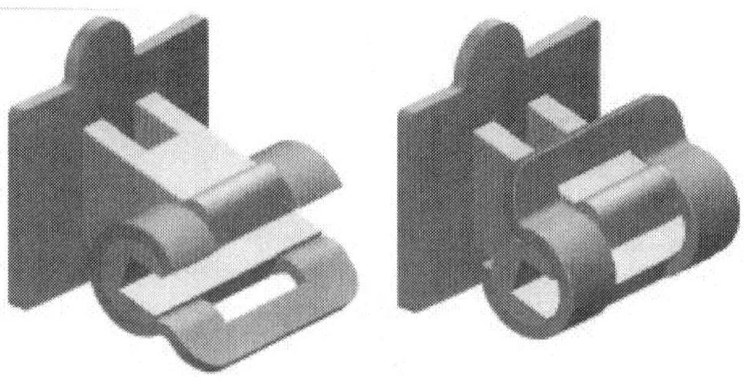

Fig. 7. Activa bracket.

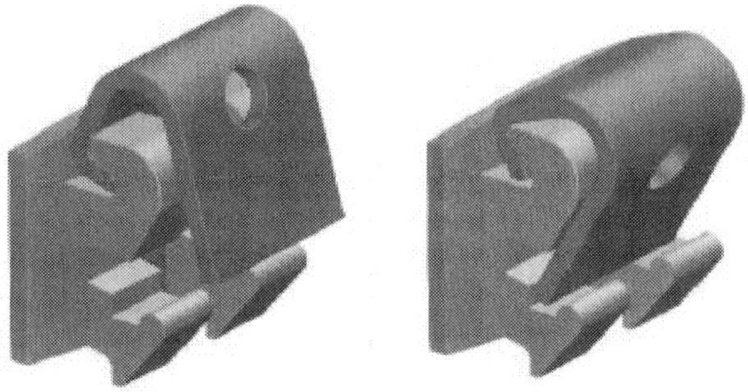

Fig. 8. Time bracket.

Perhaps the most renowned self-ligating bracket system was introduced by Dr. Dwight Damon in 1996. The Damon™ SL I is an edgewise twin bracket with a metal labial cover that straddles the tie wings. In 1999, the next generation Damon™ SL II was brought to the market (Fig. 9). It differed from the original Damon™ SL I by incorporating a flat rectangular slide between the tie wings. A special plier is used to open the metal gates incisally in the maxillary arch and gingivally in the mandibular. Once the slides are closed, the bracket becomes a passive tube. The Damon™ SL bracket system was designed to satisfy the following major criteria (Damon 1998):

a. Andrews Straight-Wire Appliance concept
b. Twin configuration
c. Slide forming a complete tube
d. Passive slide on the outside face of bracket
e. Bracket opening inferiorly in both arches

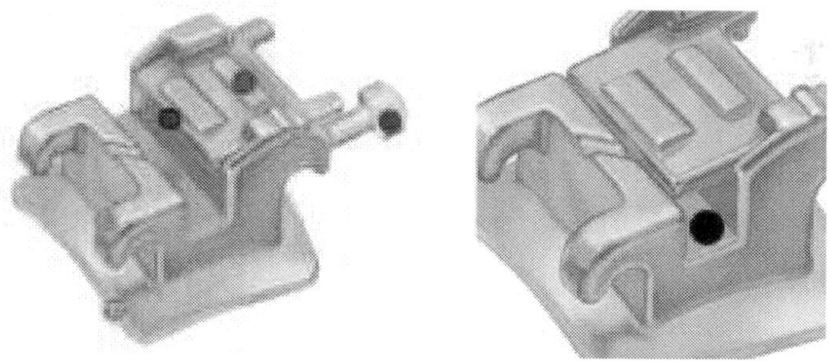

Fig. 9. Damon™ SL II brackets in open and closed positions.

In 2002, the In-Ovation R™ by GAC was introduced. This bracket features an interactive clip because it can provide both passive and active control depending on the archwires used. Round leveling wires can freely move to correct rotations during the initial leveling and aligning phase, while full size rectangular wires are fully engaged into the base of the bracket by the clip in the later stages of treatment for better torque control. A new In-Ovation C™ is now available which has a partial ceramic face for better esthetics (Figure 10).

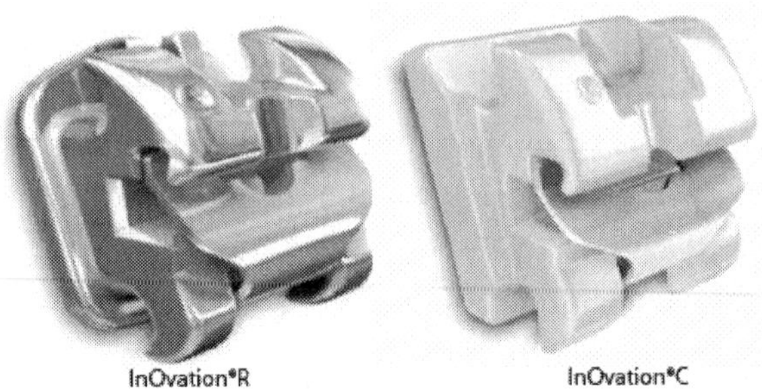

Fig. 10. The GAC In-Ovation R™ and In-Ovation C™ bracket.

In 2004, 3M Unitek introduced the SmartClip™ self-ligating bracket, which is different from other self-ligating brackets in that it does not have a slide or clip to hold the wires (Fig.11). Instead it contains a nickel-titanium clip on each side of the twin bracket that locks in the wire. The archwire is inserted by using finger pressure to push it past the flexible clip. Remove requires a special instrument from 3M Unitek™.

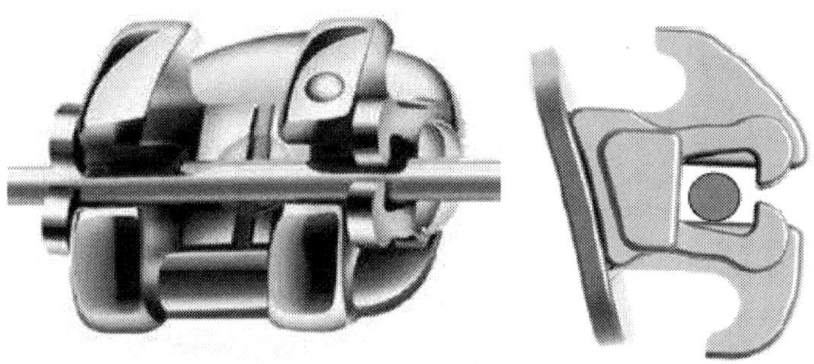

Fig. 11. The unitek smart clip™ bracket.

With the increasing popularity of self-ligating brackets, many different bracket designs are brought to the orthodontic marketplace each year. Consequently, the use of SLBs has increased exponentially; over 42% of American practitioners surveyed reported using at least one system of self-ligating brackets in 2008 (Keim et al., 2008). This figure was just 8.7%in 2002 (Keim et al., 2002). When choosing a self-ligating bracket system, it is important to understand the different types of systems (active vs. passive) in order to obtain the best and most efficient orthodontic results.

4. Clinical performance of self-ligating brackets

Recent advances in bracket technology have resulted in a number of new selfligating bracket systems and greater interest in their use. Much of this interest is in response to information comparing the benefits of self-ligating systems with conventional edgewise brackets and claiming that self-ligating bracket systems provide superior treatment efficiency and efficacy. The proposed benefits include reduced friction between archwire and bracket, reduced clinical forces, reduced treatment time, faster alignment, faster space closure, different arch dimensions, better alignment and occlusal outcomes, less patient pain, and more hygienic. However, these data come from marketing materials, nonrefereed sources, or refereed journals. The purpose of this section is to review the clinically significant effects of self-ligating brackets on orthodontic treatment with respect to the quality of available scientific evidence. Comparing between self-ligating and conventional brackets in different aspects will be addressed as well. These include:

4.1 Subjective pain experience

It is well documented that discomfort is a potential side effect during fixed appliance orthodontic therapy and this can negatively influence the desire to undergo treatment, compliance, and treatment outcome (Patel, 1992; Scheurer et al., 1996). A potentially significant variable that influences treatment-related discomfort is the amount of force applied to the dentition by the orthodontic archwire, particularly during the early stages of treatment. Classical histological studies suggest that light forces are more biologically efficient and less traumatic during orthodontic tooth movement (Reitan, 1956). Therefore, the use of increased force levels might be expected to be associated with increased discomfort. One of the factors affecting prospective tooth movement and hence the amount of force required is the degree of friction that exists between the archwire and bracket; this frictional resistance being influenced primarily by the physical characteristics of the archwire and bracket materials (Ireland et al., 1991), archwire dimensions (Taylor & Ison, 1996), and the method of archwire ligation (Ireland et al., 1991; Shivapuja & Berger, 1994). Indeed, a number of self-ligating bracket systems have been developed in recent years, including Damon ™ , In-Ovation ™ , and SmartClip ™ with the proposed benefit of reduced frictional properties (Read-Ward et al. , 1997 ; Thorstenson & Kusy, 2001 ; Henao & Kusy, 2004). Proponents and manufacturers of these systems suggest that their physical properties produce lower force levels during tooth alignment and sliding mechanics, a more biologically compatible force level and, therefore, a possible reduction in pain associated with orthodontic tooth movement (Berger & Byloff, 2001; http://www.damonbraces.com). To date (March, 2011), there have been four published clinical trials investigating degree and differences in perceived pain using self-ligating and conventional brackets (Pringle et al., 2010; Mile et al., 2006; Scott et al., 2008; Fleming et al., 2009). Of these, one split-mouth study considered pain reports after both the first and second visits, with patients indicating which system was associated with the greatest discomfort (Mile et al., 2006). Data in three of the trials are presented as continuous pain scores from 0 to 100 on a 100-mm visual analogue scale (VAS) which is one of the most commonly used tools in the measurement of perceived discomfort during orthodontic treatment (Pringle et al., 2010; Scott et al., 2008; Fleming et al., 2009). One trial reported pain scores at 15 time intervals (Pringle et al., 2010), while two trials used four time points: 4 hours, 24 hours, 3 days, and 7 days after appliance placement (Scott et al., 2008; Fleming et al., 2009). The findings from these studies conflicted slightly with one study reporting a tendency to less pain experience with Damon 3 SLBs, although this finding did not reach statistical significance (Pringle et al., 2010). Three studies (Pringle et al., 2010; Scott et al., 2008; Fleming et al., 2009) were regarded as being at low risk of bias, and they reported similar outcomes permitting statistical comparison; pain scores at four analogous time intervals were extracted from each study to facilitate this. Pain intensity over the first 7 days was reported in these three studies involving 160 patients, with 83 in the SLB group and 77 in the conventional bracket group. Patients in the SLB group reported a mean difference in pain intensity of 0.99 to 5.66 points lower than in the conventional bracket group, the greatest difference being reported 3 days after appliance placement. However, differences were not of statistical significance.

Two studies, (Mile et al., 2006; Fleming et al., 2009), reported greater pain experience during chairside manipulation of self-ligating appliances. However, as the mechanisms of archwire engagement and disengagement are very different using SmartClip (Fleming et al., 2009) and Damon 2 (Mile et al., 2006), it was felt that direct statistical comparison of this research finding would be invalid.

4.2 Bond failure rate

Treatment efficiency involves several factors including breakages. A higher bracket failure rate results in extra visits for the patient and additional clinical time required for repairs. The higher bracket failure rate demonstrated by any bracket system would need to be offset by any time saving in ligation time as well as overall treatment time.

Two studies have considered failure of bonded attachments over 20 weeks (Miles et al., 2006) and 12 months (Pandis et al., 2006) using Damon 2. The date used for assessing failure or time taken for failure to occur was not reported, and only first-time failures for each tooth were recorded. Miles et al., 2006, reported significantly more Damon brackets deboned during the study. This higher failure rate could be due to operator inexperience with the slide mechanism and also due to the bracket design because a shear force can be inadvertently applied when operating the slide. The Damon 2 (as most self ligating bracket designs) is also larger incisogingivally than the conventional twin bracket used and so more likely to interfere with the occlusion.

Pandis et al., 2006, assessed the failure rate of self-ligating and edgewise brackets bonded with a self-etching adhesive and conventional phosphoric acid etching in patients followed for 12 months of active treatment. Similar treatment plans, and mechanotherapy were selected for the study. GAC Microarch edgewise brackets and Oromco Damon 2 brackets were bonded using a split mouth design, using the 3M Transbond Plus Self-etching primer (SEP) and Transbond XT paste; and conventional acid etching, with Orthosolo primer and Enlight paste, applied at an alternate sequence so that the adhesives were equally distributed on the maxillary and mandibular right and left quadrants. No difference was found for the failure rate of self-ligating vs. conventional bracket and between the two bonding modes used. Also, no difference was identified between maxillary and mandibular arch in failure incidence whereas a statistically significant difference was shown for right-sided appliance which may be assigned to masticatory habits.

4.3 Plaque retention and periodontal health

Iatrogenic decalcification of tooth enamel and the development of visible white spot lesions are undesirable and unfortunate consequences of fixed orthodontic therapy, potentially undermining the esthetic benefits often achieved through correction of the malocclusion. It is well documented that fixed appliances increase bacterial plaque accumulation and the risk for white spot lesions (Gorelick et al., 1982; Geiger et al., 1983). During treatment, there is demonstrated increased retention in the amounts of Streptococcus mutans and lactobacilli in saliva and dental plaque (Forsberg et al., 1991). Bonded orthodontic brackets hinder access for good oral hygiene and create microbial shelters, resulting in the accumulation of plaque. The appliance architecture specifically, the archwire ligation method is an additional factor influencing bacterial colonization. Two trials have compared the impact of SLBs and elastomeric ligation on plaque retention (Pellegrini et al., 2009, Pandis et al., 2010). Longer term effects of bracket system on periodontal health and accumulation of debris has also been assessed (Pandis et al., 2008).

Pellegrini et al., 2009, performed randomized clinical study to enumerate and compare plaque bacteria surrounding 2 bracket types, self-ligating vs. elastomeric ligating using a split-mouth design. Patients were recalled and assessed 1 week and 5 weeks after bonding. Results showed that most patients bonded with self-ligating brackets had fewer bacteria in plaque than did teeth bonded with elastomeric legated brackets both at 1 and 5 weeks after bonding.

The oral cavity is a rich ecosystem with a plethora of microorganisms. While both periodontal disease and caries are considered multifactorial diseases, plaque bacteria are the major factor in their onset and progression. However, there are situations which comprise what has been termed 'ecological stress', referring to the shift of the microbiological balance, creating conditions conducive to the growth, and appearance of cariogenic and/or periodontopathic bacteria (Marsh, 2003). The different components of the fixed orthodontic system may contribute to a shift in the balance of the oral ecology. The presence of brackets and ligatures has been shown to be been mainly associated with increased risk of Streptococcus mutans and lactobacilli colonization, among other species, thus initiating a series of events, which may lead to the development of pathology of the hard tissues such as decalcification and, in specific cases, caries development. Moreover, the accumulation of plaque and the resultant alteration of the local microbial milieu may expose the tissues to the risk of developing periodontal inflammation (Øgaard et al., 1988; Fournier et al., 1998 ; Naranjo et al. , 2006).

It has been proposed at bracket ligation mode has an effect on the microbiological profile of the patients' oral environment. Pandis et al., 2010, investigated the effect of bracket type (conventional and selfligating) on the levels of streptococcus mutans and total bacterial counts in whole saliva of , fixed orthodontic patients at the age range of 11-17 years. The patients were subdivided into two groups with random allocation of bracket type (conventional or selfligating). An initial saliva sample was obtained before the initiation of treatment (T1) and a second sample 2 - 3 months following appliance bonding (T2). Salivary streptococcus mutans and total bacteria were enumerated and analysed after growth in culture. The levels of S. mutans in whole saliva of orthodontically treated patients do not seem to be significantly different between conventional and self-ligating brackets. However, the pre-treatment levels of S. mutans are significant predictors of the levels of S. mutans after placement of orthodontic appliances.

Pandis et al., 2008, conducted a cohort study to determine values of periodontal indices for patients treated with self-ligating and conventional brackets. All patients were 12-17 years with aligned mandibular arches, and absence of oral habits and anterior crossbites. Outcome variables were plaque index, gingival index, calculus index, and probing depth for the two bracket cohorts and the results showed that under these conditions the self-ligating brackets do not have an advantage over conventional brackets with respect to the periodontal status.

4.4 Torque expression and arch dimensional change

Correct buccolingual inclination of anterior teeth is considered essential to provide good occlusal relationships in orthodontic treatment. Inclination of the maxillary anterior teeth is particularly critical in establishing an esthetic smile line, proper anterior guidance, and a Class I canine and molar relationship. Undertorqued maxillary anterior teeth affect the arch length and the space requirements. It has been shown that for every 5° of anterior inclination, about 1 mm of arch length is generated. (O'Higgins et al., 1999) Undertorqued posterior teeth have a constricting effect on the maxillary arch, since they do not allow appropriate cusp-to fossa relationships between maxillary and mandibular teeth (Gioka & Iliades, 2004). The manufacturing process of brackets results in some variation in sizes and characteristics, including dimensional accuracy and torque prescription consistency. Various bracket manufacturing processes such as injection-molding, casting, and milling can affect the accuracy of the prescribed torque values, and this has been reported to be about 5% to 10% (Gioka & Iliades, 2004). Huang et al., 2009, reported that torque angle/torque moment behavior is determined by the characteristics of the archwire. The effect of the bracket system is of minor importance, with the exception of self-ligating brackets with an active clip (eg. Speed), which had the lowest torquing moments of all wires.

In relation to the mandibular arch, Pandis et al., 2007; Fleming et al., 2009; and Pandis et al., 2010, reported similar increase in the proclination of mandibular incisors associated with both appliance systems during arch alignment. In general, lateral cephalograms were traced, and mandibular incisor position and inclination were assessed for patients by using angular measurements of mandibular incisor to mandibular plane, mandibular incisor to nasion-Point B line, and mandibular incisor to Point A-pogonion line. Garino & Favero, 2003, stated that satisfactory control of tooth positions during the horizontal, mesio-distal, and torque movements, both in the extraction and non-extraction cases were observed in Speed bracket system

Self-ligating brackets seem to be equally efficient in delivering torque to maxillary incisors relative to conventional brackets in extraction and non-extraction cases. Pandis et al., 2006, conducted a randomized clinical trial employing a random distribution of variables among the studied populations. Similar buccolingual inclination of maxillary incisors in extraction and non-extraction treatment with self-ligating and conventional brackets was reported.

Treatment of a crowded dental arch on a non-extraction basis, without tooth size reduction requires an increase in arch perimeter to allow resolution of crowding and achievement of optimum arch alignment and leveling. Without active distal movement, changes typically involve both transverse expansion and proclination. The ideal scenario would involve little incisor proclination and intercanine expansion, with most of the arch perimeter increase generated by expansion across the molars and premolars. The nature and magnitude of these arch dimensional changes have implications on the long-term stability. Marked expansion of the intercanine dimension and excessive proclination of the mandibular incisors are considered to be particularly unstable (Mills, 1966; Burke et al., 1998). Relapse in such cases may develop due to constriction of the expanded intercanine dimension and uprighting of the mandibular incisors during the post-treatment phase, and is likely to manifest as mandibular incisor irregularity.

Three studies investigated arch dimensions in conventional and self-ligating brackets (All used Damon brackets). Jiang & Fu, 2008, and Pandis et al., 2009, reported the changes after treatment in their prospective studies on non-extraction basis. For intercanine and intermolar widths, there was no significant difference between the two groups. On other hand, Scott et al., 2008, reported the change after progressing to 0.019 x 0.025-in stainless steel archwires in a randomized controlled trial on extraction patients with greater incisor irregularity at the beginning of the treatment. They reported greater increase in intercanine width, probably because the canines were retracted to a wider part of the arch. Intermolar width was not increased with self-ligating brackets in that study, and, according to the authors, it was probably related to forward sliding of the molars into a narrower part of the arch in the extraction patients. In addition, different archwire sequences were used for the two groups in the studies of Jiang & Fu, 2008, and Pandis et al., 2009, whereas Scott et al., 2008, used the same archwires for both groups. The claims that self-ligating brackets facilitate greater and more physiologic arch expansion and, therefore, allow more non-extraction treatment require more evidence.

4.5 Orthodontic space closure

Only two studies considered the rate of orthodontic space closure. Miles, 2007, tested the rate of space closure at intervals of 5 weeks until complete closure was achieved. This was a prospective cohort study using a split-mouth design with moderate risk of bias. Miles concluded that there was no significant difference in the rate of en-masse space closure between SmartClip brackets and conventional brackets tied with stainless steel ligatures. However, the sample size was small, and the possibility that any true difference could be obscured in a split-mouth design should be considered. In a very recent study, Mezomo et al., 2011, conducted a randomized clinical trial to measure space closure during the retraction of upper permanent canines after first premolar extraction with self-ligating and conventional brackets. In a random split-mouth design, the retraction of upper canines was performed using an elastomeric chain with 150 g of force. The evaluations were performed on dental casts at time intervals (T0, initial; T1, 4 weeks; T2, 8 weeks; T3, 12 weeks). The amount of movement and the rotation of the canines as well as anchorage loss of the upper first molars were evaluated. Results showed that distal movement of the upper canines and anchorage loss of the first molars were similar with both conventional and self-ligating brackets. However, rotation of the upper canines was minimized with self-ligating brackets ($P < .05$). Existing evidence does not support the claim that lower friction in a self-ligating system permits more rapid space closure in a clinical setting.

4.6 Efficiency of initial orthodontic alignment

Five studies with low to moderate risk of bias, including two randomized controlled trials and three prospective cohort studies, investigated the rate of mandibular incisor alignment (Fleming et al., 2009; Miles et al., 2006; Scott et al., 2008; Miles, 2008; Pandis et al., 2007). Mandibular crowding was selected as a model for examining the efficiency of brackets because correction of this discrepancy largely depends on the "free play" or clearance of the archwire inside the slot walls. All self-ligating brackets were the passive type (Damon, Ormco; SmartClip, 3M Unitek). Pandis et al., 2007, and Scott et al., 2008, reported days needed for alignment but used different end points: visual inspection of correction of proximal contacts and changing to 0.019 x 0.025-in stainless steel archwire. Pandis et al., 2007, enrolled non-extraction patients (Fig. 12 & 13), whereas Scott et al., 2008, enrolled extraction patients. Miles, 2008, and Fleming et al., 2009, reported reduction of irregularity at various times of alignment. A standardized mean difference was calculated, and no significant difference in efficiency of alignment in the mandibular arch was found between both bracket systems. The efficiency of alignment was found to be associated with initial irregularity only. The study of Fleming et al., 2009, used a 3-dimensional analysis, thus making comparison unfeasible. However, they also concluded that, for non-extraction patients with mild mandibular incisor crowding, self-ligating brackets were no more effective at relieving irregularity.

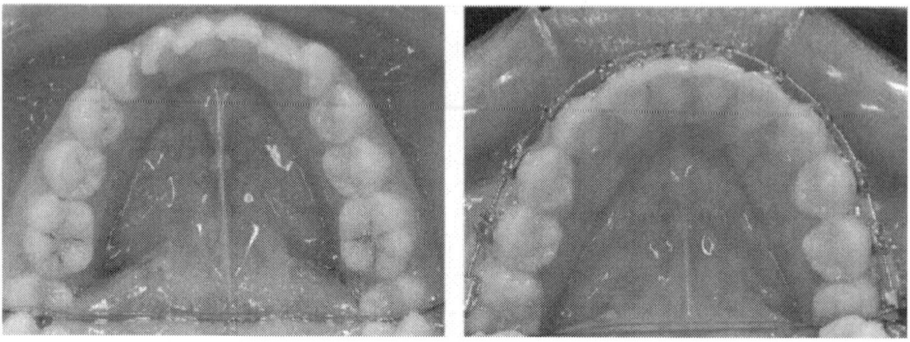

Fig. 12. Alignment of crowded mandibular anterior teeth (canine to canine) with a conventional edgewise brackets (Pandis et al., 2007)

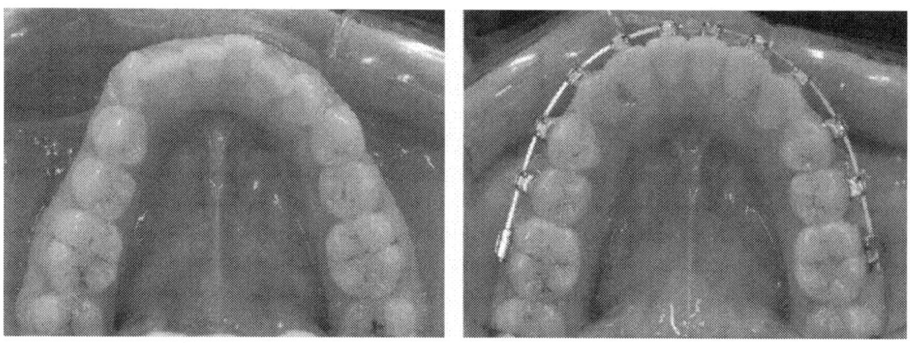

Fig. 13. Alignment of crowded mandibular anterior teeth (canine to canine) with self-ligating brackets (Pandis et al., 2007)

4.7 Apical root resorption

Apical root resorption (ARR) can be defined as blunting or shortening of the root apex, a condition often associated with orthodontic treatment. The teeth more susceptible to ARR are the maxillary and mandibular incisors, and especially the maxillary lateral incisors (Linge & Linge, 1983; Mirabella & Artun, 1995).

The introduction of self-ligating brackets provoked the investigation of archwire ligation on ARR. One of the first reports on the subject was by Blake et al., 1995, who tested the hypothesis that an active self-ligating bracket with an active clip might induce more ARR; their findings, however, did not confirm that hypothesis. The introduction of passive self-ligating systems, with no active spring and alignment performed by wires engaged in a passive tube, with more play, jiggling, and less friction raises again the question of their effect on ARR. Pandis et al., 2008, using panoramic radiographs, reported no mean difference in the amount of apical root resorption of the maxillary incisors with Microarch and Damon 2 systems. Similar results were obtained by Scott et al., 2008, who assessed changes in root lengths of mandibular incisors on periapical radiographs following arch alignment. The mean amount of resorption was slightly greater with the Damon 3 appliance (2.26 vs. 1.21 mm), although the difference failed to reach statistical significance.

4.8 Total treatment time and occlusal indices

One prospective randomized clinical trial and three retrospective cohort studies compared total treatment times between both systems. The very recent (February, 2011) multi-center randomized clinical trial was carried out to compare the effect of bracket type (Damon3 self-ligated or the Synthesis conventional ligated preadjusted bracket systems, both, Ormco, Glendora, Calif) on the duration of orthodontic treatment and the occlusal outcome as measured by the peer assessment rating (PAR). The use of the Damon3 bracket did not reduce overall treatment time or total number of visits, or result in a better occlusal outcome when compared with conventional ligated brackets in the treatment of extraction cases with crowding. For the other retrospective studies, Eberting et al., 2001, and Harradine, 2001, found significantly decreased treatment times of 4 to 6 months and 4 to 7 fewer visits with self-ligating brackets, whereas Hamilton et al., 2008, found that self-ligating brackets appear to offer no measurable advantages in orthodontic treatment time, number of treatment visits, and time spent in initial alignment over conventional pre-adjusted orthodontic brackets. However, the mean treatment times varied in the 3 studies, and the decision regarding when treatment goals had been attained might have differed among the investigators. The same 3 studies also compared the occlusal outcome after treatment. Eberting et al., 2001, used American Board of Orthodontics scores, Hamilton et al., 2008, used the index of complexity, outcome, and need, and Harradine, 2001, used the peer assessment rating. Interestingly, an almost identical pattern was observed in the 2 forest plots. The 2 smaller studies with passive self-ligating brackets (Damon, Ormco) favored self-ligation (Eberting et al., 2001; Harradine, 2001); whereas the larger study with active self-ligating brackets (In-Ovation, GAC) found no significant difference (Hamilton et al., 2008). The results in occlusal quality showed no significant difference at the end of treatment. However, caution should be used regarding these results, since the heterogeneity was high and the 3 studies might have been susceptible to bias from their retrospective designs. Studies with randomized or consecutive assignment are needed to provide further information with more valid comparisons of treatment durations.

4.9 Stability

Some claim that lower forces produced by selfligating bracket systems might result in more physiologic tooth movement and more stable treatment results. However, studies on stability after treatment with self-ligating brackets are lacking at this time.

5. Active vs. passive self-ligating brackets

The Time, In-Ovation, and Speed brackets all have what is called a "spring clip" that encroaches on the slot from the labial/buccal aspect providing an active seating force on the archwire (Fig. 14). The debate over whether a self-ligating bracket should have an active or passive ligation mechanism has been around since their development. Proponents of an active clip claim that it provides a "homing action" on the wire when deflected, providing more control with the appliance (Hanson, 1980). Such brackets have a flexible clip that creates a passive slot depth of 0.0175" to 0.020". With small round wires, the bracket is passive, but with larger wires the flexible clip is defected labially and provides an active seating force on the archwire. Passive self-ligating brackets have a slot depth of 0.028" and do not exert an active force on the wire. Those who advocate a passive clip state that there is less friction in the appliance during sliding mechanics because the slot provides more room for the archwire and they provide no active seating force (Damon, 1998). Several studies have tried to determine how a self-ligating mechanism affects friction during sliding mechanics. Active and passive self-ligating brackets showed different behavior with regard to their resistance to sliding (Brauchli et al., 2011). These studies have all consistently found that when a small round wire lies passively in the slot, the self-ligating brackets produce significantly less friction than conventionally ligated brackets (Berger, 1990; Thorstenson & Kusy, 2001). This is presumably due to the absence of the ligation that provides a seating force against the archwire. When wires of 0.018" or larger were tested, differences in friction have been found between various self-ligating brackets. Therefore, it might be concluded that low friction can be achieved with the use of passive self-ligating brackets or the combination of low-dimension archwires and active self-ligating appliances.

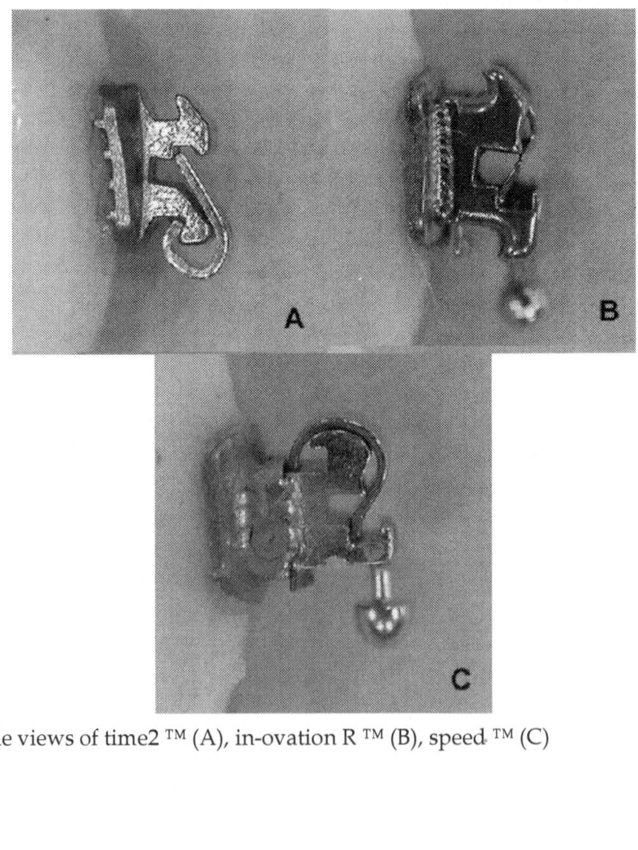

Fig. 14. Profile views of time2 ™ (A), in-ovation R ™ (B), speed ™ (C)

Redlich et al., 2003, found that the Discovery (Dentaurum; Espringen, Germany) and Time (American Orthodontics; Sheboygan, WI) brackets produced about twice as much friction as the control twin bracket with wire sizes greater than 0.018″. The authors attribute the higher frictional forces in the Time brackets to the clip exerting excessive force on the wire. Read-Ward et al., 1997, compared friction between three self-ligating brackets; SPEED (Strite Industries, Ontario, Canada), Activa ('A' Company, San Diego, CA), Mobil-Lock Variable-Slot (Forestadent, Strasbourg, France), and a conventional twin bracket Ultratrimm (Dentaurum, Germany). Three stainless steel wires were tested; 0.020″, 0.019 x 0.025″ and 0.021 x 0.025″. They found that with the 0.020″ wire, the Mobil-Lock had the least amount of friction, which was statistically less than the SPEED and Ultratrimm brackets. No significant difference was found between the Mobil-Lock and Activa. It is important to note that the Mobil-Lock and Activa have a passive ligation mechanism and that the SPEED bracket is active with a 0.020″ wire. With a 0.021 x 0.025″ wire, the SPEED bracket produced significantly greater friction than either the Mobil-Lock or Activa brackets. In a similar study, Pizzoni et al.,1998, compared the Damon SL bracket to the SPEED bracket with an active clip and two conventionally ligated brackets. The two self-ligating brackets were not statistically different for a 0.018″ wire, but when 0.017 x 0.025″ wires were used, the active clip on the SPEED bracket produced significantly greater friction than the passive Damon bracket. The literature supports the claim that when using larger wires, passive self-ligating brackets produce less friction than active self-ligating brackets.

The self-ligation design (passive versus active) appears to be the primary variable responsible for the frictional resistance generated by self-ligating brackets during translation. Passively ligated brackets produce less frictional resistance; however, this decreased friction may result in decreased control compared with actively ligated systems. Badawi et al., 2008, measured the torque expressed from two passive (Damon 2 and SmartClip) and two active (In-Ovation and Speed) self-ligating orthodontic brackets. Results showed that active self-ligating brackets demonstrated better torque control due to their active clip forcing the wire into the bracket slot. The active self-ligating brackets expressed higher torque values than the passive self-ligating brackets at clinically usable torsion angles as well. Moreover, the clinically applicable range of torque activation was greater for the active self-ligating brackets than for the passive self-ligating brackets.

Pandis et al., 2010, conducted a randomized clinical trial to compare the time required to complete the alignment of crowded maxillary anterior teeth (canine to canine) between passive (Damon MX, Ormco, Glendora, Calif) and active (In-Ovation R, GAC, Central Islip, NY) self-ligating brackets. The results showed that active and passive self-ligating brackets have no difference in treatment duration in the correction of maxillary anterior crowding, in contrast to the extent of crowding, which had an effect on the duration of treatment.

6. Clinical tips in application of self-ligating brackets

6.1 Archwire engagement with self-ligating brackets

With self-ligating brackets, it is much more important to fully engage the wire before clip closure. The wire can be held into the slot base with a variety of tools such as ligature tucker, or Mitchell's trimmer. However, these only push on one side of the bracket and may fail to fully engage the wire across the whole width of the slot. For this purpose, various instruments were developed for engagement of wires, via balanced pressure on both sides of the bracket such as the Cool Tool (Damon) which is rather akin to a torquing key, and the

R tool (GAC) which resembles a double ligature tucker and works in the same way. These specific tools work very well and can reassure the clinician that slide closure is not being attempted over an incompletely seated wire. They can also assist cheek/lip retraction during slide closure and such a tool is recommended as a routine part of slide closure on teeth where the wire requires lingual pressure for full engagement. In cases where teeth are severely rotated and one end of the slot is too close to the adjacent tooth for an instrument to be used to seat the wire, dental floss or a ligature wire looped over the archwire can be used to fully engage the wire on that side. Harradine, 2003, suggested another useful manoeuvre to engage very rotated or displaced tooth with any self-ligating bracket by closing the clip or slide first, and then threading the aligning wire through the closed bracket before engaging the other brackets, i.e. to first convert it to a 'molar' tube.

6.2 Opening clips/slides

In-Ovation brackets are opened by pushing in an occlusal direction on the tail of the clip behind the bracket. An important point is to avoid getting excess composite resin near this tail during bracket placement as it may can hinder or prevent clip opening particularly in the lower arch, where the tail is not visible from the operator's position. Time and Speed brackets are opened with a probe or other fairly sharp instrument, such as a Mitchell's trimmer using the hole in the clip. Very specific and extremely effective pliers for Damon brackets are called Kasso Damon pliers. These pliers are recommended for all first-time users since they make all slides very easy to open.

6.3 Prevention of wire pokes

Low friction increases wire displacement. Even with very irregular teeth, the very low friction with self-ligating brackets enables aligning archwires to slip through the brackets and an archwire end to protrude. This is clearly a potential nuisance which can be avoided by using tie-backs with flexible wires over extraction sites to lessen the effects of occlusal forces on unprotected spans of wire. Another way is thorough turning in the ends of flexible archwires. An interesting innovation in this respect is the Bendistal plier described by Khouri, 1998. This was designed to place an effective distal end bend in a super-elastic wire without the need for over-bending which can be difficult and uncomfortable and also risks the loss of a bonded molar tube.

Other options include the use of the crimp-on split tubes available from manufactures such as Unitek and Oromco which can be squeezed onto almost all wires, require no fabrication, are unobtrusive, and effective. It is recommended that these stops are not placed on a significantly active part of the archwire as this would diminish the range of action of the wire where it is most needed. Others suggested selective locking of individual brackets to the archwire with elastomerics to resolve this drawback particularly in those designs which have a full conventional tie-wing assembly.

6.4 Alterations in treatment mechanics

The combination of low friction and full, secure bracket engagement may help in some alteration in treatment mechanics during the progress of treatment.

6.4.1 Longer appointment intervals

Full and secure wire engagement of self-ligating brackets along with the use of low modulus wires makes an extension of the interval between appointments a logical step. Harradine, 2003, proposed patients' follow-up on an eight- to ten-week interval basis.

6.4.2 Initial traction on lighter wires

The increased control of light forces enables more mesio-distal tooth movement to be sensible on lighter, more flexible wires. Moreover, compressed coil springs to move teeth apart can appropriately be placed from initial visits in many instances.

6.4.3 Separate movement of individual teeth

The control of rotation during traction on an individual tooth makes this option much more feasible when required and with more anchorage conservation.

6.5 Bracket placement and bonding

Bracket placement and bonding is a curial step for the long-tem success of treatment. Preferably, both arches should be bonded at the same session and from second molar to second molar in each arch. For teeth that are well displaced from the arch line or where there is insufficient space to place a bracket in ideal position, it is helpful to use a traction hook to gain some initial control of these teeth. For rotated teeth, it is helpful to offset the traction hook so that it is on the part of the crown furthest from the line of the line of the arch to gain some spontaneous derotation.

6.6 Appliance debonding

Debonding of self-ligating brackets may occur by direct failure of the bracket adhesive interface, cohesive failure of the adhesive, direct failure of the adhesive enamel interface or combination of any of these. In Damon system, the best way to debond self-ligating bracket systems is by squeezing two tiewings only with a conventional debonding plier as the bracket will silently float off the adhesive. 3M Unitek™ has Distinguished debonding tool designed for the 3M Unitek Self-Ligating Bracket Systems (Clarity SL Self-Ligating Brackets and SmartClip Self-Ligating Brackets) which may be used with or without the archwire engaged in the bracket slot.

However, the risk of enamel fracture has always been present with stainless steel and ceramic brackets, particularly in teeth where the integrity of the crown is compromised. Alternative methods of debonding metals and ceramic brackets have been designed to minimize the potential for enamel surface. The main purpose of these new methods is to reduce the force levels during the debonding process. Three debonding techniques have been proposed (ultrasonic, electrothermal, and laser).

1. Ultrasonic Debonding

The ultrasonic technique uses specially designed tips applied at the bracket-adhesive interface to erode the adhesive layer between the enamel surface and bracket base. The resulting force magnitudes needed with the ultrasonic approach are significantly lower than those required for the conventional methods of bracket removal (Englehardt et al., 1993; Krell et al., 1993). However, the ultrasonic technique has a major disadvantage. Debonding time using this technique is 30 to 60 seconds per bracket, compared with 1 to 5 seconds for other bracket removal methods (Bishara and Trulove, 1990). In addition, there is excessive wear of the relatively expensive ultrasonic tips. Consequently, this method of bracket removal is not yet recommended for clinical use.

2. Electrothermal Debonding

Electrothermal debonding instruments are essentially rechargeable, cordless heating devices that are placed in contact with the bracket. The instrument transfers heat through the bracket, softening the adhesive and allowing bond failure between the bracket base and the adhesive resin (Sheridan et al., 1986; Scott, 1988). This method is a quick and effective way to debond a bracket. Its major disadvantage is related to the relatively high temperatures generated at the heated tip. Pulpal damage and mucosal burns are possible.

3. Laser debonding

Debonding ceramic brackets was attempted using both CO2 and YAG lasers 5s in combination with mechanical torque. The use of a laser is conceptually similar to the use of the electrothermal approach, that is, through heat generation to soften the adhesive. The laser approach, although still experimental, is more precise with regard to time and amount of heat application, and therefore would have better control of the amount of heat transmitted to the tooth (Hayakawa, 2005; Feldon et al., 2010). A major disadvantage, in addition to the effects of the thermal energy on the pulp, is the high cost of the instrument

6.7 Retention

Retention is one of the controversies of modern orthodontics, with uncertainty being the only certainty. Angle, 1907, stated that "the problem involved in retention is so great, often being greater than the difficulties being encountered in the treatment of the case up to this point". Bramante, 1990, attempted to rationalize the problem and demonstrated that teeth moved through bone by orthodontic appliances often have a tendency to return to their former positions. Moreover, arch form, particularly mandibular arch form, cannot be permanently altered by appliance therapy which means that bone and adjacent tissues must be allowed time to reorganize after treatment. Thus, definite retention is necessary if the finished result of active orthodontic treatment is to be maintained. There is no agreement in the literature of a uniform system of retention, and the clinical orthodontist, in consultation with each patient, must determine the appropriate retention regime for each case. (Zachrisson, 1986). Many appliance types have been used for the retention of post-orthodontic treatment. The first appliances proposed were based on banded fixed appliances (Angle, 1907), then removable retainers were advocated as Hawley retainer, clear overlay removable retainer. Most recently, the use of bonded fixed retainers has been introduced (Kneiflm, 1973; Rubenstein, 1976). These retainers have employed multistrand wire include different wire types with differing diameters. The proposed advantages of the use of multistrand wire are that the irregular surface offers increased mechanical retention for the composite without the need for the placement of retentive loops, and that the flexibility of the wire allows physiologic movement of the teeth, even when several adjacent teeth are bonded (Artun, 1984).

Relapse is a long-term problem and long-term follow-up of patients is practically difficult and financially demanding. The literature demonstrates that, at the time of writing, evidence that addresses the effectiveness of different retention strategies used to maintain tooth position after treatment by Self-ligating orthodontic appliances is lacking. However, Dr. Dwight Damon proposed the use of bonded upper retainer (lateral incisor to lateral incisor) made from 0.16"* 0.022" flat braided archwire and placed on the cingulae of upper incisors to prevent spontaneous debonding. In the lower arch, bonded lower retainer (from canine to canine) using 0.025 single strand stainless steel is recommended as well. Clear overlay retainers are to be used in addition on a night time basis.

7. Limitations of self-ligating brackets

Full archwire engagement, low friction between bracket and archwire, and faster archwire removal and ligation are inherent features of self-ligation brackets which have been clearly demonstrated and quantified in work by various authors. However, self-ligating brackets have some drawbacks that may hinder the wide spread in their use. First: is a clip that is designed to flex, more prone to breakage or permanent deformation or to inadvertent opening or closing? This question has not been formally investigated. Studies involving the use of different self-ligating brackets in the same patient or randomly assigned to different patients are needed to test such hypotheses. Second: the higher profile in self-ligating brackets, due to the complicated mechanical design, potentially causes more occlusal interferences and lip discomfort. Moreover, currently available self-ligating brackets are more expensive than most good quality tie-wing brackets. However, this significant extra cost must be measured against savings in time—an expensive commodity. If self-ligating brackets save any appreciable chairside time as some studies suggest this would provide an offsetting saving.

8. Conclusion

Self-ligating brackets (SLBs) are not new conceptually, having been pioneered in the 1930s. They have undergone a revival over the past 30 years with a variety of new appliances being developed. It is divided into 2 main categories, active and passive, according to the mechanism in which they interact with the archwire (encroaching on the slot lumen or not). Self-ligating bracket systems were built on the philosophy of delivering light forces on a low-friction basis, thus insuring more physiologic tooth movement and at balanced oral interplay.

These systems have been gaining popularity in recent years with a host of claimed advantages over conventional appliance systems relating to reduced overall treatment time, less associated subjective discomfort, promotion of periodontal health, superior torque expression, and more favorable arch -dimensional change. Other claimed advantages include possible anchorage conservation, greater amounts of expansion, less proclination of anterior teeth, less need for extractions, and better infection control. However, many of these claims were based on retrospective studies which are potentially biased as there are many uncontrolled factors which may affect the outcome. These include greater experience, differing archwires, altered wire sequences, changes in treatment mechanics, and modified appointment intervals. Observer bias may inadvertently affect the outcome as the practitioner may unknowingly be doing "a bit more" due to enthusiasm with the new product. In this regard, more prospective clinical trials with randomized or consecutive assignment and using identical wire sequences and mechanics are preferred.

While Advocates claim that low-friction SL brackets coupled with light forces enhance the treatment efficiency and address the clinical superiority of self-ligating brackets, other team believes that bracket type does not appear to have a significant influence on treatment efficiency. Treatment efficiency is the product of many mechanical and biologic factors. It is unlikely that any one factor is responsible for the efficiency and rate of tooth movement. The biology of tooth movement is a complex and highly coordinated process at the cellular, molecular, and genetic levels. Individual variation undoubtedly has a fundamental underlying role in tooth movement and treatment efficiency. SL bracket systems are only a tool that we use today; therefore, they are just a component of orthodontics. Among other things, orthodontics deals with science/ evidence, psychosocial issues, record taking, diagnoses, treatment, treatment outcomes, artistry, enhancements, and quality-of-life issues.

9. References

Angle E. A. (1907). *Treatment of malocclusion of the teeth.* 7th ed, SS White Manufacturing Co., ISBN-13: 9781152084049, Philadelphia.

Artun, J. (1984). Caries and periodontal reactions associated with long-term use of different types of bonded lingual retainers. *American Journal of Orthodontics*, Vol. 86, No. 2, pp. 112-118, ISSN 0638-0296.

Badawi, H. M.; Toogood, R.W.; Carey, J. P.; Heo, G. & Major, P. W. (2008). Torque expression of self- ligating brackets. *American Journal of Orthodontics and Dentofacial Orthopedics*, Vol. 133, No. 5, pp. 721-728. ISSN 1147-5540.

Bendar, D. & Gruendeman, G. (1993). The influence of bracket design on moment production during axial rotation. *American Journal of Orthodontics*, Vol. 104, No. 3, pp. 245-61, ISSN 0836-2787.

Berger, J. L. (1990). The influence of the SPEED bracket's selfligating design on force levels in tooth movement: A comparative in vitro study. *American Journal of Orthodontics and Dentofacial Orthopedics*, Vol. 97, No. 3, pp. 219-228, ISSN 0230-9669.

Berger, J. L. & Byloff M. (2001). Damon System. *http://www.damonbraces.com*

Berger, J. L. & Byloff, F. K. (2001). The clinical efficiency of self-ligated brackets. *Journal of Clinical Orthodontics*, Vol. 35, No. 5, pp. 304–308, ISSN 1147-5540.

Bishara, S. E. & Trulove, T. S. (1990). Comparisons of different debonding techniques for ceramic brackets: An in vitro study. Parts I and II. *American Journal of Orthodontics and Dentofacial Orthopedics*, Vol. 98, No. 3, pp. 145-153, 263-273, ISSN 0220-6042.

Blake, M.; Woodside, D. J. & Pharoah, M. J. (1995). A radiographic comparison of apical root resorption after orthodontic treatment with the edgewise and speed appliances. *American Journal of Orthodontics and Dentofacial Orthopedics*, Vol. 108, No. 1, pp. 76-84, ISSN 0759-8108.

Bramante, M. A. (1990). Controversies in orthodontics. *Dent Clin North Am*, Vol. 34, No. 1, pp. 91-102, ISSN 0345-1478.

Brauchli, L. M; Senn, C. & Wichelhaus, A. (2011). Active and passive self-ligation-a myth?. *Angle Orthodontist*, Vol. 81, No. 2, pp. 312-318, ISSN 2120-8085.

Burke, S. P.; Silveira, A. M.; Goldsmith, L. J.; Yancey, J. M.; Van Stewart, A. & Scarfe, W. C. (1998). A meta-analysis of mandibular intercanine width in treatment and postretention. Angle Orthodontist, Vol. 68, No. 1, pp. 53-60, ISSN 0950-3135.

Damon, D.H. The Damon low-friction bracket: A biologically compatible straight-wire system. (1998). *Journal of Clinical Orthodontics*, Vol. 32, No. 11, pp. 670-680, ISSN 1038-8398.

Eberting, J. J.; Straja, S. R. & Tuncay, O. C. (2001). Treatment time, outcome, and patient satisfactioncomparisons of Damon and conventional brackets. *Clin Orthod Res*, Vol. 4, No. 4, pp. 228-234, ISSN 1168-3812.

Echols, P. M. (1975). Elastic ligatures: Binding forces and anchorage taxation. *American Journal of Orthodontics*, Vol. 67, No. 6, pp. 219-220, ISSN 0105-6140.

Englehardt, G.; Boyer, D. & Bishara, S. (1993). Debonding orthodontic ceramic brackets by ultrasonic instrumentation. *Journal of Dental Research*, Vol. 72, No. 3, pp. 139-145, ISSN 0766-1142.

Feldon, P. J.; Murray, P. E.; Burch, J. G,; Meister, M. & Freedman, M. A. (2010). Diode laser debonding of ceramic brackets. *American Journal of Orthodontics and Dentofacial Orthopedics*, Vol. 138, No. 4, pp. 458-462 ISSN 2088-9051.

Fleming, P. S.; DiBiase, A. T.; Sarri, G. & Lee, R. T. (2009). Pain experience during initial alignment with a self-ligating and a conventional fixed orthodontic appliance system. A randomized controlled clinical trial. *Angle Orthodontist*, Vol. 79, No. 1, pp. 46–50, ISSN 1912-3718.

Fleming, P. S.; DiBiase, A. T.; Sarri, G. & Lee, R. T. (2009). Mandibular arch dimensional changes with 2 preadjusted edgewise appliances. American Journal of Orthodontics and Dentofacial Orthopedics, Vol. 136, No. 3, pp. 340–347, ISSN 1973-2667.

Forsberg, C. M.; Brattstro¨m, V.; Malmberg, E. & Nord, C. E. (1991). Ligature wires and elastomeric rings: two methods of ligation, and their association with microbial colonization of streptococcus mutans and lactobacilli. *European Journal of Orthodontics*, Vol. 13, No. 5, pp. 416- 420, ISSN 0174-8191.

Fournier, A.; Payant, L. & Bouclin, R. (1998). Adherence of Streptococcus mutans to orthodontic brackets. *American Journal of Orthodontics and Dentofacial Orthopedics*, Vol. 114, No. 4, pp. 414 - 417, ISSN 0979-0325.

Garino, F. & Favero, L. (2003). Control of tooth movements with the Speed system. *Prog Orthod*, Vol. 4, pp. 23-30, ISSN 1288-7576.

Geiger, A. M.; Gorelick, J. &, Gwinnett, A. J. (1983). Bond failure rates of facial and lingual attachments. *Journal of Clinical Orthodontics*, Vol. 17, No. 3, pp.165-169, ISSN 0635-0356.

Gioka, C. & Eliades, T. (2004). Materials-induced variation in the torque expression of preadjusted appliances. *American Journal of Orthodontics and Dentofacial Orthopedics*, Vol. 125, No. 3, pp. 323-328, ISSN 1501-4409.

Gorelick, L.; Geiger, A. M. & Gwinnett, A. J. (1982). Incidence of white spot formation after bonding and banding. *American Journal of Orthodontics*, Vol. 81, No. 2, pp. 93-98, ISSN 0675-8594.

Hamilton, R.; Goonewardene, M. S. & Murray, K. (2008). Comparison of active self-ligating brackets and conventional pre-adjusted brackets. *Australian Orthodontic Journal*, Vol. 24, No. 2, pp. 102-109, ISSN 1911-3074.

Hanson, G. H. (1980). The SPEED system: a report on the development of a new edgewise appliance. *American Journal of Orthodontics*, Vol. 78, No. 3, pp. 243-265, ISSN 0699-6488.

Harradine, N. W. (2001). Self-ligating brackets and treatment efficiency. *Clin Orthod Res*, Vol. 4, No. 4, pp. 220-227, ISSN 1168-3811.

Harradine, N. W. (2003). Current Products and Practices Self-ligating brackets: where are we now? Journal of Orthodontics, Vol. 30, No. 3, pp. 262–273, ISSN 1453-0427.

Hawley, C. A. (1919). A removable retainer. *International Journal of Orthodontics*, Vol. 2, pp. 291-298.

Hayakawa, K. (2005). Nd: YAG laser for debonding ceramic orthodontic brackets. *American Journal of Orthodontics and Dentofacial Orthopedics*, Vol. 128, No. 5, pp. 638-647, ISSN 1628-6212.

Henao, S. P. & Kusy, R. P. (2004). Evaluation of the frictional resistance of conventional and self-ligating bracket designs using standardized archwires and dental typodonts . *Angle Orthodontist*, Vol. 74, No. 2, pp. 202–211, ISSN 1513-2446.

Huang, Y.; Keilig, L.; Rahimi, A.; Reimann, S.; Eliades, T.; Ja¨ger, A. & Bourauel, C. (2009). Numeric modeling of torque capabilities of self-ligating and conventional brackets. *American Journal of Orthodontics and Dentofacial Orthopedics*, Vol. 136, No. 5, pp. 638-643, ISSN 1989-2278.

Ireland, A. J.; Sherriff, M. & McDonald, F. (1991). Effect of bracket and wire composition on frictional forces . *European Journal of Orthodontics*, Vol. 13, No. 4, pp. 322-328, ISSN 0191-5622.

Jiang, R. P. & Fu, M. K. (2008). Non-extraction treatment with self-ligating and conventional brackets. *Zhonghua Kou Qiang Yi Xue Za Zhi*, Vol. 43, No. 8, pp. 459-463, ISSN 1908-7583.

Khambay, B.; Millett, D. & McHugh, S. (2004). Evaluation of methods of archwire ligation on frictional resistance. *European Journal of Orthodontics*, Vol. 26, No. 3, pp. 327-332, ISSN 1522-2719.

Keim, R. G.; Gottlieb, E. L.; Nelson, A. H. & Vogels, D. S. (2008). Study of orthodontic diagnosis and treatment procedures. Part 1: results and trends. *Journal of Clinical Orthodontics*, Vol. 42, no. 11, pp. 625–640, ISSN 1907-5377.

Keim, R. G.; Gottlieb, E. L.; Nelson, A. H. & Vogels, D. S. (2002). Study of orthodontic diagnosis and treatment procedures. Part 1. Results and trends. *Journal of Clinical Orthodontics*, Vol. 36, No. 1, pp. 553-568, ISSN 0168-0786.

Khouri, S. A. (1998). The Bendistal pliers: a solution for distal end bending of super-elastic wires. *American Journal of Orthodontics and Dentofacial Orthopedics*, Vol. 114, No. 6, pp. 675–676, ISSN 0984-4207.

Kneiflm, R. W. (1973). Invisible lower cuspid to cuspid retainer. *Annie Orthod*, Vol. 43, No. 2, pp. 218- 219, ISSN 0457-1745.

Krell, K. V.; Coury, J. M. & Bishara, S. E. (1993). Orthodontic bracket removal using conventional and ultrasonic debondingtechniques: Enamel loss and time requirements. *American Journal of Orthodontics and Dentofacial Orthopedics*, Vol. 103, No. 3, pp. 258-265, 0845-6784.

Linge, B.O. & Linge, L. (1983). Apical root resorption in upper and anterior teeth. *European Journal of Orthodontics*, Vol. 5, No. 3, pp. 173-83, ISSN 0657-8039.

Maijer, R. & Smith, D. C. (1990). Time saving with self-ligating brackets. *Journal of Clinical Orthodontics*, Vol. 24, No. 1, pp. 29-31, ISSN 0238-7895.

Marsh, P. D. (2003). Are dental diseases examples of ecological catastrophes? *Microbiology*, Vol. 149, No. 2, pp. 279-294, ISSN 0002-6082.

Mezomo, M.; de Lima, E. S.; de Menezes, L. M.; Weissheimer, A. & Allgayer, S. (2011). Maxillary canine retraction with self-ligating and conventional brackets. *Angle Orthodontist*, Vol. 81, No. 2, pp. 292-297, ISSN 2120-8082.

Miles, P. G. (2005). SmartClip versus conventional twin brackets for initial alignment: is there a difference? *Austrialn Orthodontic Journal*, Vol. 21, No. 2, pp. 123-127, ISSN 1642-9868.

Miles, P. G.; Weyant, R. J. & Rustveld, L. (2006). A clinical trial of Damon 2 vs conventional twin brackets during initial alignment. Angle Orthod, Vol. 76, No. 3, pp. 480-485, ISSN 1663-7731.

Miles, P. G. (2007). Self-ligating vs conventional twin brackets during en-masse space closure with sliding mechanics. *American Journal of Orthodontics and Dentofacial Orthopedics*, Vol. 132, No. 2, pp. 223-225, ISSN 1769-3373.

Mills, J. R. (1966). The long-term results of the proclination of lower incisors. *Br Dent J*, Vol. 120, No. 8, pp. 355-363, ISSN 0521-8208.

Mirabella, A. D. & Årtun, J. (1995). Prevalence and severity of apical root resorption in upper anterior teeth in adult orthodontic patients. *European Journal of Orthodontics*, Vol. 17, No. 2, pp. 93-99, ISSN 0778-1726.

Naranjo, A. A.; Trivino, M. L.; Jaramillo, A.; Betancourth, M. & Botero, J. E. (2006). Changes in the subgingival microbiota and periodontal parameters before and 3 months after bracket placement. *American Journal of Orthodontics and Dentofacial Orthopedics*, Vol. 130, No. 3, pp. 275-281, ISSN 1697-9483.

O'Higgins, E. A.; Kirschen, R. H. & Lee R. T. (1999). The influence of maxillary incisor inclination on arch length. Br J Orthod, Vol. 26, No. 2, pp. 97-102, ISSN 1042-0243.

Pandis, N.; Polychronopoulou, A. & Eliades, T. (2006). Failure rate of self-ligating and edgewise brackets bonded with conventional acid etching and a self-etching primer: a prospective in vivo study. *Angle Orthodontist*, Vol. 76, No. 4, pp. 119-122, ISSN 1895-0317.

Pandis, N.; Polychronopoulou, A. & Eliades, T. (2007). Self-ligating vs conventional brackets in the treatment of mandibular crowding: a prospective clinical trial of treatment duration and dental effects. *American Journal of Orthodontics and Dentofacial Orthopedics*, Vol. 132, No. 2, pp. 208-215, ISSN 1769-3371.

Pandis, N.; Vlachopoulos, K.; Polychronopoulou, A.; Madianos, P. & Eliades, T. (2008). Periodontal condition of the mandibular anterior dentition in patients with conventional and Selfligating brackets. *Orthod Craniofac Res*, Vol. 11, No. 4, pp. 211-215, ISSN 1895-0317.

Pandis, N.; Nasika, M.; Polychronopoulou, A. & Eliades, T. (2008). External apical root resorption in patients treated with conventional and self-ligating brackets. *American Journal of Orthodontics and Dentofacial Orthopedics*, Vol. 134, No. 5, pp. 646-651, ISSN 0889-5406.

Pandis, N.; Papaioannou, W.; Kontou, E.; Nakou, M.; Makou, M. & Eliades, T. (2010). Salivary Streptococcus mutans in patients with conventional and self-ligating brackets. European Journal of Orthodontics, Vol. 32, No. 1, pp. 94-99, ISSN 1947-4229.

Pandis, N.; Polychronopoulou, A.; Makou, M. & Eliades, T. (2010). Mandibular dental arch changes associated with treatment of crowding using self-ligating and conventional brackets. *European Journal of Orthodontics*, Vol. 32, No. 3, pp. 248-253, ISSN 1995-9610.

Pandis, N.; Polychronopoulou, A.; Eliades, T. (2010). Active or passive self-ligating brackets? A randomized controlled trial of comparative efficiency in resolving maxillary anterior crowding in adolescents. American Journal of Orthodontics and Dentofacial Orthopedics, Vol. 137, No.1, pp. 12-16, ISSN 0889-5406.

Patel, V. (1992). Non-completion of active orthodontic treatment. *British Journal of Orthodontics*, Vol. 19, No. 1, pp. 47–54, ISSN 0156-2578.

Pellegrini, P.; Sauerwein, R.; Finlayson, T.; McLeod, J.; Covell, D. A.; Maier, T. & Machida, C. A. (2009).

Plaque retention by Selfligating vs elastomeric orthodontic brackets: quantitative comparison of oral bacteria and detection with adenosine triphosphate–driven bioluminescence. *American Journal of Orthodontics and Dentofacial Orthopedics*, Vol. 135, No. 4, pp. 426-429, ISSN 1936-1723.

Pizzoni, L.; Ravnholt, G.; Melsen, B. (1998). Frictional forces related to self-ligating brackets. European Journal of Orthodontics, Vol. 20, No. 3, pp. 283-291, ISSN 0969-9406.

Pringle, A.M.; Petrie, A.; Cunningham, S. J. & McKnight, H. (2009). Prospective randomized clinical trial to compare pain levels associated with 2 orthodontic fixed bracket systems. *American Journal of Orthodontics and Dentofacial Orthopedics*, Vol.136, No. 2, pp. 160-167, ISSN 1965-1344.

Proffit, W. R. (2000). *Contemporary Orthodontics*, third edition, Mosby, ISBN 0-323-04046-2, St. Louis.

Øgaard, B.; Rølla, G. & Arends, J. (1988). Orthodontic appliances and enamel demineralization. Part 1. Lesion development . *American Journal of Orthodontics*, Vol. 94, No. 1, pp. 68–73, ISSN 0316-4585.

Read-Ward, G. E.; Jones, S. P. & Davies, E. H. (1997). A comparison of self-ligating and conventional orthodontic bracket systems. *British Journal of Orthodontics*, Vol. 24, No. 4, pp. 309-317, ISSN 0301-228.

Redlich, M.; Mayer, Y.; Harari, D. & Lewinstein, I. (2003). In vitro study of frictional forces during sliding mechanics of "reduced-friction" brackets. *American Journal of Orthodontics and Dentofacial Orthopedics*, Vol. 124, No. 1, pp. 69-73, ISSN 1286-7900.

Reitan, K. (1956). Selecting forces in orthodontics. *Transactions of the European Orthodontic Society*, Vol. 32, pp. 108–125.

Ridley, J.; Garret, S. & Moon, P. (1979). Frictional forces of ligated plastic and metal edgewise brackets,

Journal of Dental research, Vol. 58, pp. 98, ISSN 0342-3452.

Rubenstein, B. M. (1976). A direct bond maxillary retainer. *Journal of Clinical Orthodontics*, Vol. 10, No. 1, pp. 43-48, ISSN 801-906.

Scheurer, P. A.; Firestone, A. R. & Bürgin, W. B. (1996). Perception of pain as a result of orthodontic treatment with fixed appliances. *European Journal of Orthodontics*, Vol. 18, No. 4, pp. 349–357, ISSN 0892-1656.

Schumacher, H.; Bourauel, C. & Drescher, D. (1990). Der einefluder ligatur auf die friktion zwishchen bracket und bogen, Fortschr. *Kieferorthop*, Vol. 51, No 2, pp. 106-116, ISSN 2345-6543.

Scott, G. E. (1988). Fracture toughness and surface cracks: The key to its understanding ceramic brackets. Angle Orthodontist, Vol. 58, No. 1, pp. 5-8, ISSN 0316-2664.

Scott, P.; DiBiase, A. T.; Sherriff, M. & Cobourne, M. T. (2008). Alignment efficiency of Damon 3 self-ligating and conventional orthodontic bracket systems: a randomized clinical trial. *American Journal of Orthodontics and Dentofacial Orthopedics*, Vol. 134, No. 4, pp. 470-478, ISSN 1892-9262.

Scott, P.; Sherriff, M.; DiBiase, A. T. & Cobourne, M. T. (2008). Perception of discomfort during initial orthodontic tooth alignment using aself-ligating or conventional bracket system: a randomized clinical trial. *European Journal of Orthodontics*, Vol. 30, No. 3, pp. 227–232, ISSN 1833-9656.

Sheridan, I.; Brawley, G. & Hastings, J. (1986). Electrothermal debracketing. Part I. An in vitro study. *American Journal of Orthodontics*, Vol. 89, No. 1, pp. 21-27, ISSN 0351-0550.

Shivapuja, P. K. & Berger, J. (1994). A comparative study of conventional ligation and self-ligation bracket systems. *American Journal of Orthodontics and Dentofacial Orthopedics*, Vol. 106, No. 5, pp. 472–480, ISSN 0797-7187.

Shivapuja, P. K. & Berger, J. (1994). A comparative study of conventional ligation and self-ligation bracket systems. *American Journal of Orthodontics and Dentofacial Orthopedics*, Vol. 106, No. 5, pp. 472-80, ISSN 0797-7187.

Sims, A.; Water, N.; Birnie, D. & Pethybridge, R. (1993). A comparison of the forces required to produce tooth movement in vitro using two self-ligating brackets and a pre-adjusted bracket employing two types of ligation. *European Journal of Orthodontics*, Vol. 15, No. 5, pp. 377-385,ISSN 0822-3972.

Taloumis, L. J.; Smith, T. M., Hondrum, S. O. & Lorton, L. (1997). Force decay and deformation of orthodontic elastomeric ligatures. *American Journal of Orthodontics and Dentofacial Orthopedics*, Vol. 111, No. 1, pp. 1-11, ISSN 0900-9917.

Taylor, N. G. & Ison, K. (1996). Frictional resistance between orthodontic brackets and archwires in the buccal segments. *Angle Orthodontist*, Vol. 66, No. 3, pp. 215–222. ISSN 0880-5917.

Thomas, S.; Sherriff, M. & Birnie, D. (1998). A comparative in vitro study of the frictional characteristics of two types of self-ligating brackets and two types of pre-adjusted edgewise brackets tied with elastomeric ligatures. *European Journal of Orthodontics*, Vol. 20, No. 5, pp. 589-596, ISSN 0982-5561.

Thorstenson, G. A. & Kusy, R. P. (2001). Resistance to sliding of selfligating brackets versusconventional stainless steel twin brackets with second-order angulation in the dry and wet (saliva) states. *American Journal of Orthodontics and Dentofacial Orthopedics*, Vol. 120, No. 4, pp.361- 370, ISSN 1160-6960.

Türkkahraman, H.; Sayin, M. O.; Bozkurt, F. Y.; Yetkin, Z.; Kaya, S. & Onal, S. (2005). Archwire ligation techniques, microbial colonization, and periodontal status in orthodontically treated patients. *Angle Orthodontist*, Vol. 75, No. 2, pp. 231-236, ISSN 1582-5788.

Wong, A. (1976). Orthodontic elastic materials. *American Journal of Orthodontics*, Vol. 46, No. 2, pp. 196- 204, ISSN 0106-4346.

Zachrisson, B. U. (1986). Excellence in finishing. *Journal of Clinical Orthodontics*, Vol. 20, No. 8, pp. 460- 482, ISSN 0346-2201.

2

Considerations in Orthodontic Bracket Adhesion to Hypomineralized Enamel

Shabtai Sapir
Department of Pediatric Dentistry, Hebrew University- Hadassah Faculty of Dental Medicine, Jerusalem, Israel

1. Introduction

Developmental defects of enamel (DDE) are frequently observed. In both pediatric and orthodontic dental practices. DDE consist mainly of hypoplasia, diffuse and demarcated opacities.[1] Often, a combination of enamel defects may be recognized in the same child (Fig. 1). Weerheijm et al. defined the term Molar Incisor Hypomineralization (MIH) to describe a more specific pattern of DDE: hypomineralization of systemic origin of one to four permanent first molars frequently associated with affected incisors (Fig. 2).[2]
Clinically, MIH can be seen as an abnormality in the translucency of the enamel. Some lesions have significant subsurface porosity, leading to posteruptive breakdown of the surface.

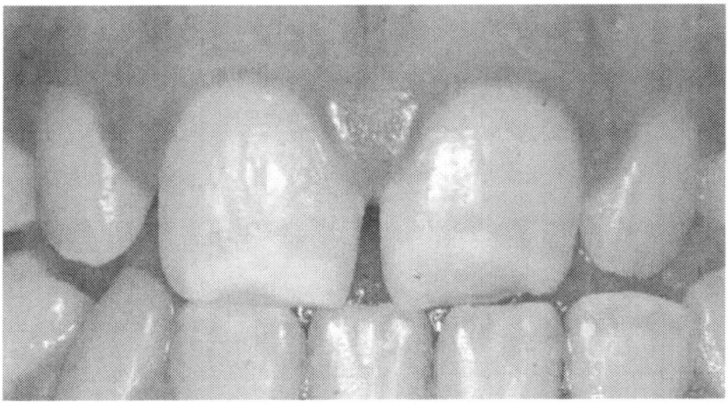

Fig. 1. Intraoral view of an 11-year-old girl at the initial examination, with hypoplasia of the incisal edges of her upper central incisors.

The opacities are usually limited to the incisal or cuspal one third of the crown, more commonly on the buccal surfaces. The enamel surface is often smooth and well mineralized, following post-eruptive maturation. The subsurface enamel is soft and porous.[3] The color of the opacities may reflect differences in hardness, porosity and mineral content. Yellow or yellow-brown demarcated opacities have lower hardness values and greater porosity. Mostly they cross the entire bulk of enamel, as opposed to white and white-creamy defects, which are usually limited to the inner enamel, closer to the Dentino-Enamel Junction (DEJ).[3,4] Patients may complain of one or more of the following: poor esthetics, thermal and mechanical sensitivity, attrition, secondary caries, tooth discoloration, malocclusion and periodontal problems.[2,5]

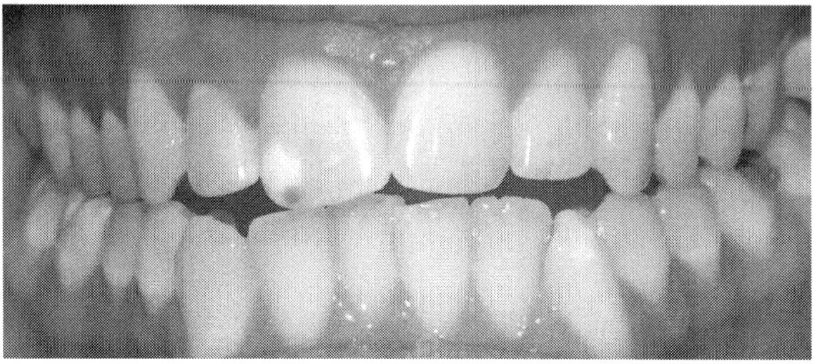

Fig. 2. Intraoral view of a 17-year old adolescent presented with MIH with low-moderate severity

Early diagnosis of DDE is important for appropriate treatment planning and for prevention of future complications. An accurate diagnosis may improve the clinician's dental care in many aspects: caries risk assessment, aesthetics, improved adhesion, retention, durability and debonding of orthodontic bands and brackets. Furthermore, financial considerations, behavioral management, and medico-legal issues can be affected by early identification of DDE.[6-11]

The purpose of this article is to discuss those pre-treatment and treatment considerations that may affect: a) The management of the young patient diagnosed with demarcated opacities; and b) Choice of adhesive material and technique used for bonding and debonding of orthodontic brackets in a patient affected by demarcated opacities.

The management of the young patient diagnosed with demarcated opacities may be divided into two parts:

1. Preliminary dental consultation and treatment prior to adhesion of fixed orthodontic appliance
2. Appliance adhesion, materials and debonding- technique.

Preliminary dental treatment prior to adhesion of fixed orthodontic appliance

May be divided into:

a. Early diagnosis and risk assessment.
b. Informed consent from the guardians/ patient
c. Post-eruption breakdown, prevention of dental caries, enhancing remineralization and desensitization.
d. Considering long-term prognosis of affected teeth and, if necessary, deciding upon extractions or restoration.

Early diagnosis and risk assessment

Children with demarcated opacities should be diagnosed early in their consultation visits. Documentation both written and photographic should be recorded in the patient's file. The patient's chief complaint, in conjunction with the biochemical and morpho-histological characteristics of the defects, may affect the prognosis and management.[3,12,13] The extent of the problem depends upon the number of the teeth involved and the severity of the defects (depth, size, color and enamel break-down). In addition, information of the patient's caries risk assessment, diet, oral hygiene and compliance can provide the clinician with an assessment of the risk for possible future complications such as: post-eruption breakdown of enamel around brackets and bands, objectionable color changes, higher risk of demineralization and caries, and the possible need to restore those lesions prior to the orthodontic treatment or shortly there after.[5,14] The orthodontist may prefer to refer the patient to other specialists for risk assessment, preventive plan and dental treatment. Nevertheless the clinician is advised to follow carefully the suggested treatment plan, to maintain the patient's compliance and document it routinely as the orthodontic treatment progresses. Some cases should be denied treatment based on enhanced risk for further deterioration of tooth substance.

Informed consent from the guardians/ patient

The informed consent prior to utilizing the orthodontic treatment should specify the problems that may arise following bonding and debonding of orthodontic appliances. This may include: post-eruption breakdown of enamel around brackets and bands, objectionable color changes, higher risk for demineralization and caries, and the possible need to restore those lesions prior to the orthodontic treatment or shortly after it is commenced or finished. An essential part of the informed consent is compliance with the preventive program and the accomplishment of the necessary dental treatment prior, during and sometimes following the orthodontic treatment.

Post-eruption breakdown, prevention of dental caries and, enhancing remineralization, and desensitization.

The recommended preventive treatment ought to be given according to the individual patient's symptoms and risk assessment. The cariogenicity and erosivity of the child's diet should be assessed and appropriate recommendations for dietary modification provided. Oral hygiene instructions may include the use of the appropriate tooth brush and desensitizing toothpaste if necessary.[14]

Weekly topical fluoride gel or varnish applications, and daily sodium fluoride rinses may improve resistance to demineralization, decrease tooth sensitivity and enhance enamel remineralization and post eruptive maturation. [15] Daily application of casein phosphor-peptide-amorphous calcium phosphate (CPP-ACP), reportedly enhances remineralization [16,17] Anecdotal reports describe surface hardening and reduced tooth sensitivity and esthetic improvement of opacities and demineralized enamel.[5,18]

Monthly follow-up visits should be scheduled for enamel surface integrity inspection and for the application of 5% sodium fluoride varnish such as Duraphat (2.26%F-Colgate-Palmolive) or the new white varnish Vanish (2.26%F-OMNII-Oral Pharmaceuticals).

Dental treatment considering long term prognosis of affected teeth and if necessary decide upon extractions.

A multidisciplinary approach that may involve other specialists such as a pediatric dentist, prosthodontics and a dental hygienist can contribute in offering a preventive program, and lead to decision on the type of restorations that may be offered prior to the orthodontic treatment.[19,20]

When a Permanent First Molar is severely hypomineralized, early orthodontic and prosthetic assessment is essential. Evaluation of the patient's and/or guardian's preferences, behavior management, financial issues, compliance, tooth vitality, restorability, dental age, skeletal relationship and growth, buccal segment crowding, occlusal relationships, presence of wisdom teeth, and the condition of other teeth, may influence the long term prognosis and dictate immediate restoration or extraction. [5,21-23]

When the molars are moderately or severely involved stainless steel crowns (SSC) may be considered. They prevent further tooth deterioration, and sensitivity, establish correct inerproximal contacts and occlusal relationship, are not as technique-sensitive or costly as cast restorations, and require little time to insert. Following orthodontic treatment, once the gingival contour is stabilized, cast adhesive crowns may be adjusted according to the final position of the tooth to provide ideal aesthetics.[5,20,22]

Appliance adhesion and debonding technique and materials

To date no research on bonding of orthodontic appliances to hypomineralized teeth has been published, however, recent research articles on different adhesives and performance of bonding materials in adhesion to normal and hypomineralized enamel may improve our knowledge of adhesion to teeth affected with MIH and help suggest educated recommendations.

The aspects that should be discussed include:

1. Type of adhesive etching, priming and bonding.
2. Enamel prophylaxis and fluoride exposure (prior to bonding).
3. Anti-cariogenic effect of adhesives and fluoride release.
4. Debonding and residual adhesive removal.
5. Modifications necessary for adhesion to hypomineralized enamel.

Type of adhesive etching, priming and bonding

The type of adhesive and the enamel conditioning chosen may determine the clinical outcome of adhesion to hypomineralized enamel. The adhesive materials used for cementing and bonding of bands and brackets commonly used in modern orthodontic practice are based on: GIC (Glass Ionomer Cement), RMGIC (Resin Modified GIC), Poly-acid modified Glass ionomer (compomer), and Resin composite.

Enamel may be conditioned in different ways: 10% Polyacrylic acid, a non-rinse conditioner, and conventional two-stage etching and priming process with 35%-37% phosphoric acid. Manufactures have simplified some adhesive systems by combining the hydrophilic primer and the adhesive, and recently introduced products with primers modified with various acidic components. The following are Non-rinse conditioners: (NRC, Dentsply De Trey), Adper Prompt L-Pop Self Etch Adhesive, 3M, St. Paul, Minn (Adper PLP), Clearfil SE Bond /Protect Bond, (Kuraray Medical Inc, Tokyo, Japan), and Transbond Plus Self Etching Primer (TSEP, 3M Unitek). The pH of these acidified or self-etching primers has been reduced to the extent that they can effectively etch enamel to the same degree as phosphoric acid.[24-28]

Anti-cariogenic effect of adhesives and fluoride release

The fluoride released from adhesives based on RMGIC (Fuji Ortho LC (GC), is significantly greater than from resin based adhesives such as Transbond XT (3M Unitek).[24] However, the values were similar between fluoride release of RMGIC (Fuji Ortho LC (GC) and resin adhesives that were enhanced with external application of fluoride.[29] Similar results were seen in prevention of demineralization.[30-32] Resin composite based adhesives with internal release capability of fluoride were found to slow down demineralization when compared to regular resin composite adhesive even though less effectively than the RMGIC based adhesives.[32]

At present there is no research to support the claims by Transbond Plus Self Etching Primer and Clearfil Protect Bond manufacturers that they are capable of releasing fluoride in substantial levels to diminish enamel demineralization. The clinical efficiency of Clearfil Protect Bond, which is claimed to possess an antibacterial effect attributed to the 12-MethacryloyloxyDodecyl Pyridinum Bromide (MDPB) molecule, is yet unproved.

Enamel prophylaxis and fluoride exposure (prior to bonding)

The hypomineralized tooth is usually characterized by well mineralized surface enamel.[3,4] The clinician should attempt to preserve it as intact as possible. Most adhesive manufactures recommend cleaning teeth of organic enamel pellicle and plaque by using prophylaxis paste or pumice prior to adhesion of orthodontic brackets. A rubber cup is preferred over a bristle brush since it causes less enamel loss.[33] The abrasive paste used is less detrimental than the type of brush.[34] Pumice prophylaxis prior to conventional acid etching and adhesion with composite resin bonding agent or with GIC/RMGIC does not seem to reduce bond failure rates.[35,36] However, omitting prophylaxis when a self etching primer is used may increase the amount of clinical bond failures.[37]

Prophylaxis pastes containing up to 13,500 ppmF were not found to adversely affect the adhesion of orthodontic brackets to normal enamel.[38]

The application of NaF fluoride varnish has not adversely affected the adhesion of orthodontic brackets to normal enamel, either when the enamel was conditioned with self etching primer or etched with 37-35% phosphoric acid.[39,40] Nevertheless, application of APF fluoride gel prior to orthodontic brackets adhesion resulted in lower adhesion.[41]

Debonding and residual adhesive removal.

The debonding of brackets and bands might cause further break-down of enamel. The amount of enamel loss depends on the bracket material, bonding and adhesive methods used and on the method of debonding. Ceramic brackets reportedly cause more enamel loss and fracture at debonding than metal brackets,[42,43] Metal bracket removal after adhesion with a resin composite resulted in 7.4 micron on average loss of enamel surface.[44] An in vitro study has not found significant differences in enamel loss between teeth with white spot lesions and teeth without white spot lesions, following orthodontic bracket debonding and polishing with low-speed finishing burs or disks.[45] However, there are no studies that examined enamel loss in more severe cases of enamel hypomineralization.

The adhesives based on RMGIC have excellent results in ease of removal, lower Adhesive Remnant Index (ARI) scores, and a lower risk of damaging enamel surface.[27,28,30] Self etching primer systems have also been reported to produce good ARI scores as compared to traditional acid-etch technique.[46-48]

The removal of the residual adhesive can be accomplished via debonding pliers, ultrasonic scaler, high-speed tungsten carbide bur or by low-speed tungsten carbide bur Debonding pliers cause the least enamel loss, however more residual adhesive remained.[48] The least enamel loss was reported to occur with self-etching primer and after enamel clean-up with a slow-speed tungsten carbide bur with water.[48]

Modifications necessary for adhesion to hypomineralized enamel

The ideal adhesive for orthodontic purpose should provide long retention, anti-cariogenic features, biocompatibility, simplicity, aesthetics, reasonable price, and easy debonding along with preservation of enamel integrity. Some of these demands are crucial for the clinician bonding a fixed appliance to hypomineralized enamel. Theoretically, self-etching primer adhesive system (SEPAS), and RMGIC based adhesives may be more advantageous when orthodontic adhesion to hypomineralized enamel is required. The use of conventional etching and priming is discouraged since phosphoric acid, may cause more enamel loss than self etching primers.[47,48] This might reduce adhesion to hypomineralized enamel, because of inadequate micro-tag formation, consequential to the formation of little intercrystal porosity.[19] Other possible effects of severe enamel loss are: increased micro leakage around brackets with potential connection between enamel surface and the subsurface opacities, which might produce either an objectionable color change following extrinsic staining or a higher risk for demineralization and postoperative sensitivity.

Moreover, All-etch single-bottle adhesive - Single Bond, (3M ESPE, St. Paul, Minn, USA), and a SEPAS-Clearfil SE Bond, did not differ significantly in their ability to bond to hypomineralized enamel.[19] Subsequently, no apparent incentive to choose phosphoric acid over SEPAS possibly will remain.

New self-etching adhesives (TSEP, Clearfil Protect Bond) may offer an alternative that meets the challenge of adhesion to hypomineralized enamel better:

1. They cause less enamel loss. [47,48]
2. They are simpler to use.
3. Rinsing is omitted. Therefore wet conditions that inhibit resin infiltration are prevented. The larger interprismatic spaces in hypomineralized enamel may promote moisture retention and structural weakness and crack propagation.[19] Also the proven efficacy of SEPBS in bonding better than conventional two-stage etching and priming systems in wet conditions may be beneficial in cases of hypomineralized enamel.[49-51]
4. Some SEPBS (Clearfil SE Bond/ Protect bond, to bond both, micromechanically and chemically to hydroxyapatite due to incorporation of the 10-Methacryloxydecyl Dihydrogen Phosphate (MDP) molecule, whereas conventional bonding relies primarily on micromechanical retention. The latter may be limited because of minimal intercrystal porosity, and microtag formation after etching hypomineralized enamel.[19]
5. Some SEPBS Clearfil SE Bond/ Protect bond, and Transbond Plus Self Etching Primer have fluoride- releasing qualities and the Protect bond also has an antibacterial component; Even though, presently no research has been published to support its clinical efficiency, this may still be an encouraging development.
6. The improved adhesion and diminished microleakage of some self-etching primers Clearfil SE Bond/ Protect bond, in adhesion to normal enamel,[52-55] might also be seen in adhesion to hypomineralized enamel, since the demineralization and resin penetration occur concurrently, therefore the etching depth and the resin penetration depth might be similar.[19]
7. SEPBS cause less postoperative sensitivity, which may be important in severely hypomineralized teeth.[56]
8. Self etching primer systems have also been reported to produce good ARI scores as compared to traditional acid-etch technique. [46-47]

Another alternative for orthodontic bracket adhesion is RMGIC, which posses the inert advantages of fluoride release[24], ease of removal, lower Adhesive Remnant Index (ARI) scores, and a lower risk of damaging enamel surface, following orthodontic bracket removal. [27,28,30]

Interestingly, the combination of self-etching primer system with RMGIC was found (in-vitro) to enhance Shear Bond Strength of orthodontic brackets to normal bovine enamel.[57] Furthermore, few clinical results indicated comparable failure rate between a composite resin adhesive when compared to Fuji Ortho LC in normal enamel.[30,58]However, to date, the effect of RMGIC bonding to hypomineralized enamel was not investigated.

Clinical recommendation (see table):

The severity of the hypomineralized enamel lesion is clinically evaluated by assessing surface enamel smoothness, hardness and color. Yellow-brown defects have a propensity to be deeper and more porous, and therefore may necessitate more cautious handling than white and white-creamy defects.[3,4]

In cases of large yellow-brown opacities that cause an esthetic problem aggressive removal of all defective enamel, and a composite resin restoration, may be considered prior to bracket adhesion.[5,22] If the clinician wishes to refrain from aggressive reduction of enamel, pretreatment with 5% sodium hypochlorite (NaOCl) to remove protein encasing the hydroxylapatite is suggested,[56,59-62] followed by a SEPBS.

In cases of white-creamy or creamy-yellow opacities that are covered with hard surface enamel (Fig. 3), definitive esthetic restoration of the defect may be postponed (if at all necessary) until the orthodontic treatment is finished. The recommended adhesive system is a SEPBS with a conventional composite resin-based adhesive. Alternatively, enamel pretreatment with SEPBS in combination with a RMGIC (Fuji Ortho LC (GC), may be considered.

Ceramic brackets reportedly cause more enamel loss and fracture at debonding than metal brackets,[42,43] and are not recommended for adhesion to hypomineralized enamel.

The removal of the residual adhesive can be accomplished via debonding pliers, and the enamel clean-up should be finished with a slow-speed tungsten carbide bur with water spray.[48]

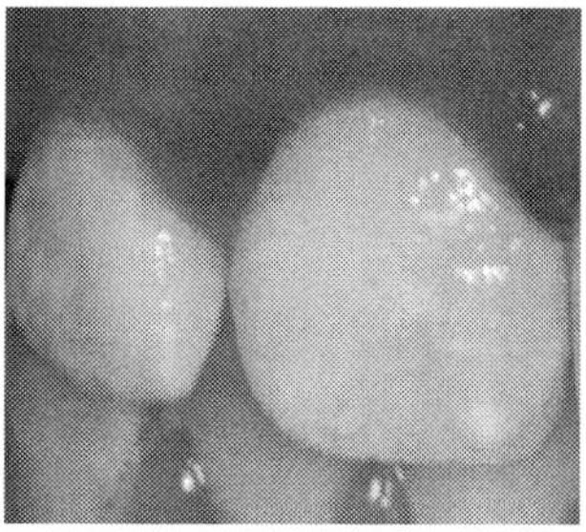

Fig. 3. Intraoral view of a 12-year-old girl with a low-severity demarcated opacities.

Discussion

Evidence-based recommendations on orthodontic adhesion to hypomineralized enamel do not exist in the dental literature. This may reflect the paucity of research investigating the adhesion of different bonding materials to hypomineralized enamel in general.[19,59,61] The few articles published on specialized topic of adhesion of resin materials to hypomineralized enamel lack standardizations of bonding and adhesive systems used, differ in storage media, testing apparatus, specimen preparation, bonded surface area (fissures, ground cut or uncut enamel surface), and the severity of enamel defects.[19] This precludes the authors of reviewing the subject in accordance with the Cochrane review system which emphasize reference containing clinically randomized controlled studies. Moreover, the conclusions drawn from investigating the adhesion of different adhesive systems to normal enamel may be inheritably tricky since the adhesion to hypomineralized enamel may posse's different charecteristics.[19]

1. Preliminary dental treatment prior to fixed orthodontic appliance adhesion
A. early diagnosis and risk assessment.
B. Informed consent from the guardians/ patient
C. prevention of dental caries and post-eruption breakdown, enhance remineralization and desensitization and maintenance Frequent recall appointments.
Active follow up and observation involving: oral hygiene instructions, dietary consultation, application of Casein phosphopeptide-amorphous calcium phosphate (CPP-ACP), and topical or systemic home and/or office fluoride regimen as indicated.
D. Considering long term prognosis of affected teeth and, if found necessary decide upon extractions or restoration.
2. Modifications necessary for adhesion to hypomineralized enamel:
A Prophylaxis with rubber cup and a paste containing up to 13,500PPM Fluoride
B. Metal brackets or ceramic brackets with metal channel that debond like metal brackets are recommended.
C. The adhesive system preferred for adhesion of orthodontic brackets to hypomineralized teeth is dependent upon the lesion hardness and color:
Large yellow-brown opacities:
Option A) removal of all defective enamel, prior to a composite resin restoration.
Option B) pre-treatment with 5% sodium hypochloride followed by a self etching primer-bonding system.
White-creamy or creamy-yellow opacities:
Option A) self etching system and adhesion of the orthodontic bracket with a conventional composite resin based adhesive.
Option B) enamel pretreatment with self etching primer may be considered in combination with a RMGIC (Fuji Ortho LC (GC).
D. Debonding of brackets with pliers followed with residual adhesive removal
by slow-speed tungsten carbide bur.

Table 1. Orthodontic management of enamel hypomineralization

Until more investigations are performed, several of our recommendations are at best educated assumptions.

The use of self-etching bonding systems may seem to yield more promising results. Nevertheless, few drawbacks should be stated:

1. They may not posses the same capacity as phosphoric acid to effectively etch uncut or unprepared enamel as is the case with orthodontic brackets adhesion to enamel.[24-28,62]
2. Auto-cure orthodontic resins (e.g., Concise, etc.) do not work well with the self-etch systems because the primer's acidity has been shown to interfere with the resins' polymerization.[64]

3. Some of those Self etching primers (e.g. Protect bond) may not work well with common LED curing light that do not cover the range of 400-515nm.

The clinician should be aware of these flaws when working with self-etching primers.

Yet, as frequently encountered in clinical situations, decision making on the management of situations as described in this text is necessary. We strongly believe that proper diagnosis and preventive management may assist the pediatric dentist as well as the orthodontist challenged by a patient with hypomineralized teeth.

Many questions are still left open and some answers to be wished for. Examples of still unanswered questions are: how does sodium hypochlorite conditioning of hypomineralized enamel affect the adhesion of RMGIC and resin adhesives, and how do the self-etching systems behave with those materials? Hopefully the uncertainties high lightened above enhance more research in this subject.

2. References

[1] Commission on Oral Health Research and Epidemiology] A review of the developmental defects of enamel index (DDE Index)] Commission on Oral Health Research and Epidemiology] Report of an FDI Working Group] Int Dent J, 1992; 42:411-426.

[2] Weerheijm KL, Jalevik B, Alaluusua S] Molar-incisor hypomineralization] Caries Res 2001; 35:390-391.

[3] Jalevik B, Odelius H, wolfram D et al] Secondary ion mass spectrometry and X-ray microanalysis of hypomineralized enamel in human permanent first molars] Arch Oral Biol 2000; 46:239-247.

[4] Suckling GW, Nelson DG, Patel MJ] Macroscopic and scanning electron microscopic appearance and hardness values of developmental defects in human of permanent teeth] Adv Dent Res 1989; 3:219-233]

[5] William V, Messer LB, Burrow MF] Molar incisor hypomineralization: review and recommendation for clinical management] Pediatr Dent 2006; 28:224-232.

[6] Ellwood RP, O'Mullane DM] Association between dental enamel opacities and dental caries in a north Wales population] Caries Res 1994; 28: 383-387.

[7] Leppaniemi A, Lukinmaa P-L, Alaluusua S] Nonfluoride hypomineralizations in the first molars and their impact on the treatment need] Caries Res 2001; 35: 36-40.

[8] Curzon MEJ, Spector PC] Enamel mottling in high strontium area of the USA] Community Dent Oral Epidem 1977; 5: 243-247.

[9] Borum MK, Andreasen JO] Sequelae of trauma to primary maxillary incisors] I] Complications in the primary dentition] Endod Dent Traumatol] 1998; 14: 31-44.

[10] Jarvinen S] Incisal overjet and traumatic injuries to upper permanent incisors] A retrospective study] Acta Odontol Scand 1978; 36:359-362.

[11] Odoi R, Croucher R, Wong F, Marcenes W] The relationship between problem behavior and traumatic dental injury amongst children aged 7-15 years old] Community Dent Oral Epidemiol] 2002; 30:392-396.

[12] Jalevik B, Klingberg G] Dental treatment, dental fear and behavior management problems in children with severe enamel hypomineralization in permanent first molars] Int J Ped Dent 2002; 12: 24-32.

[13] Jalevik B, Noren JG] Enamel hypomineralization of permanent first molars: a morphological study and survey of possible etiological factors] Int J Ped Dent 2000; 10:278-289.

[14] American Academy of Pediatric Dentistry Council on Clinical Affairs: Use of a caries-risk assessment tool (CAT) for infants, children, and adolescents] Pediatr Dent 2007-2008:29 (7 Reference Manual):29-33.

[15] Adair SM] Evidence-based use of fluoride in contemporary pediatric dental practice] Pediatr Dent 2006; 28:133-142.

[16] Giniger M, MacDonald J, Ziemba S, et al] The clinical performance of professionally dispensed bleaching gel with added amorphous calcium phosphate] JADA 2005; 136: 383-392.

[17] Iijima Y, Cai F, Shen P, et al] Acid resistance of enamel subsurface lesions remineralized by a sugar-free chewing gum containing casein phosphopeptide-amorphous calcium phosphate] Caries Res 2004; 38: 551-556.

[18] Kilpatrick N, Mahoney EK] Dental erosion: Part 2] The management of dental erosion] N Z Dent J 2004; 100:42-47.

[19] William V, Burrow MF, Palamara JEA, Messer LB] Microshear bond strength of resin composite to teeth affected by Molar hypomineralization using 2 adhesive systems] Pediatr Dent 2006; 28:233-241.

[20] Fayle SA] Molar-incisor hypomineralization: restorative management] European J Pediatr Dent 2003; 121-126.

[21] Penchas J, Peretz B, Becker A] The dilemma of treating severely decayed first permanent molars in children: To restore or to extract] ASDC J Dent Child 1994; 61:199-205.

[22] Zagdwon AM, Fayle SA, Pollard MA] A prospective clinical trial comparing metal crowns and cast restorations for defective first permanent molars] Eur J Paediatr Dent 2003; 4:138-142.

[23] Reddy L, Marker VA, Ellis E 3rd] Bond strength for orthodontic brackets contaminated by blood, composite versus resin-modified glass ionomer cements] J Oral Maxillofac Surg] 2003; 61(2): 206-213.

[24] Bishara SE, Gordan VV, Von Wald Let al] Shear bond strength of composite, glass ionomer, and acidic adhesive systems] Am J Orthod Dentofacial Orthop.1999; 115(1): 24-28.

[25] Buyukyilmaz T, Usumez S, Karaman AI] Effect of self-etching primers on bond strength-are the reliable?] Angle Orthod 2003; 73(1): 64-70.

[26] Grubisa HS, Heo G, Raboud D et al] An evaluation and comparision of orthodontic bracket bond strength achieved with self etching primer] Am J Orthod Dentofacial Orthop.2004; 126(2): 213-219.

[27] Bishara SE, Oonsombat C, Soliman MM et al] Comparison of bonding time and shear bond strength between a conventional and a new integrated bonding system] Angle Orthod] 2005; 75(2): 237-242.

[28] Aljubouri YD, Millett DT, Gilmour WH] Six and 12 months evaluation of a self-etching primer versus two-stage etch and prime for orthodontic bonding: a randomized clinical trial] Eur J Orthod 2004; 26(6):565-571.

[29] Corry A, Millett DT, Creanor SL et al] Effect of fluoride exposure on cariostatic potential of orthodontic bonding agents: an in vitro evaluation] J Orthod 2003; 30(4): 298-299.

[30] Hegarty DJ, Macfarlane TV] In vivo bracket retention comparision of a resin-modified glass ionomer cement and a resin based bracket adhesive system after a year] Am J Orthod Dentofacial Orthop.2002; 121(5): 496-501.

[31] Wilson RM, Donly KJ] Demineralization around orthodontic brackets bonded with a modified glass ionomer cement and fluoride-releasing resin composite] Pediatr Dent 2001; 23(3): 255-259.

[32] Pascotto RC, Navarro MF, Capelozza Filho L et al] In vivo effect of a resin-modified glass ionomer cement on enamel demineralization around orthodontic brackets] Am J Orthod Dentofacial Orthop.2004;125(1): 36-41.

[33] Pus MD, Way DC] Enamel loss due to orthodontic bonding with filled and unfilled resin using various clean-up techniques] Am J Orthod 1980; 77:269-283.

[34] Thompson RE, Way DC] Enamel loss due to prophylaxis and multiple bonding/debonding oforthodontic brackets] Am J Orthod 1981; 79:282-295.

[35] Barry GRP] A clinical investigation of the effect of omission of pumice prophylaxis on band and bond failure] Br J Orthod 1995; 22:245-248.

[36] Ireland AJ, Sherriff M: The effect of pumicing on the in vivo use of a resin modified glass poly (alkenoate) cement and a conventional no-mix composite for bonding orthodontic brackets] 2002; 29: 217-220.

[37] Ireland AJ, Knight H, Sherriff M] An in vivo investigation into bond failure rates with a new self-etching primer system] Am J Orthod Dentofacial Orthop 2003; 124:323-326.

[38] Damon PL, Bishara SE, Olsen ME et al] Effects of fluoride application on shear bond strength of orthodontic brackets] Angle Orthod] 1996; 66(1): 61-64.

[39] Ng'ang'a PM, Ogaard B, Cruz R et al] Tensile strength of orthodontic brackets bonded directly to fluorotic and nonfluorotic teeth: an in vitro comparative study] Am J Orthod Dentofacial Orthop.1992; 102(3): 244-250

[40] Kimura T, Dunn WJ, Taloumis LJ] Effect of fluoride varnish on the in vitro bond strength of orthodontic brackets using a self-etching primer system] Am J Orthod Dentofacial Orthop.2004; 125(3): 351-356.

[41] Meng CL, Li CH, Wang WN] Bond strength with APF applied after acid etching] Am J Orthod Dentofacial Orthop.1998; 114(5): 510-513.

[42] Joseph VP, Rossouw PE] The shear bond strengths of stainless steel orthodontic brackets bonded to teeth with orthodontic composite resin and various fissure sealants] Am J Orthod Dentofacial Orthop.1990; 98: 66-71.

[43] Jeroudi MT] Enamel fracture caused by ceramic brackets] Am J Orthod Dentofacial Orthop.1991; 99: 97-99.

[44] van Waes H, Matter T, Krejci I] Three-dimensional measurement of enamel loss caused by bonding and debonding of orthodontic brackets] Am J Orthod Dentofacial Orthop.1997; 112: 666-669.

[45] Tufekci E, Merrill TE, Pintado MR, Beyer JP, Brantley WA: Enamel loss associated with orthodontic adhesive removal on teeth with white spot lesions: An invitro study] Am J Orthod Dentofacial Orthop 2004; 125: 733-740]

[46] Vicente A, Bravo LA, Romero M] Self-etching primer and a non-rinse conditioner versus phosphoric acid: alternative methods for bonding brackets] Eur J Orthod 2006; 28:173-178.

[47] Vicente A, Bravo LA, Romero M, Ortiz AJ, Canteras M] Shear bond strength of orthodontic brackets bonded with self-etching primers] Am J Dent 2005; 18:256-260.

[48] Hosein I, Sherriff M, Ireland AJ] Enamel loss during bonding, debonding, and clean-up with use of a self-etching primer] Am J Orthod Dentofacial Orthop 2004; 126:717-724.

[49] Valente RM, De Rijk WG, Drummond JL et al] Etching conditions for resin-modified glass ionomer cement for orthodontic brackets] Am J Orthod Dentofacial Orthop.2002; 121;(25): 516-520.

[50] Cacciafesta V, Sfondrini MF, De Angelis et al] Effect of water and saliva contamination on shear bond strength of brackets bonded with conventional, hydrophilic and self-etching primers] Am J Orthod Dentofacial Orthop.2003; 123(4): 633-640.

[51] Cacciafesta V, Sfondrini MF, Scrbante A et al] Effect of blood contamination on shear bond strength of brackets bonded with a self-etching primer combined with a resin-modified glass ionomer] Am J Orthod Dentofacial Orthop.2004; 126(6): 703-708.

[52] Brandt PD Arhun N, Arman A, Sesen C, Karabulut E, Korkmaz Y, Gokalp S] Shear bond strength of orthodontic brackets with 3 self-etch adhesives] Am J Orthod Dentofacial Orthop.2006; 129: 547-550.

[53] Arhun N, Arman A, Sesen C, et al] Shear bond strength of orthodontic brackets with 3 self-etch adhesives] Am J Orthod Dentofacial Orthop.2006; 129: 547-550.

[54] Eminkahyagil N, Korkmaz Y, Gokalp S, et al] Shear bond strength of orthodontic brackets with newly developed self-etch adhesive] Angle Orthod 2005; 75: 843-848.

[55] Korbmacher H, Huck L, Adam T, Kahl-Nieke B] Evaluation of an antimicrobial and fluoride-releasing self-etching primer on the shear bond strength of orthodontic brackets] Eur Orthod 2006;

[56] Suda R, Andoh Y, Shionome M, et al] Clinical evaluation of the sedative effect of HEMA solution on the hypersensitivity of dentin] Dent Mater J 1990;9: 163-166.

[57] Cacciafesta V, Sfondrini MF, Baluga L et al] Use of a self-etching primer in combination with a resin-modified glass ionomer: effect of water and saliva contamination on shear bond strength] Am J Orthod Dentofacial Orthop.2003; 124(4): 420-426.

[58] Summers A, Kao E, Gilmore J et al] Comparision of bond strength between a conventional resin adhesive and a resin- modified glass ionomer adhesive: an in vitro and in vivo study] Am J Orthod Dentofacial Orthop.2004; 126(2): 200-206.

[59] Venezie RD, Vadiakas G, Christensen JR et.al] Enamel pretreatment with sodium hypochlorite to enhance bonding in hypocalcified amelogenesis imperfecta: case report and SEM analysis] Pediatr Dent 1994; 16: 433-436.

3

External Apical Root Resorption in Patients Treated with Passive Self-Ligating System

Masaru Yamaguchi[1] and Yasuhiro Tanimoto[2]
[1]Department of Orthodontics,
[2]Dental Biomaterials,
Nihon University School of Dentistry at Matsudo
Japan

1. Introduction

External apical root resorption (EARR) is an unavoidable pathologic consequence of orthodontic tooth movement. It can be defined as an iatrogenic disorder that unpredictably occurs after orthodontic treatment, whereby the resorbed apical root portion is replaced with normal bone. EARR is a sterile inflammatory process that is extremely complex and involves various disparate components, including mechanical forces, tooth roots, bone, cells, surrounding matrix, and certain known biologic messengers (Krishnan & Davidovitch, 2006; Meikle, 2006). In the relationship between EARR and inflammatory cytokines, Zhang et al. (2003) indicated that interleukin (IL)-1 and tumour necrosis factor (TNF)-alpha are important for the induction and the further processing of mechanically-induced root resorption in the rat. Receptor activator of nuclear factor κB ligand (RANKL) is a cytokine that belongs to the TNF family and is essential for the induction of osteoclastogenesis. Osteoblasts and bone marrow stromal cells produce this cytokine, and its signals are transduced by the specific receptor RANK, which is localized on the cell surface of osteoclast progenitors. The RANKL/RANK system has been suggested to play an integral role in osteoclast activation during orthodontic tooth movement. Shiotani et al. (2001) observed RANKL in osteoblasts, osteocytes, fibroblasts, and osteoclasts during the application of orthodontic forces. The RANKL/RANK system may regulate the natural process of root resorption in deciduous primary teeth (Lossdörfer et al., 2002). Therefore, these inflammatory cytokines contribute to alveolar bone remodeling and to resorption during orthodontic tooth movement and EARR.

The wire friction influences the forces acting in a continuous arch system. Damon (2006a) suggested that the nearly friction-free system, using the self-ligation brackets and high-tech wires, may not cause periodontal problems, including alveolar bone loss. Other studies reported that static friction measured in vitro is much less with a passive self-ligating system than with any other type of fixed appliance (Berger, 1990; Sims et al., 1993). The friction force disturb orthodontic tooth movement, thus, it is expected that influence for the periodontal tissue is different from the self-ligating brackets in the conventional appliances. We reported that GCF levels of substance P (SP), one of neuropeptides which cause the local inflammation, SP for the passive self-ligating system sites were significantly lower than for the teeth with conventional brackets at 24 hours (Yamaguchi et al., 2009). Thus, the passive self-ligating system is useful to reduce the inflammation and pain resulting from orthodontic forces.

The purposes of this study were to measure EARR and the levels of RANKL in GCF in patients undergoing with self-ligating brackets compared with conventional appliances, and to compare them.

2. Materials and methods

2.1 Subject selection

Forty subjects were selected from patients seeking treatment in the Department of Orthodontics at the Nihon University School of Dentistry at Matsudo. Forty orthodontic patients (9 males, 31 females, mean age of 18.5 ± 4.6 years) were enrolled in the study, after meeting the following criteria: (1) good general health; (2) lack of antibiotic therapy during the previous 6 months; (3) absence of anti-inflammatory drug administration in the month preceding the study; (4) healthy periodontal tissues with generalized probing depths ≦3 mm and no radiographic evidence of periodontal bone loss. Informed consent from the subjects was obtained after an explanation of the study protocol, which was reviewed by the ethic committee of Nihon University School of Dentistry at Matsudo (#10-019).

Two groups were set up, one 'conventional bracket' (CB) and another 'self-ligation bracket' (SL) groups. Twenty patients (4 males, 16 females) were treated with self-ligating brackets (Damon 3; Ormco, Japan, Tokyo, Japan). A matched control group of 20 patients (5 males, 15 females) was selected from the same registry and treated with the conventional brackets (.022-inch slot; Ormco. These controls were matched with the group for age, sex, and ANB, overjet, and overbite values before orthodontic treatment (T1).

The selection criteria for the subjects were the following.

1. Class I crowded malocclusion.
2. Four premolar extractions.
3. Excellent quality records.
4. Only patients with no history or evidence of tooth injury or wear, as shown on the charts and diagnostic records, were included.

2.2 Measurement of EARR and tooth position

To record the above parameters, the following measurements and evaluations were executed.

Tooth length: Tooth length of the maxillary central incisor at T1 and T2 was measured on the cephalogras from the incisal edge to the apex. When a difference in the length of the 2 adjacent maxillary central incisors was evident, the shorter root length was recorded. Baseline measurements of ANB angle, overjet (along the occlusal line), and overbite (perpendicular to the occlusal line) at T1 were made on the cephalograms.

Measurement of root length (EARR) and tooth position were performed according to the method of Brin and Bollen (2011).

Change in root length (EARR) of the maxillary central incisor was record as the difference between tooth lengths from T1 to T2.

Maxillary incisor movements were measured as the following. (1) The axial inclination of the maxillary central incisor to SN (1/SN) between T1 and T2. (2) The vertical and horizontal distances that the maxillary central incisor root was moved during orthodontic treatment (Table 1).

Parameter	CB group	SL group	*P* value
Male/female ratio	5/15	4/16	0.505
Mean age at T1 (y)	18.8 ± 4.5	18.3 ± 4.8	0.643
ANB (°)	3.3 ±1.2	3.2 ±1.3	0.544
Overjet (mm)	3.5 ±1.4	3.4 ±1.5	0.478
Overbite (mm)	3.3 ±1.4	3.5 ±1.3	0.377
Tooth length (mm)	26.8 ±1.6	27.0 ±1.7	0.682

Table 1. Descriptive parameters of the 2 groups at T1 (± SD)

2.3 GCF collection

GCF was collected from the mesial and distal sides of the upper central and lateral incisors. GCF sampling was performed using the method of Yamaguchi et al. (2006a), and collected at before (T1) and after (T2) orthodontic treatment. The tooth was gently washed with water, and then the sites under study were isolated with cotton rolls (to minimize saliva contamination) and gently dried with an air syringe. Paper strips (Periopaper, Harco, Tustin, CA, USA) were carefully inserted 1 mm into the gingival crevice and allowed to remain there for 1 minute, after which a second strip was placed at the same site. Care was taken to avoid mechanical injury. The contents were eluted out into 1x phosphate buffer saline (PBS) containing 0.1mM phenylmethylsulphonyfluoride and stored at -80°C until further processing (Fig. 1).

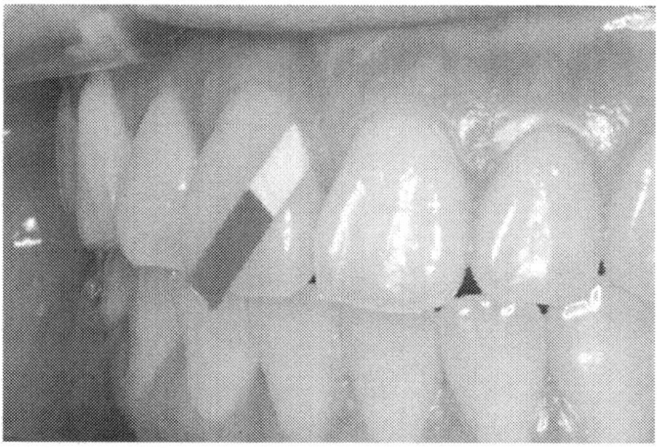

Fig. 1. GCF was collected from the mesial and distal sides of the upper central and lateral incisors.

2.4 Enzyme immunoassay

The s of RANKL and OPG level were measured in duplicate using a commercial ELISA kit (Quantikine, R&D Systems, Inc., Minneapolis, MN, USA), with the results expressed as pg/µg of total protein in the GCF.

2.5 Statistical methods

Statistical analysis among the groups was performed using one-way ANOVA and Scheffe test to evaluate the statistical difference between each pair of groups.

3. Results

3.1 Measurement of EARR and tooth position

The 2 groups were matched for sex (P = 0.505) and chronologic age at T1 (P = 0.643). Good agreement was also found for the ANB angle (P = 0.544), overjet (P = 0.478) and overbite (P = 0.377) at T1. The tooth lengths at T1 in both groups were similar: 26.8 ±1.6 in the CB group and 27.0 ±1.7 in the SL group (P = 0.6312) (Table 1).

Table 2 showed that the duration of treatment was not significant between the CB group and the SL group (P = 0.891).In both groups, the lengths were reduced at T2 (Table 2): 24.6 mm ± 2.0 in the CB group and 26.2 mm ±1.5 in the SL group. Tooth lengths in the 2 groups were statistically different at T2 (P = 0.05).

	CB	SL	*P* value
Duration of treatment (mo)	24.4 ± 2.1	24.8 ± 1.3	0.891
EARR (mm)	2.2 ± 1.4	0.80 ± 0.7	0.005 *
Change in 1/SN (°)	−6.5 ± 6.7	−6.1 ± 7.2	0.901
Apex (á) vertical movement (mm)	−0.6 ± 1.0	−0.5 ±1.3	0.883
Apex (á) horizontal movement (mm)	2.2 ± 1.6	2.5± 1.8	0.750

Table 2. Comparison of changes (± SD) during mechanotherapy (T1-T2) in EARR and tooth position in the Conventional bracket and Self-ligation bracket groups (absolute values in parentheses)

The mean amount of root resorption of the maxillary central incisor measured on the lateral cephalogram was significantly greater in the CB group than the SL group at T2. This mean difference in EARR between the groups did reach statistical significance.

In Table 2, the axial movements of the central incisor—vertical and horizontal apical movements—are presented.
The 1/SN change between T1 and T2 indicated an increase in the axial inclination in the CB and SL groups (about 6°). Change in the axial inclination of the maxillary central incisor (1/SN) was not significant difference between the CB group and the SL group ($P = 0.901$). The amounts of vertical movement of the apex were also not significant difference in both groups ($P = 0.883$). For the horizontal movements of the apex, similar ($P = 0.750$) amounts of distal palatal root movement were observed in both groups (Table 2).

3.2 GCF study

GCF volume has been correlated with inflammatory state, however, there was no statistically significant difference in the mean as for the volume of GCF between CB group and SL group at T1 (CB: 0.41 ± 0.06 µl, SL: 0.39 ± 0.09 µl) and T2 (CB:0.40 ± 0.07 µl, SL: 0.42 ± 0.05 µl), respectively. In all of the patients, probing depths remained less than 2 mm and gingival health was excellent, with no gingival bleeding.
At T1, there were no significant differences in the mean RANKL value between the CB and the SL. However, the mean RANKL value in the CB was significantly higher in the SL at T2 ($p<0.05$). While, the mean OPG values for the CB and SL were not significantly difference between T1 and T2. (Fig. 2)

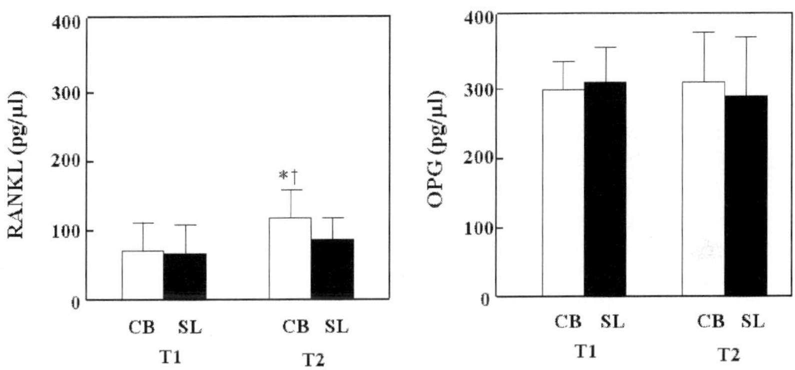

Fig. 2. Changes in RANKL and OPG concentrations in the GCF samples from the conventional brackets (CB) and self-ligating bracket (SL). Significant differences in concentrations between T1 and T2 are indicated with an * ($p < 0.05$) , and between CB and SL with an †($p < 0.05$), correspondingly.

4. Discussion

In this study, the mean amount of root resorption of the maxillary central incisor measured on the lateral cephalogram was significantly greater in the CB group than the SL group at T2 (Table 2).
Considering to risk factor of EARR, according to Weltman et al. (2010) it are divided into the treatment-related and patient-related factors. Orthodontic treatment-related risk factors

include treatment duration (Segal et al., 2004; Sameshima & Sinclair, 2004; Fox, 2005), magnitude of applied force (Harris et al., 2006; Chan & Darendeliler, 2006; Barbagallo et al., 2008), direction of tooth movement (Costopoulos & Nanda, 1996; Parker & Harris, 1998; Han et al., 2005), amount of apical displacement (Segal et al., 2004; Fox, 2005), and method of force application [continuous vs intermittent (Weiland, 2003; Brezniak & Wasserstein, 2002), type of appliance (Brezniak & Wasserstein, 1993; Pandis et al., 2008), and treatment technique (McNab et al., 2000; Scott et al., 2008).

Previous studies found that heavy forces produced significantly more EARR than light forces or controls (Harris et al., 2006; Chan & Darendeliler, 2006; Barbagallo et al., 2008). Chan and Darendeliler (2006) found that the mean volume of the resorption craters was 11.59 times greater in the heavy-force group than in the control group (significant). Heavy forces in both compression and tension areas produced significantly more RR than in regions under light compression and light tension forces. Barbagallo et al. (2008) also found that heavy force produced significantly more RR (9 times greater than the control) than light force (5 times greater than the control). Therefore, light force may have the advantage of prevention of occurrence of EARR.

According to Chen et al. (2010), the claim of reduced friction with self-ligating brackets is often cited as a primary advantage over conventional brackets (Damon, 1998b; Griffiths et al., 2005; Kim et al., 2008). This occurs because the usual steel or elastomeric ligatures are not necessary, and it is claimed that passive designs generate even less friction than active ones (Budd et al., 2008). Beger (1990) demonstrated that a significant decrease in the force level required for the self-ligating bracket when compared with elastomeric and steel-tie ligation in both metal and plastic bracket systems, and concluded that self-ligating bracket is less force needed to produce tooth movement by reduced friction (Beger, 1990).

During the process of root resorption, organic matrix proteins and cytokines are released into the gingival crevice. In this GCF study, the mean RANKL value in the CB was significantly higher in the SL at T2 ($p<0.05$) (Fig. 2). A recent study demonstrated that mRNA of RANK was detected in tissues involved in root resorption following subjection to orthodontic forces (Low et al., 2005). Furthermore, our laboratory reported that RANKL expression was increased by compression force *in vitro* and *in vivo*. Yamaguchi et al. (2006b) demonstrated that compressed PDL cells obtained from tissues with severe external apical root resorption may produce a large amount of RANKL and upregulate osteoclastogenesis *in vitro*. Nakano et al. (2011) observed RANKL immunoreactivity in rat odontoclasts with an orthodontic force of 50 g (heavy force) on day 7 *in vivo*. Nishijima et al. (2006) found an increased concentration of RANKL in GCF during orthodontic tooth movement, and the ratio of concentration of RANKL to that of OPG in the GCF was significantly higher than at the control sites. These studies suggest that during orthodontic tooth movement, OPG/RANKL/RANK system in the periodontal tissues is an important determinant regulating balanced alveolar bone resorption. Taken together, those findings and the present results, suggest that OPG/ RANKL/RANK system may play an important role in orthodontically root resorption. Furthermore, George and Evans (2009) demonstrated that the consentration of RANKL in GCF in severe and mild resorption were significant higher than that of no loss of root structure. Therefore, these findings and our present results, taken together, the self-ligating brackets may be a useful system for reduction of remarkable inflammation and EARR.

Despite claims regarding the clinical superiority of self-ligating brackets, evidence is generally lacking. Pandis et al (2008) and Scott et al. (2008) reported that there was no significant difference in EARR between CB and SL groups. Further studies should be carried out to investigate the advantage and disadvantage of self-ligating brackets in orthodontic treatment.

5. Conclusion

These results show that the mean amount of EARR and the GCF levels of RANKL were significant lower in the Damon 3 appliance than conventional brackets. Therefore, self-ligating brackets may be a useful system for reduction of remarkable inflammation and EARR.

6. Acknowledgements

This research was supported, in part, by a Grant-in-Aid for Scientific Research from the Japan Society for the Promotion of Science (C:22592297).

7. References

Barbagallo, L.J., Jones, A.S., Petocz, P. & Darendeliler, M.A. (2008). Physical properties of root cementum: Part 10. Comparison of the effects of invisible removable thermoplastic appliances with light and heavy orthodontic forces on premolar cementum. A microcomputed-tomography study. *Am J Orthod Dentofacial Orthop,* Vol.133, No.2, pp. 218-227, ISSN 0002-9416.

Berger, J.L. (1990). The influence of the SPEED bracket's self-ligating design on force levels in tooth movement: a comparative in vitro study. *Am J Orthod Dentofac Orthop,* Vol.97, No. 3, pp. 219-228, ISSN 0002-9416.

Brezniak, N. & Wasserstein, A. (1993). Root resorption after orthodontic treatment: Part 1. Literature review. *Am J Orthod Dentofacial Orthop,* Vol.103, No.1, pp. 62-66, ISSN 0002-9416.

Brezniak, N. & Wasserstein, A. (2002). Orthodontically induced inflammatory root resorption. Part II: The clinical aspects. *Angle Orthod,* Vol.72, No.2, pp.180-184, ISSN 0003-3219.

Brin, I. & Bollen, A.M. (2011). External apical root resorption in patients treated by serial extractions followed by mechanotherapy. *Am J Orthod Dentofacial Orthop.* Vol.139, No.2, e129-134, ISSN 0002-9416.

Budd, S., Daskalogiannakis, J. & Tompson B.D. (2008). A study of the frictional characteristics of four commercially available self-ligating bracket systems. *Eur J Orthod,* Vol.30, No.6, pp. 645-653, ISSN 0141-5387.

Chan, E. & Darendeliler, M.A. (2006). Physical properties of root cementum: part 7. Extent of root resorption under areas of compression and tension. *Am J Orthod Dentofacial Orthop,* Vol.129, No.4, pp. 504-510, ISSN 0002-9416.

Chen, S.S., Greenlee, G.M., Kim, J.E., Smith, C.L. & Huang, G.J. (2010). Systematic review of self-ligating brackets. *Am J Orthod Dentofacial Orthop,* Vol.137, No.6, 726.e1-726, ISSN 0002-9416.

Costopoulos, G. & Nanda, R. (1996). An evaluation of root resorption incident to orthodontic intrusion. *Am J Orthod Dentofacial Orthop,* Vol.109, No.5, pp. 543-548, ISSN 0002-9416.

Damon, D.H. (1998a). The Damon low-friction bracket: a biologically compatible straight-wire system. *J Clin Orthod,* Vol.32, No.11, pp. 670-680, ISSN 0889-5406.

Damon, D.H. (1998b). The rationale, evolution and clinical application of the self-ligating bracket. *Clin Orthod Res,* Vol.1, No.1, pp. 52-61, ISSN 1397-5927.

Fox, N. (2005). Longer orthodontic treatment may result in greater external apical root resorption. *Evid Based Dent,* Vol.6, No.1, pp. 21, ISSN 1532-3382.

George A, & Evans CA. (2009). Detection of root resorption using dentin and bone markers. *Orthod Craniofac Res,* 12(3), pp. 229-235, ISSN 1601-6335.

Griffiths, H.S., Sherriff, M. & Ireland, A.J. (2005). Resistance to sliding with 3 types of elastomeric modules. *Am J Orthod Dentofacial Orthop,* Vol.127, No.6, pp. 670-675, ISSN 0002-9416.

Han, G., Huang, S., Von den Hoff, J.W., Zeng, X. & Kuijpers-Jagtman, A.M. (2005). Root resorption after orthodontic intrusion and extrusion: an intraindividual study. *Angle Orthod,* Vol.75, No.6, pp. 912-918, ISSN 0003-3219.

Harris, D.A., Jones, A.S. & Darendeliler, M.A. (2006). Physical properties of root cementum: part 8. Volumetric analysis of root resorption craters after application of controlled intrusive light and heavy orthodontic forces: a microcomputed tomography scan study. *Am J Orthod Dentofacial Orthop,* Vol.130, No.5, pp. 639-647, ISSN 0002-9416.

Kim, T.K., Kim, K.D. & Baek, S.H. (2008). Comparison of frictional forces during the initial leveling stage in various combinations of self-ligating brackets and archwires with a custom-designed typodont system. *Am J Orthod Dentofacial Orthop,* Vol.133, No.2, 187.e15-24, ISSN 0002-9416.

Krishnan, V. & Davidovitch, Z. (2006). Cellular, molecular, and tissue-level reactions to orthodontic force. *Am J Orthod Dentofacial Orthop,* Vol.129, No.4, 469.e1-32, ISSN 0002-9416.

Lossdörfer, S., Götz, W. & Jäger, A. (2002). Immunohistochemical localization of receptor activator of nuclear factor kappaB (RANK) and its ligand (RANKL) in human deciduous teeth. *Calcif Tissue Int,* Vol.71, No.1, pp. 45-52, ISSN 0171-967X.

Low, E., Zoellner, H., Kharbanda, O.P. & Darendeliler, M.A. (2005). Expression of mRNA for osteoprotegerin and receptor activator of nuclear factor kappa beta ligand (RANKL) during root resorption induced by the application of heavy orthodontic forces on rat molars. *Am J Orthod Dentofacial Orthop,* Vol.128, No.4, pp. 497-503, ISSN 0002-9416.

McNab, S., Battistutta, D., Taverne, A. & Symons, A.L. (2000). External apical root resorption following orthodontic treatment. *Angle Orthod,* Vol.70, No.3, pp. 227-232, ISSN 0003-3219.

Meikle, M.C. (2006). The tissue, cellular, and molecular regulation of orthodontic tooth movement: 100 years after Carl Sandstedt. *Eur J Orthod,* Vol.28, No.3, pp. 221-240, ISSN 0141-5387.

Nakano, Y., Yamaguchi, M., Fujita, S., Asano, M., Saito, K. & Kasai, K. (2011). Expressions of RANKL/RANK and M-CSF/c-fms in root resorption lacunae in rat molar by heavy orthodontic force. *Eur J Orthod,* in press, ISSN 0141-5387.

Nishijima, Y., Yamaguchi, M., Kojima, T., Aihara, N., Nakajima, R. & Kasai K. (2006). Levels of RANKL and OPG in gingival crevicular fluid during orthodontic tooth movement and effect of compression force on releases from periodontal ligament cells in vitro. Orthod Craniofac Res, Vol.9, No,2, pp. 63-70, ISSN 1601-6335.

Pandis, N., Nasika, M., Polychronopoulou, A. & Eliades, T. (2008). External apical root resorption in patients treated with conventional and self-ligating brackets. *Am J Orthod Dentofacial Orthop,* Vol.134, No.5, 646-651, ISSN 0002-9416.

Parker, R.J. & Harris, E.F. (1998). Directions of orthodontic tooth movements associated with external apical root resorption of the maxillary central incisor. *Am J Orthod Dentofacial Orthop,* Vol.114, No.6, pp. 677-683, ISSN 0002-9416.

Sameshima, G.T. & Sinclair, P.M. (2004). Characteristics of patients with severe root resorption. *Orthod Craniofac Res,* Vol.7, No.2, pp. 108-114, ISSN 1601-6335.

Scott, P., DiBiase, A.T., Sherriff, M. & Cobourne, M.T. (2008). Alignment efficiency of Damon3 self-ligating and conventional orthodontic bracket systems: a randomized clinical trial. *Am J Orthod Dentofacial Orthop,* Vol.134, No.4, 470.e1-8, ISSN 0002-9416.

Segal, G.R., Schiffman, P.H. & Tuncay, O.C. (2004). Meta analysis of the treatment-related factors of external apical root resorption. *Orthod Craniofac Res,* Vol.7, No.2, pp. 71-78, ISSN 1601-6335.

Shiotani, A., Shibasaki, Y. & Sasaki, T. (2001). Localization of receptor activator of NF-kappaB ligand, RANKL, in periodontal tissues during experimental movement of rat molars. *J Electron Microsc (Tokyo),* Vol.50, No.4, pp. 365-369, ISSN 0022-0744.

Sims, A.P., Waters, N.E., Birnie, D.J. & Pethybridge, R.J. (1993). A comparison of the forces required to produce tooth movement in vitro using two self-ligating brackets and a pre-adjusted bracket employing two types of ligation. *Eur J Orthod,* Vol.15, No.5, pp. 377-385, ISSN 0141-5387.

Weiland, F. (2003). Constant versus dissipating forces in orthodontics: the effect on initial tooth movement and root resorption. *Eur J Orthod,* Vol.25, No.4, pp. 335-342, ISSN 0141-5387.

Weltman, B., Vig, K.W., Fields, H.W., Shanker, S. & Kaizar, E.E. (2010). Root resorption associated with orthodontic tooth movement: a systematic review. *Am J Orthod Dentofacial Orthop,* Vo.137, No.4, pp. 462-476, ISSN 0002-9416.

Yamaguchi, M., Yoshii, M. & Kasai, K. (2006a). Relationship between substance P and interleukin-1beta in gingival crevicular fluid during orthodontic tooth movement in adults. *Eur J Orthod,* Vol.28, No.3, pp. 241-246, ISSN 0141-5387.

Yamaguchi, M., Aihara, N., Kojima, T. & Kasai, K. (2006b). RANKL increase in compressed periodontal ligament cells from root resorption. *J Dent Res,* Vol.85, No.8, 751-756, ISSN 0022-0345.

Yamaguchi, M., Takizawa, T., Nakajima, R., Imamura, R. & Kasai, K. (2009). The damon system and release of substance p in gingival crevicular fluid during orthodontic tooth movement in adults. *World J Orthod*, Vol.10, No.2, pp.141-146, ISSN 1530-5678.

Zhang, D., Goetz., W, Braumann, B., Bourauel, C. & Jaeger, A. (2003). Effect of soluble receptors to interleukin-1 and tumor necrosis factor alpha on experimentally induced root resorption in rats. *J Periodont Res*, Vol.38, No.3, pp. 324-332, ISSN 0022-3484.

Part 2

Technique

4

Treatment of Class II Deep Overbite with Multiloop Edgewise Arch-Wire (MEAW) Therapy

Paulo Beltrão
French Board Of Orthodontics
Portugal

1. Introduction

The deepbite occlusion together with a deepbite skeletal pattern is difficult to treat, and the time needed for treatment is long because of patient`s strong muscle pattern.

Apart from genetic factors some of the reasons for the frequent appearance of class II anomalies of the bone structure are mouth breathing and muscular malfunctioning in the environment of the oral cavity. However, 3 factors of class II are likely to be the most important ones associated with the adaptation of the mandible and the occlusal function. The 3 factors are:

1. Insufficient height of bite
2. Strong inclination of the occlusal plane
3. Lacking of occlusal support and pressure of mandibular joint

The upper dentition of people who have class II malocclusion have insufficient vertical dimension on the molar area and steepening of the upper posterior occlusal plane. Due to these occlusal interferences in the molar area, the mandible cannot adapt anteriorly. Instead, it adapts posteriorly, aggravating the distocclusion. The loss of the posterior support causes the condyle to be compressed and decreasing or suppressing condylar growth.

Sassouni and Nanda (1964) proved the vertical disproportion were, in many cases, at the origin of anteroposterior dysplasias. Therefore, treatment strategies should focus on vertical control in order to correct anteroposterior disharmony.

Actually, 70% of the class II malocclusion does not imply the protrusion of the maxilla but it is known to be caused by retrusion of the mandible (McNamara 1982).

Mandibular growth is possible by allowing the functional anterior adaptation of the mandible (Carlson 1985, Moss 1971, McNamara 1979 and 1987).

Morphological characteristics of the class II deep overbite are: the mandible is small and retruded; small vertical dimension and insufficient occlusal support; accentuated curved of spee with two occlusal plane (flat occlusal plane in the upper anterior area and steepening of the occlusal plane in the upper posterior area); occlusal interference in the molar area, labial tipping of the upper anterior tooth; functional failure due to poor anterior guidance. The skeletal feature of the class II deep overbite malocclusions are closely related to the deviation in the vertical aspect of the occlusion. According to this, correcting the occlusal plane by controlling the vertical dimension is extremely important in the treatment of class II deepbite malocclusion. The treatment's purposes for class II deepbite are: Eliminate pernicious habits and respiratory problems; Increase the vertical dimension (upper and lower molar eruption); To rebuild and flatten the upper posterior occlusal plane; Eliminate the discrepancy in the upper and lower dental arch width; Reposition the mandible forward; Improve overbite (deepbite) and obtain an appropriate occlusal and anterior guidance; Obtain normal intercuspidation and acquire an excellent profile.

The treatment of low-angle class II malocclusions must prevent occlusal interference and extrude the upper molars to increase their vertical height and flatten the occlusal plane. The lower dentition, especially the premolars are extruded to increase vertical height and to reduce the excessive curve of spee. As result, the mandible readapts to the physiological position and the occlusal function is restored. This kind of treatment will help to overcome many of the existing problems when we treat class II malocclusion in non-growing patients and provide the means to establishing functional occlusion in cases that are difficult to treat.

The steps of the class II deep overbite malocclusion are: Levelling; Eliminate of occlusal interference; Establishing mandibular position; Reconstruction of the occlusal plane; Achieving a physiological occlusion.

2. The multiloop edgewise arch wire (MEAW)

The MEAW was developed in 1967 by Young H. KIM as a mean for correcting marked open bite malocclusion and has been found to be extremely effective.

Further development of MEAW Technique extends its applications to treat any type of malocclusion, especially during the final stage of the treatment.

The MEAW's are constructed with .016x.022 stainless steel (bracket 0.018 - inch slot) or .017x.025 ss (bracket 0.022 – inch slot).

The arches have ideal arch form with five loops on each side of the arch.

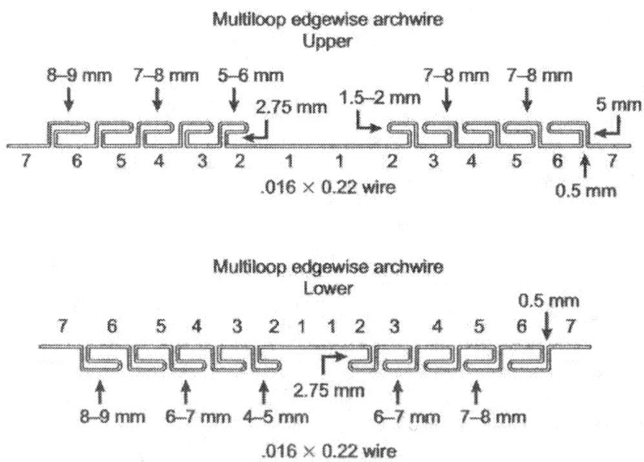

Fig. 1. Upper and lower multiloop edgewise archwire (MEAWs)

2.1 Functions of the loops on each side of the archwire

a. The loops between the teeth reduce the load deflection rate (LDR) of the wire significantly, providing a low but continuous orthodontic force of the teeth. The relative

LDR of the MEAW compared to a stainless steel wire without loops is 40%, 32% for TMA, 28% for sentalloy and 20% for nitinol.

b. The horizontal loop allows an easier control of movement for each tooth.
c. The vertical component serves as a "breaker" between the teeth and allows teeth to move independently.
d. Makes the alignment and intrusion of the supra erupted tooth as well as the torque adjustment easy.
e. The tip back activation in the posterior segment of the wire produces the uprighting of the posterior teeth. Fifteen degrees of molar uprighting produce as much as 4,5mm of distalization of the teeth.
f. With the aid of the elastics, it can reconstruct the occlusal plane.

An experimental study developed by Lee and Co-Workers (1995) of Seoul National University using the MEAW on Rhesus monkeys showed that marked tooth movement occurred along with considerable bone remodelling cellular activity, while on a control group of monkeys with a standard ideal arch-wire of the same size showed insignificant cellular activity with signs of root resorption.

To create an ideal arch with multiloops extended from the distal of lateral incisors to mesial of second molars, the ideal arch wire length is 2,5 - 3 x the length of the usual arch wire. This would decrease the orthodontic force by 1/5 and at the same time continuously applies an orthodontic force to the teeth. Activation of the wire involves the incorporation of progressive reverse curve onto the arch wire (second order bend). The tip back activation creates side effects; which must be counteracted by adding progressive buccal root torque and toe in. To incorporate the torque in upper arch, it is necessary to grab the wire at the distal portion of the canine with KIM plier and tilt the second loop 3 degrees laterally. It is necessary to do the same for the third, the fourth and the fifth loop to provide a gradual torque and to keep the loops away from the gingival tissue.

The progressive buccal root torque (third order bend) and the toe in (first order bend) are important to counteract the side effects of the tip back activation.

The tip back activation produces an intrusive force which is buccal of the centre of resistance of the posterior teeth and can create flaring of the posterior teeth and deformation of the arch wire. The use of vertical short class II elastics is necessary to produce the desired vertical and distal movement of the tooth segment in order to rebuild the occlusal plane and the sagittal relationship of the dentition. Since the wire is a relatively soft stainless steel , it should be heat treated, approximately at 500°, with the use of an electro-polishing treatment (to increase the resiliency), before the MEAW being inserted into the patient's mouth.

In the absence of a furnace, an alcohol lamp can be used. Heat the wire until the colour changes to golden brown. The colour must be even.

3. Cephalometric analysis

KIM'S METHOD ANALYSIS

- ODI (overbite depth indicator)
- APDI (anteroposterior dysplasia indicator)
- CF (combination factor)

3.1 ODI- Overbite depth indicator

In 1978 Dr. KIM after studying cephalograms of 119 patients with normal occlusion and 500 various malocclusions, he selected fifteens cephalometric measurements to determine which

produced the highest correlation with the incisal overbite depth. The ODI is a combined measurement of two angles: the A-B plane to the mandibular plane (MP) and the palatal plane(PP) to the Frankfort horizontal (FH) plane. When the palatal plane slopes upward and forward in relation to the FH plane, it is read as a negative angle and this value is subtracted from the A-B to the mandibular plane angle.
When the palatal plane slopes downward and forward in relation to the FH plane, it is read as a positive angle and this value is added to the A-B to the mandibular plane angle. There is a norm of 74.5 degrees and with a standard deviation of 6.07. A value of 68° or less indicates a skeletal openbite tendency. A value of 80° or more indicates a deepbite skeletal pattern, and extraction of permanent teeth should be avoided, if possible, due to the strong potential to deepbite relapse. This skeletal pattern needs as much dental support as possible.

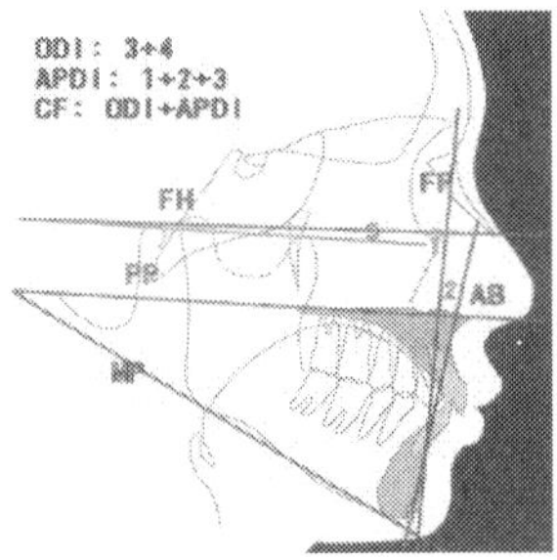

Fig. 2. Kim analysis (4-MP-AB angle)

3.2 APDI-anteroposterior dysplasia index

The APDI is determined from three angles: the facial plane angle (HF/FP (Na-Pog)), plus or minus the A-B plane angle (Downs), and plus or minus the palatal plane angle in relation to the FH plane, which is geometrically equivalent to the PP-AB.
PP-AB is apparently the antero-posterior relationship of the maxillary and mandible.
The normal mean of the APDI is 81, 4 degrees. The smaller the APDI value becomes in relation to the normal mean (81.4 degrees) the greater the probability of a distocclusion exists. Conversely, as the APDI value increases above the normal mean, the greater the probability of a mesiocclusion being present. The APDI is a measure of skeletal class II or III tendency, and reflects the horizontal discrepancies of a malocclusion.
The APDI reflects the treatment potential of a patient, because the APDI can be changed by growth and treatment. According to Kim (Kim and Vietas, 1978) APDI must be near 81° at the end of treatment, unless a strong relapse tendency will be present.

3.3 Combination factor

The combination factor (CF) is a combination of ODI and APDI.
A high CF (>155°) indicates a tendency for low angle and a skeletal pattern that has the potential to accommodate all of the teeth.
A low CF (<155°) shows the tendency for high angle and the need for tooth extraction is higher.
When the CF falls below 150° that indicates the teeth cannot be retracted due to a lack of posterior vertical space and indicates that extraction of some teeth is probable.

The CF factor indicates if a patient has the potential to be treated with an extraction or non-extraction protocol.

4. The dynamic mechanism of the skeleton and the growth of the maxilla

The craniofacial bones are joined together by sutures or synchondrosis. These sutures allow slight relative movements.

The sphenoid is the principal central bone of the cranial base and makes the synchondrosis ethmosphenoidal with the ethmoid (fuses at 7-8 years old) and synchondrosis spheno occipital (fuses in late puberty 18-20 years old) with the occipital.

According to Hooper (1986) the sphenobasilar articulation is the most important among the cranial bones and it is where the movement of flexion-extension occurs.

The degree of basicranial flexion differs in the various types of malocclusion. The cranial base angles (Na-S-Ar) comes to approximately 124,2 ± 5,2 in class I patterns.

From this average value a more obtuse (extension) angle indicates skeletal Class II and a more acute (flexion) angle means skeletal Class III.The rotating movement of the cranialbase (flexion/extension) occurs at the spheno-occipital articulation and it is transmitted to the maxilla through the Vomer. This dynamic mechanism has a great influence on the growth pattern of an individual during the growth period.

When the sphenoid makes flexion the rotating force of the vomer is posteroinferior and the maxilla is strongly pushed inferiorly. This causes vertical elongation of the maxillary complex, short antero posterior dimension and posterior crowding. This is related to the development of a class III skeletal frame (Sato 2001).

When the rotating movement of the sphenoid is extension the vomer will rotate anteriorly and the maxilla will be strongly pushed anteriorly. This movement of the maxilla causes anterosuperior tipping of the palatal surface and labial tipping in the anterior teeth, long anteroposterior dimension due growth of the posterior area of the maxillary tuberosity . This creates space for the downward movement of the tooth buds and eliminates the posterior crowding. This is typically seen in the development of Class II skeletal frame (Sato 2001).

According to precious et al (1987) there are three types of maxillary growth and each growth pattern is closely related to the development of malocclusion: 1) translation with the frontal bone; 2) vertical elongation and 3) anterior rotation, which both advances and elongates the inferior part of the maxilla.

The maxillary also laterally rotates (internal and external rotation). In the internal rotation, the incisive bone is pushed forward because the length of the dental arch is increased and the width is decreased. This results in a deep palate typical of the Class II division malocclusion.

External rotation of the maxilla decreases the length and increases the width of the dental arch and creates a shallow palate. This is typical in class III malocclusion.

5. Occlusal function and mandibular growth

In the 1970's several studies (Petrovic, Carlson, McNamara, Woodside) showed the possibility of modifying the mandibular growth pattern if it was related with its function - Mc Namara, Graber, Harvold, Bass (1970's) showed that the amount of mandibular growth changes due to cell proliferation in the condyles was related to occlusal function changes.

Petrovic (1975) created his cybernetic model of mandibular growth with the concept of Moss's functional Matrix Theory as its basis. The most important aspect in the cybernetic model was that occlusal function was an important factor in mandibular growth. According to him the maxillary antero inferior growth functionally "shifts" the mandibula and the TMJ adapts to the new position by secondary growth of the condyles.

In the pubertal and post pubertal period the principal factor that influences the skeletal craniofacial growth is the occlusal function, rather than the heredity. According to this, it's important to improve the occlusal function to prevent the abnormal growth.

Therefore, the early orthodontic treatment is important to take advantage of the benefits of the period of growth, in order to obtain the harmony of maxilla facial skeleton growth.

6. Relation of the vertical dimension with mandibular growth

The increase in the vertical dimension and mandibular growth are closely related. When there is an increase or decrease in vertical dimension, the mandible adapts through functional displacement. If the functional displacement is persistent the TMJ adapts by secondary growth of the condyle and produces a displacement of the skeletal morphology.

Shudy (1964) reported the relationship of the vertical growth of the craniofacial skeleton and mandibular rotation.

When the increase of the vertical dimension is bigger than the growth of condyle the result is backward rotation of the mandible and anterior openbite. When the increase of the vertical dimension is lesser than the growth of the condyle, the result is forward rotation of the mandible and anterior deepbite.

7. The development process of skeletal class II low angle malocclusion

The craniofacial skeleton is a dynamic mechanism.

The functional force due to mandibular function like mastication, swallowing etc...is transmitted by the neuromuscular system and temporomandibular joint (TMJ) to the temporal bone. The temporal bone reacts with internal or external rotation and affects the rotating movement of the sphenotemporal articulation and the temporal-occipital articulation. The rotation movement of the sphenoid is transmitted through the Vomer to the maxillary and then the mandible will functionally adapts to the upper occlusal surface.

The whole facial bone is secondarily affected once the mandibular movement is transmitted to the temporal bone.

This produces a cycle (feedback regulatory mechanism).

When the degree of the cranial base is extension, the sphenoid bone through the vomer will strongly push the maxilla protrusively. The protrusive rotation of the maxilla will stimulate the anteroposterior growth of the maxilla.

The growth in the tuberosity area allows the elimination of the posterior discrepancy. According to this the maxilla has a good anteroposterior growth and a feeble vertical growth. The protrusive rotation of the maxilla secondarily produces the labial tipping of the maxillary anterior teeth axis and space between them (typical in class II division one malocclusion).

The consequence of a poor maxillary vertical height is:

- Insufficient height of bite
- Lacking of occlusal support

- Strong inclination of the posterior occlusal plane

The inclination of the upper occlusal plane is determined by:

a. Growth and rotation of the sphenoid and maxillary bone
b. Vertical growth of the maxillary alveolar bone (Hyun-Sook Kim 2004)

A lesser increase in vertical dimension than the growth of the mandibular ramus results in anterior rotation of the mandible (increasing the deepbite). In this condition, the posterior occlusal plane of the maxilla always shows a strong tipping and the mandible usually adapts posteriorly aggravating the distocclusion.

The mandibular distocclusion increases the pressure in the TMJ and decreases the condylar growth. The occlusion consequently becomes deep, increases the occlusal force and the pressure to the temporal bone increases too.

The temporal bone reacts with internal rotation, which increases the extension of the neurocranial base. The treatment objective of class II deepbite is to break this vicious cycle, rebuilding the occlusal plane.

8. General characterization of low angle class II malocclusion

McNamara and Moyers et al have suggested that the fundamental problems in the balance of craniofacial skeletal structures in class II malocclusion are due to mandibular retrognatism rather than maxillary prognathism.

The skeletal features of class II malocclusion are not characterized by overgrowth of the maxilla, but rather by restrained growth of the mandible.

The mandible is small with short corpus length and retruded, accentuated curve of spee with two occlusal planes (flat occlusal plane in the upper anterior area and steep occlusal plane in the upper posterior area), occlusal interference in the molar area, labial tipping of the upper anterior teeth, lip incompetence, small vertical dimension and insufficient occlusal support , insufficient eruption of the molar teeth (infraeruption), anterior inclination of the condyle (class II high angle has posterior inclination of the condyle), deep overbite; small gonial angle (GOA), small LFH(lower facial height).

Sadao Sato et al in a study (2004) about morphological characterization of different types of class II malocclusion, selected three groups of twenty adults in each group (10 males and 10 females). One group with normal occlusion and no missing teeth and two other groups of untreated high and low angle class II malocclusion subjects.

The results of skeletal features of the low angle class II groups were: LFH (lower facial height), gonial angle (GOA) and APDI were significantly smaller than those of the normal group. The ODI (overbite depth indicator) were significantly larger than the same measures in the normal group and the high angle class II group.

The corpus length were significantly smaller than those of the normal group, indicating that small and retruded mandibles are typical of class II group (high-angle and low-angle). The condylar axis in the low-angle class II group was inclined upward from back to front.

The anterior and posterior cranial base length were both long and the cranial angle base was long (extension) too. The morphology of pterygopalatine fosse was curve, the floor of maxillary sinus was high, the floor of nasal cavity was flat, the palatal plane (PP) had posterior tipping, the anteroposterior dimension of maxilla was long, and steepening of the posterior occlusal plane.

The results of dental pattern of the low angle class II group were: the vertical height of every upper teeth were significantly smaller than those of the normal group and the vertical

height of incisors canines and premolars were significantly smaller than those of the high angle class II group.
The values of vertical height of the lower teeth of the low angle class II were: short vertical height of incisors, canines and premolars, especially the first premolar, were always short and it causes an excessive curve of spee.
The skeletal features of the class II malocclusion are closely related to the deviation in the vertical aspect of the occlusion.
In the treatment of class II malocclusion the correction of the occlusal plane by controlling the vertical dimension is very important.

9. Treatment of class II low angle based on the dynamics of the craniofacial skeleton

The skeletal features of class II malocclusion are closely related to the handicaps in the vertical aspect of the occlusion.
FUSHIMA el AL (1989) measured the vertical height of posterior teeth in subjects with mandibular asymmetry. He found that the vertical height of posterior teeth on the side toward which the mandible had shifted was lower than the contralateral dental height.
The treatment of low angle class II malocclusion must prevent occlusal interferences and extrude upper molars to increase the vertical dimension and flatten the occlusal plane. Once vertical dimension changes the mandible adapts through functional displacement.
According to Dawson (1989) the inclination of the occlusal plane must match the anteroposterior inclination of the condylar trajectory and the guidance of lingual concavity of the upper incisors.
The lower dentition, especially the premolars are extruded to increase the vertical dimension and to level the curve of spee. As a result, the mandible moves forward to the physiological position and the occlusal function is improved.
The advancement of the mandible followed by condylar growth and adaptive remodelling of the TMJ are desirable in order to improve the profile. This kind of treatment is very useful when we treat non-growing patients with class II low angle malocclusion.
However, it is very important to treat the patients during the period of good growth and development to increase the results. According to this, we use a double arch wire (DAW) to control the vertical dimension from the mixed dentition period to the permanent dentition.

9.1 The treatment goals for class II deepbite are

- Elimination of the pernicious habits and respiratory problems
- Increase vertical dimension
- Rebuild and flatten the upper posterior occlusal plane
- Eliminate the discrepancy in upper and lower dental arch width
- Reposition the mandible forward in a physiological position
- Inhibition of the VICIOUS CYCLE
- Improve overbite (deepbite)
- Obtain normal intercuspidation and excellent profile

9.2 The treatment steps of class II deepbite malocclusion are

1. Levelling;
2. Elimination of occlusal interferences;

3. Establishing mandibular position;
4. Reconstruction of the occlusal plane;
5. Achieving a physiological occlusion .

9.2.1 The first step is the leveling (0.016 round wire SS) to start the correction of the mandibular curve of spee.

9.2.2 Elimination of occlusal interferences (cuspal and occlusal interferences) with 017x.025 MEAWS arch wire (bracket with slot 0.022 inch) step down bend (premolars) for maxillary bite rising and step up bend (premolars) for mandibular bite rising, with reverse curve in the mandible. The reverse curve in the mandibular arch wire is to eliminate the posterior molar interference with the alignment of lower second molar.

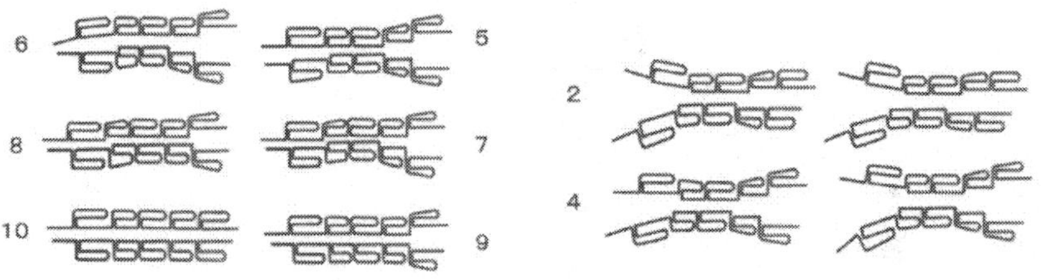

Fig. 3. Sequence of class II deep bite treatment

Case report 1

Patient male 13 years old and 5 months of age, with skeletal class II and dental class II/1 on a hypodivergent face pattern, mandibular retrognathism, deepbite (10mm), overjet (12mm), curve of spee deep with steep occlusal plane in the molar area producing interference in the posterior area, insufficient occlusal support due to absence of 46 and 36.The patient began the treatment with 13years old and 5 months and the duration of the treatment was 27 months. The type of appliance was a edgewise multi-bracket 0,022x0,028 slot, 0° torque, 0° angulation, high pull head gear (HPHG) and MEAWs arch wires. The appliance was removed in July 2008 (15Y+9M).

The purpose of this treatment for this patient with class II deepite malocclusion was the elimination of the posterior interference and bite raising to produce anterior adaptation of the mandible and secondarily to induce mandibular growth.

The steps of the treatment:

a-Leveling; b-Elimination of occlusal interferences ; c-Establishing mandibular position ;

d- Reconstruction of the occlusal plane; e- Achieving a physiological occlusion.

Step one - Leveling (alignment, mesialization of 47 e 37, use of HPHG with j hooks with application point in the anterior zone (to produce intrusion of the upper incisors), upper arch 0,017x0,025 ss, 0.016 ss lower arch followed by 0.018x0,025 ss with "shoe horn" to mesialize 37 and 47.

Step two - Elimination of occlusal interferences, use of the same lower arch and 0,017x0,025 multiloop edgewise arch wire (MEAW) in the maxillary, use of short class II ,3/16 inch, 6oz elastics on both side and the HPHG was discontinued.

Step three - Establishing mandibular position: the space in the mandible was closed and step down bend (in the premolars) was done in the upper MEAW to bite rising (use of short class II 3/16 inch, 6oz elastics). Step up bend in the lower arch was done. At the end of this phase the molar occlusion was in class one.

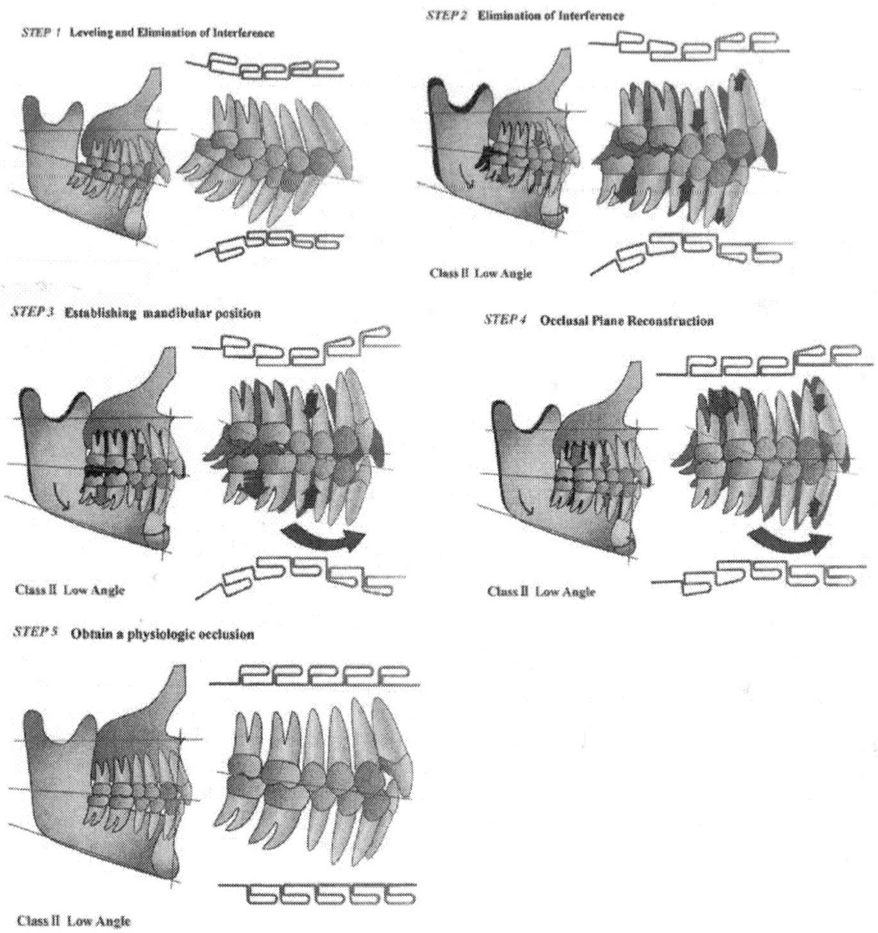

Fig. 4. Sequence of class II deep bite treatment (Sato 2008)

Step four/five - Reconstruction of the occlusal plane and achieving a physiological occlusion: flatten the occlusal plane in the molar area - "artistics bends" in the anterior upper area.

The retention phase was done with maxillary Hawley plate for night time use (6months) and bonded lingual wire from 33 to 43.

Post-treatment results show a well balanced face, nice profile and a pleasant smile. The intra-oral photo show a good class I relationship, overbite and overjet have been corrected. The mandibular superposition shows a slight protusion of the lower incisors. The APDI of 81° is a guarantee of stability.

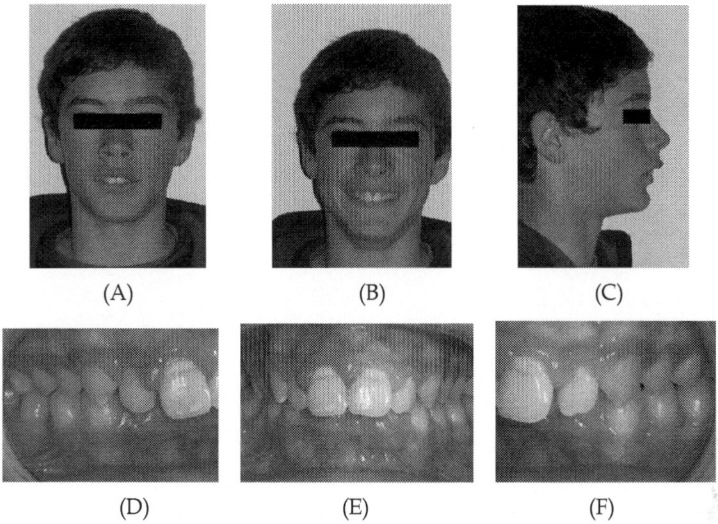

Fig. 5. Pre-treatment extraoral (A - B) and intraoral (D - F) photographs

	Range	Beginning	End of treatment	End of retention
FMIA	67°+- 3	65	60	61
FMA	25°+- 3	20	21	21
IMPA	88°+- 3	95	99	98
SNA	82°+- 2	78	76	76
SNB	80°+- 2	70	73	73
ANB	2°-+ 2	8	3	3
Ao-Bo	2mm	8mm	4mm	4mm
OP	10°-14°	7	4	4
Z	75°+-5	67	74	74
PFH	45mm	46	52	52
AFH	65mm	66	75	75
INDEX	0,69	0,69	0,69	0,69

Table 1. Cephalometric analysis (Tweed- Merrifield)

<table>
<tr><th></th><th colspan="2">Beginning</th><th colspan="2">End of treatment</th><th colspan="2">End of retention</th></tr>
<tr><td rowspan="2">ODI</td><td>MP/AB 87</td><td rowspan="2">84</td><td>78</td><td rowspan="2">77</td><td>80</td><td rowspan="2">79</td></tr>
<tr><td>FH/PP -3</td><td>-1</td><td>-1</td></tr>
<tr><td rowspan="3">APDI</td><td>HF/FP 88</td><td rowspan="3">70</td><td>90</td><td rowspan="3">81</td><td>90</td><td rowspan="3">80</td></tr>
<tr><td>FP/AB -15</td><td>-8</td><td>-9</td></tr>
<tr><td>HF/PP -3</td><td>-1</td><td>-1</td></tr>
<tr><td>CF</td><td>ODI+APDI</td><td>154</td><td></td><td>158</td><td></td><td>159</td></tr>
</table>

Table 2. Cephalometric analysis (Kim

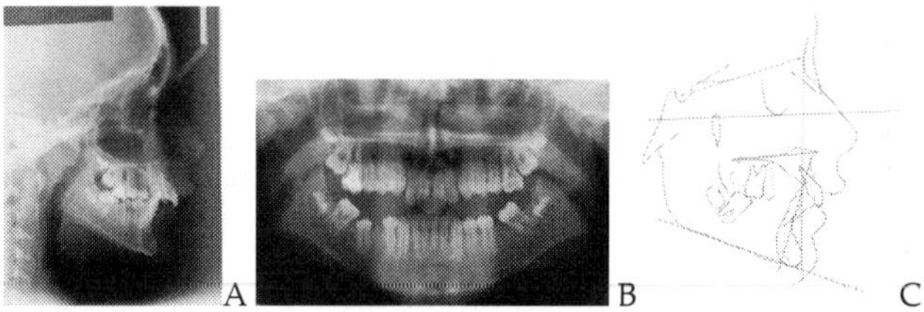

Fig. 6. Pre-treatment records

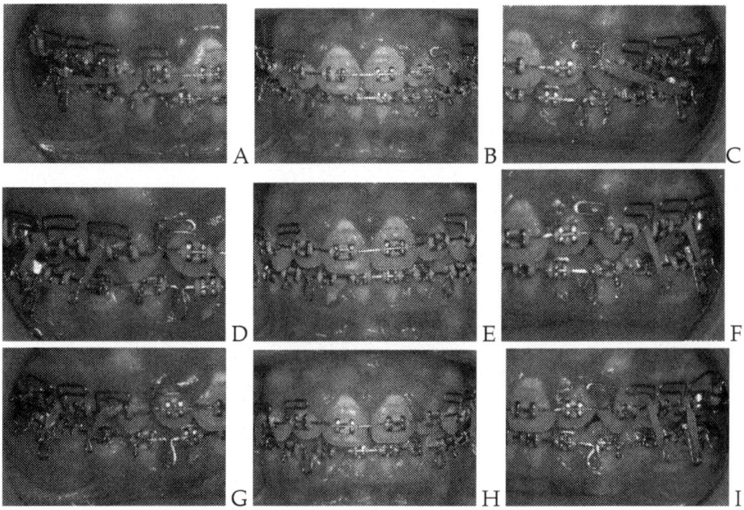

Fig. 7. Photos during the treatment (A -I)

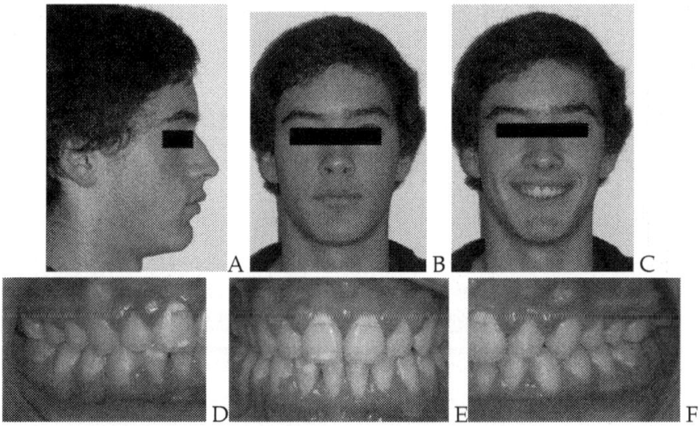

Fig. 8. Post-treatment extraoral (A-C) and intraoral (D-F) photos

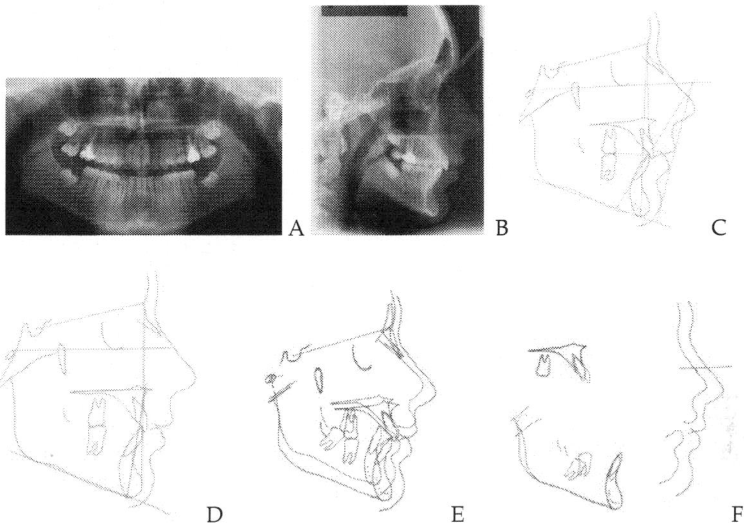

Fig. 9. Post-treatment records (A-D),superimpositions (E-F)

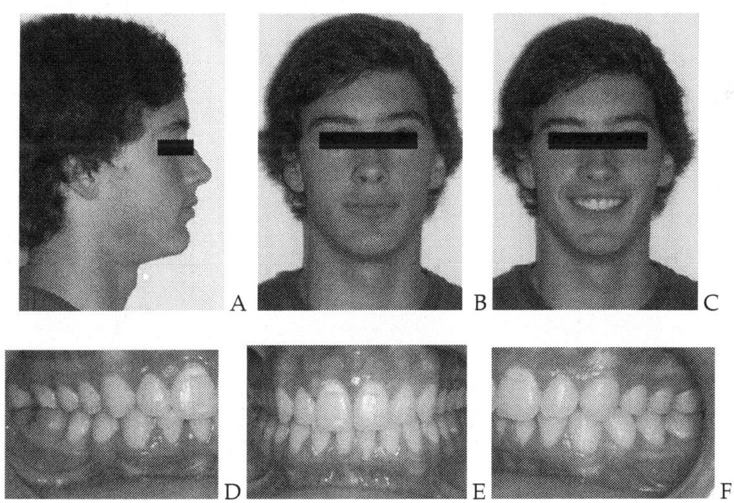

Fig. 10. Post-retention extra oral photos (A - C) and intraoral photos (D-F)

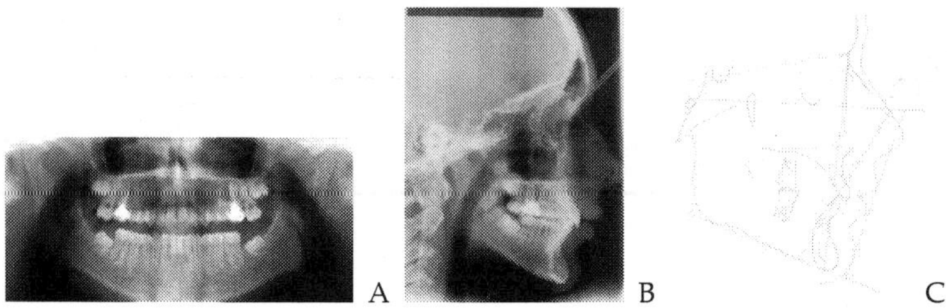

Fig. 11. Post-retention records (A - C)

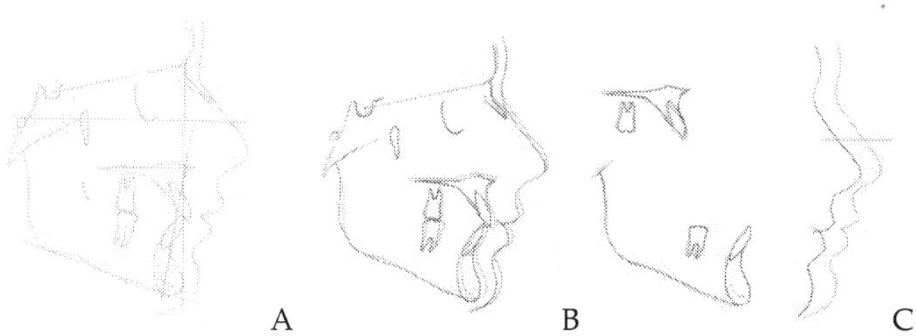

Fig. 12. Superimpositions (A- C)

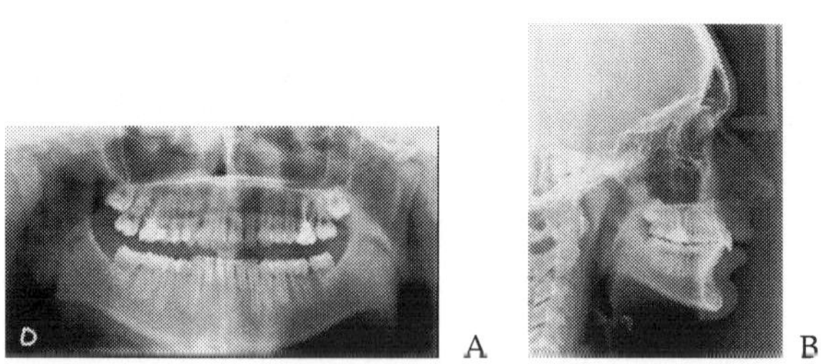

Fig. 13. 30 months post-treatment radiographs

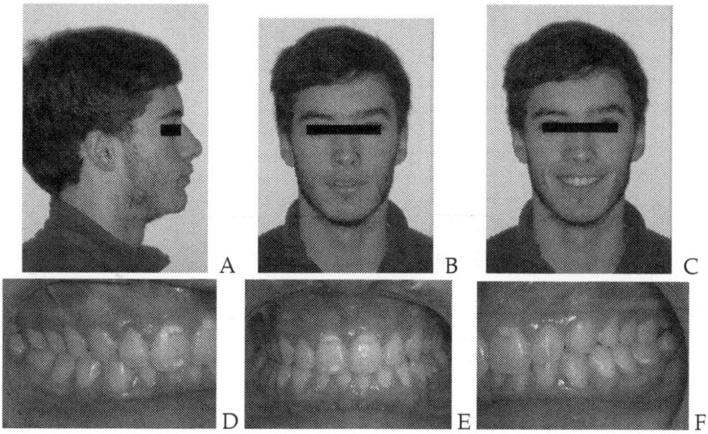

Fig. 14. 30 months post-treatment extraoral (A-B-C) and intraoral (D-E-F) photos

Case Report 2

Patient male (13 years old/10 months), short anterior facial height with skeletal class II and dental class II/1 on a hypodivergent face pattern, mandibular retrognathism, deep bite (7mm); overjet (10mm), curve of spee with steep occlusal plane in the molar area producing

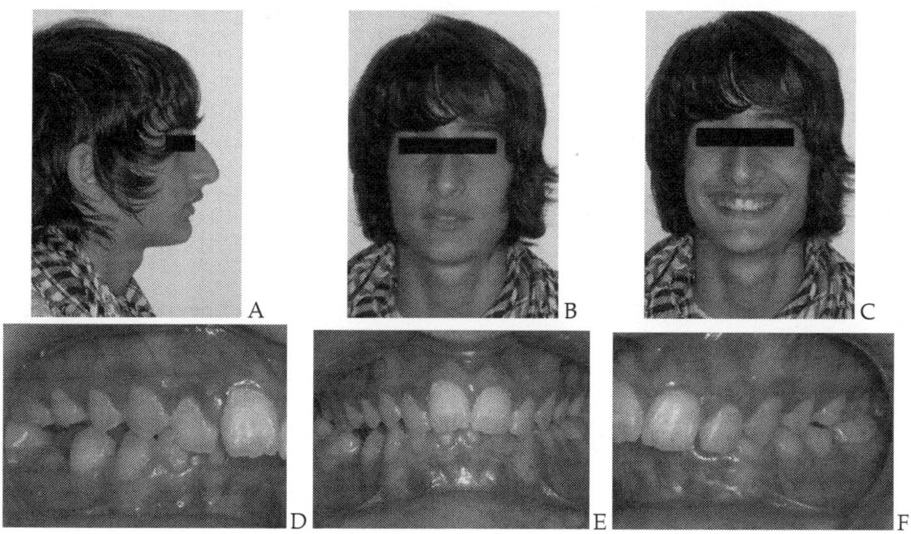

Fig. 15. Pre-treatment extraoral A-B-C) and intraoral (D-E-F) photos

Interference in the posterior area, insufficient occlusal support.
The z angle of 66° confirms an unbalanced face which is based on a retrognathic chin. There is no crowding. Arches forms are different because of an old habit of thumb sucking.

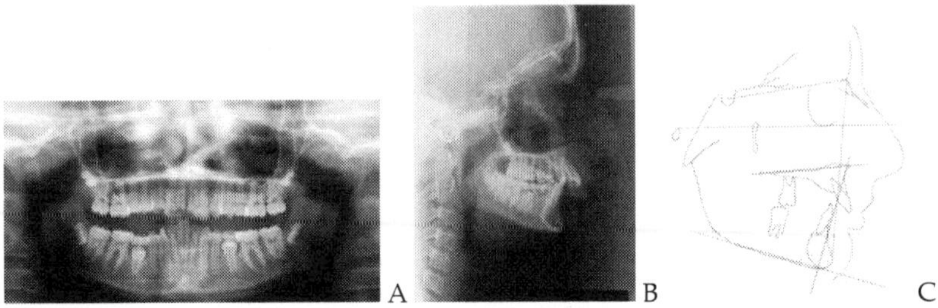

Fig. 16. Pre-treatment records (A-C)

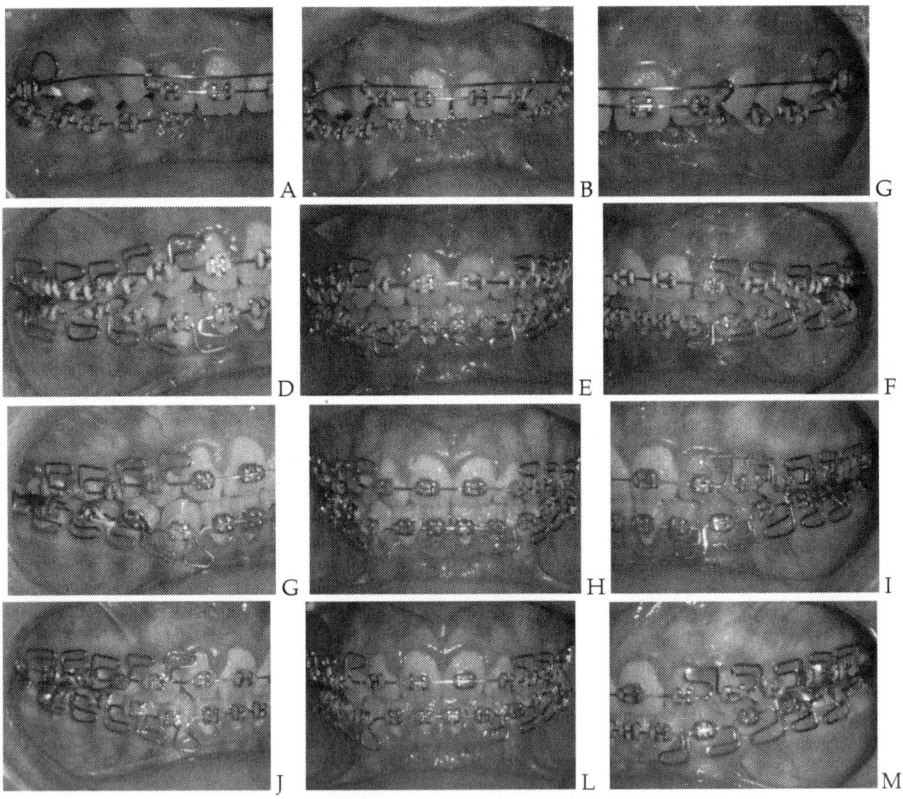

Fig. 17. Photos during the treatment.(A-C) after two months of treatment DAW(double arch wire) was inserted and was kept for five months. (D-F) twelve months of treatment (five months with MEAW upper and lower and short class II elastics (6 oz, 3/16 inch)). (G-I) 18 months of treatment.(J-M) 22 months of treatment

According to Kym's analysis, the ODI (86°) indicates a deepbite skeletal pattern and extraction of permanent teeth should be avoided if possible, due to the strong potential for deepbite relapse. The APDI (70°).indicates a class II skeletal pattern and the CF (combination factor of 156) indicates a skeletal pattern with potential to accommodate all the teeth.
Treatment began with age (13/7), after 2 months a DAW (double arch wire) was inserted to erupt upper molars and alignment, intrusion of the upper anterior teeth.
After 5 months, the use of MEAW and short class II elastics (3/16 inch, 6 oz) started.
This treatment lasts for 24 months. At the end of the treatment, the photographs (figure n°18.) illustrate a balanced face, a better profile and a pleasant smile, a good class I relationship, the overbite and overjet have been corrected.
The lower incisor remains in its pre-treatment position.
The general superimposition shows the total mandibular response in height and length.
The post-treatment APDI is 80°, this value shows the stability of the treatment and counteract the tendency of relapse.

	Range	Beginning	End of treatment	End of retention
FMIA	67°+- 3	64	58	
FMA	25°+- 3	18	20	
IMPA	88°+- 3	98	102	
SNA	82°+- 2	79	76	
SNB	80°+- 2	74	73	
ANB	2°-+ 2	5	3	
Ao-Bo	2mm	7mm	2mm	
OP	10°-14°	7	8	
Z	75°+-5	67	73	
PFH	45mm	45	50	
AFH	65mm	60	65	
INDEX	0,69	0,75	0,77	

Table 3. Cephalometric analysis (Tweed- Merrifield)

	Beginning		End of treatment		End of retention	
ODI	MP/AB 82	80	82	80		
	FH/PP -2		-2			
APDI	HF/FP 80	73	82	80		
	FP/AB -5		-4			
	HF/PP -2		2			
CF	ODI+APDI	153		160		

Table 4. Cephalometric analysis (Kim)

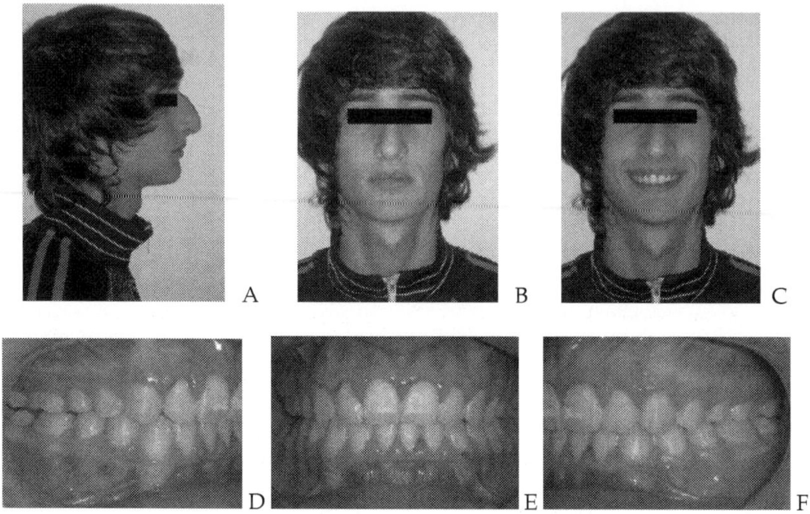

Fig. 18. Post-treatment extraoral photos (A-C) and intraoral photos (D-F)

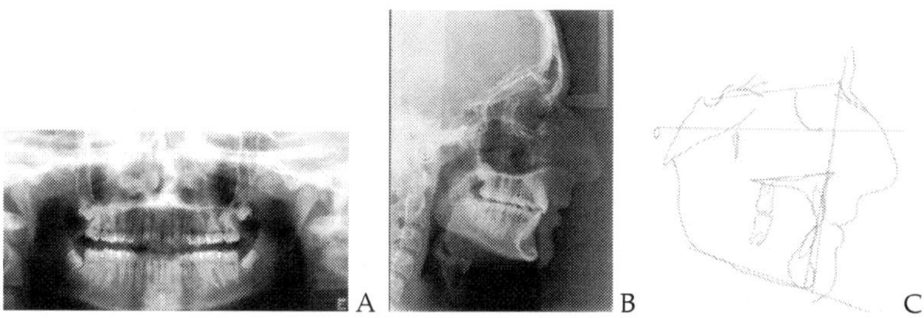

Fig. 19. Post-treatment records

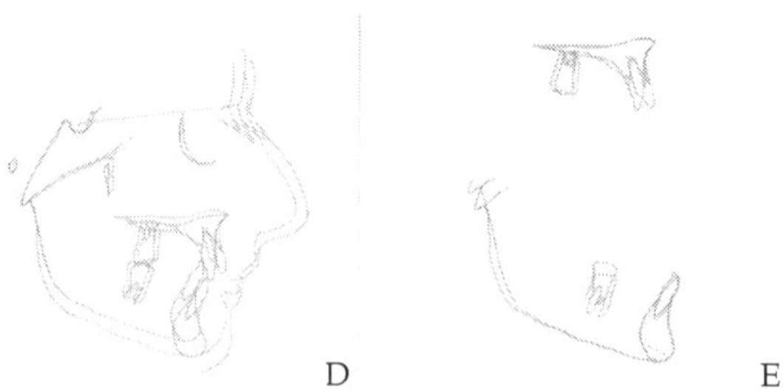

Fig. 20. Superimpositions

Case Report 3

Patient male (13 years, 4 months), short anterior facial height, skeletal class II and dental class II/1 on a hypodivergent face pattern, mandibular retrusion , thin lips, deep overbite (7mm), overjet (7mm) curve of spee deep with steep occlusal plane in the molar area, insufficient occlusal support. (2mm of crowding).

According to KYM's analysis the ODI=88 indicates a deep bite skeletal pattern and extraction of permanent teeth should be avoided if possible.

The APDI (66) indicates a class II skeletal pattern and the CF of 154 indicates a skeletal pattern that has a potential to accommodate all of the teeth.

Treatment goals: a- increase the vertical dimension , b- rebuild and flatten the upper posterior occlusal plane; c- reposition the mandible forward ; d- correction the crowding.

Treatment plane (steps): a - Leveling ; b-Elimination of interferences and crowding ; c - Establishing mandibular position; d- Occlusal plane reconstruction ; e- Obtain a physiologic occlusion.Treatment began with levelling using .0016 ss round wire, (brackets with 0.022 inch slot).Three months after the beginning of the treatment, MEAW's (multiloop edgewise arch wires .0017x.0025 inch/ss) were applied to upper and lower arches. A reverse curve was done in the mandibular MEAW. Then step down bends were done in the upper arch and step up bends in the lower arch to bite rising. Short class II 3/16 inch elastics, 6 oz were used. 14 months after the beginning of the treatment the malocclusion was corrected. The retention phase was done with maxillary Hawley plate for night time use (6months) and bonded lingual wire from 43 to 33.The post-treatment photos show a well balanced face, a better smile, a good class I molar relationship, overbite and overjet correct. The mandibular superimposition shows a slight protrusion of the lower incisors (the IMPA was increased from 108 to 111).The APDI was increased from 69 to 77 .

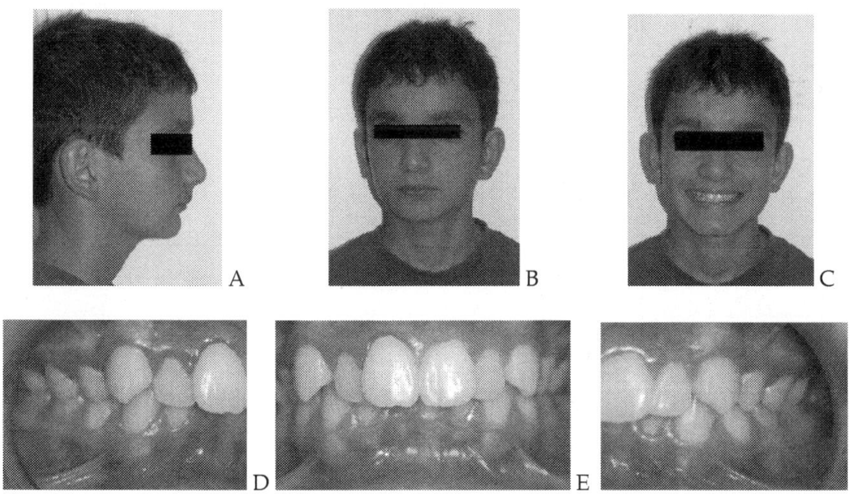

Fig. 21. Pre-treatment Photos A-F

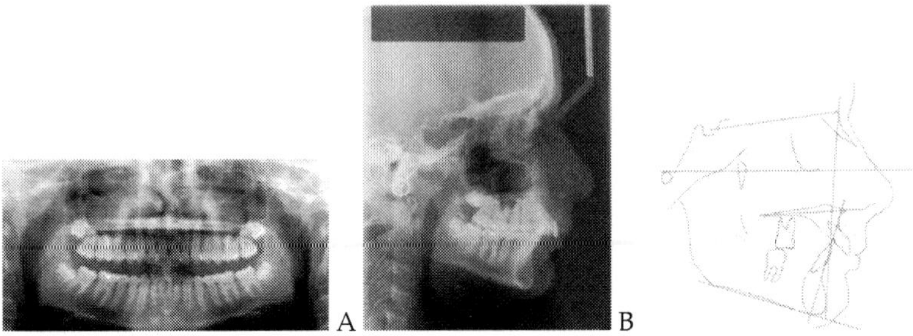

Fig. 22. Pre-treatment records

	Beginning		End of treatment		End of retention	
ODI	MP/AB 90	88	87	85		
	FH/PP -2		-2			
APDI	HF/FP 84	69	85	77		
	FP/AB -13		-7			
	HF/PP -2		-1			
CF	ODI+APDI	157		162		

Table 5. Cephalometric analysis (Kim)

	Range	Beginning	End of treatment	End of retention
FMIA	67°+- 3	55	52	
FMA	25°+- 3	17	17	
IMPA	88°+- 3	108	111	
SNA	82°+- 2	83	82	
SNB	80°+- 2	76	78	
ANB	2°-+ 2	7	4	
Ao-Bo	2mm	8mm	6mm	
OP	10°-14°	6	3	
Z	75°+-5	70	73	
PFH	45mm	49	51	
AFH	65mm	61	63	
INDEX	0,69	0,80	0,80	

Table 6. Cephalometric analysis (Tweed- Merrifield)

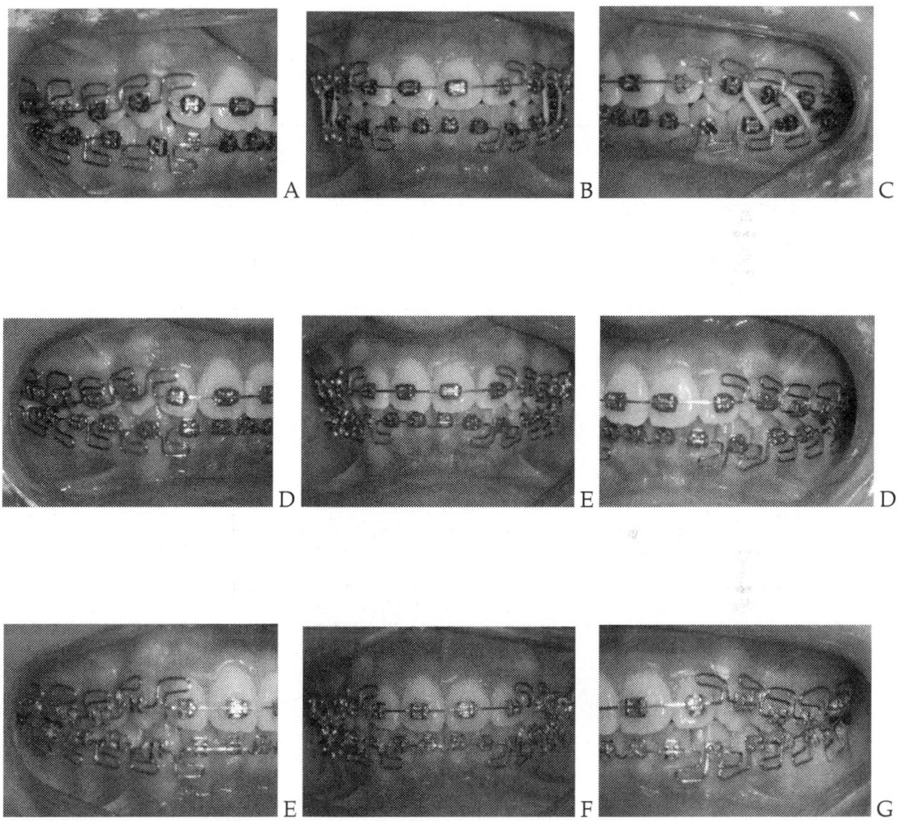

Fig. 23. Photos during the treatment (A - G)

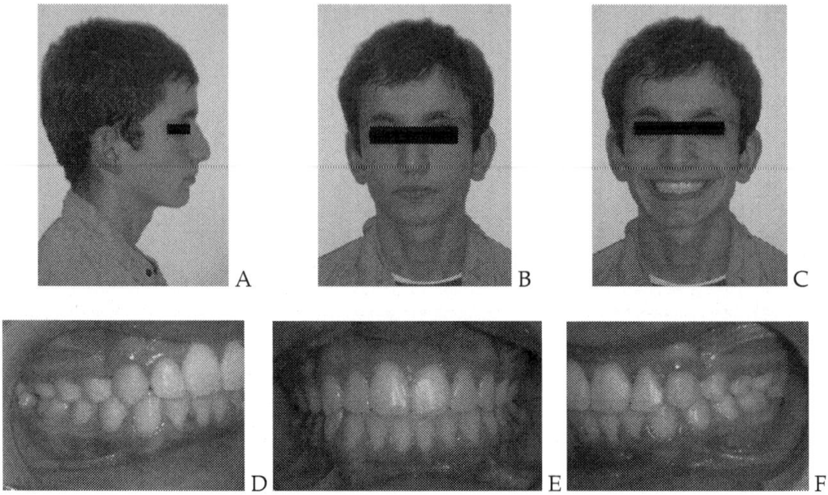

Fig. 24. Post-treatment extraoral (A-C) and intraoral (D-F) photos

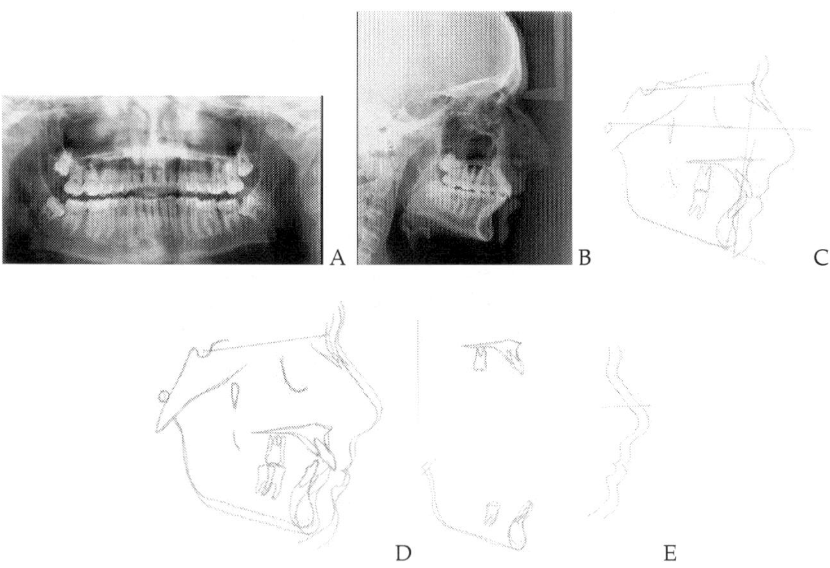

Fig. 25. Post-treatment records

10. Conclusion

The MEAW technique proved to be effective in the treatment of class II deepbite malocclusion, correcting the posterior occlusal plane and increasing the vertical dimension, allowing a stable mandibular advancement.

11. References

Dawson, P.E.(1989) *Evaluation, diagnosis and treatment of occlusal problems, Dawson, P.E.*(ed), The C.V. Mosby company

Decker, A (1989). Le traitement des classes II sans extractions de prémolaires, *journal de l`Edgewise* - vol 20 : 89-112

Fushima, K ; Kitamura, Y; Mita, H ; Sato, S; Kim, Y (1996).The significance of the cant of occlusal plane in class II/1 malocclusion. *European journal of orthodontics*, 18, 27-40

Hyun-Sook Kim, Seon-Young Kim (2004).Compensatory changes of a occlusal plane angles in relation to a skeletal factors; *Korea journal of orthodontics*:34 (3) :229-40

Kato, Sae; Chung, Woo-Nahm; Sato, Sadao (2002), Morphological Characterization of different types of class II malocclusion; *bulletim of Kanagawa dental college*; vol 30, n°2, September, pp 93-98

Kim, Young H, (1974)overbite depth indicator with particular reference to anterior openbite, *AJO*, 65:586-611

Kim, YH; Vietas JJ(1978) Anteroposterior dysplasia indicator; *American journal of orthodontics ; 73:619-33*

Kim, YH, (1979), ODI/APDI combination factor, *Angle orthodontics, 49:77-84*

Kim, YH; (1999); Treatment of anterior openbite and deepbite malocclusions with MEAW therapy; *The enigma of vertical dimension-craniofacial growth series vol 36 Ann Arbor (edited by James McNamara Jr): center for Human growth and development-* University of Michigan

Knierim, RW (1999).diagnosis of openbite and deepbite problems: a clinician`s perspective on the Kim approach; ; *The enigma of vertical dimension-craniofacial growth series vol 36 Ann Arbor (edited by James McNamara Jr): center for Human growth and development-* Univ.Michigan

Mc Namara, J.A. jr and Carlson, D.S. (1979)Quantitative analysis of temporomandibular joint adaptations to protrusive function; *American journal of orthodontics*, 76, 593-611

Merrifield, LL.(1966)The profile line as an aid to critical evaluation of facial esthetics; *American journal of orthodontics, 804-822*

Ortial, J.P(1989), Les modifications faciales par l`orthodontie, *journal de l`edgewise*, vol.20, 53-86

Petrovic, A.G. and Stutzaman, J.(1975) Control process in the postnatal growth of the condylar cartilage, in *McNamara J.A.jr, ed.determinants of mandibular growth, monograph 4:craniofacial growth series, Ann Arbor-Center for Human growth and development,* University of Michigan

Sassouni, V, (1969)A classification of skeletal facial types, *AJODO*, 55, 109-123

Sato, Sadao(2001) -*A treatment approach to malocclusions under the consideration of craniofacial dynamics,* Grace printing press, inc

Sato, Sadao.(2002)Morphological characterization of different types of class II malocclusion; *Bulletin of Kanagawa dental College*, vol.30, n°2, September, pp, 93-98
Sato, Sadao (2008), orthodontic marathon course at Kanagawa dental college -Japan

5

Sagittal Skeletal and Occlusal Changes of Class II, Division 1 Postadolescent Cases in the Herbst and Activator Therapy

Nenad Nedeljkovic
Clinic of Orthodontics, School of Dentistry, University of Belgrade
Serbia

1. Introduction

Class II malocclusions are common orthodontic irregularities (they account for 27% of all orthodontic irregularities) and they are considered a major reason for consulting an orthodontist. The positive outcome of Class II malocclusion treatment has some significant advantages: the prevention of traumatic injuries of upper incisors associated with large overjet and hard palate injuries with lower incisors, prevention of trauma of temporomandibular joints resulting from excessive load during the performance of orofacial functions, prevention of the development of dysfunctions (breading, speech...) and psycho-social adaptation for children during the important process of personality development.

In the treatment of skeletal Class II malocclusions, the objective is often to stimulate sagittal mandibular growth since the sagittal mandibular deficiency is the most common cause of this orthodontic irregularity. An appliance for affecting mandibular position and growth was first designed in 1877. It was introduced by Norman W. Kingsley and this treatment method was called "Jumping the bite" (Pancherz, 2008). This term denotes a treatment with an orthodontic appliance for the direction of bite mesially, advancement of the mandible. The appliance comprised of an upper plate furnished with an inclined plane that held the lower incisors and forced the mandible anteriorly.

The principle of bite jumping has led to the development of the different removable functional appliances that we use today such as the Activator by Andersen and Häupl, bionator according to Balters, Fränkel appliance etc. (Graber et al., 1997). The effect of the activator on mandibular growth has been a subject of debate for many years (Bjork, 1951; Korkhaus, 1960; Harvold & Vargervik, 1971; Ahlgren & Laurin, 1976, Pancherz, 1979, 1984; Wieslander L & Lagerstrom, 1979; Luder, 1982; Jacobsson & Paulin, 1990). Some researchers claim that mandibular condylar growth can be stimulated by removable functional appliances treatment while others state that the changes in the occlusion are a result of dentoalveolar remodeling processes. This disagreement between the scientists is mainly due to the difficulties in the evaluation of treatment results as the activator, like all other removable functional appliances, has several disadvantages: 1) the appliance is mostly used only part of the day. This implies that in certain individuals the threshold for condylar growth adaptation to forward displacement of the mandible will never be reached. 2)

Patient compliance can also present a moot point. In case of undetected insufficient appliance wear, the interpretation of the treatment outcome could be biased. 3) Treatment time is relatively long (over 2 years) and often there is no suitable control group of untreated patients. This is the reason for arising difficulties to differentiate between physiological growth changes and changes induced by treatment (Pancherz, 2008).

With the modification of dentofacial growth direction, alongside with dentoalveolar harmonization of the occlusion, the usage of functional orthodontic appliances can provide a possibility to change or prevent morphogenetic abnormalities (Graber et al., 1997; Harvold & Vargervik, 1971). Optimal timing, i.e., the age of patients for treatment with removable functional appliances is the period of adolescence or period just before the pubertal growth spurt. After this period, the growth progresses slowly until adulthood, when it continues but in smaller amount. This period of postadolescence (after pubertal peak of growth) which chronologically lasts several years, is very important in functional orthodontics. This age of patients with Class II irregularities is considered to be very respectable, aesthetically and psychologically as well as functionally, since the majority of patients tend to consult an orthodontist during this period for aesthetic reasons. An orthodontist has several possible treatment solutions at his disposal: removable and fixed functional appliances treatment, camouflage orthodontics and orthognatic surgery. Surgery with previous orthodontic preparation gives satisfactory results, however, patients should wait until the end of growth, and commonly, they refuse this type of intervention. The camouflage orthodontics of Class II, Division 1 malocclusion includes the reduction of number of teeth in order to accomplish normal occlusion with questionable skeletal-soft tissue results at the end of treatment. As regards removable functional appliances, we cannot adhere to the terms stimulation or redirection of growth at this age, but we will mainly speak about dentoalveolar effects, taking into account a very important fact - patient compliance. The similar problem appears in fixed multibracket appliance therapy with class II intermaxillary elastics.

The purpose of fixed functional appliances is to overcome the shortcomings of removable functional appliances. In recent years, functional appliances are more frequently divided into fixed and removable appliances. The Herbst appliance is one of the most used fixed appliances in treatment of Class II malocclusions that is effective even after the period of adolescence.

Taking into account age and growth development, the dominant current concept of Class II treatment is: 1. Growth adaptation in children and adolescents, 2. Camouflage orthodontics in postadolescents and 3. Surgical correction in adults.

However, when considering the fact that skeleto-facial growth continues many years after the cessation of body height growth and that the TMJ in adults is capable of remodeling, it seems logical to revise the above treatment concept. Therefore, with respect to age and growth development, the following modified new concept for the treatment of Class II irregularities is proposed (Pancherz & Ruf, 2000): 1. Growth adaptation in children, adolescents, postadolescents and young adults, 2. Camouflage orthodontics in older adults and 3. Surgical correction in older adults.

The aim of investigation was to establish the sagittal skeletal, dentoalveolar and occlusal changes that occurring during the Herbst treatment of patients with Class II/1 malocclusion in the late puberty, and to compare them with those that occurred during the Activator treatment.

2. Material and method

The sample for this study comprised 50 patients with skeletal Class II, division 1 malocclusion (treated at the Clinic of Orthodontics, School of Dentistry, University of Belgrade), of both sexes, aged 14 - 17 years. The previous careful functional analysis eliminated the possibility of functional distal occlusion. The cases with minimal ANB angle of 5.5° and minimal overjet of 6.5mm were enrolled in this study. The minimal age of the patients was 14 years, which provided the basis for the assumption that they had passed maximal pubertal growth, and thus, the optimal period for functional therapy. This was confirmed by the assessment of skeletal maturity (Fig 3.1), so the sample comprised postadolescents and distribution according to sex was not performed.

The patients were divided into two groups: 1. Herbst treatment group (25 patients treated with the Herbst appliance) and 2. Activator treatment group (25 patients treated with the Activator appliance). The Herbst group consisted of 11 male and 14 female patients, aged 14 - 17 years at the beginning of treatment. The Activator group consisted of 13 male and 12 female patients, aged 14 - 16 years. After the treatment plan has been prepared, the patients in the Activator group, like those in the Herbst group, were first offered the Herbst therapy. The Activator patients refused this type of treatment mainly for reasons related to comfort or financial reasons. For similar reasons, they denied alternative solutions of camouflage therapy or preparation for orthognatic surgery, which again suggested the use of fixed multibracket orthodontic appliances. Finally, they accepted the therapy option using the Activator, with detailed explanation of the treatment and possible treatment effects related to their age. All of the Class II, division 1 patients in the Herbst group were treated successfully (Class I molar relationship, normal overjet and overbite) at the end of treatment. In the Activator group, most of the patients were treated without complete achievement. Success at the end of treatment has observed in 5 (20%) patients only. Six patients in the Activator group switched the group (they accepted the Herbst appliance treatment), mostly because they were not satisfied with the course of the Activator treatment and its progress. Other patients without desirable results continued with camouflage orthodontic treatment and multibracket appliance.

The therapy with the Herbst appliance and therapy effects are considered as combined, because the Herbst appliance is used in the combination with multibracket appliance. The Herbst appliance was removed after 6-8 months and then multibracket fixed appliance was used so the mean overall treatment time was 17.5 months.

The Activator therapy lasted 12-25 months depending on the amount of progress observed during control visits. The patients' compliance was not monitored. Both subject groups were longitudinally monitored pre- and post treatment. At the start of treatment, the age of the Herbst patients approximately matched the age of the Activator patients. Pretreatment and post treatment study models, orthopantomographic images and standard profile cephalograms were obtained for each patient. The Ethical committee of the School of Dentistry in Belgrade approved the study, pointing out that the patients and their parents should sign the consent to the entire procedure related to the therapy. Since the examinations were conducted before and after treatment, both groups were additionally divided into two subgroups: pretreatment Herbst and pretreatment Activator group (before the treatment) and post treatment Herbst and post treatment Activator group (after the treatment).

2.1 Appliance characteristics

2.1.1 The Herbst appliance

The first phase in the usage of this appliance in treatment is obtaining the construction bite in incisal relationship, with careful attention to the middle of the jaws.

The Herbst appliance used in this study was type 1, manufactured in the German company Dentaurum (Fig. 1.1 - 1.6). The Herbst appliance can be compared to an artificial joint working between the maxilla and mandible. A bilateral telescope mechanism attached to orthodontic bands of the Herbst appliance keeps the mandible in an anterior jumped position (Fig. 1.5 and Fig. 1.6). Each telescope mechanism consists of a tube, a plunger, two pivots and two screws, which enable the telescoping parts to make additional lateral movements over the pivots and prevent the telescoping parts from slipping of the pivots (Fig. 1.1).

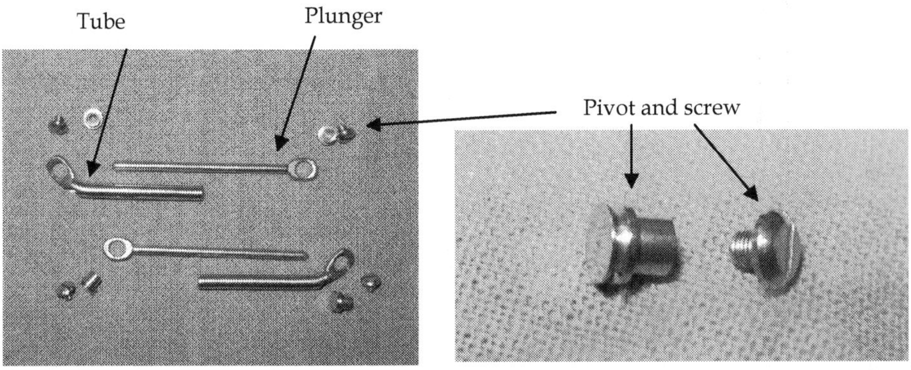

Fig. 1.1. Parts of the Herbst appliance: tube, plunger, pivot and screw.

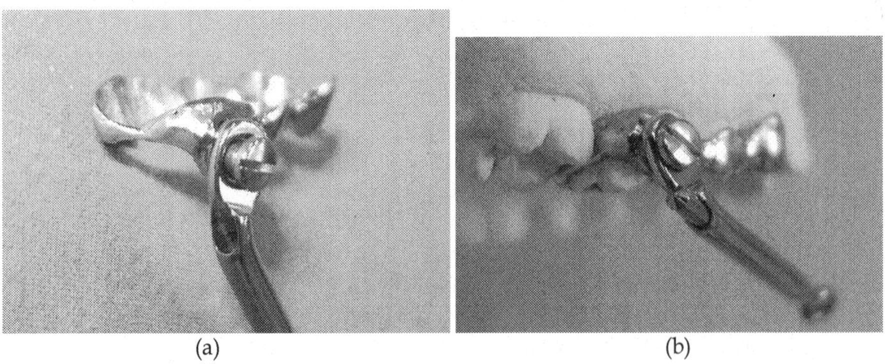

Fig. 1.2. a) fixing the tube on the pivot using the screw, b) the plunger in the tube of the Herbst appliance.

The pivot for the tube is usually soldered to the maxillary first molar band and the pivot for the plunger to the mandibular first premolar band (Figures 1.2, 1.3 and 1.4). The length of the tube determines the amount of sagittal activation, i.e. bite jumping. The mandible is usually retained in an incisal edge-to-edge position, which is determined by the construction bite (Fig. 1.5).

A large interpivot distance prevents the plunger from slipping out of the tube when the mouth is wide open. Therefore, the upper pivot should be placed distally on the molar band and the lower pivot mesially on the premolar band (Fig. 1.5). The length of the plunger should be kept at a maximum in order to prevent it from disengaging from the tube.

The entire system is held on the splints of the Herbst appliance in the upper and lower jaw. The splints are cemented to the teeth and can be prepared in two ways (both types of splints are used in the study):

1. The cast splint Herbst appliance manufactured on double study models by casting it from CoCrMo alloy, the procedure similar to the construction of prosthetic denture with metal framework. It was constructed in the technical dental laboratory of the Clinic for Prosthodontics, School of Dentistry in Belgrade. In the upper jaw, the splint engaged both premolars and permanent first molars, and it is, basically, constructed separately for right and left side. In the lower jaw, because of the greater anchorage required, the splint incorporated the premolars and permanent first molars interconnected with a lingual arch wire behind the lower front teeth (Fig. 1.3.a and Fig. 1.4).

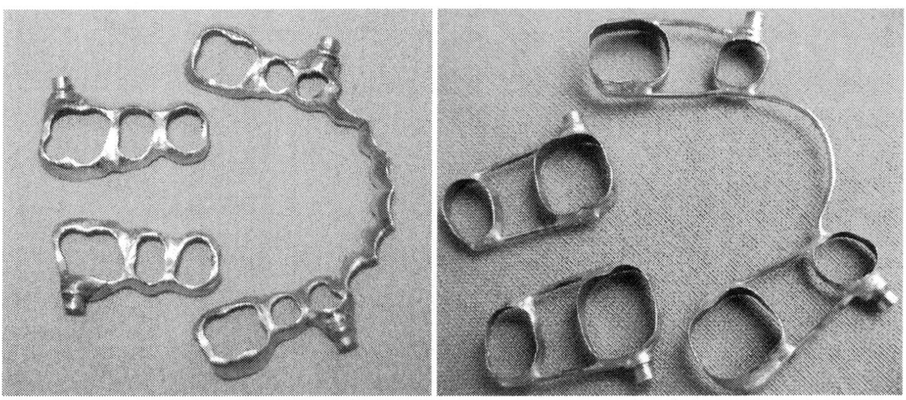

(a) (b)

Fig. 1.3. a) cast splint of the Herbst appliance, b) standard banded splint of the Herbst appliance.

2. The banded Herbst appliance, constructed on study models; first, the adjacent teeth that will not be banded are etched. Then, the bands for the first premolars and permanent first molars in both jaws are chosen and adjusted. In the upper dental arch, the splint is paired and reinforced with 1.0-1.2 mm wire on the vestibular and palatal side. The reinforcements are first punctured and then soldered. The process is similar in the lower dental arch, except that on the lingual side, a lingual arch is modeled from wire of the same diameter, which extends from the permanent first molar on one side to the same tooth on the other side, behind the lingual surfaces of the front teeth (Fig. 1.3b).

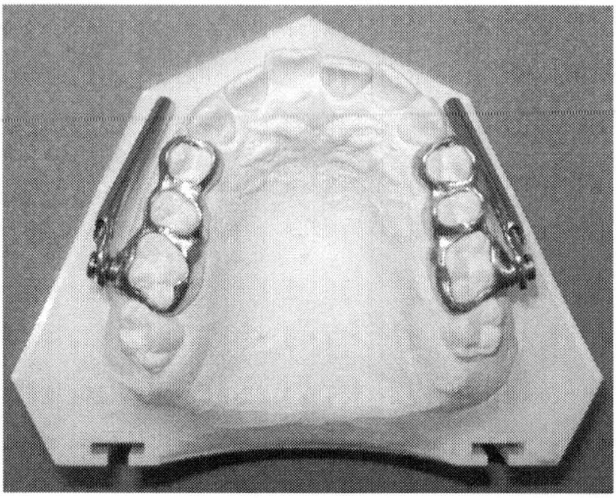

a)

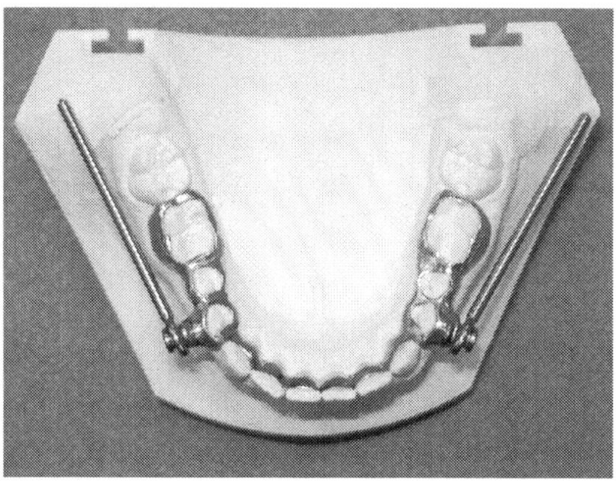

b)

Fig. 1.4. The Herbst appliance a) on the upper and b) lower study model.

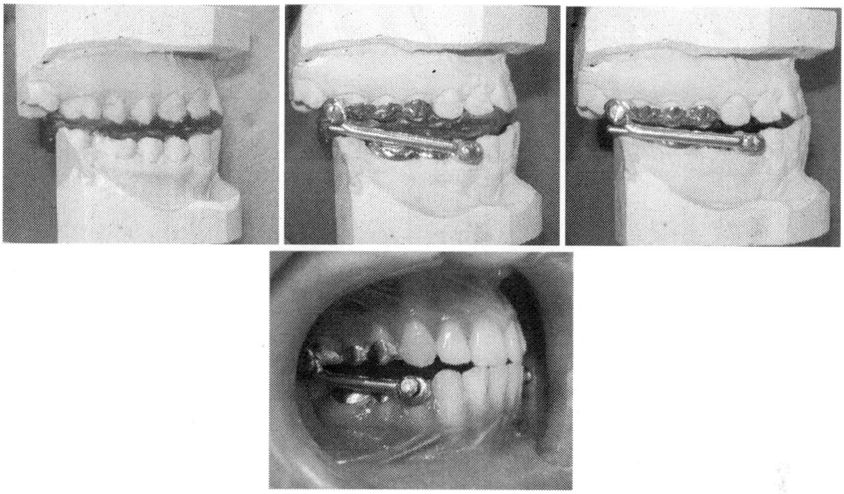

Fig. 1.5. Construction bite, adjusted Herbst appliance on a study model, cemented Herbst appliance.

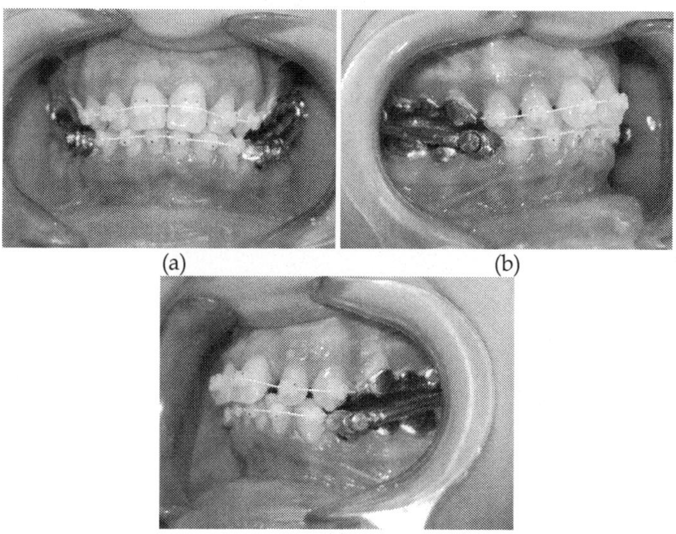

(a) (b)

(c)

Fig. 1.6. The Herbst appliance and segmented multibracket appliance: a) front view, b) lateral right, and c) lateral left view.

2.1.2 The activator appliance

In the first phase of the activator construction, after the common clinical procedure, the construction bite in the eugnathic relationship (I class dentoalveolar relationship) was taken, with the mandible forced forward until the upper canine between the lower canine and the first lower premolar relationship was achieved. The construction bite was taken with the mandible protruded 4-6 mm and interocclusal space of 2-3 mm above physiological rest in the molar region. During the procedure of construction bite taking, the great care was exercised regarding the middles of the jaws. After this, the trial of the wax activator followed to check the relationship between the jaws and possible corrections (Fig. 2.1).

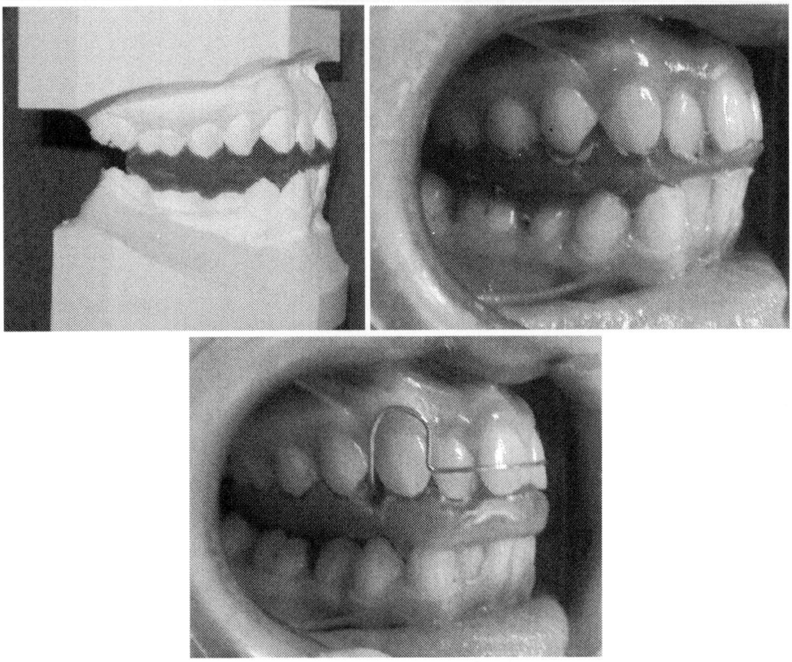

Fig. 2.1. Constructions bite and wax trial.

The activator appliance used in this study (Fig. 2.2) consisted of an acrylic intermaxillary block with upper labial arch (0.8 mm) which passively touched the incisal third of the upper incisors. The acrylic was extended to cover the incisal third of the mandibular incisors in order to prevent the labial tipping of these teeth. The acrylic extended to the lower lingual sulcus to provide stability and anchorage. The appliance was constructed in technical dental laboratory at the Clinic of Orthodontics, School of Dentistry in Belgrade. At control visits, the acrylic was trimmed behind the upper front teeth, which was in concordance with treatment of protruded incisors in the sense of their retrusion and overjet reduction. The interocclusal acrylic in the molar and premolar region was not trimmed until the improvement of the sagittal jaw relationship was achieved, in cases with associated deep bite. In the last phase, the acrylic was trimmed selectively according to the occlusal needs of the lateral teeth. Patients were advised to wear the appliance 15 hours a day, but their compliance was not monitored.

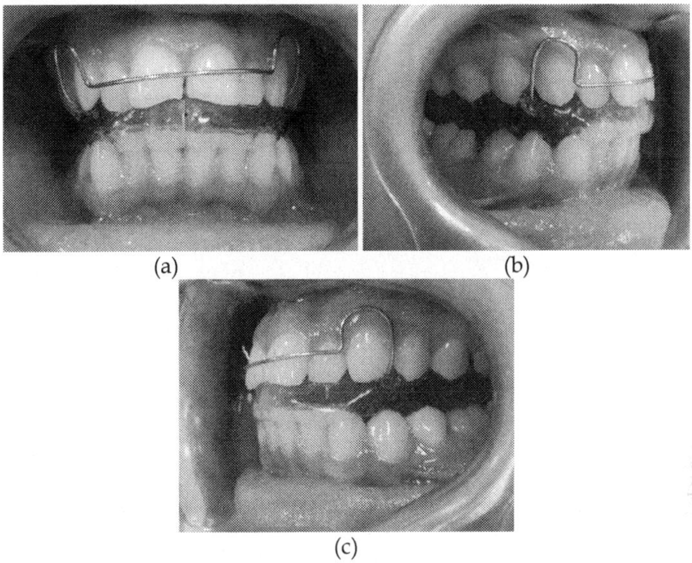

Fig. 2.2. The Activator supplied to the patient: a) frontal view, b) lateral right, and c) lateral left view.

2.2 Skeletal maturity assessment

Chronological maturity was determined for each patient on the date of the profile cephalometric imaging.

On these images, skeletal maturity was first determined for each patient according to the stages of the cervical vertebral maturation (Fig. 3.1 and Fig. 3.2):

- Stage 1 (CvS 1). The inferior borders of the bodies of all cervical vertebrae are flat. The superior borders are tapered from posterior to anterior.
- Stage 2 (CvS 2). A concavity develops in the inferior border of the second vertebra. The anterior vertical height of the bodies increases.
- Stage 3 (CvS 3). A concavity develops in the inferior border of the third vertebra.
- Stage 4 (CvS 4). A concavity develops in the inferior border of the fourth vertebra. Concavities in the lower borders of the fifth and sixth vertebrae are beginning to form. The bodies of all cervical vertebrae are rectangular in shape.
- Stage 5 (CvS 5). Concavities are well defined in the lower borders of the bodies of all six vertebrae. The bodies have become nearly square in shape and the spaces between the bodies are reduced.
- Stage 6 (CvS 6). All concavities have deepened. The bodies of vertebrae are now higher than they are wide.

The stages CvS 1 - CvS 2 represent the periods of prepubertal growth. The stages CvS 3 - CvS 4 are the period of maximal growth (pubertal growth spurt), while the stages CvS 5 - CvS 6 indicate the stage when the maximal growth has passed and the puberty is finished.

All of the patients at the beginning of this study were in the stages from CvS 4 to CvS 6. The middle stage in both subjects was CvS 5, which means, they had passed maximal pubertal growth.

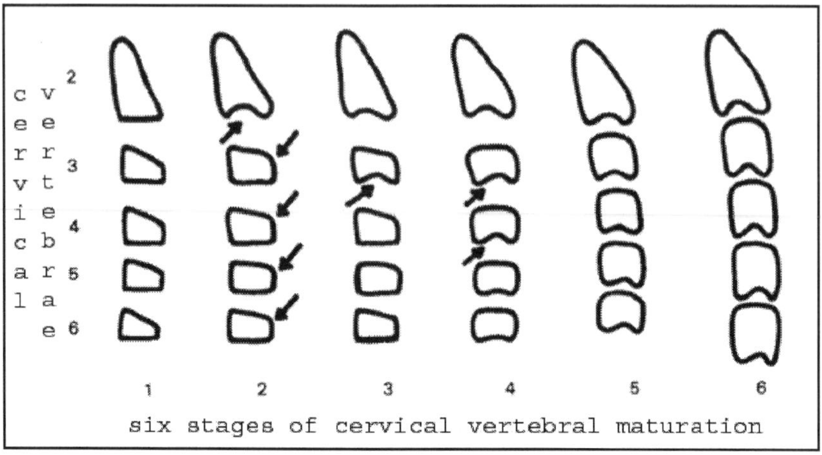

Fig. 3.1. Six stages of cervical vertebral maturation (O'Relly & Yanneillo, 1988).

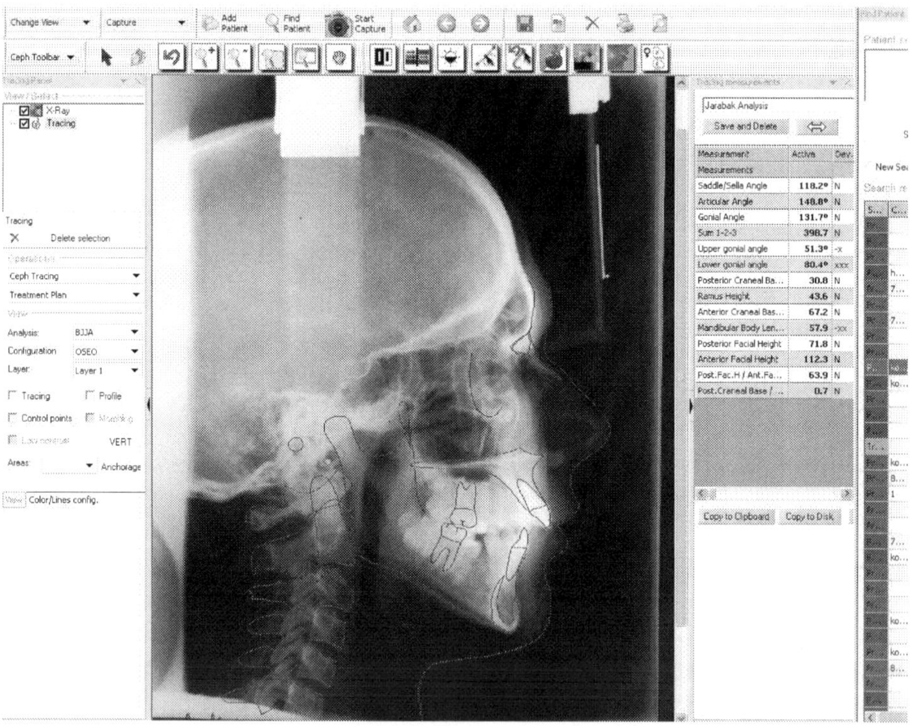

Fig. 3.2. Assessment of cervical vertebral maturation stages using computerized cephalometric analysis.

2.3 Profile cephalometric analysis

The profile cephalometric analysis was performed using the computer program Nemotec Dental Studio NX 2006 to assess sagittal skeletal and dentoalveolar changes. The sagittal occlusal changes were analyzed as well. Pretreatment and post treatment cephalometric images were first superimposed, in relation to nasion-sella line (NSL). Then, maxillary occlusal plane - RL (occlusal reference line passing through the incisal edge of the upper incisor and the most distal point of molar contact in the occlusion) was determined. A line perpendicular to RL through sella (point S) i.e. RLp was used in measurement (Fig. 4). Linear measurements are performed parallel with RL to RLp for each patient and selected in a table 1. of SO-Analysis (Analysis of changes in sagittal occlusion):

SO ANALYSIS	Variable (measurements to RLp)	Before	After	After - Before (D)	Correction Max.+ Mand.
Skeletal + Dental	ms mi				Molar relation
Skeletal + Dental	is ii				Overjet
Skeletal	ss Pg				Skeletal
Dental (Molars)	ms(D)-ss(D) mi(D)-Pg(D)	- -	- -		Molars
Dental (Incisors)	is(D)-ss(D) ii(D)-Pg(D)	- -	- -		Incisors

Table 1. Analysis of sagittal skeletal and occlusal changes before and after treatment (SO-Analysis by Pancherz H).

1. ms-RLp - position of the maxillary permanent first molar (the shortest distance of the most mesial point of the approximal surface of the upper first molar to RLp),
2. mi-RLp - position of the mandibular permanent first molar (the shortest distance of the most mesial point of the approximal surface of the lower first molar to RLp),
3. (ms-RLp) - (mi- RLp) the molar relationship correction,
4. is-RLp - position of the maxillary central incisor (the shortest distance of the incisal edge of the upper incisor to RLp)
5. ii-RLp - position of the mandibular central incisor (the shortest distance of the incisal edge of the lower incisor to RLp),
6. (is-RLp) - (ii-RLp) the overjet correction,
7. ss-RLp - position of the maxilary base (the shortest distance of the most recessed point of the anterior side of the maxilla to RLp),
8. Pg-RLp - position of the mandibular base (the shortest distance of the most prominent point of the chin profile to RLp),

9. (ss-RLp) - (Pg-RLp) the skeletal correction,
10. (ms-RLp) - (ss-RLp) the correction of the permanent first maxillary molar position within the maxilla,
11. (mi-RLp) - (Pg-RLp) the correction of the permanent first mandibular molar position within the mandible,
12. (ms-ss) - (mi-Pg) the molar correction,
13. (is-RLp) - (ss-RLp) the correction of the upper incisor position within the maxilla,
14. (ii-RLp) - (Pg-RLp) the correction of the lower incisor position within the mandible,
15. (is-ss) - (ii-Pg) the incisor correction.

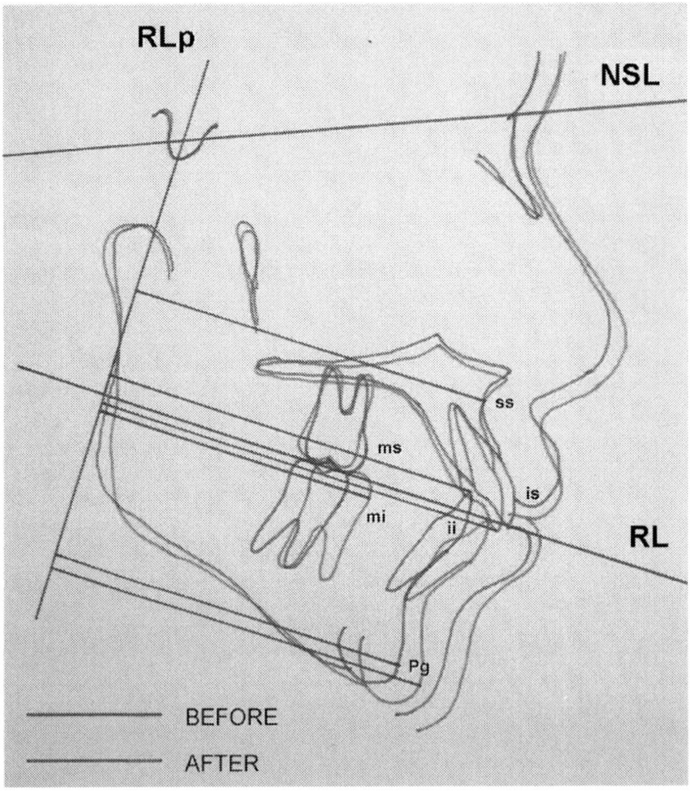

Fig. 4. Superposition of cephalometric images before (blue) and after (red) treatment with visible skeletal and dentoalveolar changes.

2.4 Statistical analysis

Statistical analysis was performed using Windows XP professional in the program Microsoft Office Excel 2003 and SPSS ver. 14. All values of the parameters are statistically evaluated using standard statistical analyses: 1. measurements of central tendency: arithmetic mean (average), 2. reliability intervals: max and min (maximal and minimal value); 3. variability measurements: SD (standard deviation), variance (average square deviation), variation coefficient; 4. statistical hypothesis testing: t test (testing of statistical differences with Student's t-test: t test for independent samples - to test significant differences within groups and between groups; and t test for paired samples - to control treatment results within the examined groups before and after treatment), correlation coefficient - to explain relations and connections between two indicators or changes within one series before and after treatment), and f test (to compare two dependent samples - test of equivalent pairs).

3. Results

Parameters of sagittal skeletal and dental changes (the method according to Pancherz):

Statistical parameters	HERBST						Correction of molar relation
	ms			mi			
	before	after	after-before	before	after	after-before	
aver	54.70	53.74	0.96	53.10	55.76	2.66	3.62
s.d.	4.62	4.52	1.48	5.02	4.70	1.47	1.00
min	44.00	43.00	-4.00	42.50	44.50	1.00	2.00
max	64.00	62.00	3.00	62.00	64.00	8.00	5.50
var	21.35	20.46	2.19	25.19	22.06	2.16	1.01
KV	8.45%	8.42%		9.45%	8.42%		
TTEST	*p < 0.01***			*p < 0.001****			
Cor	*0.9479*			*0.9564*			
Ftest	*0.9175*			*0.7484*			
Statistical parameters	**ACTIVATOR**						**Correction of molar relation**
	ms			**mi**			
	before	**after**	**after-before**	**before**	**after**	**after-before**	
aver	52.80	52.98	-0.18	51.14	52.98	1.84	1.66
s.d.	5.58	5.81	1.58	6.08	6.08	1.44	1.07
min	39.00	39.00	-4.50	38.00	39.00	0.00	0.00
max	64.00	65.00	1.50	63.50	66.50	6.50	3.00
var	31.17	33.78	2.50	36.93	36.97	2.08	1.14
KV	10.57%	10.97%		11.88%	11.48%		
TTEST	*0.5743*			*p < 0.001****			
Cor	*0.9623*			*0.9719*			
Ftest	*0.8452*			*0.9979*			

Table 2. The upper and lower first permanent molar positions and molar relation.

The upper and lower first permanent molar position showed statistical significance in both groups (Table 2.). In the Herbst subjects, the maxillary permanent first molar was distalized (p<0.01), whereas the mandibular first molar shows mesial position (p<0.001) in both subject groups. Molar relation correction during Herbst treatment (3.62 mm) was more than two times larger than in the Activator group (1.66mm).

Statistical parameters	Pancherz analysis: comparison between groups					
	ms			mi		
	before	after	after - before	before	after	after - before
TTEST Activator-Herbst	0.1961	0.6083	*$p < 0.01$***	0.2197	*$p < 0.05$**	*$p < 0.05$**
Cor Activator-Herbst	0.1086	0.1555	-0.2083	0.0955	0.1133	-0.3709
Ftest Activator-Herbst	0.3608	0.2266	0.7467	0.3551	0.2134	0.9240

Table 3. The upper and lower first permanent molar positions - comparison between the Herbst and Activator group.

The upper and lower first permanent molar positions, showed statistical significance of treatment effects between the groups. Compared with the Activator subjects, the maxillary ($p<0.01$) and mandibular ($p<0.05$) permanent first molar changes during Herbst treatment were significantly pronounced (Table 3.).

Statistical parameters	HERBST						Overjet correction
	is			ii			
	before	after	after-before	before	after	after-before	
aver	86.90	83.82	3.32	75.60	80.46	4.86	8.18
s.d.	5.62	5.42	2.70	5.31	5.26	2.65	2.80
min	74.00	71.00	-5.00	63.00	68.50	0.00	3.50
max	95.00	94.00	7.00	84.50	90.50	10.00	14.00
var	31.63	29.41	7.29	28.23	27.62	7.03	7.83
KV	6.47%	6.47%		7.03%	6.53%		
TTEST herbst	*$p < 0.001$****			*$p < 0.001$****			
Cor herbst	*0.8959*			*0.8742*			
Ftest herbst	*0.8606*			*0.9581*			
Statistical parameters	**ACTIVATOR**						**Overjet correction**
	is			**ii**			
	before	**after**	**after-before**	**before**	**after**	**after-before**	
aver	85.86	84.62	1.24	76.56	78.66	2.10	3.34
s.d.	7.83	8.00	1.67	6.79	6.09	1.43	2.16
min	74.00	72.50	-2.50	65.50	67.00	0.00	0.00
max	99.00	97.00	4.00	89.00	90.50	5.00	6.50
var	61.32	63.92	2.77	46.09	37.12	2.04	4.68
KV	9.12%	9.45%		8.87%	7.75%		
TTEST activator	*$p < 0.01$***			*$p < 0.001$****			
Cor activator	*0.9781*			*0.9769*			
Ftest activator	*0.9198*			*0.6001*			

Table 4. The position of the upper and lower incisor and overjet.

The upper and lower incisors, showed statistical significance in both subjects (Table 4.). Maxillary incisors shows retroinclination (Herbst subjects, $p<0.001$ and Activator, $p<0.01$), whereas mandibular incisors show proclination ($p<0.001$) in both subjects. Overjet correction during Herbst treatment (8.18 mm) was more extensive than in Activator group (3.34mm).

Statistical parameters	Pancherz analysis: comparison between groups					
	is			ii		
	before	after	after - before	before	after	after - before
TTEST Activator-Herbst	0.5921	0.6807	*p<0.001****	0.5803	0.2689	*p<0.001****
Cor Activator-Herbst	-0.0346	0.0760	0.2347	-0.0363	-0.0047	-0.5350
Ftest Activator-Herbst	0.1116	0.0630	0.0215	0.2370	0.4746	0.0036

Table 5. The position of the upper and lower incisor – testing between the Herbst and Activator group.

The upper and lower incisors, showed statistical significance of treatment effects between the subjects (Table 5.). Compared with the Activator subjects, the maxillary and mandibular incisor changes during Herbst treatment were significantly pronounced (p<0.001).

Statistical parameters	HERBST						Skeletal correction
	ss			Pg			
	before	after	after-before	before	after	after-before	
aver	77.28	76.72	0.52	76.80	79.98	3.18	3.70
s.d.	4.49	4.14	1.29	5.72	4.83	2.43	1.78
min	67.0	67.0	-3.5	66.0	69.0	0.5	1.0
max	85.0	84.0	2.0	89.5	91.0	9.0	9.0
var	20.14	17.14	1.65	32.66	23.34	5.89	3.16
KV	5.81%	5.40%		7.44%	6.04%		
TTEST	*p < 0.05**			*p < 0.001****			
Cor	*0.9666*			*0.9074*			
Ftest	*0.6961*			*0.4164*			
Statistical parameters	**ACTIVATOR**						**Skeletal correction**
	ss			**Pg**			
	before	**after**	**after-before**	**before**	**after**	**after-before**	
aver	77.04	77.40	-0.36	77.76	79.26	1.5	1.14
s.d.	6.28	6.44	0.81	8.97	8.72	1.46	1.38
min	65.5	66.4	-2	59.5	61	0	-0.5
max	88.2	89.0	1.0	96.5	98.0	6.5	5.5
var	39.4775	41.583	0.65	80.52	75.98	2.14	1.90
KV	8.16%	8.33%		11.54%	11.00%		
TTEST	*p < 0.05**			*p < 0.01***			
Co r	*0.9922*			*0.9867*			
Ftest	*0.8998*			*0.8881*			

Table 6. The position of the upper and lower jaw and skeletal correction.

The upper and lower jaw position, showed statistical significance in both groups (Table 6.). In the Herbst group, point ss changed its position slightly backward (p<0.05), while in the Activator group shows anterior position (p<0.05). Point Pg changed its position anteriorly in both groups, but the amount of change was more extensive in the Herbst group (p<0.001). Skeletal correction during Herbst treatment (3.70mm) was about three times larger than in Activator group (1.14mm).

Statistical parameters	Pancherz analysis: comparison between groups					
	ss			Pg		
	before	after	after - before	before	after	after - before
TTEST Activator-Herbst	0.8772	0.6593	*p<0.01***	0.6539	0.7195	*p<0.01***
Cor Activator-Herbst	0.0820	0.0886	0.1570	-0.2577	-0.2732	-0.0264
Ftest Activator-Herbst	0.1061	0.0345	0.0275	0.0314	0.0054	0.0164

Table 7. The position of the upper and lower jaw – testing between the Herbst and Activator group.

The upper and lower jaw position parameters, showed statistical significance of treatment effects between the groups. Herbst treatment seemed to have some greater influence on maxillary and mandibular jaw base position. For both parameters: ss ($p<0.01$) and Pg ($p<0.01$) were significantly greater in the Herbst subject (Table 7.).

	HERBST					
	ms(D)-ss(D) after-before	mi(D)-Pg(D) after-before	Molars	is(D)-ss(D) after-before	ii(D)-Pg(D) after-before	Incisors
aver	0.44	-0.52	-0.08	2.80	1.68	4.48
s.d.	1.00	1.87	1.75	2.12	2.08	2.67
min	-1.00	-5.00	-3.50	-1.50	-2.00	-1.50
max	2.50	3.00	3.50	6.50	7.50	9.00
var	1.01	3.49	3.06	4.50	4.33	7.14
	ACTIVATOR					
	ms(D)-ss(D) after-before	mi(D)-Pg(D) after-before	Molars	is(D)-ss(D) after-before	ii(D)-Pg(D) after-before	Incisors
aver	0.18	0.34	0.52	1.60	0.60	2.20
s.d.	1.24	1.24	1.34	1.23	0.93	1.79
min	-3.50	-1.00	-3.50	-0.50	-1.50	-1.00
max	2.00	2.50	2.50	4.00	2.00	6.00
var	-3.50	-1.00	-3.50	-0.50	-1.50	-1.00

Table 8. The correction of the position of the molars and incisors.

The correction of the incisor position showes greater amount in the Herbst subjects (Table 8.).

Significance Herbst - Activator	Molar relation	Overjet	Skeletal relation	Molars	Incisors
TTEST Activator-Herbst	*p<0.001****	*p<0.001****	*p<0.001****	0.1798	*p<0.001****
Cor Activator-Herbst	-0.0868	0.0799	0.0008	-0.0792	0.1825
Ftest Activator-Herbst	0.7616	0.2147	0.2212	0.2028	0.0540

Table 9. Treatment effects (the correction of the molar relation, the overjet correction, the skeletal relationship correction, the correction of the molars and incisors).

The treatment effects parameters (the correction of the molar relationship, the overjet correction, the skeletal relationship correction, the correction of the molars and incisors), showed the statistical significance between the subjects. For parameters: the correction of the molar relationship, the overjet correction, the skeletal relationship correction, the correction of the incisors, the greater statistical significance was found ($p<0.001$) because of the bigger changes during the Herbst treatment (Table 9.).

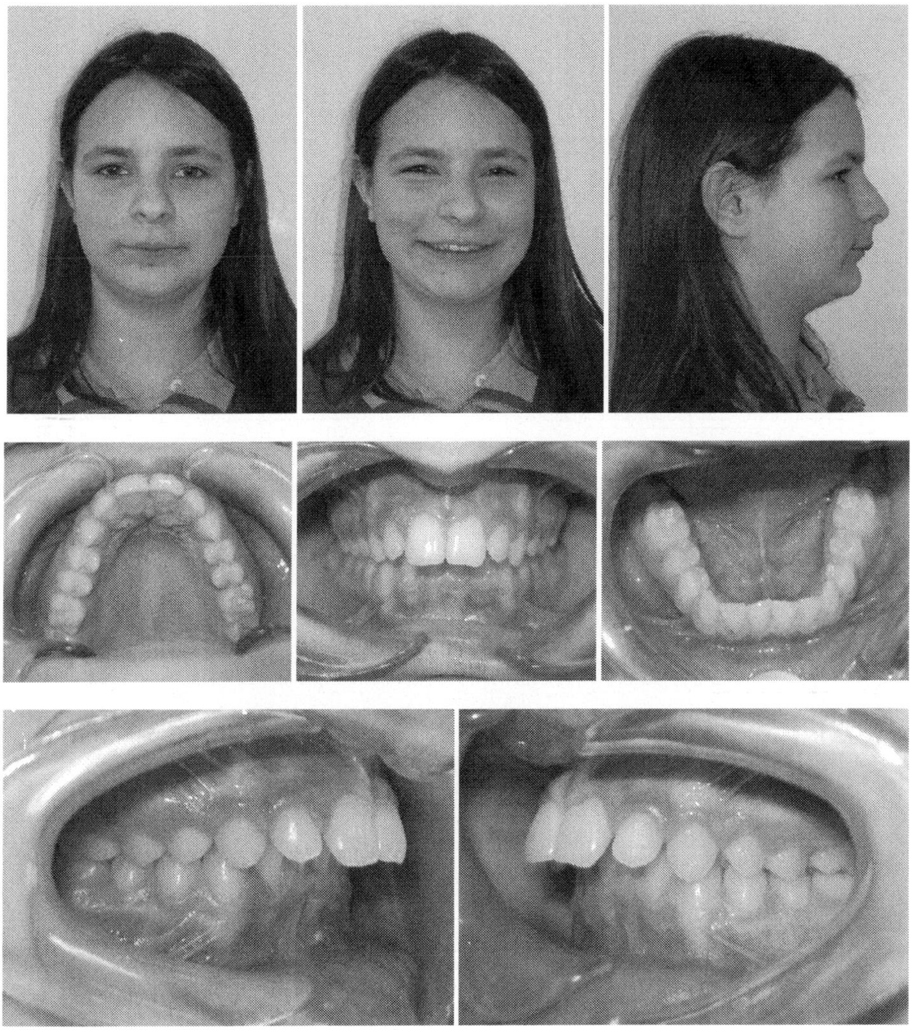

Fig. 5.1. Class II, division 1 patient before treatment (15 years old, female). Extraoral and intraoral photos.

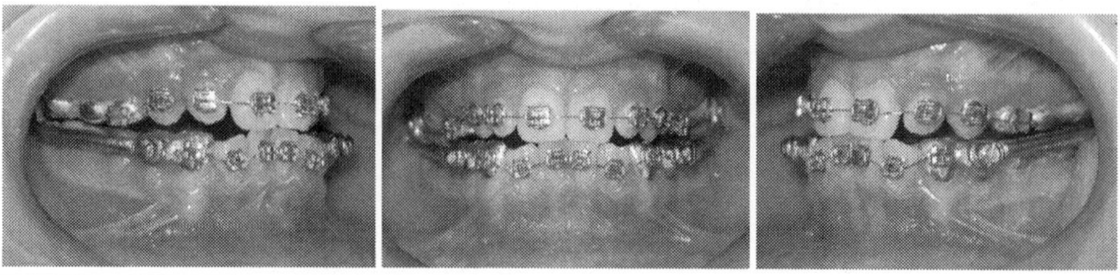

Fig. 5.2. The Herbst appliance and segmented multibracket appliance.

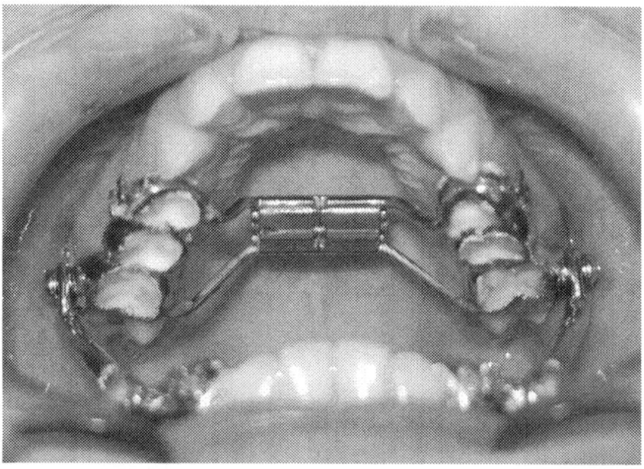

a)

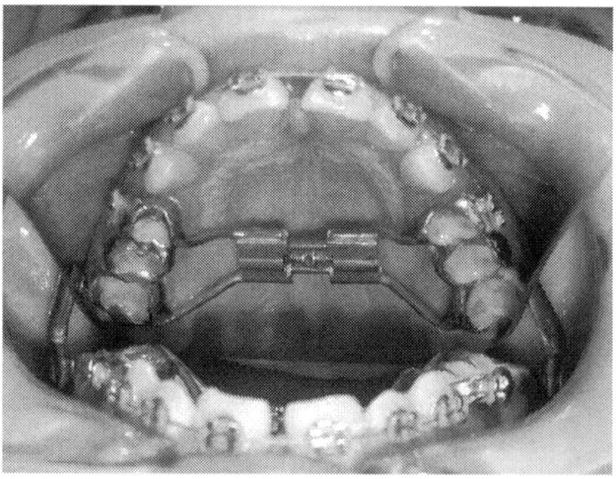

b)

Fig. 5.3. Sagittal and transversal treatment effects: a) The cast splint Herbst appliance with Rapid palatal expander (RPE), b) Headgear effect of Herbst appliance (diastema between canine and first premolar) and transversal RPE effect (diastema mediana).

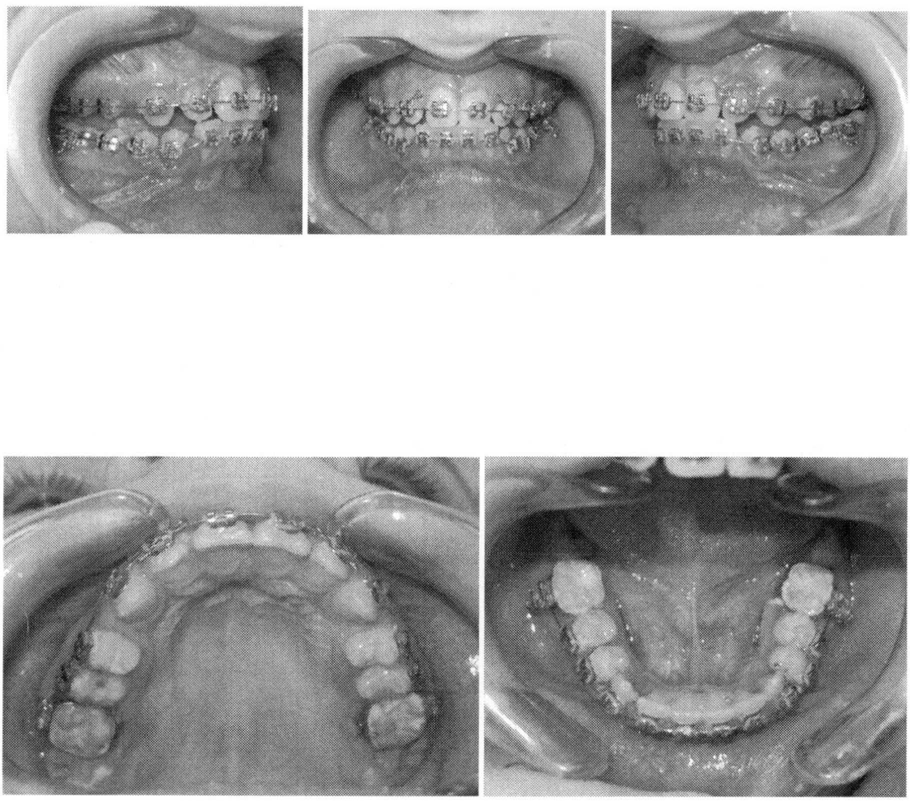

Fig. 5.4. Removed Herbst appliance (after 7 months) and completed multibracket appliance.

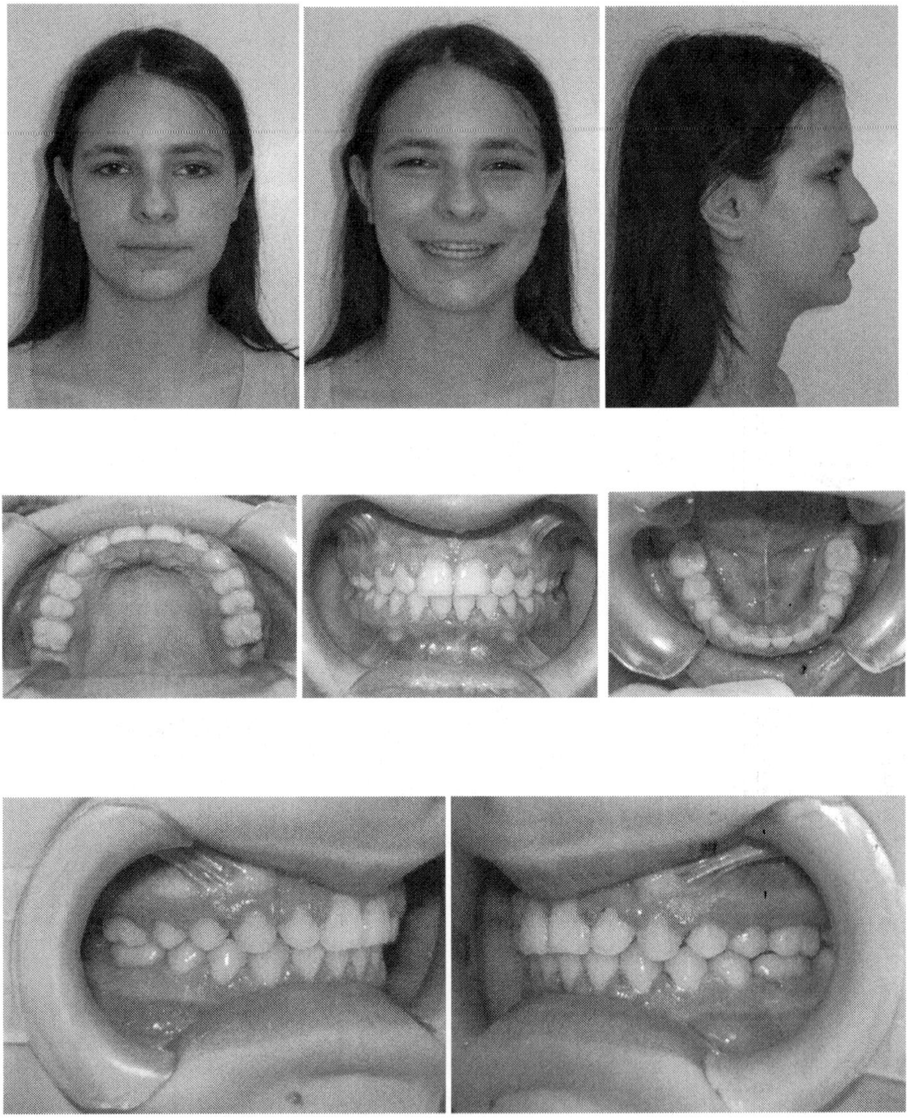

Fig. 5.5. The end of treatment (patient after 15 months of treatment). Extraoral and intraoral photos.

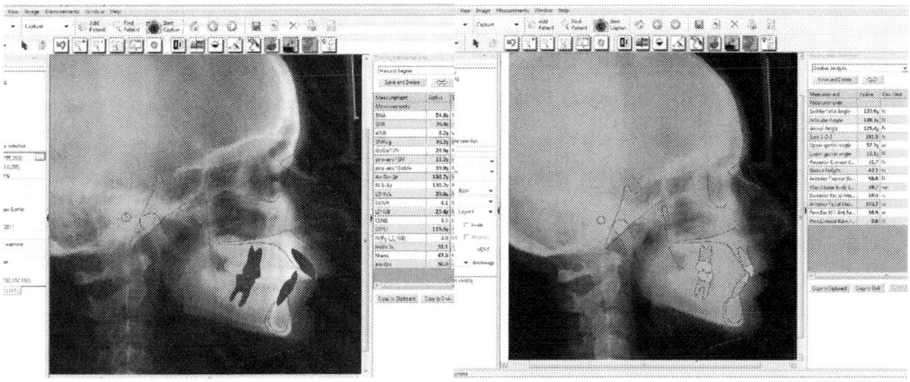

(a) (b)

Fig. 5.6. Cephalometric diagnostic records: a) before treatment and b) after treatment.

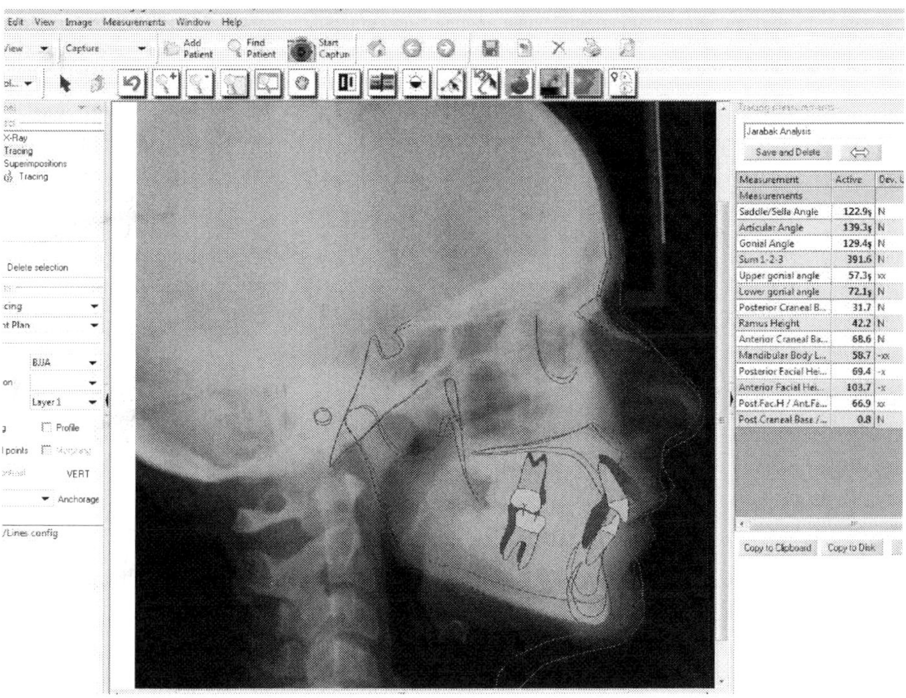

Fig. 5.7. Superimposition of cephalograms before (brown) and after (blue) treatment.

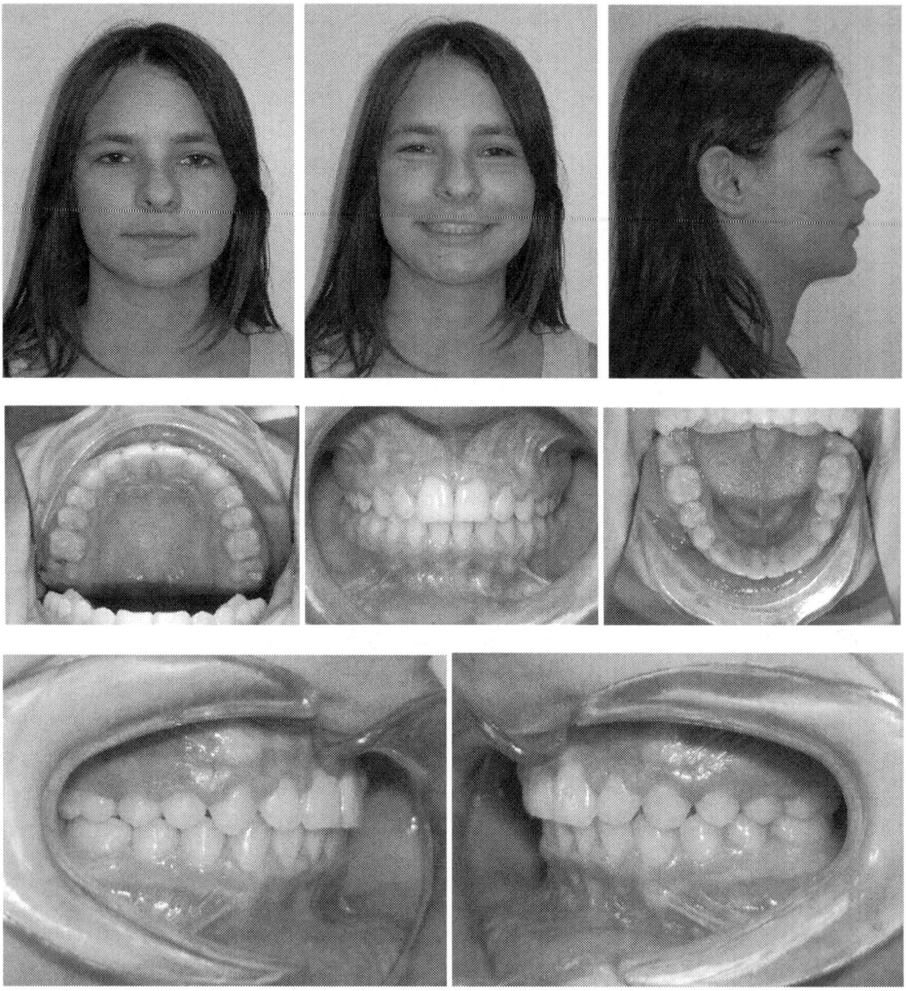

Fig. 5.8. Ten months in retention period after the end of treatment. Extraoral and intraoral photos.

4. Discussion

In the recent years, Pancherz analysis has been accepted by numerous orthodontists as a very reliable method of assessment of sagittal skeletal and dentoalveolar changes in longitudinal studies (Pancherz, 1981, 1982, 1989, 1991, 1994, 1997; Pancherz & Anehus-Pancherz 1993; Pancherz & Michailidou, 2004; Ruf & Pancherz, 1996, 1998, 1999, 2000, 2004; O'Brien et al., 2002, 2004; You & Hagg, 2002, Konik et al., 1997; Cura et al., 1996; Chen & Shen, 2003; Paulsen, 1997; Lin & Gu, 2005; Hansen & Pancherz, 1992; Hansen et al., 1997;

etc.). It is particualarly used to monitor treatment effects in patients before and after treatment.

1. ms-RLp: The analysis of sagittal position of the upper molar before and after treatment showed statistically significant difference (p<0.01). Before treatment, ms–RLp amounted to 54.70mm, and after treatment 53.74mm. The average total movement of point ms distally was 0.96mm. Namely, distalization of this tooth occurred as a result of headgear effect of the Herbst appliance on the upper molars (Table 2., Fig. 5.3., 5.7.). There was no significant difference for this parameter in the Activator group before and after treatment (p=ns). The total movement of ms point was slightly mesially and amounted to 0.18 mm on average.

2. mi-RLp: The analysis of sagittal position of the lower molar before and after treatment showed statistically significant difference (p<0.001) in both groups, due to mesial movement of the lower molars. The average mi–RLp in the Herbst group before treatment was 53.10mm, and after treatment 55.76 mm, and in the Activator group it was 51.14mm before treatment, and 52.98mm after treatment. The overall average movement of mi point mesially was 2.66mm in the Herbst group, and 1.84mm in the Activator group. In the treatment of skeletal Class II malocclusion using functional appliances, this is a common finding. It is usually explained by the loss of mandibular anchorage for skeletal bite correction associated with dentoalveolar changes and occlusal compensation (Table 2., Fig. 5.6., 5.7.).

3. (ms-RLp) - (mi-RLp): molar relationship correction: There was an overall change in molar sagittal relationship amounting to average 3.62 mm in the Hersbt group, due to the distalization of the upper molars and mesial movement of the lower molars (Fig. 5.7.). In the Activator group, this change was significantly smaller - 1.66mm.

The comparison between the Herbst and Activator group for parameters of the sagittal position of the upper and lower molar showed statistical difference for both parameters (p<0.01), which suggests greater molar movement during Herbst treatment (Table 3.).

4. is-RLp: The analysis of sagittal position of the upper incisor before and after treatment showed statistically significant difference (p<0.001) in the Herbst group. Before treatment, mi-RLp amounted to 86.90mm, and after treatment 83.82mm. The overall average movement of is point posteriorly was 3.32mm. Namely, the retrusion of the front teeth occurred as a result of headgear effect of the Herbst appliance on the upper molars and fixed multibracket appliance on the front teeth (Table 4., Fig. 5.6., 5.7.). This is a common finding with this type of treatment. The retrusion of the upper incisors occurred in the Activator group as well, with somewhat smaller statistical significance (p<0.01). The mean pretreatment is-RLp was 85.86 mm and post treatment 84.62 mm. The average overall movement of point is distally was 1.24mm.

5. ii-RLp: The analysis of sagittal position of the lower incisor before and after treatment showed statistically significant difference (p<0.001) in both examined groups, because of mesial movement of the lower lateral teeth and protrusion of the incisor teeth. The mean pretreatment and post treatment value of ii-RLp was 75.60 mm and 80.46 mm in the Herbst group, respectively 76.56 mm and 78.66 mm in the Activator group. The overall average movement of ii point mesialy was 4.86mm in the Herbst group, and 2.10 mm in the Activator group. This treatment effect on the lower incisors can be explained by the loss of mandibular anchorage for skeletal bite correction (Table 4., Fig. 5.6., 5.7.).

6. (is-RLp) - (ii-RLp): overjet correction: In the Herbst group, there was an overall change in incisor position and overjet correction by 8.18 mm, as a result of the upper incisor retrusion and lower incisor protrusion (Fig. 5.1.-5.8.). In the Activator group, the average overjet reduction was only 3.34 mm (Table 4.).

The comparison between the Herbst and Activator group for parameters of the sagittal position of the upper and lower front teeth showed statistical difference for both parameters ($p<0.001$), which suggests greater incisor movement in the sense of the upper incisor retrusion and lower incisor protrusion during Herbst treatment (Table 5.). Prominent lower incisor protrusion is not always desirable since there is a higher risk of relapse in the lower front teeth after treatment.

7.ss-RLp: The analysis of sagittal position of the upper jaw (ss point) in the Herbst group before and after treatment showed statistically significant difference ($p<0.05$). Namely, the ss point (in cephalometric analysis frequently marked as point A) moved backward due to the headgear effect of the Herbst appliance and fixed multibracket appliance on the maxillary front teeth retrusion (Fig. 5.7.). The average pretreatment and post treatment distance from point ss to RLp was 77.28 mm and 76.72 mm. The average overall backward movement of ss point was 0.52 mm. This therapeutic effect can be explained as a consequence of the headgear effect of the Herbst appliance, as well as the headgear appliance too, that occurs due to the influence of orthopedic forces. They lead to maxillary growth disabling. The front teeth retrusion and their correct torque that cause the anterior part of the apical base (the anterior side of the maxilla) to follow the backward movement of the upper front teeth roots, leads to backward movement of the ss point too. In the Activator group, there was statistically significant difference regarding the position of ss point before and after treatment ($p<0.05$). In this case, however, ss point was 77.04 mm before treatment and 77.40 mm after treatment, which implies that it moved forward (Table 6.). The average overall forward movement of ss point was 0.36 mm. This finding is associated with mild forward sagittal growth of the maxilla.

8. Pg-RLp: The analysis of sagittal position of the lower jaw (Pg point) in the Herbst group before and after treatment showed statistically significant difference ($p<0.001$). Namely, Pg point moved forward, which means that the position of the mandible became more mesial (Fig. 5.7.). The average pretreatment and post treatment distance from point Pg to RLp was 76.80 mm and 79.98 mm. The average overall forward movement of Pg point was 3.18 mm. The treatment effect of functional appliance on mandibular growth and anterior displacement is a debatable issue. Namely, this claim is difficult to confirm since the treatment is provided mainly in the ideal treatment period of prepubertal growth spurt. In this study, however, the patients were in a declining growth phase with little residual growth. As we said, Herbst treatment effects come from the fact that skeleto-facial growth continues many years after the cessation of body height growth and that the TMJ in adults is capable of remodeling too. Also, in the Activator group, there was statistical difference regarding the position of Pg point before and after treatment with smaller statistical significance ($p<0.01$). In this case, the average distance from point Pg to RLp was 77.76 mm before treatment and 79.26 mm after treatment. The average overall forward movement of Pg point was 1.50 mm (Table 6.).

9.(ss-RLp) - (Pg-RLp): skeletal correction: In the Herbst group, there was the overall skeletal change - correction of 3.70 mm due to the backward movement of ss point by 0.52 mm and mesial movement of Pg point by 3.18 mm. In the Activator group, the skeletal correction was only 1.14 mm (Table 6.).

The comparison between the Herbst and Activator group for the parameters of maxillary and mandibular sagittal position, the points ss and Pg, showed statistical significance for both parameters ($p<0.01$), which implied greater skeletal changes during Herbst treatment

(Table 7.), in the sense of backward movement of ss point due to headgear effect of the Herbst appliance and greater mesial movement of Pg point due to anterior displacement of the mandible.

The parameters of the upper and lower molar correction: 10. **(ms-RLp) - (ss-RLp)** and 11. **(mi-RLp) - (Pg-RLp)** provide the data on the overall molar position in relation to the skeletal changes: 12. **(ms-ss) - (mi-Pg).** The results suggest that the overall molar position correction in the Herbst group was 0.08 mm and in the Activator group 0.52mm (Table 8.).

The parameters of the upper and lower incisor correction: 13. **(is-RLp) - (ss-RLp)** and 14. **(ii-RLp) - (Pg-RLp)** provide the data on the overall incisor position in relation to the skeletal changes: 15. **(is-ss) - (ii-Pg).** The results suggest that the overall incisor position correction in the Herbst group was 4.48 mm and in the Activator group 2.20 mm (Table 8.).

The last part of Pancherz analysis provides very important information on the comparable analysis of the treatment effects of Herbst and Activator appliance (Table 9.). The testing of statistical differences of treatment effects parameters (molar relationship correction, overjet correction, skeletal relationship correction, molar correction and incisor correction) between the examined groups confirmed the following:

1. a high level of statistical significance ($p<0.001$) was established in the comparison of molar relationship correction as a result of greater changes occurring during Herbst treatment,
2. a high level of statistical significance ($p<0.001$) was established in the comparison of overjet correction as a result of greater changes occurring during Herbst treatment,
3. a high level of statistical significance ($p<0.001$) was established in the comparison of skeletal relationship correction as a result of greater changes occurring during Herbst treatment,
4. no statistical significance was established between the examined groups (p=ns) in the comparison of molar correction,
5. a high level of statistical significance ($p<0.001$) was established in the comparison of incisor correction as a result of greater changes occurring during Herbst treatment.

Konik et al. (1997) investigated the Herbst effects in older patients, i.e. the patients that had passed the ideal period for functional therapy. They compared the effects of the Herbst appliance in older patients (late Herbst treatment - 21 subjects in stages MP3-E and F) and younger patients that are in prepubertal growth spurt period (early Herbst treatment - 22 subjects in stages MP3-H and I). They concluded that the Herbst appliance is equally effective both in adolescents and in young adults. This finding is in accordance with the findings by Pancherz & Ruf (2000) and Pancherz (2008). Also, conclusion of Von Bremen et al., (2009) research was: Herbst treatment can be considered equally efficient in adolescent and in adult Class II, division 1 subjects.

Sagittal skeletal changes in Herbst treatment were reported by many authors (Pancherz, 1981, 1982, 1989, 1991, 1994, 1997; Pancherz & Ruf, 1999, 2000, 2008; Pancherz et al., 1989; Pancherz & Fischer, 2003; Ruf & Pancherz, 1996, 1998, 1999, 2000, 2004; Ruf et al., 2001; White, 1994; Paulsen, 1997; Shen & Hagg, 2005; Smith, 1998, 2000; Graber et al., 1997; Windmiller, 1993; Weschler & Pancherz, 2005; Baltromejus et al., 2002; Dischinger, 1995, 1998; Du et al., 2002; Hansen et al., 1997; Hanks, 2003; Howe & McNamara, 1983; McNamara et al., 1990; O'Brien et al., 2003; Siara-Olds et al. 2010). These changes mainly relate to a more anterior position of the mandible as a result of mandibular growth stimulation and adaptation combined with TMJ remodelation. The headgear effect of the Herbst appliance on the upper jaw and upper molars combined with multibracket fixed appliance effect on the frontal teeth retrusion can lead to the maxillary growth restriction and movement of point ss posteriorly. This Herbst effect was mostly examined by Pancherz (1982, 1987) and Ruf & Pancherz (2008). Valant & Sinclair (1989) state that the reduction of ANB angle at the end of treatment was achieved by mesial movement of the mandible by 1.3 mm as a result of growth stimulation and maxillary growth restriction and posterior movement of point A by 0.7 mm. This finding is concurrent with results from our study. The similar conclusion was reached by Creekmore & Radney (1983) in a investigation on Fränkel regulator treatment effects in patients with Class II malocclusion. Konik et al. (1997) compared the effects of the Herbst appliance in older patients (late Herbst treatment) and younger patients that are in prepubertal growth spurt period (early Herbst treatment). They concluded that the Herbst appliance had led to the maxillary growth restriction (the movement of point ss-OLP after treatment amounted to 0.1mm with SD±1.2). The movement of point Pg anteriorly was 2.4mm ± 2.2. Siara-Olds et al. (2010) found that the Herbst appliance significantly restricted maxillary growth, comparing to other functional appliances in the treatment of skeletal Class II malocclusion.

Examining the effects of removable functional appliances during pubertal growth spurt, in Class II, division 1 treatment, some authors concluded that changes on the maxilla occurred as well. In Activator treatment these findings were reported by Harvold & Vargervik (1971), Baltromejus et al. (2002), Pancherz (1984), Cozza et al. (2006), Jakobson (1967) and Moreira et al. (2003) achieved maxillary growth restriction by Bionator treatment. Milosavljevic (2006) examined the effects of the Twin block appliance in Class II, division 1 treatment and reported the similar result. Fränkel (1969) confirmed slowed maxillary growth by means of a function regulator. McNamara et al. (1990) did not point out the similar result. Many research studies investigated whether functional appliance treatment produced a stimulation effect on mandibular growth or resulted in mesial movement only, i.e. whether skeletal or dentoalveolar changes occurred Chen et al. (2002), De Vincenzo (1991), Bascifci et al. (2003) and Nelson et al. (1993) in their studies on the Activator effects observed the increased growth of the mandible. In treatment of distal bite with Balters Bionator, the increased mandibular growth was reported by Moreira et al. (2003). However, other authors have found that there was only mesial movement of the mandible without any significant growth changes (Jorgensen, 1974; Wieslander & Lagerström, 1979; Pancherz, 1979, 1984; Cozza et al., 2006; Milosavljevic, 2006).

Comparing treatment effects of the Herbst and Activator appliance and monitoring changes of point Pg during treatment, Baltromejus et al. (2002) found great variations in both groups. In the Activator group Pg point moved anteriorly and caudally ($p<0.001$). In the Herbst group Pg point also moved anteriorly and caudally ($p<0.001$). Compared with the Activator group, the amount of changes in Pg point during Herbst treatment was smaller in both sagittal ($p<0{,}001$) and vertical direction ($p<0{,}001$). The mean age of Herbst and Activator subjects was 12.6 years and 10.3 years, respectively. There were no sex differences found in any group concerning the direction of Pg point changes.

The headgear effect of the Herbst appliance on the maxilla produces dentolaveolar effect on the upper molars. This can be seen in the upper molar distalization, which is a common finding in studies. The headgear effect of the Herbst appliance alongside with the effect of the multibracket fixed appliance produces dentoalveolar effect on the front teeth, which is reflected in the upper incisor retrusion. In addition, activation forces on the lower jaw and the anchorage incorporating the lower first molars can lead to mesial bodily movement of of these teeth. The strong activation forces on the mandible and the movement of the entire lower dental arch mesially particularly are reflected on the lower front teeth (Allen-Noble, 2003; Baltromejus et al., 2002; Dischinger, 1995, 1998; Du et al., 2002; Hansen et al., 1997; Hanks, 2003; Howe, 1982; McNamara et al., 1990; O'Brien et al., 2003; Pancherz, 1981, 1982, 1989, 1991, 1994, 1997; Pancherz & Ruf, 1999, 2000, 2008; Pancherz et al., 1989; Pancherz & Fischer, 2003; Ruf & Pancherz, 1996, 1998, 1999, 2000, 2004; Ruf et al., 2001; White, 1994; Schavioni et al., 1992; Shen & Hagg, 2005; Smith, 1998, 2000; Valant & Sinclair, 1989; Graber et al., 1997; Windmiller, 1993; Weschler & Pancherz, 2005). In essence, the entire lower arch moved mesially, excluding skeletal movements. The lower front teeth protrusion occurs, which is preferable when the lower incisors are retruded. However, the protrusion of the lower incisors frequently occurs when it is undesirable. It is mainly due to the loss of anchorage in the mandible. Konik et al. (1997) state that dentoalveolar movements such as distalization of the upper molars and mesial movement of the lower molars are more prominent in older patients with Class II, division 1 malocclusion treated with the Herbst appliance than in adolescent patients. Protrusion of the lower incisors and retrusion of the upper incisors, induced by the Herbst treatment in older patients with Class II, division 1 malocclusion, are more prominent than in adolescents. In older patients, the anchorage system includes the upper front teeth, while this can not be done in adolescents due to their mixed dentition. The lower front teeth were more protruded during Herbst treatment in adults, mainly because of stronger forces induced by the telescopic mechanism on the lower dental arch and relative loss of anchorage in the lower jaw. O'Brien et al. (2003) state that the Herbst appliance was more effective in overjet reduction in phase I of treatment in comparison with the Twin block appliance. In the study by Voudouris et al. (2003) on monkeys treated with the Herbst appliances, cephalometric superimposition on maxillary implants showed that in experimental animals the first permanent molars moved distally and were slightly intruded, and mandibular first molars moved mesially and slightly inferiorly, which was in accordance with the findings in humans. The upper incisors moved palatally and were extruded, but the mandibular incisors moved labially, inferiorly and tipped mesially. The incisors moved minimally in untreated animal control group but without statistical significance. Scepan (1997) in research on the effects of the Activator treatment states that the upper molars inclined distally while the lower molars moved mesially. McNamara et al. (1990) report greater distal movement of the upper molars in patients treated with the Herbst appliance in comparison with the removable Fränkel appliance. The similar was reported by O'Brien et al. (2003) who compared treatment effects of the Herbst and Twin block appliance.

5. The future

Based on the literature review, results of this study and clinical experience, early treatment of patients with Class II malocclusions should be provided with removable functional appliances since these appliances are more efficient and easier to manipulate in younger children (adolescents). On the other hand, treatment with the Herbst appliance should be provided mainly in patients who are in post pubertal stage of development and have their permanent dentition; in this age and dental-alveolar-skeletal developmental phase, removable appliances are less efficient and patient compliance is decreased.

As mentioned above, a recent clinical cephalometric roentgenographic investigation and MRI investigation has shown that the Herbst appliance is very effective in patients with Class II malocclusion at the end of their growth (radius union: Deicke & Pancherz, 2005). Therefore, we consider this method to be an alternative to orthognatic surgery in many adult patients with Class II malocclusions. The findings from the study of Ruf & Pancherz (2004) comparing young adults with Class II malocclluison either treated with the Herbst appliance or with mandibular sagittal split osteotomy support our opinion. Comparable changes in sagittal maxillary/mandibular jaw base relationship and skeletal profile convexity can be observed in both groups at the end of treatment (after final teeth alignment with a fixed appliance). Furthermore, in comparison with surgery, Herbst treatment implies lower costs and lower risks for the patient without increasing total treatment time (Pancherz & Ruf, 2000). Growth adaptation should be performed with removable functional appliances in children and adolescents with mixed dentition since these appliances are more effective and easier to handle in younger children. However, in adolescents who have their permanent dentition, postadolescents and in young adults, fixed functional appliances, such as the Herbst appliance, are usually indicated. The approximate age for young adulthood would be 18 to 24 years in females and 20 to 25 years in males. An upper age limit for successful Herbst treatment is, however, difficult to define. Konik et al. (1997) have concluded that the optimal timing for treatment of Class II, division 1 subjects with the Herbst appliance is the period after the pubertal growth spurt (in young adults with the permanent dentition) since the results are the most stable in Class I occlusion. The late Herbst treatment reduces the need for prolonged retention period after treatment and the possibility of relapse.

Camouflage orthodontics mainly comprises tooth sacrifice in the maxillary dental arch to create space for retraction of the anterior teeth. However, by this approach the skeletal Class II problem (mandibular retrusion) remains. Surgical correction implies that that the mandible is advanced to a Class I skeletal jaw relationship using either sagittal split osteotomy or mandibular distraction osteogenesis. Occasionally, mandibular advancement is combined with maxillary setback surgery (Le Fort I). The philosophical question is based on potential iatrogenic sequelae for primarily cosmetic problem: "What price surgery?" (Pancherz & Ruf, 2000).

The mechanism of growth modification is critical because a specific soft tissue mechanism might guide clinicians to plan appropriate future treatments. Some day treatment could include genetic therapies for condylar growth modification. These technologies could be directed to the soft or hard tissues. This might lead to stable condyle-fossa growth modification in the long term that has been elusive so far. Voudouris et al. (2003) claim that the general functional matrix theory was vague and largely unproven. Their results indicate a more specific mechanism from the connective tissues and the fluids in the growth relativity concept that uses more than muscle function alone to explain and achieve the clinical results of Herbst therapy. Nowadays, at the beginning of the 21st century, we can claim the following: Fixed functional appliances (Herbst) produce consistent changes in the condyl-fossa complex that can be reproduced in comparison with the inconsistent results reported in the literature for removable functional appliances (Voudouris et al., 2003).

As for the future design of the Herbst appliance, there are three goals (Hanks, 2003): to reduce the number of emergency appointments (breakage, particularly with banded splints, disengagement), to increase patient comfort (hygiene, possible ulcerations of the mucosa on the distal assembly) and to transform the Herbst into a more user-friendly appliance (easier access, particularly to distal assemblies).

6. Conclusion

The clinical effect of the Herbst appliance and Activator in treatment of Class II, division 1 malocclusions shows significant improvement of the occlusal relationships because of sagittal skeletal and dentoalveolar changes in both jaws.

Class II molar correction in patients treated by the Herbst appliance and Class II molar improvement in patients treated by the Activator, are results of forward mandibular movement and posterior movement of the maxillary molars.

Overjet correction in patients treated by the Herbst appliance and overjet reduction in patients treated by the Activator, result from the mandibular advancement, proclination of mandibular incisors and retroinclination of maxillary incisors.

The Herbst appliance is more efficient in the correction of Class II, division 1 malocclusion in the patients after pubertal peak of growth, compared to the Activator, due to more prominent skeletal, dentoalveolar and combined changes.

7. References

Ahlgren, J. & Laurin, C. (1976). Late results of activator treatment: a cephalometric study. *Bri J Orthod, Vol.* 3, pp. 181–187.

Allen-Noble, P. (2003). Multifunctional Herbst Solutions. *Clinical Impressions,* Vol. 12, No. 2, pp. 26-27.

Bastiftici, A.F.; Uysal, T.; Buyukerkmen, A. & San, Z. (2003). The effects of activator treatment on the craniofacial structures of class II/1 patients. *Eur J Orthod,* Vol. 25, No. 1, pp. 87-94.

Baltromejus, S.; Ruf, S. & Pancherz, H. (2002). Effective Temporomandibular joint growth and chin position changes: Activator versus Herbst treatment. A Cephalometric roentgenographic study. *Eur J Orthod,* Vol. 24, No. 6, pp. 627–637.

Bjork, A. (1951). The principle of the Andresen method of orthodontic treatment, a discussion based on cephalometric X-ray analysis of treated cases. *Am J Orthod,* Vol. 37, pp. 437–458.

Chen, R.J.; Will, L. & Niederman, R. (2002). Analysis of efficacy of functional appliances on mandibular growth. *Am J Orthod Dentofacial Orthop,* Vol. 122, pp. 470–476.

Chen, R.J. & Shen, G. (2003). The feasibility and reliability of Pancherz's analysis in evaluating the treatment effects of bite-jumping on skeletal class II malocclusion. *Shang J Stom,* Vol. 12, No. 4, pp. 256–259. *Am J Orthod Dentofacial Orthop,* Vol. 122, pp. 470–476.

Cozza, P.; Bracceti, T.; Franchi, L.; De Toffol, T. & McNamara J.A. (2006). Mandibular changes produced by functional appliances in Class II malocclusion: a sistematic review. *Am J Orthod Dentofacial Orthop,* Vol. 129, pp. 599- 12.

Creekmore, T.D. & Radney, L.J. (1983). Fränkel appliance therapy: Orthopedic or orthodontic? *Am J Orthod,* Vol. 82, pp. 89-108.

Cura, N.; Sarac, M.; Ozturk, Y. & Surmeli N. (1996). Orthodontic and orthopedic effects of Activator, Activator-HG combination and Bass appliances: A comparative study. *Am J Orthod Dentofac Orthop*, Vol. 110, pp. 36–45.

Deicke, M. & Pancherz, H. (2005). Is Radius-Union an indicator for completed facial growth? *Angle Orthod*, Vol. 75, No. 3, pp. 287–291.

DeVincenzo, J. (1991). Changes in mandibular lenght before, during and after successful orthopedic correction of Class II malocclusions, using a functional appliance. *Am J Orthod Dentofac Orthop*, Vol. 99, pp. 241–257.

Dischinger, T. (1995). Edgewise Herbst appliance. J Clin Orthod, Vol. 29, No. 12, pp. 738–742.

Dischinger, T. (1998). Full-face Orthopedic with One Multifunctional Appliance - No Cooperation Required. *Clinical impressions*, Vol. 4, No. 7, pp. 2-7.

Du, X.; Hagg, U. & Rabie, B. (2002). Effects of headgear Herbst and mandibular step - by - step advancement versus conventional herbst appliance and maximal jumping of the mandible. *Eur J Orthod*, Vol. 24, No. 2, pp. 167–174.

Fränkel, R. (1969). The treatment of Class II, division 1 malocclusion with functional correctors. *Am J Orthod*, Vol. 54, pp. 265-275.

Graber, T.; Rakosi, T. & Petrovic, A. (1997). *Dentofacial orthopedics with Functional appliances*. Mosby.

Hansen, K. & Pancherz, H. (1992). Long-term effects of Herbst treatment in relation to normal growth development: a cephalometric study. *Eur J Orthod*, Vol. 14, pp. 285-295.

Hansen, K.; Koutsonas, K.T. & Pancherz, H. (1997). Long-term effects of Herbst treatment on the mandibular incisor segment: A cephalometric and biometric investigation. *Am J Orthod Dentofac Orthop*, Vol. 112, pp. 92-103.

Hanks, S. (2003). Herbst therapy: Trying to get out of the 20th Century. *Good practice*, Vol. 4, No. 1, pp. 2–4.

Harvold, E.P. & Vargervik, K. (1971). Morphogenetic responce to activator treatment. *Am J Orthod*, Vol. 60, pp. 478–490.

Howe, R.P. (1982). The bonded Herbst appliance. *J Clin Orthod*, Vol. 10, pp. 663–667.

Howe, R.P. & McNamara, J.A. (1983). Clinical management of the bonded Herbst appliance. *J Clin Orthod*, Vol. 17, No. 7, pp. 456–463.

Jacobsson, S.O. (1967). Cephalometric evaluation of treatment effect on Class II, Division 1 malocclusions. *Am J Orthod*, Vol. 6, pp. 446-457.

Jacobsson, S.O. & Paulin, G. (1990). The influence of activator treatment on skeletal growth in Angle II, 1 cases. A roentgenocephalometric study. *Eur J Orthod*, Vol. 12, pp. 174–184.

Jorgensen, S.E. (1974). Activators in orthodontic treatment: Indications and advantages. *Am J Orthod*, Vol. 65, pp. 260-269.

Konik, M.; Pancherz, H. & Hansen, K. (1997). The mechanism of Class II correction in late Herbst treatment, *Am J Orthod Dentofac Orthop*, Vol. 112, pp. 87-91.

Korkhaus, G. (1960). Present orthodontic thought in Germany. *Am J Orthod*, Vol. 46, pp. 270–287.

Lin, J. & Gu, Y. (2005). Lower second molar extraction in correction of severe skeletal class III maloclusion. *Angle Orthod*, Vol. 76, No. 2, pp. 217–225.

Luder, H.U. (1982). Skeletal profile changes related to two patterns of activator effects. *Am J Orthod*, Vol. 80, pp. 390-396.

McNamara, J.A.; Howe, R.P. & Dischinger T.G. (1990). A comparison of the Herbst and Frankel appliances in the treatment of Class II malocclusion. *Am J Orthod Dentofacial Orthop*, Vol. 98, pp. 134-144.

Milosavljevic, Z. (2006). *Treatment effects of Twin Block appliance in the therapy of Class II malocclusion*. Doctoral thesis, Belgrade, Serbia.

Moreira, M.C.; Santos-Pinto, A.; Rosa Martins, C.; Martins, P. & Sakima T. (2003). Orthopedic and orthodontic components of Class II, division 1 malocclusion correction with Balters Bionator: A cephalometric study with metallic implants. *World J Orthod*, Vol. 4, pp. 237-242.

Nelson, C.; Harkness, M. & Herbison P. (1993). Mandibular changes during functional appliance treatment. *Am J Orthod Dentofacial Orthop*, Vol. 104, pp. 153-161.

O'Brien, K. at all. (2003). Effectiveness of treatment for Class II malocclusion with the Herbst or twin-block appliances: A randomized, controlled trial. *Am J Orthod Dentofacial Orthop*, Vol. 124, No. 2, pp. 128-137.

O'Brien, K. at all. (2003). Effectiveness of early orthodontic treatment with the Twin-block appliance: A multicenter, randomized, controlled trial. Part 1: Dental and skeletal effects. *Am J Orthod Dentofacial Orthop*, Vol. 124, No. 3, pp. 234-243.

O'Brien, K. & Wright, J. (2002). How to write a protocol. J Orthod, Vol. 29, No. 1, pp. 58–61.

O'Relly, T. & Yanneillo, G. (1988). Mandibular growth changes and maturation of cervical vertebrae - A longitudinal cephalometric study. Angle Orthod, Vol. 4, pp. 179–184.

Pancherz, H. (1979). The mandibular plane angle in activator treatment. *Angle Orthod*, Vol. 49, pp. 11–20.

Pancherz, H. & Stickel, A. (1980). Can 'articulare' be used in the cephalometric analysis of mandibular lenght? A methodologic study. *Eur J Orthod*, Vol. 10, No. 1, pp. 362–368.

Pancherz, H. (1981). The effect of continuous bite jumping on the dentofacial complex: A follow-up study after Herbst appliance treatment of Class II malocclusions. *Eur J Orthod*, Vol. 3, pp. 49–60.

Pancherz, H. (1982). The mechanism of Class II correction in Herbst appliance treatment. A cephalometric investigation. *Am J Orthod*, Vol. 82, pp. 104-113.

Pancherz, H. (1984). A cephalometric analysis of skeletal and dental changes contributing to Class II correction in activator treatment. Am J Orthod, Vol. 85, pp. 125–134.

Pancherz, H.; Malmgren, O. & Haag, U. (1989). Class II correction in Herbst and Bass therapy. *Eur J Orthod*, Vol. 11, pp. 17–30.

Pancherz, H. (1989). Die Herbst-Apparatur in der modernen Kiferorthopadie, *Informationen*, Vol. 4, pp. 467-490.

Pancherz, H. (1991). The nature of Class II relapse after Herbst appliance treatment: A cephalometric long-term investigation. *Am J Orthod Dentofacial Orthop*, Vol. 100, pp. 220–233.

Pancherz, H. & Anehus-Pancherz, M. (1993). The headgear effect of the Herbst appliance: A cephalometric long-term study. *Am J Orthod Dentofacial Orthop*, Vol. 103, No. 6, pp. 510–520.

Pancherz, H. (1994). Das Herbstsche Scharnier, *Kieferorthop*, Vol. 8, pp. 125-131.

Pancherz, H. (1997). The effects, limitations, and long-term dentofacial adaptations to treatment with the Herbst appliance. Semin Orthod, Vol. 3, No. 4, pp. 232–243.

Pancherz, H.; Zeiber, K. & Hoyer, B. (1997). Cephalometric characteristics of Class II division 1 and Class II division 2malocclusions: A comparative study in children. *Angle Orthod*, Vol. 2, pp. 111-20.

Pancherz, H. & Ruf, S. (1999). Thomalske-Faubert C.: Mandibular articular disk position changes during Herbst treatment: a prospective longitudinal MRI study. *Am J Orthod Dentofacial Orthop,* Vol. 116, pp. 207-214.

Pancherz, H. & Ruf, S. (2000). The Herbst Appliance: Research - based updated clinical possibilities. *World J Orthod*, Vol. 1, No. 1, pp. 17-31.

Pancherz, H. & Fischer, S. (2003). Amount and direction of temporomandibular joint growth changes in Herbst treatment: A cephalometric long-term investigation. *Angle Orthod*, Vol. 73, pp. 493–501.

Pancherz, H. & Michailidou, C. (2004). Temporoandibular joint growth changes in hyperdivergent and hypodivergent Herbst subjects. A long-term roentgenographic study. *Am J Orthod Dentofacial Orthop, Vol. 126, No. 2, pp. 153–161.*

Pancherz, H.; Ruf, S.; Erbe, C. & Hansen K. (2004). The mechanism of Class II correction in Surgical Orthodontic treatment of Adult Class II, Division 1 malocclusion. *Angle Orthod*, Vol. 74, pp. 800–809.

Pancherz, H. & Ruf, S. (2008). *The Herbst appliance*. Quintessence Publishing Co Ltd, Grafton Road, Great Britain.

Paulsen, H.U. (1997). Morphological changes of the TMJ condyles of 100 patients treated with the Herbst appliance in the period of puberty to adulthood: a long-term radiographic study. *Eur J Orthod*, Vol. 19, pp. 657–688.

Ruf, S. & Pancherz, H. (1996). Development of the frontal sinus in relation to somatic and skeletal maturity. A cephalometric roentgenographic study at puberty. *Eur J Orthod*, Vol. 18, pp. 491–497.

Ruf, S. & Pancherz, H. (1998). Long-term TMJ effects of Herbst treatment: A clinical and MRI study. *Am J Orthod Dentofacial Orthop*, Vol. 114, No. 5, pp. 475–483.

Ruf, S. & Pancherz, H. (1999). Temporomandibular joint remodeling in adolescents and young adults during Herbst treatment: A prospective longitudinal magnetic resonance imaging and cephalometric radiographic investigation. *Am J Orthod Dentofacial Orthop*, Vol. 115, pp. 607-618.

Ruf, S. & Pancherz, H. (1999). Dentoskeletal effects and facial profile changes in young adults treated with the Herbst appliance. Angle Orthod, Vol. 69, pp. 239-246.

Ruf, S. & Pancherz, H. (2000). Does Bite Jumping Damage the TMJ? A Orospective Longitudinal Clinical and MRI Study of Herbst Patients. *Angle Orthod,* Vol. 70, pp. 183-199.

Ruf, S.; Baltromejus, S. & Pancherz, H. (2001). Effective condylar growth and chin position changes in Activator treatment: A cephalometric roentgenographic study. *Angle Orthod,* Vol. 71, No. 1, pp. 4–11.

Ruf, S. & Pancherz, H. (2004). Ortognatic surgery and dentofacial orthopedics in adult Class II division 1 treatment: mandibular sagital split osteotomy versus Herbst appliance. *Am J Orthod Dentofacial Orthop,* Vol. 126, pp. 140–152.

Schavioni, R.; Grenga, V. & Macri, V. (1992). Treatment of Class II high angle malocclusion with the Herbst appliance: A cephalometric investigation. *Am J Orthod Dentofacial Orthop,* Vol. 102, No. 5, pp. 393–409.

Shen, G. & Hagg, U. (2005). Darendeliler MA.: Skeletal effects of bite jumping therapy on the mandible - Removable vs. Fixed functional appliances. *Orthod Craniofacial Res,* Vol. 8, pp. 2–10.

Siara-Olds, N.J.; Pangrazio-Kulbersh, V; Berger, J & Bayirli, B. (2010). Long-Term Dentoskeletal Changes with the Bionator, Herbst, Twin Block, and MARA Functional Appliances. *Angle Orthod,* Vol. 80, No. 1, pp. 18-29.

Smith, R.J. (1998). Matching the Herbst to the malocclusion. *Clinical impressions,* Vol. 2, No. 7, pp. 6-12.

Smith, R.J. (2000). How to improve practice efficiency and profitability. *Clinical Impressions,* Vol. 4, No. 4, pp. 6-21.

Scepan I. (1997). *Functional appliances treatment effects of Class II malocclusions.* Doctoral thesis. Belgrade, Serbia.

Valant, J.R. & Sinclair, P.M. (1989). Treatment effects of the Herbst appliance. *Am J Orthod Dentofacial Orthop,* Vol. 95, pp. 138–147.

Von Bremen, J.; Bock, N. & Ruf, S. (2009). Is Herbst-Multibracket Appliance Treatment More Efficient in Adolescents than in Adults?. Angle Orthod, Vol. 79, No. 1, pp. 173-177.

Voudouris, C.J.; Woodside, G.D. & Kuftinec, M.M. (2003). Condyle-fossa modifications and muscle interactions during Herbst treatment, Part 1. New technological methods. *Am J Orthod Dentofacial Orthop,* Vol. 123, No. 6, pp. 604–613.

Voudouris, J.Ç. at all (2003). Condyle-fosa modifikations and muscle interactions during Herbst treatment, Part 2. Results and conclusions. *Am J Orthod Dentofacial Orthop,* Vol. 124, No. 1, pp. 13–29.

White, L. (1994). Current Herbst appliance therapy. *J Clin Orthod,* Vol. 28, No. 5, pp. 296–309.

Wieslander, L. & Lagerstrom, L. (1979). The effect of activator treatment on Class II malocclusions. *Am J Orthod,* Vol. 1, pp. 20-26.

Windmiller, E. (1993). The acrylic-splint herbst appliance: A cephalometric evaluation. *Am J Orthod Dentofac Orthop,* Vol. 104, pp. 73–84.

Weschler, D. & Pancherz, H. (2005). Efficiency of three mandibular anchorage forms in Herbst treatment: A cephalometric investigation. *Angle Orthod*, Vol. 75, No. 1, pp. 23-27.

You, Q.L. & Hagg, U. (2002). A comparison of three cephalometric analysis on the evaluation of orthodontic treatment. J Stomatol, Vol. 11, No. 2, pp. 97-100.

6

Sterilization and Disinfection in Orthodontics

Alev Aksoy, Gulcın Kılıç, Emad Hussein and Darleen Aboukhalil
Suleyman Demirel University. Faculty of Dentistry. Department of Orthodontics. Isparta Turkey

Devoted for the memory of my beloved father Okay Aksoy who passed away suddenly on 25th of March

1. Introduction

On a daily basis, the practicing dentist and his personnel are at risk of being exposed to a wide range of patients with blood borne diseases such as HIV/AIDS, hepatitis B, hepatitis C, and airborne diseases such as Influenza and Tuberculosis (Değer, 2004; Ozer, 2005). Infection can be directly transmitted by oral fluids, blood, contaminated instruments and surfaces or via the respiratory system (Toroglu et al., 2001; Shah et al., 2009). To accomplish infection control accurately and to reduce the risk of cross contamination, all patients have to be treated while practicing universal precautions, the latter including the imperative steps of disinfection and sterilization (Değer, 2004; Akcam and Ozdiler, 1999).

Orthodontists do not perform oral surgery, but come in direct contact with blood and oral fluids of healthy patients or infectious diseases patients when placing or removing fixed appliances (Toroglu et al., 2001). Some orthodontic instruments used regularly have hinges and cutting edges, and this makes disinfection prior to sterilization a sensitive procedure (Holht et al., 1998). Instruments have to be cleaned and dried prior to sterilization in order to minimize damage and corrosion when applicable, and to increase lifespan.

Various dental supplies and instruments that are used every day make specific studies about infection control necessary, as their components and/or their maintenance procedures might differ. The standards of infection control and universal precautions remain generally unchanged, but technologic advancements, new products, new material and new data require constant evaluation and adjustments of the techniques accordingly (Deger, 2004). It is therefore our obligation to apply the most recent disinfection and sterilization practices to achieve the best results (Akcam and Ozdiler, 1999; Ozer, 2005, Haydar, 2000).

The first general infection control instructions for dentistry were published by Center for Disease Control and Prevention (CDC) in 1986 and are being updated every year in this respect. The main principle is to consider each patient as being infected because many infectious diseases can be present in one individual without any signs and symptoms, especially at an early stage (Külekçi, 2000b). The American Dentist Association recommends to all staff part of the dental team to apply the universal precautions prevent infection and cross-contamination. The universal precautions suggest standard application of infection control and sterilization techniques for each patient. (Külekçi, 2000a; Acar, 2007).

1.1 Flora of the human body

In normal conditions, microorganisms are living inside our body, in different regions and different cavities, and on our skin. The external microorganisms are in continuous contact with living things whereas microbial flora interacts with organisms in our body. Most of the time, the interaction of body flora with organisms continues throughout the person's lifetime without causing any damage. (Değer, 2004)

One of the easiest ways for a microorganism to enter the body is via the oral cavity during respiration and/or eating. (Değer, 2004)

1.1.1 Normal microbial flora

The microorganisms living in harmony in the human body are called "normal microbial flora". Human body flora is part of the normal resistance mechanism of the body, hence it begins to establish as early as birth. Most of its microorganisms are bacteria, although viruses, fungi and protozoa can be present in minority. (Değer, 2004)

1.1.2 Permanent flora

Microorganisms are stabilizing in specific regions at different times. They can be modified for a short period but are reestablished not too long afterwards via the permanent flora. (Değer, 2004)

1.1.3 Oral and upper airway normal flora

Mouth flora is established between six and eight hours after birth. The development of oral flora happens throughout the following stages: birth, childhood and adulthood. Oral hygiene and nutrition play an important role as well. Virulent Streptococcus is present in large numbers in the permanent flora, between four to twelve hours after birth. Aerobic and anaerobic staphylococcus, gram (-) diplococci and dyphtheroids manifest during infancy before the eruption of the primary teeth. After eruption, Streptococcus Viridans takes over. (Değer 2004)

The microorganisms in the oral flora can be listed as:

- Streptococci
- Anaerobics (Bacteroides, Porphyromonas, Prevotella, Fusobacterium, Capnocytophaga, Peptostreptococcus, Salmonella, Leptotrichia, Eubacterium, Veillonella, Helicobacter, Spirochetes)
- Actinobacilli
- Gram negative bacteria
- Staphylococci (Külekçi, 2000a)

1.1.4 Pathogenesis in oral flora

Pathogenesis of bacteria depends on various factors. Microorganisms spread out vigorously when changes in the mucosal barrier occur, when systemic and local factors might impair tissue congestion and when there is a lack of tissue oxygenation.

Normal oral flora is usually the cause of dental, gingival and bone infections. Frequently, anaerobic bacteria (Bacteroides, Porphyromonas, Prevotella, Fusobacterium, Capnocytophaga, Peptostreptococcus, Salmonella, Leptotrichia, Eubacterium, Veillonella, Helicobacter, Spirochetes) are involved. (Külekçi, 2000a, Değer, 2004)

1.2 Infection and contamination

Infection is the settlement of microorganisms in any of the tissues of a living body for living and proliferation. Disease is the reaction of the tissues exposed to these harmful agents that are called microbes (Georgescu, 2002).

The transfer of pathogens materializes by the way of direct and indirect contact, inhalation and inoculation. Microorganisms that participate in contamination and cross infection during dental procedures, affected areas in the body and associated illnesses are summarized in table 1 (Georgescu, 2002).

For infection to occur four factors are needed and they define the "infection chain". These factors are:

1. Organism that is sensitive to infection
2. Microorganism that is virulent and pathogenic enough to cause infection
3. Infection carrier
4. Port of entry to the organism

No sickness will take place if not all four are present. An effective infection control strategy aims to break any of the rings of this chain in order to avoid disease (Georgescu, 2002; ADA, 2003).

1.3 Cross-infection in dentistry

Microorganisms are easily transferred between patients, dentists and dental staff in private offices. Infection involving these people is called cross-infection (Mutlu et al., 1996)

Oral cavity harbors the microorganisms that carry the risk of infection by contamination. Infection control is the most common subject that is discussed. Infection risk encloses wide range of area from patient to patient, patient to doctor, patient to dental staff and to laboratory technicians. All employers are responsible to protect their staff and patients from cross infection by applying high standard sterilization and disinfection precautions. (Mutlu et al., 1996, Georgescu, 2002)

1.3.1 Infectious microorganisms in dentistry

1.3.1.1 Hepatitis viruses

Hepatitis Virus is highly important in the field of dentistry. Six hepatitis viruses have been found in the last 35 years. They are identified as A, B, C, D, E and G. B, C, D and G carry heavy importance in dentistry as far as cross-infection is concerned (Bulut, 2009).

Hepatitis B Virus: Infection with Hepatitis B virus (HBV) usually occurs via the parenteral route but also through skin or mucosal cracks. Probability of infection following an injury with a contaminated needle stick or sharp instrument lies between 25 and 30%. Contaminated blood and secretions are the main sources for transmission of infection. In the same order of ideas, saliva on its own is not a problem but since it generally carries blood or blood products it has the potential to infect. Moreover, there is no evidence to prove virus transmission via inhalation or aerosols. It is also known that blood spatter in the eyes, although should not be occurring often, may cause infection. The incubation period for HBV is 45-160 days. Infection begins after the incubation period and lasts during the acute phase. Nevertheless, the acute disease is not always obvious; 50% of the HBV infection is subclinical and the infected people are not always aware of their illnesses (Kocabaş, 2004).

Hepatitis C Virus: Hepatitis C virus (HCV) has been defined in 1988 by modern colonization techniques. This virus is an RNA virus that has 6 types and 40 subtypes. HCV infection is transmitted by the parenteral route. No sexual transmission has been proven up to date. HCV can be found in many of the body fluids. Its ratio in the saliva is generally low and

Herpes Simplex Virus Type I (HSV I)	Nasopharynx	Direct contact	Oral Herpetic lesions Conjunctivitis
Hepatitis B Hepatitis C Hepatitis D Hepatitis G	Liver	Inoculation	Hepatitis B Hepatitis C Hepatitis D Hepatitis G
Human Immunodeficiency Virus (HIV)	T4 lymphocytes (CD4+ lymphocytes)	Blood and body fluids	HIV infection Acquired Immunodeficiency Syndrome (AIDS)
Mycobacterium Tuberculosis	Pharynx	Inhalation of droplets and aerosols born from oropharyngeal secretions	Tuberculosis
Pseudomonas Aeruginosa	Dental chair water	Aerosol inhalation and swallowing of contaminated water	Pneumonia Wound infection Dental abscess
Methicillin-resistant Staphylococcus aureus (MRSA)	Mouth, skin, nasopharynx	Direct contact with hand/skin	Dental abscess
Candida Albicans	Mouth and skin	Saliva or direct contact with nasopharyngial secretions	Candidiasis Cutaneous infections
Escherichia coli	Gastrointestinal Tract	Aspiration of droplets originating from Oropharyngeal secretions	Wound infection Sinusitis Upper Airway infections
Epstein Barr Virus (EBV)	Lymphoid nodules Nasopharynx		Infectious Mononucleosis, Burkitt Lymphoma

Table 1. Microorganisms that participate in contamination and cross infection during dental procedures, affected areas in the body and associated illnesses (Değer, 2004)

shows correlation with hepatic functions. No HCV transmission is reported in vivo. Incubation period is 15-150 days after viral contact. Many infected persons cannot realize it because of the slow clinical course of development. People having acute infection are 70-80% asymptomatic. After one has been wounded by an HCV contaminated instrument, there is no specific treatment. Immunoglobulin treatment or short term Interferon treatment can be recommended. Retrospective studies show the HCV incidence in healthcare personnel is as high as 4.1% (Dolar, 2006).

Hepatitis D virus or Delta Agent: Hepatitis D virus (HDV) was discovered in 1977. This RNA virus needs HBV for existence, replication and infection. Therefore HDV is found in individuals having either acute Hepatitis B infection or are chronic Hepatitis B carriers. The incubation period after contact is 15-150 days. Hepatitis B vaccination includes immunization for Hepatitis B and D (Kocabaş, 2004).

Hepatitis G Virus: Hepatitis G virus (HGV) discovered lately is a highly infective virus affecting the liver. The ratio of positivity is high in opiate users and in patients who receive dialysis and/or are hemophilic. Studies on the effect of this virus for chronic hepatitis are still going on. Nevertheless it has been proposed that it does not have a highly toxic effect on the liver depending on the studies conducted so far. HGV from the flavi virus is a type of RNA virus. HGV can be transmitted by blood and blood products. Prevention of HGV is possible and highly successful by effective sterilization techniques (Erensoy, 2001).

1.3.1.2 Herpes Simplex Virus (HSV)

Herpes Simplex virus (HSV), having two antigenic types, is responsible for oral or genital infections. HSV-1 is responsible for oral mucosal infections, whereas HSV-2 is responsible for genital herpetic lesions. HSV infections are generally asymptomatic. Antibodies are found in most of the adults. Prevalence of HSV antibodies is related with the socio-economical state and age of the infected patients. Contamination by HSV occurs by mucosal contact, thus not spreading by air. Agent enters from small skin and mucosal wounds in oropharynx, cervices and conjunctiva and begins to reproduce. As a result of this proliferation, focal necrosis, epithelial cell degeneration and multiple vesicular eruptions develop (Bulut, 2009).

Avoiding direct contact with the ulcerated tissue is the most effective protection.

1.3.1.3 Epstein - Barr virus (EBV)

The first infection by Epstein-Barr virus (EBV) is generally asymptomatic. It may cause nonspecific illness during infancy. Fever, weakness, exudative angina and regional or general lymphadenopathy are seen in symptomatic (infective Mononucleosis) adults.

Viral diffusion and contamination occurs by the way of saliva and oropharyngeal secretions. EBV exists in lymphoid nodules primarily but also can be colonized on pharyngeal epithelial tissue where it can be hidden (Denizci and Çankal, 2006)

Standard precautions are sufficient to prevent contamination from EBV.

1.3.1.4 Human Immunodeficiency Virus (HIV)

Human Immunodeficiency Virus (HIV) is a member of Retroviridae that contain two identical RNA in a single spiral carrying interesting virology characteristic. Virus attaches to its receptor on the surface of the CD4 lymphocyte. HIV can be contracted via the parenteral route, mucosal contact or contact with broken skin. Viral load can also be found in other body secretions. Therefore, it can be transmitted via sexual contact with an infected partner. In spite of some available data, HIV is a fairly weak virus that can be inactivated at 56°C for 10 minutes using appropriate disinfectants and its spread is not as easy as expected. Thus the risk of HIV transmission following a needle stick is 0.3% (0.2-0.5%). HIV can also be transmitted from an infected mother giving birth to her child (Bakır ve Babayiğit, 2004). The risk of mortality in dentistry is 1.7 times greater for HBV than it is for HIV. If HIV penetrates broken skin, it can be held by the macrophages up to 24 hours in a human body and up to 36 hours in animals. This time interval is of utmost importance and can be favorably used by health officials. Immediately following contamination, the area in question needs to be cleaned and washed with warm water and soap; the use of antiseptics in such cases is still controversial. Mucosal membranes, if contaminated, are also to be washed. And so, antiretroviral therapy is to be initiated within two hours following exposure for optimal effect (Bulut, 2009).

1.3.1.5 Influenza Virus

Influenza virus causes flu, the most common epidemic worldwide. It is transmitted via body droplets. The incubation period for the illness varies between one and four days, but symptoms usually display after two days. Fever, fatigue, headache, diffuse muscle pain and characteristic spasmodic cough and sore throat are the main signs and symptoms of the illness. Symptoms usually last for four days whereas fatigue can last longer. Three antigenic types of Influenza virus are classified as A, B and C. The most variable antigenic type that causes pandemic is the A type. Vaccination can help in preventing Influenza infection. Moreover, in-office precautions must be taken to prevent the spread of the flu virus.

Chlorine, hydrogen peroxide, antiseptics with iodine and alcohol are to be used in addition to standard cleaning procedures.

Coughing and sneezing to be done in a paper tissue that will be discarded after use and the hands washed.

Eyes, nose and mouth must not be touched when hands are unclean.

During illness, one must stay away from others.

The location must be air-conditioned frequently.

Hands must be washed with water and soap for 15-20 seconds and alcohol-based hand rub can be used in inaccessible areas of water and soap or if hands are not soiled (Ergönül, 2009).

1.4 Infection control in dentistry

1.4.1 Medical anamnesis

During the initial appointment, a detailed and complete medical history has to be taken from the patient, and in subsequent visits, updated accordingly. Although general health problems will affect the nature of the dental treatment, medical anamnesis is not the reliable way of determining individuals who are asymptomatic carriers and are unaware of their illness (Mutlu et al.1996). Hence, a social history is often useful.

1.4.2 Vaccination

Dentists and dental staff are always recommended to be vaccinated against tuberculosis, rubella, diphtheria, tetanus and most importantly, against HBV (Değer, 2004).

Hepatitis B vaccine consists of 3 injections to the deltoid muscle. Side effects are minimal and not common. Some people do not have sufficient level of antibodies (anti-HBs Ag) after the third injection. This is mostly seen in immunosuppressive patients, the elderly and overweight individuals. Five years after vaccination, immunity remains only in 7% of the individuals. Therefore, booster doses are required. Booster doses are given at 3-5 year intervals after vaccination. (Kocabaş, 2004)

1.4.3 Personnel protective equipment

Dental personnel should wear gloves during cleaning and touching contaminated instruments and surfaces. Hands should be washed after removal of gloves after each patient. Changing or washing the gloves will disturb the structure of the gloves as a barrier and is not an accepted practice (Külekçi, 2000b).

Surgical masks, protective glasses and plastic face masks should be worn during oral procedures that are likely to splash blood, saliva and oral fluids. When there is a risk of contamination of blood or saliva disposable gowns or laboratory clothing should be worn. Such aprons should be changed when contaminated with blood (ADA, 2003; Değer 2004)

Plastic stretch, single use waterproof coatings such as aluminum foil can be used to coat surfaces that are difficult to clean. Coatings should be removed without removing the gloves and contaminated gloves must be disposed of together with (Mutlu et al, 1996, Chris 1996).

1.4.4 Protection of hands and skin

Skin care and protection is required to kept the risk of viral cross-infection to a minimum level. Hand and finger infections occur frequently and can cause cross-infection with other patients. Wearing gloves reduces the possibility of transmission of viral infections from dentists to patients and accumulation of blood and microorganisms in finger nails. Latex and vinyl non-sterile gloves prevent blood and saliva-borne micro-organisms entering from cuts, abrasions and wounds in hand. But the hands and nails should be cleaned with appropriate skin antiseptics both before wearing and after removing gloves (Mutlu et al., 1996; ADA 2003).

1.4.5 Clinical and laboratory coats

Daily clothes can be protected from contamination by wearing uniforms or clothes on them. Clothes contaminated with blood, saliva and oral secretions should be washed with water and chlorine if possible. Normal washing and drying system appropriate to manufacturers recommendations is sufficient to eliminate harmful microorganisms including the viruses (Mutlu et al., 1996; ADA 2003).

1.4.6 Protection of eyes

Protective apparatus are utulized to protect eyes and mucous membranes from macroscopic particles, chemical injury and from losses caused by microbial infections. Googles might be used for the patients as well to protect eyes in addition to physicians and ancillary staff (Mutlu et al., 1996, Chris 1996).

The eyes can be protected by different types of glasses but ideally they should be plastic and both sides must have protective properties. They can be used alone but also can be used on-grade goggles. These glasses can easily be cleaned and disinfected without deformation if necessary (Mutlu et al., 1996, Chris 1996).

Plastic masks completely covering the face can also be used instead of glasses (viewfinder). Glutarahdehyde can be used for cleaning glasses. İodoforms were reported to cause coloration. There is currently no information on the effects of hypochlorite solutions. Autoclaving of plastics was reported to impair the optical properties of these kinds of glasses (Georgescu 2002, ADA 2003).

1.4.7 Hand Instruments

The hand instruments must be sterilized by heat, and water channels must be cleaned with the help of pressurized water at the beginning and end of each day in between each patient because the instruments used in dentistry are in contact with mucous membranes and their complex structures limits cleaning, disinfection and sterilization of the internal and external surfaces. Hand tools should be sterilized between patients by appropriate methods. Sterilization, lubricating and storing recommendations of manufacturers should be strongly followed so that the tools to be durable. Today all high-speed and low-speed hand tools are said to be heat-resistant by the manufacturers. Surface deletion or disinfection by using chemical antiseptics of the hand instruments on the dental units which are in contact with air and waterways are not the proposed methods of cleaning for using the instrument again. These instruments have replaceable parts and therefore after each patient, disposable parts are recommended to be changed after each use (Chris 1996, ADA 2003).

1.4.8 Removal of sharp Instruments and infectious wastes

The patient's blood and saliva-contaminated sharp instruments should be considered as infected and necessary precautions should be taken for preventing injuries. To avoid needle accidence the use of disposable syringes should be preferred and sharp tools must be placed in boxes that are puncture-resistant and this box should be left to an area nearby (Chris 1996, ADA, 2003; Değer 2004).

Precautions that should be taken when using sharp instruments are as follows:

All of the personel must wear protective clothing during clinical operations and cleaning.

Whole staff that contact with body fluids should be vaccinated.

Sharp instruments should not be left around and should not be passed from hand to hand.

Needles should be placed in their cover with the help of a suitable tool and they should be discarded immediately after usage.

Sharp instrument boxes must be sufficient amount and when 3/4 of the boxes are full, waste should be discarded.

There must be someone responsible to change the full boxes with the empty ones.

All staff should have a detailed knowledge with the use and the getting rid of sharp tools.

Gauze, cotton rolls, disposable waste, that are contaminated with blood, must be placed in waterproof plastic bags and removed.

It is a low probability of any kind of transfer of microorganisms by clothes. Therefore, normal washing and drying of dirty clothes is a good method for cleaning and is sufficient. Gloves should be worn during processing with blood, saliva-absorbing tube fluid and other liquid waste. Liquids must be poured to a channel connected to sewage with care. (Chris 1996, ADA 2003, Değer 2004)

1.5 Sterilization and disinfection procedures in orthodontics: Definitions

Sterilization: Sterilization destroys all forms of microorganisms including viruses and bacterial and mycotic spores. An instrument will be either sterile or not sterile. There is no in between (Saniç, 2003).

Disinfection: Disinfection is the process of destroying or inhibiting most pathogenic microorganisms and inactivating some viruses, hence reducing microbial contamination to safety levels (Saniç, 2003).

Antisepsis: Application of chemicals on living tissue to avoid infection.

Asepsi: It means an environment free of germs. That is the destruction of all disease-forming microorganisms in the working environment.

Dekontamination: work against all kinds of germs to reduce the microbial source in number for protection from, unexpected contamination and infection is called decontamination. (Miller 1991; Değer 2004).

The tools used in the hospital varies according to the risk of infection. The method of disinfection is selected according to the level of risk of infection. (Mullick, 1986; ADA, 2003). Sterilization of all tools and equipment used in dentistry is extremely important, but it is not always possible to apply the most effective method. In such cases, any proper method of disinfection should be used (Mutlu, 1996; ADA, 2003).

1.5.1 Sterilization techniques

Foundations of modern medicine were laid on the possibility of contamination of the wound or physician by microorganisms.

This process began with the description of Pasteur 'the presence of the microorganism germs on the surfaces of all the items commonly found in hospitals' in the French Academy of Medicine on April 30, 1878.
One of the oldest records of sterilization is the work of a physicist in 1832, from Manchester named William Henry about the effect of heated water pressure in a container on infectious bacteria (Akçam and Özdiler, 1999)

1.5.1.1 Sterilization stages

a. Cleaning
b. Packaging- loading
c. Sterilization
d. Unloading- registration
e. Storage- distribution

1.6 Sterilization and disinfection of orthodontic instruments and material

Orthodontists generally do not make very intensive operations on tissues and they do not treat infectious diseases. Despite this, however, patients can carry germs that may infect other people. The use of proper sterilization techniques are important today because of the professional, ethical and legal aspects. Although it is not possible to obtain a complete sterilization in orthodontics clinics, it is possible to approache ideal sterilization by using new techniques (Akcam and Ozdiler, 1999).
A study conducted by Starnbach have shown that in the fields of dentistry the orthodontists are in second raw fort he incidence of having hepatitis B. HTLV-III (AIDS) virus is weaker and less infectious. Orthodontists became more conscious of the need of surface decontamination of the tools they are using with the increase of the incidence of AIDS, like hepatitis B (Kirchoff, 1987; Mc Carthy et al.1997).

1.6.1 Sterilization of orthodontic pliers

Prior to dry-heat sterilization, if water drops or excess disinfectant is left on the pliers they can be severely damaged (Ozer, 2005). Corrosion of these instruments is one of the few sterilization consequences that orthodontists face. Corrosion is an electrochemical event that metals undergo when reacting with an oxidant as a result of oxidation and reduction reactions (Uzel and Haydar 1989).
To prevent corrosion, orthodontic pliers should be dried with pressured air prior to sterilization. If they are not dried well, ions' reaction will create a loose layer of rust. Corrosion can also be prevented by oiling the joint surfaces with appropriate solutions (Haydar, 2000). Autoclaving will negatively affect orthodontic instruments causing blunting and corrosion of their sharp cutting edges. And one of its major disadvantages is that it is time consuming. Hence, soaking in 1% sodium nitrate can be recommended as an alternative. Unsaturated chemical vapor sterilization of pliers is appropriate to minimize corrosion, but this method requires a well ventilated area to eliminate noxious odors (Haydar, 2000).
In a study, Mazzocchi et al. evaluated the effects of autoclaving, dry-heat and chemical sterilization for 500 cycle's usage, on hardness, degradation and nitrification in the surface color. The maximum increase in hardness was observed when the autoclave was used, and the least amount when dry-heat sterilization was used. Degradation in the surface color was observed in each group but mostly when the chemical sterilization was used. Briefly, clinical and metallurgical modifications in every group in this study, after 500 cycle sterilization, are really minimal. Hence, they can be omitted (Mazzochi, 1996).

Glass bead sterilization is another viable method in which pliers are left inside the sterilizer at 218oC (450oF) for 15 seconds only. Note that large instruments can not be sterilized with this method (Deger, 2004).
In another study, Wichelhaus et al. evaluated corrosion resistances of orthodontic pliers after chemical sterilization with surface disinfectants. According to their findings, dry-heat sterilization does not corrode the instruments as much as chemical sterilization (Wichelhaus et al., 2004). Once the orthodontic pliers have been used clinically and thus contaminated with oral fluids and plaque, the efficiency of different disinfection methods were evaluated. Thus, spray disinfection such as (Incidur or Iso - Septol) was found to be insufficient for reducing the amount of the microorganisms. For this reason, disinfecting orthodontic pliers with spray disinfectants is proscribed. Soaking the instruments in a disinfecting solution was also found to be insufficient for decreasing the amount of the microorganisms. A successful high level disinfection can be obtained by using an ultrasonic bath (Sekusept 5%). Successful results can be achieved from thermal disinfection; the amount of microorganisms is hence decreased (Wichelhaus et al., 2004).

1.6.2 Disinfection of orthodontic brackets

Chlorhexidine is an appropriate disinfectant to be used on metal or ceramic brackets. In a study that evaluated the effect of 0.01 % chlorhexidine solution on metal and ceramic brackets, it was found that chlorhexidine does not have a significant effect on the metal brackets' adhesion ability (Speera et al., 2005). On the other hand, the attachment ability of ceramic brackets is significantly affected from this disinfecting solution, but the clinical effect does not reach levels below 6-8 Mpa (Wichelhaus et al., 2006).

1.6.3 Decontamination of orthodontic bands

Stainless steel bands of various sizes are frequently used on molars during fixed orthodontic treatment. Choosing the appropriate size requires often several trials. If trying of the bands is attempted inside the patient's mouth and determined that the size is not appropriate, the band should be decontaminated from saliva and blood, and autoclaved for future use (Benson and Douglas, 2007).
There is currently little information about the contamination level and the disinfection procedure's success of the bands that are to be reused. Fulford et al, (2003) suggested that bacterial multiplication is not observed on the bands that are exposed to enzymatic disinfectant prior to autoclave sterilization (Fulford et al., 2003).

1.6.4 Sterilization of orthodontic wires

Studies on the effect of sterilization on orthodontic wires have been going on since the 1980's. The results are in contradiction with one another. Some of the studies report mechanical alterations whereas the others defend the opposite (Buckthal et al., 1986).
Pernier et al (2005) observed the sterilization of 6 different arch wires by autoclaving them for 18 minutes in 134°C via surface analysis techniques. No significant change was observed on the alloys surface characteristics that would effect their utilization.

1.6.5 Disinfection of elastomeric ligatures

Polyurethane elastomers are frequently used in orthodontics as ligature and chain. The unused parts of elastomeric ligatures are generally sterilized via cold sterilization since they are not heat-resistant. Disinfection of these materials in a 5% gluteraldehyde solution for a period of 10 minutes is recommended. Various studies showed that repeated disinfection of the same elastic can accelerate the destruction of the cross links available in the long chain molecules of polyurethane polyesters. Sterilization of elastomeric ligatures inside the autoclave at 121°C does not lead to permanent deformations or to increased shrinkage whereas in the case of dry-heat, their manipulation becomes more difficult (Mayberry et al., 1996).

Based on two different disinfectants, tensile strength and glass transformation temperature of elastomeric ligatures that are not disinfected are found significantly different than those that are exposed to phenol and glutaraldehyde (Evangelista et al., 2007).

A parallel observation was detected between the decrease in tensile strength as a result of exposure to disinfectants in Evangelista et al's study and the decrease in tensile strength in Jeffries and Fraunhofer's study. Breakage of intermolecular links and glass transformation temperatures are decreased as a result of prolonged contact with disinfectants. Polyurethanes are not inert materials, and when they are exposed to enzymes, water, moisture and heat, they will absorb water and get destroyed. As a result of the plasticizer effect of disinfection solutions on polymer ligatures, decrease in tensile force and glass transformation temperature will occur (Mayberry et al., 1996; Evangelista et al., 2007).

1.6.6 Bacterial contamination and disinfection of removable acrylic appliances

When using removable appliances, there is an excessive formation of a biofilm layer that is observed on the retentive areas of hooks and springs, and on the smooth acrylic surfaces of the appliance (Uzel and Haydar; 1989; Lessa et al., 2007).

Studies showed that Lactobacillus and Streptococcus mutans levels are increased inside dental biofilm as a result of changing oral micro flora during orthodontic therapy with active removable appliances. Toothbrushes were not efficient enough to remove the microorganisms on the retentive areas of the appliances. Hence, it is recommended to use antimicrobial agents to eliminate the bacterial biofilm. Disinfection methods of acrylic orthodontic appliances should inactivate pathogenic microorganisms immediately, without damaging the composition of the appliance. Soaking the appliance in a chemical solution could cause decomposition of the acrylic resin molecules (Amitha ve Munshi, 1995).

In Lessa et al's study, chlorhexidine gluconate, cetilpyridinium chloridine and sterile water were compared in terms of their eliminating action on Streptococcus mutans. Antimicrobial solutions in spray form were used, and they were examined for causing any changes in the composition of acrylic or not. The results of this study suggested that both of the previously mentioned antimicrobial agents reduced contamination compared to sterile water, but chlorhexidine gluconate was found to be significantly more effective than cetilpyridinium chloridine (Lessa et al., 2007).

1.6.7 Surface disinfection

Surfaces that can not be sterilized must be disinfected effectively. These surfaces include the air-water sprayers, aspirator heads, reflector arms, cuspidors, drawers, head rest and arms. Suitable clinic and instrument setting will reduce the surfaces to be disinfected. If the chair's positions can be controlled using a pedal and cuspidors controlled by buttons at the level of the elbow or the knee, hand contact is therefore minimized (Uzel, 1989).

Sodium hypochlorite 1% or solutions including 70% alcohol are used for surface disinfection in orthodontic clinics. Iodine solutions used for disinfection are cheap, easily stored and highly effective. The only disadvantage is the staining characteristic of iodine. There are types that can be diluted in water or in 70% isopropyl alcohol (Özer, 2005).

1.7 Antibacterial agents in orthodontics

In a healthy oral cavity, microbial flora is in equilibrium with its surroundings. This equilibrium could be disrupted by application of orthodontic appliances which can then result in disease. The most common adverse effects of fixed orthodontic appliances are periodontal disease and decalcifications caused by bacteria. The surface features and designs of orthodontic appliances and bonding materials affect the formation of the biofilm layer (Maruo et al., 2008).

Inside the oral cavity, an increase in the levels of *Streptococcus mutans* and *Lactobacillus* strains is detected once the orthodontic appliances have been bonded. In many studies, a correlation existed between this bacterial growth and tooth decay. When carious activity increases, increasing the frequency of teeth brushing or high level topical fluoride application is not enough to arrest the demineralization process. Thus, individuals that are treated with orthodontic therapy and individuals that are at high risk need not only to improve their oral hygiene habits but also use chemotherapeutic agents that will act as caries suppressors. Chlorhexidine is an antimicrobial agent that is very efficient against *Streptococcus mutans*. Many applications are recommended to maximize caries prevention. In patients receiving fixed orthodontic therapy, there are a number of studies suggesting that the use of chlorhexidine solution significantly decreases *Streptococcus mutans* levels and bacterial levels in dental plaque and saliva (Dogan et al., 2009; Kuvvetli and Sadallı, 2006).

In a two group study, the effect of 0.2% chlorhexidine and fluoride toothpaste on plaque development is compared clinically and microbiologically in orthodontic patients. In the 0.2% chlorhexidine group, a decrease of the bacterial content is detected and it is shown that majority of *Streptococcus mutans* are eliminated. During fixed orthodontic treatment, 0.2% chlorhexidine mouth rinse can be used to reduce plaque accumulation, thus increasing the efficiency of oral hygiene. For an improved oral health, patient education and regular professional recalls are mandatory (Kuvvetli and Sadallı, 2006).

Sterling Winthrop Research Institute has developed a topical antimicrobial agent: Octenidine di hydrochloride. In early studies, it was shown that this solution prevented formation of biofilm in experimental animal and human models (Tazegül et al., 2006). Octenidine di hydrochloride is an antimicrobial effective against bacterial plaque formation (Dogan, 2008). Rosin et al (2002) evaluated the antibacterial and antiplaque efficiency of using polyhexamethylen biguanid hydrochloride, chlorhexidine gluconate and Listerine after teeth brushing. 0.12% biguanid hydrochloride was found to be more effective than Listerine, however, after 5 days, chlorhexidine was found to be more effective than polyhexamethylen biguanid hydrochloride (Decker et al., 2003)

2. Conclusion

Dentists face with many kinds and amounth of micro-organisms because of their professions that require intemate contact with their patients. These microorganisms may lead either a simple illness such as influenza or a serious one such as hepatitis infection or AIDS. For this reason, Keeping in mind that every patient is potentially infectious, all the measures must be taken during dental practice. Sterilization and disinfection methods should be implemented meticulously and their effectiveness carry crucial importance for the physician and the patient's health.

Although orthodontists usually do not work on tissues and treat infectious diseases patients may still carry germs that infect other people. Thus today, the use of proper sterilization techniques are important because of professional, ethical and legal aspects. Although it is not possible to obtain a complete sterilization in orthodontic clinics, it may be approachable by using new techniques.

In the orthodontic practice, providing full range sterilization requires serious effort. The presence of transmissible diseases like HIV/AIDS and Hepatitis B & C make it an absolute necessity to protect clinic staff and patients from cross contamination, by using effective disinfection and sterilization techniques.

Sterilization of instruments used in orthodontics brings some special problems together, because of the hinge regions and cutting edges that are difficult to clean and sterilize. In addition, there is a need to avoid damage during cleaning operations, because the repair or renewal of the equipments are expensive.

Orthodontic clinics running with a limited number of instruments and appliances, prefers fast methods for sterilization for effective working. To ensure this, in addition to planning the sterilization area in ortodontic clinics, new sterilization-disinfection techniques and solutions must be learned.

As a result in the orthodontic practice, providing full range sterilization requires serious effort. The presence of transmissible diseases like HIV/AIDS and Hepatitis B & C make it an absolute necessity to protect clinic staff and patients from cross contamination, by using effective disinfection and sterilization techniques.

3. References

Acar N. Diş Hekimliğinde Sterilizasyon Kontrolü ve Önemi. 5. Ulusal Sterilizasyon Dezenfeksiyon Kongresi. Sivas, 2007.

Akçam M.O, Özdiler E. Ortodontide Sterilizasyon ve Dezenfeksiyon. Cumhuriyet Üniversitesi Diş Hekimliği Fakültesi Dergisi. 1999; 2: 129-133.

Amitha H, Munshi AK. Effect of Chlorhexidine Gluconate Mouthwash on the Plaque Microflora in Children Using Intraoral Appliances. J Clin Pediatr Dent 1995;20:23-9.

Bakır B, Babayiğit M. HIV Enfeksiyonu ve AIDS: Epidemiyoloji ve Korunma Yolları. TSK Koruyucu Hekimlik Bülteni, 2004; 3 (11).

Benson P.E., Douglas C.W.I. Decontamination of Orthodontic Bands following Size Determination and Cleaning. Journal of Orthodontics, 2007; 34:18–24.

Buckthal JE, Mayhew MJ, Kusy Rp, Crawford JJ. Survey of Sterilization and Disinfection Procedures. Journal of Clinical Orthodontics, 1986; 20:759-765.

Bulut ÖE. Diş Hekimliği Pratiğini İlgilendiren İnfeksiyöz Hastalıklar. Başkent Üniversitesi Ağız-Diş-Çene Hastalıkları ve Cerrahisi. Ankara, 2009.

Campbell PM, Phenix N. Sterilization in the Orthodontic Office. J Clin Orthod. Oct. 684-686, 1998.

Chris H Miller. Infectious Diseases and Dentistry Infection Control. Dent. Clin. North Am. 1996; 40:434-455.

Decker EM, Weiger R, Wiech I, Heide PE, Brecx M. Comparison of Antiadhesive and Antibacterial Effects of Antiseptics on Streptococcus Sanguinis. Eur J Oral Sci. 2003;111:144–148.

Değer Y. Ölçü Maddelerinin Dezenfeksiyonunda Kullanılan Sprey Dezenfektanların Farklı Mikroorganizmalar Üzerindeki Mikrobiyolojik Etkinliklerinin Karşılaştırmalı

Olarak İncelenmesi. T. C. Dicle Üniversitesi Sağlık Bilimleri Enstitüsü. Doktora Tezi. Diyarbakır, 2004.

Denizci S, Çankal D. Ebstein Barr Virüsün Oral Hastalıklarla İlişkisi ve Diş Hekimliği Açısından Önemi. EÜ Dişhek Fak Derg 2006; 27: 125-133.

Doğan A.A, Adiloğlu A, Onal S, Çetin ES, Polat E, Uskun E, Koksal F. Short-term Relative Antibacterial effect of Octenidine dihydrochloride on the Oral Microflora in Orthodontically Treated Patients. International Journal of Infectious Diseases, 2008, 12: e19 – e25.

Dogan A.A, Cetin ES, Hussein E, Adiloglu A. Microbiological Evaluation of Octenidine Dihydrochloride Mouth Rinse after 5 Days, Use in Orthodontic Patients. Angle Orthodontist, 2009; 79.

Dolar ME. Hepatit B ve C Virüs Bulaş Yolları ve Korunma. Uludağ Üniversitesi Gastroenteroloji Bilim Dalı. Bursa, 2006.

Erensoy S. Hepatit Etiyolojisinde Sorgulanan Yeni Virüsler. Viral Hepatit 2001, 1. Baskı. Viral Hepatitle Savaşım Derneği 2001; 259-273.

Ergönül Ö. Pandemik İnfluenza A H1N1 ve Korunma Yolları. Marmara Üniversitesi Tıp Fakültesi Enfeksiyon Hastalıkları ve Klinik Mikrobiyoloji Anabilim Dalı. İstanbul, 2009.

Erverdi N, Biren S, Kadir T, Acar A. Investigation of Bacteremia following orthodontic debanding. Angle Orthod, 2000, 70:11-14.

Evangelista MB., Berzins DW, Monaghan P. Effect of Disinfecting Solutions on the Mechanical Properties of Orthodontic Elastomeric Ligatures. Angle Orthod. Vol 77, No 4, 2007; 681-687.

Fulford MR, Ireland AJ, Main BG. Decontamination of Tried-in Orthodontic Molar Bands. Eur J Orthod 2003; 25:621-22.

Georgescu CE, Skang N, Patrascu I. Cross Infection in Dentistry. Roum Biotechmol. Lett.2002; 7: 861-868.

Haydar S.G. Ortodontide Sterilizasyon ve Dezenfeksiyon TDBD 58. 2000.

Holht WF, Miller CH, Neeb JM, Sheldrake MA. Sterilization of orthodontic instruments and bands in cassettes. Am J Orthod. 98:411-6, 1998

Hussein EA, Acar A, Aksoy Doğan A, Tanju Kadir, Caldemir S, Erverdi N. Investigation of bacteremia after toothbrushing in orthodontic patients. Korean J Orthod 2009;39(3):177-184.

Hussein EA, Aksoy Dogan A. Distribution of Mutans Streptococci in Orthodontic Patients: Pilot Study. Turkish Journal of Orthodontics. 2009;22 (1):26-36.

Infection Control Recommendations for the Dental Office and Dental Laboratory. ADA Council on Scientific Affairs and ADA Council on Dental Practice. May 2003; 1-7.

Infection Control Recommendations for the Dental Office and the Dental Laboratory. ADA Council on Scientific Affairs and ADA Council on Dental Practice. May. 2004.

Jeffries CL, von Fraunhofer JA. The Effects of %2 Alkaline Glutaraldehyde Solution on the Elastic Properties of Elastomeric Chain. Angle Orthod.1991;61:25-3.

Kirchoff ST. Sterilization in Orthodontics. J Clin Orthod. Mayıs 1987; 326-336.

Kocabaş E. Hepatit B Hastalığı ve Aşıları, Çukurova Üniversitesi Tıp Fakültesi Çocuk Enfeksiyon Hastalıkları Bilim Dalı, Adana, 2004.

Kohn WG, Collins AS, Cleveland JL, Harte JA, Eklund KJ, Malvitz DM. Guidelines for Infection Control in Dental Health-Care Settings 2003.

Kuvvetli SS, Sandallı N. Sabit Ortodontik Tedavi Gören Hastalarda Ağız Hijyeninin Sağlanması ve Diş Çürüklerinin Önlenmesi. EÜ Diş Hek Fak Derg 2006; 27: 135-144: 766-772.

Külekçi G. Ağız Mikrobiyolojisi, Diş Hekimliğinde İnfeksiyon Kontrolü, TDBD Özel Sayısı, 58, 2000a; 10-2.

Külekçi G. Diş Hekimliği Açısından Adım Adım Enfeksiyon Kontrolü.TDBD Özel Sayı 58, 2000b;91-3.

Külekçi G, Dülger O, Ergin U. Diş Hekimliğinde Otoklav. TDBD 2005; 91:74-86

Külekçi G. Diş Hekimliğinde Sterilizasyon Öncesi Alet Temizliği. IDO Dergi, 2008, 113 (Mart/Nisan); 55-7.

Lessa FCR, Enoki C, YokoIto I, Faria G, Matsumoto MAN, Filho PN. In-vivo Evaluation of the Bacterial Contamination and Disinfection of Acrylic Baseplates of Removable Orthodontic Appliances. Am J Orthod Dentofacial Orthop 2007; 131:705.e11-705.e17.

Maruo IT, Rosa EAR, Maruo H, Tanaka O, Guariza Filho O,Ignacio SA, Camargo ES. Effect of Chlorhexidine Mouth Rinse on Streptococci Counts of Tooth-tissue-borne Palatal Expander Biofilm. Orthod Craniofac Res 2008; 11:136–142.

Mayberry D, Allen R, Close J Kinney DA. Effects of Disinfecting Procedures on Elastomeric Ligatures. J Clin Orthod. 1996; 3:49-51.

Mazzochi A., Orthodontic Pliers and Sterilization Procedures. Virtuel Journal of Clinical Orthodontics 1996.

McCarthy GM, Mamandras AH. MacDonald JK. Infection Control in the Orthodontic Office in Canada. Am J Orthod.112:275-281, 1997.

Miller CH. Sterilization Diciplined Microbial Control, Dent. Clin. North. Am Vol:35,No:2 April, 1991; 339-355 .

Miller CH, Tan CM, Beiswanger MA, Gaines DJ, Setcos JC, Palenik CJ. Cleaning Dental Instruments: Measuring the Effectiveness of an Instrument Washer/Disinfector. Am J Dent. 2000; 13:39-43.

Mulick JF. Upgrading Sterilization in the Orthodontic Office. Am J Orthod. 89: 1986; 346-351.

Mutlu S,Porter S, Scully C. Diş Hekimliğinde Çapraz Enfeksiyon Kontrolü.1996;51-59.

Özer M. Diş Hekimliğinde Sterilizasyon Kontrol Yöntemleri. 4. Ulusal Sterilizasyon Dezenfeksiyon Kongresi. Samsun, 2005.

Pernier C., Grosgogeat B., Ponsonnet L., Benay G., Lissac M. Influence of Autoclave Sterilization on the Surface Parameters and Mechanical Properties of Six Orthodontic Wires. European J of Orthodontics 2005; 27:72-81.

Renick MR, Brantley WA, Beck FM, Vig KW, Webb CS. Studies of Orthodontic Elastomeric Modules. Part 1:Glass Transition Temperatures for Representative Pigmented Products in the as- recieved Condition after Orthodontic Use. Am J Orthod Dentofacial Orthop. 2004; 126:337-343.

Rosin M, Welk A, Kocher T, Majic-Todt A, Kramer A, Pitten FA. The effect of a Polyhexamethylene biguanide mouthrinse compared to an Essential Oil Rinse and a Chlorhexidine Rinse on Bacterial Counts and 4-day Plaque Regrowth. J Clin Periodontol. 2002; 29:392–399.

Saniç A. Sterilizasyon Uygulamaları ve Problemler. Turkiye Klinikleri J Microbiol-Infec. 2003;2(2)

Shah R, Collins M, Hodge TM., Laing E.R. A national study of cross infection control: 'are we clean enough?' British Dental Journal 2009;207:267-274.

Speera C, Zimny D, Hopfenmueller W, Holtgrave EA. Bond Strength of Disinfected Metal and Ceramic Brackets. Angle Orthod 2005; 75:836–842.

Starnbach H, Biddle P. A pragmathic Approach to Asepsis in the Orthodontic Office. Angle Orthod. 50, 1980, 63-66.

Tazegül S, Koçak MM, Topuz Ö, Özcan S, Çekiç A, Erten H. Üç Farklı Solüsyonun Streptococcus Mutans ve Entrecoccus Faecalis Üzerine Antimikrobiyal Etkinliklerinin Değerlendirilmesi. EÜ Diş. Hek. Fak. Der. 2006; 27:153-158.

Toroğlu SM., Haytaç C, Köksal F. Evaluation of Aerosol Contamination During Debonding Proceduresb. Angle Orthodontist, 2001; 71: 299-306.

Uzel İ, Haydar B. Klinik Ortodontide Sterilizasyon ve Dezenfeksiyon. Türk Ort Der. 1989, 2(2): 328-333.

Wichelhaus A, Brauchle G, Mertmann M, Sander FG. Corrosion of Orthodontic Pliers Using Different Sterilization Procedures. J Orofac Orthop 2004; 65:501–11.

Wichelhaus A, Bader F, Sander FG, Krieger D, Mertens T. Effective Disinfection of Orthodontic Pliers. J Orofac Orthop 2006; 67:316–36.

7

Laser in Orthodontics

Fekrazad Reza[1], Kalhori A.M. Katayoun[2],
Ahrari Farzaneh[3] and Tadayon Nikoo[4]
[1]Periodontist, Dental Department, AJA University of Medical Sciences, Laser Research Centre of Dentistry, Tehran University of Medical Sciences, Tehran,
[2]Oral & Maxillofacial Pathologist, Laser Research Centre of Dentistry, Tehran University of Medical Sciences, Tehran,
[3]Orthodontist, Department of Orthodontics, Mashhad University of Medical Sciences, Mashhad,
[4]Pedodontist, Private Practice, Tehran,
Iran

1. Introduction

1.1 Preface

For many years research in Laser supported therapies in Dental Sciences is progressing steadily. There is no field of dentistry where development took place at such a tearing pace in recent years as in the field of laser dentistry. In the beginning it was only in some branches of this scientific field where significant therapeutic advantages compared to conventional forms of treatment could be reached, but by now this development already includes all branches of dentistry and integrates them into the spectrum of laser supported dental treatment. A great variety of different wavelengths always presents new possibilities of use with constantly new partly almost unbelievable -accomplishments. Everyone who wants to conduct conscientious dentistry in the future inevitably has to integrate the advantages of laser substitution into his or her therapeutic strategy.

1.2 History

Laser' is an acronym for 'light amplification by the stimulation emission of radiation'. Its theoretical basis was postulated by Albert Einstein. In explaining the photoelectric effect, Einstein assumed that a photon could penetrate matter, where it would collide with an atom. Since all atoms have electrons, an electron would be ejected from the atom by the energy of the photon, with great velocity. Einstein also predicted in 1917 in Zur Theorie der Strahlung (Theory of Wavelength), that when there exists the population inversion between the upper and lower energy levels among the atom systems, it was possible to realize amplified stimulated radiation, ie laser light. Stimulated electromagnetic radiation emission has the same frequency (wavelength) and phase (coherence) as the incident radiation. (Einstein, 1905, 1917)
The laser was demonstrated for the first time in 1960 by Maiman after the pioneering the oretical work of Basov, Prokhorov and Townes (Schawlow &Townes, 1940, 1949, 1958, 1994) Many other kinds of laser were invented soon after the solid ruby laser – the first uranium

laser by IBM Laboratories (in November 1960), the first helium-neon laser by Bell Laboratories in 1961 (Javan et al)and the first semiconductor laser by Robert Hall at General Electric Laboratories in 1962; the first working neodymium-doped yttrium aluminium garnet (Nd:YAG) laser and CO2 laser by Bell Laboratories in 1964, argon ion laser in 1964, chemical laser in 1965 and metal vapour laser in 1966. In each case, the 'name' of the laser was annotated with regard to the active medium (source of laser photons) used.
There is a specific and fundamental relationship between light wavelength and absorption by an 'illuminated' target material. Thus, the unique nature of laser light and its specific absorption, led to an expansion of its use in medicine. Within a year of the invention, pioneers such as Dr Leon Goldman began research on the interaction of laser light on biologic systems, including early clinical studies on humans (Goldman et al., 1964)
Although Maiman(1960) had exposed an extracted tooth to his ruby laser in 1960, the possibilities for laser use in dentistry did not occur until 1989, with the production of the American Dental Laser for commercial use. This laser, using an active medium of Nd:YAG, emitted pulsed light and was developed and marketed by Terry Myers(1989), an American dentist. Though low-powered and due to its emission wavelength, inappropriate for use on dental hard tissue, the availability of a dedicated laser for oral use gained popularity amongst dentists. This laser was first sold in the UK in 1990.In 1989, experimental work by Keller and Hibst (1989) using a pulsed Erbium YAG (2,940 nm) laser, demonstrated its effectiveness in cutting enamel, dentine and bone. This laser became commercially available in the UK in 1995 and, shortly followed by a similar Er,Cr:YSGG (erbium chromium: yttrium scandium gallium garnet) laser in 1997, amounted to a laser armamentarium that would address the surgical needs of clinical dentistry in general practice .

1.3 Laser definition

As explained before the word laser is an acronym for Light Amplification by Stimulated Emission of Radiation. The scientific rationale for the use of lasers in dentistry can be reviewed in that context. Light is a form of energy that travels in a wave and exists as a particle.[1] this particle is called a photon.
Laser is an acronym which completely describes the whole physical process of the generation of light. The laser is in fact energy transformer. Different kinds of energy, such as light, kinetic of electrical energy, are transformed into a new kind of optical energy with special properties. This new kind of optical energy is completely artificial and cannot be found anywhere in nature. Based on this consideration, it can be stated that a laser transforms energy of "low quality" into a kind of energy which has "high quality" (Meister, 2007).Special materials with well defined properties must be used to transform the energy during the simultaneous generation of light. These materials can be gases, Liquids, Semiconductor materials, glasses or artificial gemstones (crystals), and moving charged particles. Therefore, the systems will be classified as gas, dye, semiconductor, solid-state and free-electron laser (Meister, 2007).
The component parts of a typical laser are:

1. Active medium

A material, either naturally occurring or man-made that when stimulated, emits laser light. This material may be a solid, liquid or gas. The first 'dental' laser used a crystal of neodymium-doped yttrium Aluminium garnet (Nd:YAG) as its active medium. 'YAG' is a complex crystal with the chemical composition Y3Al5O12. During crystal growth, 1% neodymium (Nd3+) ions are doped into the YAG crystal (Parker,2007).The active medium is positioned within the laser cavity, an internally-polished tube, with mirrors co-axially positioned at each end and surrounded by the external energizing input, or pumping mechanism.

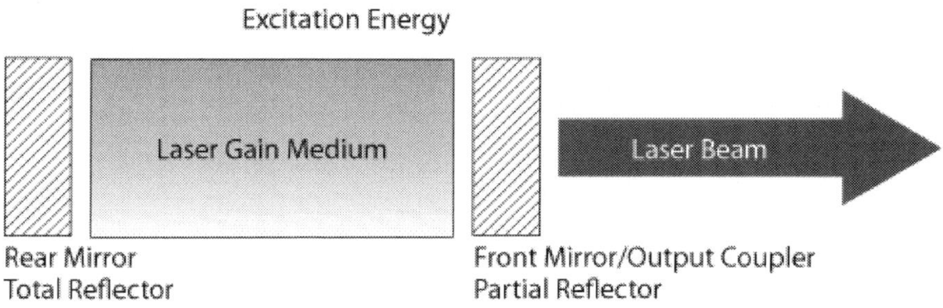

Fig. 1. The component parts of a typical laser

2. Pumping mechanism

This represents a man-made source of primary energy that excites the active medium. This is usually a light source, either a flashlight or arc-light, but can be a diode laser unit or an electromagnetic coil. Energy from this primary source is absorbed by the active medium, resulting in the production of laser light. This process is very inefficient, with only some 3-10% of incident energy resulting in laser light,9 the rest being converted to heat energy.

3. Optical resonator

Laser light produced by the stimulated active medium is bounced back and forth through the axis of the laser cavity, using two mirrors placed at either end, thus amplifying the power. The distal mirror is totally reflective and the proximal mirror is partly transmissive, so that at a given energy density, laser light will escape to be transmitted to the target tissue(Parker,2007). (Fig.1)

1.4 Delivery system

Dependant upon the emitted wavelength, the delivery system may be a quartz fiber-optic, a flexible hollow waveguide, an articulated arm (incorporating mirrors), or a hand-piece containing the laser unit (at present only for low-powered lasers). Early attempts to produce delivery systems relied upon the use of fixed mirror and/or lens apparatus. Therefore, shorter wavelengths such as argon, diodes and Nd:YAG can enjoy such fiber delivery, whereas longer wavelengths (Er,Cr:YSGG, Er:YAG and carbon dioxide) give rise to severe power losses through quartz fiber and hence require alternative delivery systems (Merberg,1993;Inberg et al.,1998;Konorov et al.,2004).

1.5 Characteristics of laser light

A wave of photons has 3 basic properties:

(1) A constant velocity (the speed of light).(2) Amplitude (the vertical measurement of the height of the wave, from top to bottom). This is a measurement of energy of that wave, expressed as a joule, or 1 unit of energy. In dental applications, a useful quantity is a mill joule, one thousandth of a joule.(3) Wavelength (the horizontal distance between any 2 corresponding points of the wave).

Both ordinary light and laser light consist of waves. However, laser light is distinguished from ordinary light by the following 2 properties :(1) Laser light is generated as only 1 colour, a property called monochromaticism. This color can be either visible or invisible to the human eye, but is described as the measurement of the wavelength, which, for dental lasers, is expressed in nanometres (one billionth of a meter).(2) The waves of laser light are coherent for all lasers. Each wave is identical in physical size and shape. This monochromatic, coherent wave of light energy emerges from the laser device as a precise, collimated beam. These properties make the laser beam a uniquely efficient source of energy (Meserendino & Pick, 1995).

1.6 Model of operation

Laser sources can emit light continuously or in pulsed fashion. The difference is related to the time -limited emission of such a system. In what is known As: continuous-wave" (CW) mode. Carbon dioxide, argon, and diode lasers operate in this manner.If the time - limited emission is less than 0.25 s. the laser emits light in so-called "pulse" mode. Free-running pulse, which has very short bursts of laser energy, with each pulse being a few 10 thousandths of a second in duration. Nd and Er:YAG, as well as Er,Cr:YSGG devices operate as free-running pulsed lasers.A special case of pulsed laser operation is the chopped mode. A continuously emitting laser beam is interrupted at regular intervals using different kinds of apertures through which the light can pass. Compared to the regular pulse operation of a laser, the apertures are placed outside the Laser Set-up where the energy is transformed.

1.7 Laser types in dentistry

A wide variety of laser systems have been established in dentistry (Wigdor et al., 1995). The available radiation is emitted from the blue spectral range up to the mid-infrared region. Numerous different applications have been developed, depending on the varying parameters of the emitted laser light. It is important to know what kind of laser is suited to a specific indication, in order to get the maximum benefit by implementing this technology in dental practice (Meister, 2007).

1.7.1 The argon ion laser

Ionized gases and vapors represent only a small segment of the range of media suitable for use in lasers. The idea of using ionized noble gases as laser media was realized technically by Gordon et al. in 1964, i. e., again in the early years of laser development. Noble - gas ion lasers using argon, krypton and xenon are among the most powerful continuous-wave lasers in the visible range of the spectrum. Especially in dentistry, the Argon ion laser is used, for example, for soft-tissue surgery, photo-polymerization and decay prevention (Mattson et al. 1998, Powell et al. 1995, Anderson et al. 2002, Hicks et al. 2004).

Argon's strongest emission lines at 488 nm and 514.5 nm are of relevance for dental applications. The 488 nm line and lines beneath are used for photo- polymerization caused by absorption in campherchinone, and the 488/514.5 nm combination is suitable for soft-tissue surgery due to the high absorption in melanin, hemoglobin and oxyhemoglobin.

1.7.2 The helium – neon laser

The Helium- neon laser was not only the first gas laser, but also the first continuous-wave laser in the history of laser development (Javan et al. 1961). It is the typical representative of the class of neutral- gas atomic lasers.Thanks to its visible emission line at 623.8nm and owing to its outstanding optical properties; this laser is commonly used as a tool for adjusting optical and mechanical systems, in holography and interfermetry, as well as in applications in biology and medicine. Its in expensive production also contributes to the worldwide use of this laser. It is thus not surprising that a laser of this kind operating at the above wavelength was also the first to be used in photodynamic therapy (Dougherty 1993) and low - level laser therapy (Saperia et al. 1986, Gomi et al. 1986, Bihari & Mester 1989).He-Ne lasers operating with various wave-lengths in single-line and multi-line dome are available commercially. Their emission range extends from intermediate and near infrared (3391, 1523, 1152, nm), red (640, 635, 632.8, 629 nm), orange (612, 604 nm) and yellow (594 nm) all the way to the green (543 nm) spectral range . The output power of these systems varies between <1 mW to several 10 Mw (3391 nm and 632.9 nm)the power generally being increased exclusively by extending the amplification path.

1.7.3 The semiconductor laser

Laser activity in semiconductor crystal was first observed in 1962 (Hall et al., Nathan et al., Holonyak et al., Quist et al.). So-called semiconductor or diode lasers emit coherent radiation in the ultraviolet (UV), visible(VIS) and infrared (IR) spectral ranges. The first semiconductor lasers were pulsed and operated at low temperatures. Not until 1970 was continuous - wave operation at room temperature achieved. Suitable semiconductor compounds are the elements of Groups II to VI the periodic table. They primarily include gallium -arsenide (GaAS) compounds, with mixed crystals including elements from Groups III to V being of particular importance. Diode lasers that are based on the elements gallium and arsenic and arsenic and emit in the range of 700-1,000 nm, i.e., in the near IR region of the spectrum, have become increasingly important in recent years. Especially in dentistry, 810 and 980 nm had become the most important wavelengths for using these lasers in endodontics and periodontics (Kimura et al. 2000, Aoki et al. 2004).

1.7.4 The neodymium: YAG laser

The Neodymium: YAG laser was developed in 1964 (Geusic et al. 1964) and is the classical and most widely used solid- state laser. Emitting its strongest fundamental wave length at 1,064 nm, the Neodymium : YAG laser is characterized by a relatively simple set - up and the generation of high output powers, both in pulsed mode at high repetition rates (up to 10 kHz) and in continuous wave mode (Geusic 1966) .The actual laser process takes place in the neodymium ion (Nd^{3+}). Neodymium belongs to the group of rare earths (lanthanides) and is embedded in a host crystal consisting of Yttrium - Aluminium -Garnet (YAG, $Y_3A_{15}O_{12}$).

1.7.5 The erbium family lasers

Since 1988 Erbium lasers are the mainly used laser systems in dentistry for cavity preparation (Paghdiwala 1988, Hibst et al. 1089, Keller 1989). Their emission wavelengths are in the spectral range from 2.6 to 3 µm and are perfectly matched to the absorption maximum of water and the OH- groups, also found as components of dental tissue. Two Erbium laser systems are preferred dentistry: first, the Erbium: YAG laser, which emits light at 2.94 µm (Zharikov et al. 1975), and second, the Erbium, chromium: YSGG laser, which emits light at 2.79 µm (Zharikov et al. 1984, Moulton et al. 1988).In general, Erbium lasers are excited by flash lamps. This implies that these lasers cannot run in continuous-wave mode due to the long lifetime of the lower laser level. In pulsed mode, however, Erbium lasers can be operated up to a pulse repetition rate of 40 Hz and average powers of 20 W at pulse energies of 1 J.

1.7.6 The carbon dioxide laser

The Carbon dioxide laser is the most powerful gas laser. Its technical realization was achieved by Patel in 1964 (1964 a,b) .In dentistry , use is generally made of low power sealed tubes with CW output powers of up to 50 W and pulsed - mode outputs of up to 300 W. The transformer or active medium of a Carbon dioxide laser is a mixture of Carbon dioxide (laser gas), nitrogen (excitation gas) and helium (cooling gas). The preferred laser transitions occur at 9.6 and 10.6 μm, with the emission at 10.6 μm describing the strongest laser transition. The Carbon dioxide laser is used for a variety of purposes in dentistry. Its strong absorption in water and hydroxyl apatite (maximum at 9.6 μm) makes it an ideal instrument for surgery on soft and hard tissue.

1.8 Light – Tissue interaction

When electromagnetic radiation hits biological tissue, different interactions occur as a function of various physical parameters. The processes occurring during the propagation of light in so- called turbid media can be divided into three cases (Hall and Girkin 2004):

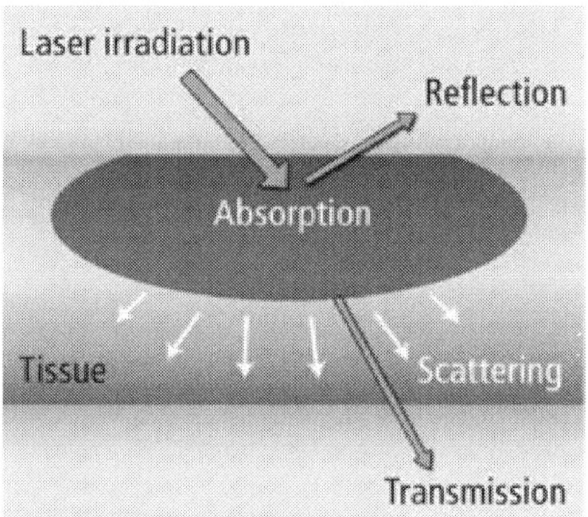

Fig. 2. What happens when Laser hits the tissue?

- Reflections on the tissue surface Reflection is a surface phenomenon (Fresnel reflection), resulting in the change in direction of the light wave caused by single interaction with a large object, the direction of the reflected wave often being opposite the incident wave. In reflection, wavelength or photon energy of the light wave is not altered.(Fig.2)
- Interactions in the tissue

Absorption

The energy of the light is absorbed by the object and then converted into a different form such as heat, for instance. An object can also absorb the energy of the light and then reemit this energy as another light which has less energy. This process is well known as florescence. (Fig.3)

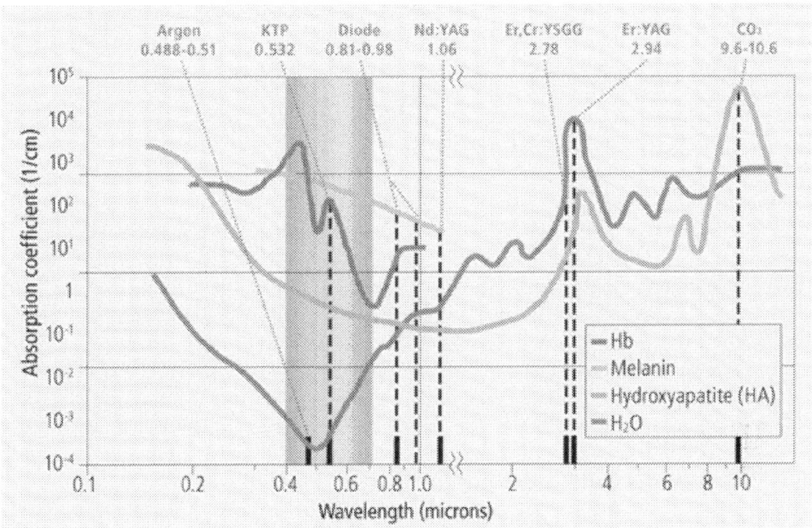

Fig. 3. Absorption curve of various tissue components.

Scattering

Scattering is the change in direction of a light wave on single or multiple occasions when it interacts with a small particle or object within inhomogeneous and/or turbid materials. The scattering of a light wave with the objects may, or may not, cause a change in the energy of the incident light wave, resulting in absorption, diffuse reflection or diffuse transmission. The angle or quantity of scattering depends on the relative sizes of the wavelength and the particles.

- Penetration of the tissue
- The wave is not influenced by the material. The energy and direction of propagation of the wave of incident is not changed during transmission. The light is transmitted as a collimated beam (Meister, 2007).

In short, laser-tissue interactions depend on the interplay of irradiation parameters: 1) wavelength or wavelength band of that particular laser source; 2) physical properties of the tissue irradiated with that particular wavelength or wavelength band; 3) irradiance or pulse energy; 4) continuous wave (CW) or pulsed irradiation; 5) laser beam size on the tissue; 6) irradiation duration or laser pulse length and repetition rate; and 7) any change in the physical properties of the tissue as a result of laser irradiation with the parameters (3-6) above(Cilesiz,2004). At low irradiances and/or energies, laser-tissue interactions are either purely optical or a combination of optical and photochemical or photobiostimulative. When laser power or pulse energy is increased, photothermal interactions start dominating. Finally, photomechanical (sometimes referred to as photoacoustic) effects become apparent when repetitive and very short laser pulses are delivered to the tissue. Therefore there are five interaction mechanisms associated with the use of lasers in biomedicine: 1) purely optical, e.g., fluorescence spectroscopy for cancer screening, optical coherence tomography (OCT) for high-resolution imaging; 2) photochemical (causes target cells to start light-induced chemical reactions.), e.g., photodynamic therapy (PDT); photobiostimulative, e.g., laser acupuncture;3) Photoablative,(causes photodissociation or breaking of the molecular bonds in tissue.) 4) photothermal(converts light energy into heat energy. This causes the tissue to heat up and vaporize.), e.g., laser-assisted refraction correction by ablation of parts of cornea, tattoo removal; and 5) photomechanical (photoacoustic),(causes dielectric breakdown in tissue caused by shock wave plasma expansion resulting in localized mechanical rupture.) e.g., laser lithotripsy.

A comparative plot of laser-tissue interactions as a function of exposure time and irradiance is given in Fig. 4. Niemz (2002) emphasizes that all laser-tissue interaction mechanisms share a common datum: characteristic energy density varies typically between 1 and 1000 J/cm^2, whereas irradiance varies over 15 orders of magnitude. Consequently, laser exposure duration is the parameter that determines the nature of laser-tissue interactions. (Cilesiz, 2004)

Niemz (2002) has also determined that all effects with near-infrared laser wavelengths at pulse durations of 1 microsecond or greater are thermal in nature. There are 5 factors to consider regarding heat generation by these lasers:(1) wavelength and optical penetration depth of the laser;(2) absorption characteristics of exposed tissue;(3) temporal mode (pulsed or continuous);(4) exposure time; and(5) power density of the laser beam.

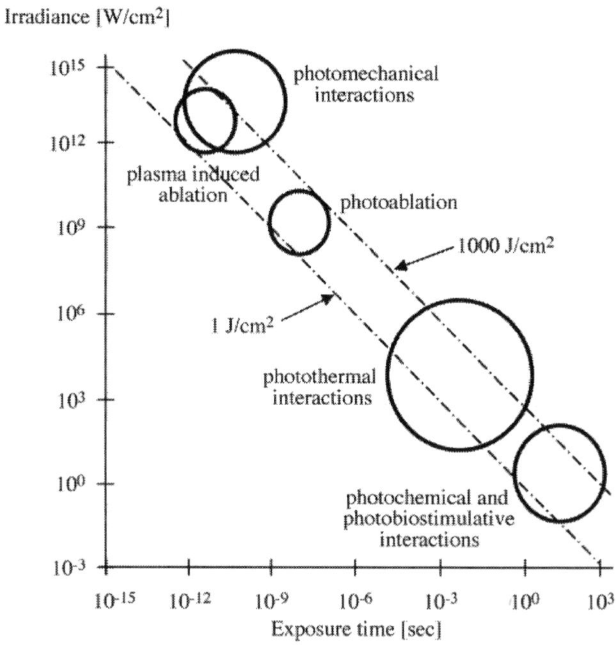

Fig. 4. Representation of laser-tissue interactions in terms of exposure time and irradiance

2. Diagnostic lasers

2.1.1 Tree-dimensional laser scanning and reconstruction (holography)

Three-dimensional (3D) laser scanners are increasingly being used in orthodontics to establish databases for normative populations (Yamada et al. 2002) and cross sectional

growth changes (Nute and Moss 2000), and also to assess clinical outcomes in orthognathic surgical (McCance et al. 1992, Ayoub et al. 1996, McCance et al. 1997, Ayoub et al. 1998, Ji et al. 2002, Khambay et al. 2002, Marmulla et al. 2003) and nonsurgical treatments (McDonagh et al. 2001, Ismail et al. 2002, Moss et al. 2003, Jang et al. 2009).
The basic concepts of the system have been described by Arridge et al (1985). The laser system consisted of two vertically fanned out low power helium-neon laser beams which were projected on to the face and viewed from an oblique angle by a television camera. In 1988 Ayoub et al. (1996) developed a video-capture stereoscopic method of imaging. Two pairs of stereo cameras ensured that the curved facial surfaces were completely imaged within 2 seconds. The system allowed photo-realistic image generation of the face that could be viewed from any direction. This polygonal facial model could be used to measure facial landmarks and volumes. Various applications of laser holography in orthodontics are:

2.1.2 Facial soft tissue analysis

The recent emphases on soft tissues as the limiting factor in treatment and on soft-tissue relationships in establishing the goals of treatment has made 3D analysis of soft tissues more important in diagnosis and treatment planning. It is equally important to be able to detect changes in the facial soft tissues produced by growth or treatment. With advancement in technology, laser-scanning devices are now smaller and can be assembled in any location for studies on facial morphology (Kau et al. 2004). The scanning process is non-invasive and normally completed within a few seconds. Furthermore, the data acquired is accurate to approximately 0.5 mm, depending on the technique used (Arridge et al., 1985; Moss et al., 1987, 1988, 2003; Nute and Moss 2000; Kau et al., 2005). These systems are valuable tools for their ease of application and creation of 3D images. It has been stated that there are many advantages of laser scanners over other types of 3D imaging technology in terms of cost, speed, and portability (Sholts et al. 2010).

2.1.3 Digital models

Orthodontic study models are usually collected by clinicians to aid diagnosis, monitor treatment, and complement the written record. Study models are also used in research, audit, and teaching. The need to retain dental casts for future reference has created storage problems for orthodontists (McGuinness and Stephens, 1992). The holograms offer a more convenient and cost-effective means of recording and maintaining this information accurately. These computer-based digital orthodontic models have the potential for assessing tooth size, arch form, and tooth-arch discrepancies (Alcaniz *et al.*, 1999; Lu *et al.*, 2000; Hirogaki *et al.*, 2001; Santoro *et al.*, 2003; Quimby *et al.*, 2004). Some investigators have performed 3D superimposition of dental casts to analyze orthodontic tooth movement (Ashmore et al. 2002, Hayashi et al. 2002, Hayashi et al.2004, Yao et al. 2005, Cha et al. 2007).
It has been claimed that most parameters on the digital models can be reliably measured, and digital models can potentially eliminate the requirement for the production and storage of dental casts (Asquith et al. 2007). In recent times the cost limitation of laser linear scanning has been addressed by high throughput commercial production.

2.2 Laser Doppler flowmetry

The laser Doppler flowmetry (LDF), developed in the 1970s as a noninvasive electro-optical technique to measure the velocity of red cells in skin capillaries, has been used for the diagnosis of pulp vitality in human teeth (Gazelius et al. 1986). The original technique utilized a light beam from a helium-neon (He-Ne) laser emitting at 632.8 nm, which, when scattered by moving red cells underwent a frequency shift according to the Doppler principle. A fraction of the light back-scattered from the illuminated area, shifted frequency in this way. This light was detected and processed to produce a signal that was a function of the red cell flux. This information was used as a measure of blood flow, the value being expressed as a percentage of full-scale deflection at a given gain. Other wavelengths of semiconductor laser have also been used: 780 nm and 780-820 nm (Kimura et al. 2000). Zang et al. (1996) demonstrated greatly improved results using forward scattering detection as opposed to conventional backward scattering detection. These results were confirmed by Sasano (1998). Odor et al. (1996) reported that the 810 nm wavelength showed good sensitivity but poor specificity and that the 633 nm wavelength showed good specificity but poor sensitivity. In general, infrared light (780-810 nm) has a greater ability to penetrate enamel and dentine than shorter wavelength red light (632.8 nm) (Vongsavan et al. 1993). The lasers used for LDF are usually at a low-power level of 1 or 2 mW and no reports on pulp injury by this method have been made. Konno et al. (2007) stated that high-powered (5 mW) transmitted laser light could be a better tool for both monitoring the pulpal blood flow of the teeth and assessing tooth-pulp vitality than the conventional back-scattered light flow meter apparatus. It was suggested that this was due to because blood-flow signals did not include flow of nonpulpal origin, and also because the output signals and responses to blood-flow changes were clear and could easily be monitored.

LDF techniques are united in their validity for pulp vitality testing as they reflect vascular rather than nervous responsiveness (Tronstad 1992). Pulpal responses to orthodontic forces or the orthopedic forces created by rapid maxillary expansion have previously been investigated by LDF (McDonald et al. 1994, Barwick & Ramsay 1996, Brodin et al. 1996, Ikawa et al. 2001, Sano et al. 2002, Konno et al. 2007, Babacan et al. 2010). LDF is also a reliable method for blood flow measurements after orthognathic surgery. Among patients who undergo a segmental maxillary osteotomy or Le fort I osteotomy, significant reduction in pulpal sensibility has been noted in teeth in the osteotomized segment or maxilla (Yoshida et al. 1996, Firestone et al. 1997, Harada et al. 2004, Emshoff et al. 2000, Emshoff et al. 2008).

2.3 Laser florescence for caries detection

The early detection and quantification of initial caries formed around orthodontic brackets is a possibility aiming to minimize the damage of caries lesions in orthodontic patients (Aljehani et al. 2004, Staudt et al. 2004). Quantitative methods would be able to detect caries lesions earlier than visual inspection would, and such methods could be used to assess the outcome of preventive interventions (Alencar et al. 2009).

The laser fluorescence (LF) device is a quantitative method based on emission of light from a diode laser at a wavelength of 655 nm and measurement of the fluorescence emitted mainly from the carious tissues. At this wavelength, clean healthy teeth exhibit little or no fluorescence. In contrast, demineralized teeth exhibit fluorescence proportionate to the degree of demineralization, resulting in elevated scale readings on the display. The fluorescence is believed to originate from protoporphyrin IX and related metabolic products of oral bacteria (Konig et al.1998, Lussi et al. 2004, Gostanian et al. 2006). The LF device may be useful for assessing the severity, progression, and depth of white spot lesions during orthodontic treatment (Benham et al. 2009).

Two versions of the LF device are currently available commercially. The older version (DIAGNOdent, Kavo, Biberach, Germany) which was introduced in 1998, is used to detect occlusal and smooth surface caries. The latest version, the DIAGNOdent pen (LFpen) (Kavo), has been designed for easier access to a proximal surfaces (Lussi et al. 2006).
The original LF device has shown good performance and reproducibility for detection and quantification of occlusal and smooth surface caries lesions in in-vitro studies, but the results of in-vivo studies have been somewhat contradictory (Rocha et al. 2003, Anttonen et al. 2004, Astvaldsdottir et al. 2004, Tranaeus et al. 2004, Bamzahim et al. 2005, Angnes et al. 2005, Akarsu and Koprulu 2006, Reis et al. 2006, Abalos et al. 2009, Chu et al. 2009, Khalife et al. 2009). A review by Bader and Shugars (2004) disclosed that although several evaluations of diagnostic performance have appeared in the literature, the range of the LF device performances is extensive. For detection of dentinal caries, sensitivity values ranged widely (0.19 to 1.0) although most tended to be high. Specificity values exhibited a similar pattern, ranging from 0.52 to 1.0. In comparison with visual assessment methods, the LF exhibited a sensitivity value that was almost always higher and a specificity value that was almost always lower. The LF pen has performed as well as the original device on occlusal surfaces in vitro (Lussi et al. 2006). To date, there is only one published study of the clinical performance of the LF pen on occlusal surfaces (Huth et al. 2008).
In general, in vivo studies of LF for occlusal caries detection indicate moderate to high sensitivity and lower specificity (Bader and Shugars 2004, Reis et al. 2006, Abalos et al. 2009, Chu et al. 2009). Therefore, the LF device should be regarded at most as a supplementary aid for detection of caries on coronal surfaces. Recently Alencar et al. (2009) proposed a new approach using the LF devices associated with fluorescent dyes and concluded these devices might be feasible options to be used in clinical association with porphyrins, in order to detect early demineralization around orthodontic brackets which cannot be estimated directly in a clinical situation.

3. High intensity laser therapy in orthodontics

3.1.1 Laser curing of light-cured materials

The application of visible light is necessary for initiating the polymerization reaction of many cements used in orthodontics, including photo-polymerized adhesive resins and some glass ionomer products. Camphorquinone, a photo initiator used in most dental adhesives, activates at wavelengths between 460 and 480 nm (blue region of the visible light spectrum), with a peak at 468 nm (Usumez et al., 2003). It has been demonstrated that at least 300 mW/cm2 of light intensity is required for optimal curing of a 2-mm thick layer of resin composite (Rueggeberg et al., 1994). There are several options for curing of orthodontic cements:

3.1.2 Conventional and fast quartz-tungsten-halogen (QTH) lights

Halogen bulbs use electric energy to heat a quartz-halogen or tungsten-halogen filament to high temperatures. This filament then glows and creates light. In a halogen bulb, only 1 % of electric energy is consumed for generation of light, and the rest is converted to heat, degrading the components of the bulb over time. Lifetime of halogen devices is less than 100 hours, and these are very sensitive to shock and vibration. The light produced by halogen devices has a wide wavelength range, including both ultraviolet and visible lights, necessitating the use of special filters to select blue light for emission. The light intensity of halogen lights may vary between 400 mW/cm2 to 800 mW/cm2. However, the output power of halogen bulbs is decreased over time, so that many halogen bulbs used in dental offices may have light intensities lower than what is considered optimal for sufficient polymerization of adhesives (Barghi et al., 1994). Curing time of 20 to 40 seconds is recommended when using conventional halogen lights for curing orthodontic adhesives and light-cured resin-modified glass ionomers, respectively (Cacciafesta et al., 2005). This may appear a time-consuming procedure for many clinicians, and therefore several attempts have been made to reduce the curing time by using devices that produce higher light intensities.

Fast halogen lamps have similar construction to conventional bulbs but they produce higher output intensities, exceeding 1000 mW/cm2. This is achieved by using higher-output lamps or application of special light guides that focus the light and concentrate it onto a smaller beam area. This way, curing times can be reduced to half of the time needed for curing with conventional halogen lights. However, limitations of filter technique and thermal problems prevent from further development in halogen devices.

3.1.3 Light emitting diodes (LEDs)

In 1995, Mills (1995) introduced solid-state light-emitting diode (LED) technology to overcome the shortcomings of halogen bulbs in polymerization of light-cured materials. When an electric current flows through junctions of semiconductors, light is generated with little energy loss as heat. LEDs have a lifetime of over 10.000 hours, and show little degradation of output power over time. They require no filters to produce blue light, consume low power for operation and are small, cordless, and resistant to hock and vibration. The curing time of 20 to 40 seconds is recommended when using LED devices for polymerization of orthodontic cements. Several studies indicated that at similar irradiation times, LED units have comparable (Dunn and Taloumis, 2002; Silta et al., 2005; Bishara et al., 2003) or higher (Carvalho Fde et al., 2010) efficiency than conventional halogen devices in polymerization of orthodontic adhesives.

3.1.4 Plasma arc units

Xenon plasma arc lamps were introduced to provide high intensity curing of adhesive materials in dentistry. The device consisted of an anode and a cathode, placed in a quartz tube which fills with xenon gas. When an electron current is passed through xenon, the gas becomes ionized (plasma condition) and generates an intense white light, which should be filtered to deliver blue wavelengths. However, the frequency bands produced by plasma arc units are much narrower than those of halogen lights and therefore less filtering is required. The process of plasma light generation requires a high voltage and generates considerable heat. The lifespan of plasma discharged tubes is several hundred hours. The light intensity is between 1400 to 2400 mW/cm2, (Wendl and Droschl, 2004) therefore less time is needed for polymerization of cements. According to manufacturer' claims, 1 to 3 seconds of irradiation with plasma arc unit is sufficient for polymerization of most dental adhesives. However, Ip and Rock (2004) reported that irradiation time of 2 seconds with plasma light resulted in significantly lower bond strength than 20 seconds of curing with conventional halogen light. It seems that at least 4 to 10 seconds of plasma irradiation should be performed to achieve comparable bond strengths to conventional halogen bulbs.

3.1.5 Argon laser

Argon laser is promising for the polymerization of dental restorative materials because one of the argon laser's emission peaks (488 nm) matches well with the absorption peak of the photoinitiator, camphorquinone (CQ) in light-curing dental restorative materials. It was claimed that the argon laser can polymerize a light-cured orthodontic adhesive 4 times faster with the same or even higher bond strength (Talbot et al 2000) and with less frequency of enamel fracture at debonding than with the conventional curing light (Lalani et al. 2000). In addition, at recommended curing times, in-vitro pulp chamber temperature increases from the laser units were significantly lower than those of the conventional curing light (Powell et al. 1999). Therefore, the argon laser should not pose a serious thermal risk to the pulp if used at the recommended energies (Cobb et al. 2000, Anic et al. 1996).

James et al (2003) presented in-vitro mean shear bond strength results using adhesive-precoated (APC) brackets for the argon laser (238.1 mW/cm2, 10 seconds) of 4.2 MPa compared with the conventional curing light (771.9 mW/cm2, 20 seconds) of 5.3 MPa. Using a higher intensity argon laser (approximately 800 mW/cm2, 10 seconds) system, Lalani et al (2000) reported similar bond strengths with their conventional curing light (approximately 400 mW/cm2, 40 seconds) group.

Kelsey et al (1989) conducted a carefully controlled laboratory study to determine the optimum power setting and polymerization cycle time to cure 4 commercially available composite resins with an argon laser. The most effective resin polymerization was achieved when Prisma APH was polymerized (310 mW) for 7 seconds, when Herculite was polymerized (160 mW) for 12 seconds, when P-50 was polymerized (525 mW) for 13 seconds, and when Silux Plus was polymerized (270 mW) for 13 seconds. The authors concluded that the exact parameters of laser power and exposure time seem to be material specific, with greater variation noted in power settings than in exposure times. Talbot et al (2000) saw a significant difference between bond strength values at 3 laser energies (200, 230, and 300 mW). Therefore, it seems that the power setting is a major factor in the outcome of bond strength values.

Elvebak et al. (2006) tested the effects of curing time and light intensity on the shear bond strength of adhesive composites for stainless-steel orthodontic brackets. An argon laser at four different power settings (100, 150, 200, and 250 mW) and four different exposure times (5, 10, 15, and 20 seconds) was used to bond APC stainless-steel brackets. They results showed the location of bond failure did not differ significantly in relation to exposure time. However, the location of bond failure was significantly different in relation to light power. They concluded that short exposure time and a low power setting produce shear bond strengths equivalent to those produced by longer exposure times and higher power settings.

To date, little has been reported on the clinical performance of argon laser for orthodontic bracket bonding. Elaut and Wehrbein (2004) completed a 14-month prospective controlled clinical trial to assess the bond failure rate and decalcification incidence with conventional curing light and argon laser curing. There was no significant difference between curing methods for decalcification, but there were statistically fewer bond failures with the argon laser. They concluded that the clinical bond strength was superior with argon laser. Hildebrand et al. (2007) compared bond strengths after curing with the argon laser (10 seconds) and the conventional curing light (40 seconds) in vivo and in vitro. They stated that the bond strength for argon laser curing is comparable to conventional light curing and is sufficient for clinical applications. Although the argon laser left more adhesive on the tooth surfaces on debonding, there was no increase in enamel surface fractures.

Although the usefulness of argon lasers has been well documented, the expense of this laser has prevented it from becoming a popular light-curing source. Recently, Kim et al. (2010) assessed the effectiveness of the diode-pumped solid-state (DPSS) laser with a wavelength of 473 nm on the bonding of orthodontic brackets to teeth. This recently developed laser is expected to show similar features to the argon laser due to the similar emission wavelength. Furthermore, since this DPSS laser is compact and much cheaper than the argon laser, it has potential applications in dentistry instead of the argon laser. They concluded that the shear bond strength value of the DPSS laser-treated groups was similar to that of the control group (QTH light) and curing with DPSS laser will reduce chair time. However, future experiment is needed to support their claim.

3.2 Enamel conditioning for bracket bonding with laser

Proper conditioning of enamel surface is necessary for bonding of orthodontic attachments to teeth. In orthodontics, as in other fields of dentistry, the most common method of enamel preparation is acid phosphoric etching. Acid etching process prepares the surface by selective removal of interprismatic mineral structure, while the organic materials are less affected. The resultant rough and microfissured surface is very useful for retention of adhesive resins, but these structures are also more vulnerable to caries formation. Acid etching removes and demineralizes the most superficial and protective layer of enamel and makes the teeth more susceptible to long-term acid attack, especially when resin monomers can not sufficiently fill the demineralized area due to saliva contamination or air bubbles (Martinez-Insua et al., 2000). Since the prevalence of white spot lesions is very high among orthodontic patients (Gorelick et al., 1982), prevention of enamel demineralization is of great importance in orthodontics.

There has been extensive research to find an alternative conditioning method to overcome the main disadvantage of phosphoric acid etching, i.e. the potential for producing decalcification. Some researchers have worked on conditioning enamel with polyacrylic acid (Maijer and Smith, 1979) or pretreatment the enamel surface with sandblast of aluminum oxide (Canay et al., 2000) to reduce the rate of enamel loss during etching. However, these methods failed to achieve adequate bond strength to resist intraoral forces.(Canay et al. 2000; Jones et al., 1999)

Laser etching has become an alternative to acid etching of enamel. Laser etching is painless and does not involve either vibration or heat; also, the easy handling of the apparatus makes this treatment highly attractive for routine clinical use (Ozer et al. 2008). Laser etching of enamel creates microcracks that are ideal for resin penetration (Visuri et al. 1996). The surface produced by laser irradiation is also acid resistant. Laser irradiation of the enamel modifies the calcium-phosphate ratio and leads to the formation of more stable and less acid soluble compounds, thus reducing the susceptibility to caries attack (Oho et al. 1990, Klein et al. 2005). Because water spraying and air drying are not needed with laser etching, time can be saved (Usümez et al. 2002, Lee et al. 2003). From a clinical standpoint, saving chair time also improves adhesion because it reduces the risk of salivary contamination.

Different types of laser such as CO2, Er:YAG, Nd:YAG, and Er,Cr:YSGG have been used in orthodontics for enamel conditioning to bond brackets. Kim et al. (2005) and Lee et al. (2003) tested the effectiveness of Er:YAG laser in etching the enamel surface for orthodontic treatment and concluded that Er:YAG laser ablation can be an alternative tool to conventional acid etching.

Fuhrmann et al. (2001) concluded that CO2 and Nd:YAG dental lasers produce enamel conditioning and tensile bond strength sufficient to meet the requirements of bracket bonding. They stated that CO2 laser produces craters of various dimensions, while the

Nd:YAG laser produces honeycomb structures regionally similar to enamel samples from the acid-etch technique. However, Ariyaratnam et al. (1997) believed that the Nd:YAG laser, when compared to 37% phosphoric acid, produces lower bond strength and alters the surface morphology of enamel. In another study, the authors claimed that dentinal surface exposed by the Nd:YAG laser exhibited microcracks and fissures, and concluded that this is not a suitable method for substituting dentinal acid etching (Ariyaratnam et al. 1999).

Ozer et al. (2008) compared Er,Cr:YSGG laser irradiation at 0.75 and 1.5 W with phosphoric acid etching and self etching primer for orthodontic bonding. They stated that varying power outputs of laser irradiation make different etching patterns: 0.75-W laser irradiation had lower shear bond strength, whereas 1.5-W power output showed comparable shear bond strengths with phosphoric acid and self etching primer. Basaran et al. (2007) reported that the mean shear bond strength and enamel surface etching obtained with an Er,Cr:YSGG laser (operated at 1 W or 2 W for 15 seconds) is comparable to that obtained with acid etching. Enamel and dentin surfaces etched with Er,Cr:YSGG lasers show microirregularities and no smear layer (Hossain et al. 1999). More recently Usümez et al.(2002) found that the results of enamel conditioning with Er,Cr:YSGG laser at 2 W of power (20Hz, 100mJ) were similar to those of acid etching. Cutting the power in half (20Hz, 50mJ) significantly decreased the bond strength of the irradiated surface compared to acid etching; however, individual results varied greatly in each case. So they suggested that Er,Cr:YSGG laser by itself cannot be counted as a successful alternative to conventional methods of increasing bond strengths to enamel. This was recently confirmed by Jaberi ansari et al. (2011,in press) who claimed that re-etching with acid phosphoric will be necessary if Er,Cr:YSGG laser is used for tooth preparation or surface treatment.

Although there are some contradicting findings about the use of lasers for enamel etching, this may be due to the different outputs and experimental designs of the studies (Ozer et al. 2008).

3.3 Bonding to porcelain

Sometimes orthodontic attachments should be bonded to porcelain surfaces, a phenomenon which is most commonly seen in adult patients. Conventional acid etching is unable to produce sufficient bond strength of orthodontic brackets to porcelain surfaces. It has been demonstrated that the application of 9.6% hydrofluoric acid for 2 minutes provides suitable surface alterations for orthodontic bonding. (Zachrisson and Buyukyilmaz, 2005) However, the use of hydrofluoric acid can damage the surrounding teeth and soft tissues, if careful isolation of the operating area is not performed. When etching with hydrofluoric acid, the surrounding teeth and soft tissues should be protected with cream, the etchant should be removed with cotton roll, and the area should be rinsed using high-volume suction. Several alternative techniques have been proposed to replace the use of hydrofluoric acid gel in bonding to porcelain surfaces, such as the application of acidulated phosphate fluoride (APF) gels or laser etching.

Li et al. (2000) prepared porcelain with 0.6, 0.9, and 1.2-W Nd:YAG lasers for bonding and concluded that this type of laser in combination with light cure composites created acceptable bond strength to porcelain. It appears that using an Nd:YAG laser not only eliminates the need to rough up the porcelain, it would also eliminate the potential gingival burns associated with HF acid and the need to repolish the porcelain at deband. Furthermore, etching time is considerably shorter with the Nd:YAG laser compared to HF acid (10 s vs. 3–5 min). The advantage of the Nd:YAG laser in improving the shear bond strength of titanium ceramic interface was also shown by Kim and Cho (2009). A 2-W CO2 laser in superpulse mode was also found to be appropriate for orthodontic bracket bonding to deglazed porcelain surfaces. Akova et al. (2005) believe that the increased bond strength observed in the laser-treated group is related to micromechanical retention.

Poosti et al. (2011) evaluated the shear bond strength of metal orthodontic brackets to porcelain following conditioning by Er:YAG (2-W for 10 s and 3-W for 10 s) and Nd:YAG (0.8-W for 10 s) lasers in comparison to conventional methods. The results revealed that Nd:YAG laser was shown to be an acceptable substitute for hydrofluoric acid while Er:YAG laser with the mentioned power and duration was not a suitable option.

3.4 Increasing the acid resistance of enamel to prevent formation of white spot lesions

One of the most important problems during orthodontic treatment is the occurrence of enamel demineralization around orthodontic appliances. Fixed orthodontic appliances facilitate the adherence of food particles and make tooth brushing more difficult, resulting in increased amount of bacterial plaque around orthodontic attachments. The organic acids produced by oral bacteria dissolve calcium and phosphorus ions from enamel surface, creating the initial sign of demineralization, namely white spots lesions. These lesions are more commonly seen in upper anterior teeth and upper and lower premolars.(Lovrov et al., 2007) The incidence of white spot lesions is significantly higher in orthodontic patients than untreated subjects.(Tufekci et al., 2011) The clinical study of Ogaard et al (1988a) indicated that white spot lesions can be seen in as early as 4 weeks under unfitted orthodontic bands, implying the rapid progression of demineralization around orthodontic attachments. White spot formation is considered a great problem in orthodontic patients, because it detracts from the aesthetic results of treatment and may compromise tooth health by progression to caries cavity. Therefore prevention of caries formation is of great importance in orthodontic patients, especially for those with poor oral hygiene.

There have been extensive attempts to find a method to reduce the incidence of demineralization in orthodontic patients. Some studies (Ogaard et al., 1988b) indicated the efficacy of using daily fluoride mouth rinse in reducing the occurrence of white spot lesions during orthodontic treatment, but excellent cooperation in using a mouth rinse can be achieved in only 13% of patients.(Geiger et al., 1992) Another method to prevent demineralization is to use fluoride releasing composite resins or conventional or resin modified glass ionomer cements for bonding orthodontic attachments,(Dubroc et al., 1994; Marcusson et al., 1997) but some studies (Cook and Youngson, 1988; Fox et al., 1991; Klockowski et al., 1989) reported lower bond strength when using these adhesives, compared to conventional composite resins. Recently, amorphous calcium phosphate (ACP) agents have been considered as promising agents for increasing enamel resistance to decalcification and also to treat white spot lesions in orthodontic patients. Rose (2000a, b) indicated that casein phosphopeptide-amorphous calcium phosphate (CPP-ACP) agent effectively binds with dental plaque, providing a large reservoir of readily available calcium to inhibit demineralization and also to assist remineralization. Despite improvements in materials and preventive measures, enamel demineralization continues to be a great concern for both orthodontists and patients. Therefore, finding new prophylactic measures to prevent demineralization may be a great step towards achieving healthy and aesthetic teeth at the end of treatment.

In 1965 Sognnaes and Stern were the first to report that when the enamel was exposed to ruby laser irradiation, the resistance of enamel to acid attack was improved. To confirm the previous report of Sognnaes and Stern, Yamamoto and Sato (1980) embedded small pieces of lased enamel into several parts of human dentures. After three months, the unlased area of the enamel showed chalky white lesions, whereas no detectable visible change was observed in the lased area. Subsequently, several investigations have demonstrated that treatment with various lasers can reduce the rate of subsurface demineralization in enamel (Nelson et al. 1986, Nelson et al. 1987, Powell et al. 1994, Qiao et al. 2005). There are several theories regarding the mechanisms by which laser irradiation enhances enamel resistance. These theories range from a surface melting through partial fusion and recrystalization of enamel prisms to changes in the enamel's organic matrix (Wigdor et al. 1995). A number of studies have also shown that combining laser irradiation with fluoride treatment could have a synergistic effect on acid resistance (Goodman & Kaufman 1977, Flaitz et al. 1995, Hicks et al. 1993, Hicks et al. 1994, Hicks et al. 1995, Hicks et al. 1997, Moslemi et al. 2009).

Using quantitative microradiography, argon laser irradiation of enamel reduced the amount of demineralization by 30-50% (Duncan et al. 1993, Powell et al. 1994). Fox, Duncan and Otsuka (1992) found that, in addition to decreasing enamel demineralization and loss of tooth structure, CO2 laser treatment reduced the threshold pH at which dissolution occurred by about a factor of five. Lenz et al. (1982) have suggested that the enamel surface is sealed by the laser and is less permeable for the subsequent diffusion of ions into and from the enamel.

In 2001, Hossain et al. used an Er,Cr:YSGG laser to irradiate the enamel or dentin samples at 6 W (67.9 J/ cm2) or 5 W (56.6 J/cm2) pulse energy, respectively, with or without water mist. The results suggested that Er,Cr:YSGG laser irradiation appears to be effective for increasing acid resistance. SEM observations showed that the lased areas were melted and seemed to be thermally degenerated. After acid demineralization, the thermally degenerated enamel or dentin surfaces were almost unchanged. In 2005 Qiao et al. irradiated the enamel and dentin samples with the Er,Cr:YSGG laser at 6 or 4 W for 6 seconds, respectively. They concluded that Er,Cr:YSGG laser irradiation is effective for increasing the acid resistance of dental hard tissue and does not cause thermal side effects.

Kim et al. (2006) compared the effects of Er:YAG laser ablation and of phosphoric acid etching on the in-vitro acid resistance of bovine enamel and found that reduction rate and reduced depth of calcium content along the subsurface was lowest in Er:YAG laser-treated enamel than the acid etched enamel. Hence, they concluded that the Er:YAG laser-treated enamels were more resistant to acid attack than phosphoric acid-etched enamels.

According to these results it may be concluded that laser treatment of enamel of caries vulnerable areas such as around brockets would be a useful strategy in orthodontic patients. However, this would demand further investigation.

3.5 Bracket debonding

Ceramic brackets were introduced in the mid 1980s to supply the demands of orthodontic patients for more aesthetic and invisible appliances. However, ceramic materials have some innate defaults that preclude easy application of them in orthodontics. The low fracture toughness of ceramics may cause partial or complete bracket fracture during removal. This precludes reuse of the same bracket at a corrected position and may result in eye damage, ingestion or aspiration of bracket fragments. In addition, removal of bracket fragment on the tooth may require the use of diamond burs, a process that is time consuming and can damage the pulp (Vukovich et al., 1991) and enamel surface.(Chen et al., 2007) Another problem with clinical application of ceramic brackets is the high incidence of enamel damage during debonding. Enamel damage, either in the form of enamel fracture or enamel crack, detracts from esthetics of the tooth and may need costly restorative treatment and also can compromise the tooth integrity by increasing the risk of eventual tooth fracture. When the required force for bracket removal exceeds the cohesive strength of the enamel, fracture of the enamel surface is inevitable. The debonding stress of ceramic brackets can exceed 20 MPa, (Theodorakopoulou et al., 2004; Gwinnett, 1988; Odegaard and Segner, 1988) and these forces may be sufficient to fracture the enamel and create severe discomfort in patients who their teeth have been mobilize by orthodontic treatment.(Tocchio et al., 1993)

For debonding of ceramic brackets, special pliers have been used conventionally to apply a sufficiently high force to fracture the bond. However, ceramic brackets are brittle and cannot be removed easily by pliers. Enamel damage and bracket fracture have been reported frequently with conventional debonding of ceramic brackets (Artun, 1997; Bishara et al., 2008; Joseph and Rossouw, 1990) due to the high bond strength combined with the low fracture toughness of ceramics. Some alternative methods have been proposed for weakening the bond immediately before debonding, including ultrasonic and electro thermal devices.(Bishara and Trulove, 1990a; Brouns et al., 1993; Bishara and Trulove, 1990b) With electrothermal method, adhesive resin is softened above a critical temperature (approximately 150 to 200° C) to allow removing the brackets at a significantly reduced force level.(Strobl et al., 1992) The main drawback of instruments that use electric heat element as a heat source is that there is no quantitative control on the amount of delivered heat energy to ceramic bracket, which in turn may excessively heat the tooth during bracket removal. Some studies reported pulp damage after use of electrothermal devices for debonding of ceramic brackets.(Dovgan et al., 1995; Jost-Brinkmann et al., 1992) and consequently these methods failed to achieve popularity among orthodontists.

Since the early 1990s, lasers have been used experimentally for debonding of ceramic brackets. The use of lasers eliminates problems such as enamel tear outs, bracket failures, and pain that are encountered during conventional ceramic bracket removal techniques. Additionally, lasers have the advantage of decreasing debonding force and operation time (Strobl et al. 1992, Tocchio et al. 1993, Mimura et al. 1995, Rickabaugh et al. 1996, Ma et al. 1997, Obata et al. 1999, Abdul-Kader et al. 1999, Hayakawa 2005, Xianglong et al. 2008).

In most previous studies, carbon dioxide lasers whose wavelength is more easily absorbed by the ceramic brackets had been preferred for debonding. Strobl et al. (1992) investigated the removal of polycrystalline and monocrystalline alumina brackets using carbon dioxide and YAG lasers. Their results showed that laser-aided debonding significantly reduced debonding force by thermal softening of the resin. It was also concluded that with the Nd:YAG laser, approximately 69-75% of the incident light reached the enamel surface, which has the potential to cause pain or damage to the tooth structure.

Mimura et al. (1995) used a carbon dioxide laser to investigate the differences in the laser-aided debonding mechanism between 2 adhesives. Unlike previous studies, they applied the force and the lasing simultaneously. They concluded that the laser-focused adhesives tended to be removed with the brackets in the Bis-GMA groups, whereas the adhesives tended to remain on the tooth surface in the MMA groups.

Rickabaugh et al. (1996) and Ma et al. (1997) used carbon dioxide lasers and modified debonding pliers to accurately position the laser beam on the ceramic bracket. In accordance with previous studies, their results showed significant differences in tensile debonding forces between the control and study groups. They also stated that the bracket could be removed from the tooth with pliers as soon as the adhesive-softening temperature had been reached, and the debonding pliers holding the bracket reduced the possibility of dropping it on the patient. Additionally, quick removal of the bracket prevented the heat energy stored in the bracket from transmitting to the tooth.

Iijima et al. (2010) suggested that the mechanical properties of tooth enamel such as hardness and elastic modulus were not affected by CO2 laser irradiation. Obata et al. (1999) debonded ceramic brackets with the aid of super and normal pulse CO2 lasers. They showed that a Super pulse CO2 laser is better than a continuous one. As they minimized the power levels of the super pulse CO2 laser, they obtained a smaller intrapulpal temperature increase compared to the normal pulse laser. The investigators concluded that using a super pulse CO2 laser for debonding did not cause a risk for the pulp. Recently, Tehranchi et al. (2010) evaluated the effect of super pulse CO2 laser (power density of 50 W, exposure time of 5 s, and duration pulse of 500 μs) on shear bond strength and adhesive remnant index during debonding of ceramic brackets. They showed less debonding force and more adhesive remnant index on the tooth surface in the laser group.

Tocchio et al (1993) used Nd:YAG laser light at wavelengths of 248, 308, and 1060 nm at power densities between 3 and 33W per square centimeter to debond 2 types of ceramic brackets by externally applied stress of either 0 or 0.8 MPa. No enamel or bracket damage was reported as a result of laser debonding. According to the investigators, laser energy can degrade the adhesive resin by thermal softening, thermal ablation, or photoablation. This mechanism causes rapid thermal expansion or burnout and vaporization of the resin, causing a small explosion. The pressure generated by the explosion functions as the debonding force. The rise in intrapulpal temperature as a result of lasing was extremely low, and the maximum temperature increase was 5.1°C.

A high peak Nd:YAG laser at 2.0 J (1.2-ms pulse duration, 5 pulse per second) was used by Hayakawa (2005) to develop an effective method for debonding ceramic brackets. Even though the Nd:YAG laser has a higher degree of enamel transmissibility than the CO2 laser, it has a lower ceramic absorption level that will directly influence the resin by enhancing the effects of thermal ablation and photoablation. In this study, very short lasing time caused an instantaneous resin reaction that produced a localized, instantaneous temperature increase. The investigator stated that the intrapulpal temperature had not increased much (maximum rise was 5.1°C), probably because of this instantaneous reaction of the adhesive resin to the laser. Although the laser energy delivered was too small compared to Strobl et al.'s (1992) application, it was effective because of the millisecond pulses with high peak powers.

Oztoprak et al. (2010) preferred the Er:YAG laser since it has a lesser thermal effect than the Nd:YAG or CO2 laser (Wigdor et al. 1993). They stated that Er:YAG laser is effective for reducing the shear bond strengths of orthodontic polycrystalline ceramic brackets from high values to levels for safe removal from the teeth. These investigators developed a new method to debond ceramic brackets by scanning thoroughly the surface of the brackets for 9 s. This was confirmed by Nalbantgil et al. (2010) which stated that 6 s lasing with the scanning method using the Er:YAG laser may be an effective and safe way to remove ceramic brackets without causing intrapulpal and enamel damage.

Ahrari et al. (2011) used ultra pulse CO2 laser (188 W, 400 Hz) for deboning of chemically-retained and mechanically-retained ceramic brackets and reported that laser-assisted debonding reduced the risk of enamel damage and bracket fracture, and produced the more desirable ARI scores, without causing thermal damage to the pulp.

Yet laser wavelength and mode of operation (continuous pulsed or modulated) should be chosen properly in order to prevent any thermal hazard given to the enamel or pulp.

3.6 Laser welding

Today, most orthodontic appliances are fabricated by joining of different individual components together. However, in-office fusion of wires or other attachments to orthodontic appliances is still a common procedure for construction or repair of appliances during orthodontic treatment to achieve optimal treatment results. In orthodontics, as in other parts of dentistry, fusion can be achieved through soldering, brazing or welding. The only difference between soldering and brazing is the liquidus temperature of intermediate alloy.

3.6.1 Soldering

In soldering, the metal parts are joined by heating them at temperatures below the solidus temperature of substrate metal. A filler metal with liquidus temperature not more than 450°C is applied. The filler metal melts and flows through the interface without affecting the dimension of the joined structure.(Chandra et al, 2000)

Two methods are used for producing the necessary heat to melt the filler: gas blow torch and electrical resistance soldering. The use of gas blow torch is less expensive, but the heat is much more localized in electrical resistance soldering. It should be noted that the interface between a silver solder and stainless steel is more mechanical than alloying, therefore adequate amount of solder should be used to reinforce the junction. (van Noort, 2002)

3.6.2 Brazing

In brazing, the liquids temperature of filler metal is above 450°C and below the solidus temperature of the base metal. Similar to soldering, the filler metal melts and flows, joining metal parts together without affecting the dimensions of the joined structure. Brazing is a common procedure to join the components of orthodontic appliances such as base and wing components of brackets. However, brazing alloys contain traces of cytotoxic cadmium, and also form a galvanic couple that can lead to ionic release of mainly copper and zinc elements. (Eliades, 2007)

3.6.3 Welding

Welding defines the joining of two metal pieces by applying heat, pressure, or both, without the use of an intermediate alloy. In welding, fusion takes place by metallic bonding through a localized union across the interface. Welding is commonly used for joining flat structures such as band or brackets. The only orthodontic wire material that is truly capable of being welded is β-Titanium. Stainless steel is also can be welded to stainless steel, but the joint is not very strong and should be reinforced with solder. Nickel titanium wires cannot be welded or soldered.(Ferracane, 2001)

There are three ways of welding in dentistry.

Pressure welding: Pressure welding is achieved by applying a sufficiently large force to the metal parts to be joined. Pure gold foils can be pressure welded by hand or mechanical condensers.

Spot (resistance) welding: Welding at a spot is called spot welding. This process is used to join flat structures, such as orthodontic bands and brackets and also to join some types of orthodontic wires. In spot welding, the parts to be joined should be pressed firmly together between two electrodes usually made of copper. Then a high electric current is passed through the system, and since the parts to be joined are less conductive of electricity than the copper electrodes, they will heat up and create a fused localized melted joint. Usually a current of 250 to 750 amperes is used, for a time of between 1/25th and 1/50th second.(Combe, 1981) Spot welding is successful in formation of overlapping joints of stainless steel or other chromium-containing alloys, but should not be used for gold alloys, since they are good conductors of electricity. Electrical resistance welding is suitable for β-Ti wire, the only orthodontic wire that has true weldability.

The strength of the welded joint is enhanced by an increase in the weld area. However, the welded area becomes brittle and susceptible to corrosion, because of precipitation of chromium carbide at temperatures above 500C, a process that is known as weld decay. Therefore, small welds are generally considered better, because fusion is achieved with minimal changes in the original grain structure.

Laser welding: Another method employed for joining metal frameworks is laser welding. To weld dental alloys, Nd:YAG laser is mainly used (Yamagishi *et al.*, 1993; Liu *et al.*, 2002; Iwasaki *et al.*, 2004; Watanabe and Topham, 2004, 2006; Srimaneepong *et al.*, 2005; Watanabe *et al.*, 2006).

In laser welding, laser light is focused on small regions, applying high energy to these areas in a very short amount of time. Heating is mainly focused at the point of application; therefore the surrounding areas do not damage. (O'Brien, 1997) In some studies, laser welded joints showed greater mechanical resistance than that achieved by traditional welding.(Fornaini et al., 2010)

Titanium alloys are commonly used in dentistry for crowns, bridges, partial denture frameworks, and also for orthodontic wires. These cannot be easily soldered by traditional torch-soldering or oven-soldering procedures. This is related to the fact that at temperatures used for soldering procedures, the thickness of the titanium oxide layer increases and it may even debond from the metal surface at higher temperatures. For effective joining of components made of pure titanium, laser welding is a preferred method, because it is associated with a lower thermal influence on the parts being joined, preserves the excellent biocompatibility potential of pure titanium and prevents the risk of galvanic corrosion. (Anusavice, 2003)

Laser welding is recently used in bracket manufacturing as an alternative to brazing. This technique eliminates the need to brazing alloy, reduces the risk of corrosion, and provides acceptable mechanical performance in association with a low risk of joint failure. (Eliades, 2007)

Solmi *et al.* (2004) analyzed the adhesion and proliferation of human gingival fibroblasts placed in direct contact with conventionally soldered and laser-welded orthodontic joints for up to 16 days. Significant differences in counts of survival fibroblasts were observed at all experimental times. The fibroblasts on both the laser-welded and control substrates showed similar patterns. By contrast, on the substrate of the soldered samples, the fibroblasts showed no sign of adaptation at any time during the study. These results highlight the superior biocompatibility of laser welding over brazing.

Testing the cell reactions of osteoblasts, fibroblasts, and keratinocytes, Sestini *et al.* (2006) found a good tolerance of electrical resistance and laser welding, while traditional silver solder was toxic for osteoblast differentiation, fibroblast viability, and keratinocyte growth.

The influence of brazing or welding on tensile strength has not been uniformly determined. In different studies, the factors affecting the mechanical strength of welded joints have been described: wavelength, peak pulse power, pulse energy, output energy, pulse duration, pulse frequency, and spot diameter of the laser welding machine and the type of metal used (McCartney and Doud, 1993; Yamagishi *et al.*, 1993; Taylor *et al.*, 1998; Watanabe *et al.*, 2001, 2003, 2004, 2006; Yan and Yang, 2006). Chai and Chou (1998) showed an equal or superior mechanical strength of the welded sites compared with the unsectioned parent metal of different Ti alloys depending on welding conditions. In contrast, the fracture load of unwelded Ti, gold, or Co–Cr alloys in different configurations of laser welding were not achieved (Watanabe *et al.*, 2001, 2003, 2004, 2006). Especially for gold and Co–Cr alloys, only 50 per cent or less of the original measurements were found. In the study by Bertrand *et al.* (2004), a small change in the chemical composition of the Ni-based alloys caused an important difference in weldability.

Rocha *et al.* (2006) compared laser and TIG welding of non-precious alloys. TIG welding increased the flexural strength of Ti, Co–Cr, and Ni–Cr as the used welded cylinders presented higher flexural strength than the non-weld cylinders. The highest means were observed for Co–Cr weld by TIG and non-welded Co–Cr. By contrast, laser welding achieved only 17.5 per cent of the flexural strength of Co–Cr alloy. When joining Co–Cr alloy specimens, Zupancic *et al.* (2006) showed significant differences between brazing and laser welding. Those authors estimated a low penetration depth, peripheral overheating, porosities, and carbon content of the alloy as possible reasons for the relative weakness of laser welding.

The evaluation of three orthodontic arch wire alloy materials, stainless steel, beta titanium, and Timolium, for their laser-weld characteristics showed significantly different tensile strength values between these materials (Krishnan and Kumar, 2004). Although a comparison with original wires was not carried out in that study, it could be assumed that laser-welded specimens showed a significantly lower tensile strength than pure metals.

More recently Bock et al. (2008) showed that small changes in laser welding parameters significantly influenced the mechanical properties of orthodontic wires. Although laser welding is a solder-free alternative for orthodontic purposes, further investigations are needed to determine the optimal parameters.

3.7 Laser minor surgery

Laser surgery offers numerous advantages compared with traditional scalpel surgery. Soft-tissue excision is more precise with a laser than a scalpel (Rossman and Cobb 1995). A laser coagulates blood vessels, seals lymphatic, and sterilizes the wound during ablation, maintaining a clear and clean surgical field. The use of soft-tissue lasers result in a shorter operative time and faster postoperative recuperation (Sarver and Yanosky 2005). Laser surgery is routinely performed by using only topical anesthetic, which is particularly beneficial in an open orthodontic clinic (Sarver 2006). There is markedly less bleeding (particularly for frenal surgery), minimal swelling, and no need for irritating sutures or unsightly periodontal dressing (Haytac and Ozcelik 2006). Post surgically, patients report less discomfort and fewer functional complications (speaking and chewing), and require fewer analgesics than do patients treated with conventional scalpei surgery (Haytac and Ozcelik 2006).

The primary disadvantage of laser surgery is its high expense. Some clinicians have reported greater tactile sense with a scalpel (which might be particularly true for noncontact soft-tissue lasers such as the erbium laser), tissue desiccation, and poor wound healing (Baker et al. 2002).

Lasers cut by thermal ablation—decomposition of tissue through an instantaneous process of absorption, melting, and vaporization. Essentially, the cells of the target tissue absorb the concentrated light energy, rapidly rise in temperature, and produce a micro-explosion known as spallation (Moritz 2006).

Surgical lasers typically have (1) a central zone of carbonization surrounded by, (2) a zone of vaporization, coagulation, and protein denaturation, and (3) a stimulating zone. This may be one reason for the improved healing with laser surgery compared with traditional scalpel surgery. During laser curettage, sufficient hemostasis and significant reduction of the initial levels of periodontal pathogens are achieved (Lioubavina-Hack 2002). Various applications of laser surgery in orthodontics are:

3.7.1 Gingival enlargements, gingival hyperplasia and reshaping gingival shape and contours

Sometimes removal of excessive gingival tissues is necessary to provide optimal display of teeth. For example, inadequate tooth display in smile in an adolescent patient may be related to altered passive eruption or gingival encroachment, making the teeth appears short. In this cases, gingivectomy may provide sufficient tooth display and appropriate tooth proportions.

Gingival hyperplasia is commonly observed during orthodontic treatment, especially in patients with poor oral hygiene. Generally, it is preferred to postpone treatment of gingival hyperplasia until the end of orthodontic treatment, unless the gingival tissue or enlargement interferes with tooth movement. If this occurs, the excess gingiva must be removed surgically during the treatment. Orthodontists should also consider gingival shape and contour of the teeth and make necessary corrections to provide optimal treatment results at the end of orthodontic treatment. Recontouring gingival shape and contour can be readily accomplished in the orthodontist's office with a diode laser. Laser gingivectomy has advantages such as minimal bleeding and postoperative pain and no swelling (Lioubavina-Hack 2002). Correction of gingival hyperplasia can also be performed easily with the aid of laser light.

3.7.2 Fibrotomy

Fibrotomy (Pericision) is frequently indicated to provide long term stability of teeth with severe rotations before treatment. This procedure is usually performed for upper and lower anterior teeth (e.g. maxillary lateral incisors in class II Div 2 patients) where maintaining treatment results is of great importance. Fibrotomy or severing of transpalatal fibers should be performed at the end of orthodontic treatment and before appliance removal.(Vanarsdall RL and Secchi AG, 2005) The teeth should be held in good alignment after fibrotomy when gingival healing occurs.

The poor patient acceptability in conventional fiberotomy, as an invasive procedure, suggests that an alternative technique needs to be considered. Kim et al. (2010) investigated the effectiveness and periodontal side effects of laser circumferential supracrestal fibrotomy (CSF) of orthodontically rotated teeth in beagles. A gallium-aluminum-arsenide (Ga-Al-As) diode laser with an 808-nm wavelength and 0.4-mm fiber diameter was used. The laser tip was inserted into the gingival sulcus to the level of the alveolar bone crest, and the incision was extended around the tooth circumference with the system configured to the soft tissue cutting mode (continuous wave; 1.2 W). The amount of relapse, sulcus depth, and gingival recession were measured at weeks 4 and 8. They concluded that laser CSF is an effective procedure to decrease relapse after tooth rotation, causing no apparent damage to the supporting periodontal structures. It was claimed that the bactericidal effect transferred by the laser within the periodontal pocket can reduce the risk of infection.

3.7.3 Frenectomy

Frenectomy is usually indicated to prevent relapse after correction of midline diastema. Before eruption of maxillary canines, small physiologic spaces usually exist between maxillary incisors, a developmental stage named "ugly duckling stage". These spaces tend to close spontaneously after eruption of maxillary canines. Therefore frenectomy is not indicated during mixed dentition treatment, unless the presence of a large diastema between central incisors causes a great aesthetic problem, or prevents the eruption of other anterior teeth. When frenectomy is indicated, it is recommended to close the space between central incisors with orthodontic treatment prior to frenectomy. Otherwise, the formation of scar tissue prevents orthodontic space closure. Of course in some occasions, the presence of a very thick frenum may prevent space closure. If this occurs, frenectomy should be performed after partial space closure, and orthodontic treatment should be resumed immediately after frenectomy to complete space closure. In the conventional surgical method a simple incision is used to allow access to the interdental area, the fibrous connection to the bone is removed, and the frenum is then sutured at a higher level.

Olivi et al. (2010) clinically evaluated the efficacy of Er,Cr:YSGG laser at a power setting of 1.5 W or less in 156 frenectomies. The reported very high patient acceptance and no postoperative adverse events. Recently diode laser frenectomy without infiltrated anesthesia was suggested by Kafas et al. (2009). They concluded that this procedure have optimum healing post-surgically. However, in severe cases of soft tissue excision the need of anesthesia may be essential (Kato and Wijeyeweera 2007).

Haytac and Ozcelik (2006) reported that CO2 laser treatment used for frenectomy operations provides better patient perception in terms of postoperative pain and function than that obtained by the scalpel technique. They suggested that CO2 laser offers a safe, effective, acceptable, and impressive alternative for frenectomy operations. The results were the same for Nd:YAG laser frenectomy. Kara (2009) compared the effects of Nd:YAG laser and conventional technique on the degree of preoperative anxiety levels, postoperative pain, discomfort, and functional complications (eating and speech) of frenectomy. The results suggested that Nd:YAG laser treatment of soft tissue disorders provides better patient perceptions of success than those seen with conventional surgery.

4. Low intensity laser therapy in orthodontics

4.1 Description of therapeutic lasers

Low level laser therapy (LLLT) is also known as "soft laser therapy" and bio-stimulation. The use of LLLT in health care has been documented in the literature for more than three decades. Numerous research studies have demonstrated that LLLT is effective for some specific applications in dentistry. The LLLT literatures are large, with more than 1,000 papers published on this topic. A problem in dissecting this literature is the variation in methodology and dosimetry between different studies. Not only have a range of different wave lengths been examined, but exposure times and the frequency of treatments also vary (Walsh et al,2006).

While broad band light can exert effects on cells, interest has been concentrated on using lasers as a light source because of their greater therapeutic effect (Karu. 1989, Laakso et al. 1993). While much of the initial work with LLLT used the helium - neon gas laser work with LLLT used the helium- neon gas laser (λ = 632.8 nm), nowadays most LLLT clinical procedures are undertaken using semiconductor diode lasers, for example, gallium arsenide based diode lasers operating at λ = 830 nm or λ = 635 nm wavelengths . Since wavelength is the most important factor in any type of phototherapy, the clinician must consider which wavelengths are capable of producing the desired effects within living tissues. The typical power output for a low level laser device used for this therapy is of the order of 10-50 mW, and total irradiances at any point are of the order of several Joules. Thermal effects of LLLT on dental tissues are not significant, and do not contribute to the therapeutic effects seen. The wavelengths use for LLLT has poor absorption in water, and thus penetrate soft and hard tissues from 3 mm to up to 15 mm (Sandford &Walsh.1994;Ohshiro & Calderhead.1998; Walsh.2003;Walsh et al.2006).

4.2 History

In 1967, a few years after the first working laser was invented, Endre Mester in Semmelweis University, Budapest, Hungary wanted to test if laser radiation might cause cancer in mice (Mester, 1968). They did not get cancer, and to his surprise the hair on the treated group grew back more quickly than the untreated group. This was the first demonstration of "laser biostimulation". In fact, light therapy is one of the oldest therapeutic methods used by humans historically as solar therapy by Egyptians, later as UV therapy for which Nils Finsen won the Nobel Prize in 1904. (Roelandts,2002).

The use of lasers and LEDs as light sources was the next step in the technological development of light therapy, which is now applied to many thousands of people worldwide each day. The reason why the technique is termed LOW-level is that the optimum levels of energy density delivered are low when compared to other forms of laser therapy as practiced for ablation, cutting, and thermally coagulating tissue. In general, the power densities used for LLLT are lower than those needed to produce heating of tissue, i.e., less than 100 mW/cm2, depending on wavelength and tissue type (Huang YY et al., 2009).

4.3 Introduction

Although laser phototherapy ("low level laser therapy") has been practiced for more than 30 years there is still controversy regarding its scientific standard. Questions still remain even though more than 400 studies with a dental focus have been reported. The biomodulative effects exerted on cells are well documented (Karu 2003, 2006, 2007), to a certain degree in animal studies. The safety of the treatment is also well documented. In spite of clinical observations for a great variety of conditions, some controversy remains.

Due to the fact that so many parameters are included, it is more difficult to reach a consensus in this area of dental laser applications than in the domain of high-intensity laser applications. Many different wavelengths, power densities, energy densities and application modes have been used and there is no current consensus about optical standards. In addition, the reporting of the actual laser parameters and dosimetry in studies is often substandard and control studies are therefore difficult to perform. Consequently the evaluation of the various applications becomes problematic. The optical properties and performance of the various commercially available lasers vary widely, adding to the problems in the evaluation process (Bradley & Tuner, 2007).

Surgical lasers are rather precise in their indications: the results are verified more easily with the naked eye as well as through subsequent lab analyses. Therapeutic lasers work on the cellular level, influencing the fundamental functions of the cells. Any pathological condition can thus theoretically be improved if the suitable wavelength and energy of light is applied. This is at the same time the beauty and the problem of laser biomodulation: how can one therapy be applied in so many situations? There is supposedly no universal method in the history of medicine and a skeptical attitude from dentists is basically a sound reaction. The results of non-dental research often have to be extrapolated into dental area when conclusions are to be attempted. It should to a high degree of probability be possible to extrapolate the effects on nerves, wound healing, pain relief, edema, etc., and in non- dental areas of the animal or human body for dental conditions. A problematic part of the existing literature is the frequent lack of understanding of laser physics and laser therapeutic approaches, whether from manufacturers, users, researchers or indeed from peer reviewers(Bradley & Tuner, 2007).

Several meta-analyses have failed to evaluate crucial dosimetric parameters such as applied energies and energy densities, and later re-evaluations using the same material have been able to turn a negative interpretation into positive on (Bjordal et al. 1998, 2001, 2003). But once published , meta analyses are irrepressible. Even Cochrane analyses of laser interventions (Bjordal 2005) have failed to observe basic analysis of doses, wavelengths and application modes. Future studies had better address the most crucial parameter of the study, namely the laser itself. Consensus is needed on how to describe these parameters.

The phenomenon of cell biomodulation is well described (Karu 2003), but the optimal clinical parameters are still little known and will have to be more accurately defined in future studies. Many positive studies were conducted within a supposed "therapeutic window" but were not necessarily close to the optimal applications. The most important fields of future research will be discussed here. Laser phototherapy is non- invasive, non-pharmaceutical, has very few side effects, is painless and enjoys a high acceptance from patients. More attention to the method's potential is therefore logical .A not so well-known fact that should be recognized, is that surgical lasers can have a biomodulatory effect, too. Furthermore, all these "surgical" lasers can be used for biomodulation purposes if the dosage is adjusted accordingly. To further emphasize this fact would increase the value of a surgical laser (Bradley & Tuner, 2007).

4.4 Mechanism of action

The mechanisms of low level laser therapy are complex, but essentially rely upon the absorption of particular visible red and near-infrared wavelengths in photoreceptors within sub-cellular components, particularly the electron transport (respiratory) chain within the membranes of mitochondria(Karu.1989a,1989b; Walsh et al,2006).

The absorption of light by the respiratory chain components causes a short- term activation of the respiratory chain, and oxidation of the NADH pool. This stimulation of oxidative phosphorylation leads to changes in the redox status of both the mitochondria and the cytoplasm of the cell. The electron transport chain is able to provide increased levels of promotive force to the cell, through increased supply of ATP, as well as an increase in the electrical potential of the mitochondria membrane, alkalization of the cytoplasm, and activation of nucleic acid synthesis. Because ATP is the "energy currency" for a cell, LLLT has a potent that results in simulation of the normal functions of the cell(Yu et al.1997;Walsh et al, 2006).

Karu.(1987,1988,1989)who has studied the bio-stimulative effects of light on cell cultures in great detail, has demonstrated that cell cultures that are initially irradiated with laser light show a range of biological effects. Of importance, is these cultures are then irradiated with non- monochromatic and incoherent light, the previous laser- produced biological effects are almost nullified. This suggests that there are more complex mechanisms at work than the simple excitation of polarization- sensitive chromophores in the cell. Considerable insight into the effect of wave length on LLLT has been gained from the work of Karu who over a period of years has conducted extensive research using cell cultures of various types. Her work has provided and action spectrum for bio-stimulation of the rate of DNA synthesis in HeLa cells, and for proliferation of bacteria and yeast colonies. These spectra show peaks in the blue (λ = 404 nm and λ = 454 nm), red (λ = 620nm), and near-infrared (λ =760 nm) and λ = 830 nm). (Karu,1987,1988,1989).The tissue response to photonic energy as well as to other energetic stimuli follows the Arndt Schultz pattern where low energies stimulated and high energies tend to inhibit.(Fig.5). It follows from this that low energies will be appropriate for the stimulation of healing while high energies may be more suitable for pain control with the aim of suppressing aberrant sensitization of nerve fibers(Bradley & Tuner, 2007).The Arndt-Schulz law thus provides a useful theoretical basis to explain the varying photobiostimulatory and photobioinhibitory effects observed in the laboratory; however it also goes some way to accounting for the apparently conflicting results that are sometimes achieved with low-intensity laser therapy. (Fig.5)

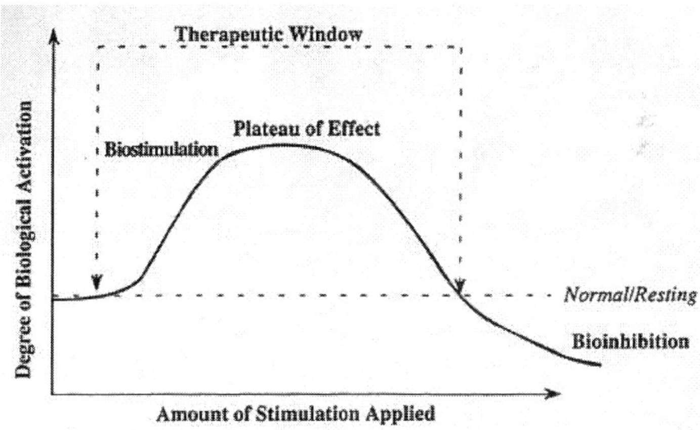

Fig. 5. Arndt-Schultz Law

This is only a generalization in that promotion of healing in an inflammatory situation may have a pain relieving action in its own right. From an extensive background of laboratory date, Dyson. (2005) has divided cellular responses in the context of healing into primary and secondary responses.

Primary responses:
1. The photons are absorbed by cytochromes.2. Singlet oxygen free radicals are generated, effecting ATP synthesis and thus increasing the energy available to the cells.3. Nitric oxide is produced.4. Reversible increase in cell membrane permeability to calcium and other ions occurs, triggering changes in cell activity, i.e. secondary responses.
Secondary responses:
1. DNA and RNA synthesis.2. Cell proliferation.3. Growth factor release.4. Collagen synthesis by fibroblasts.5. Changes in nerve conduction, neurotransmitter release etc.
Potential mechanisms of pain relief:
The potential mechanisms involved in pain relief (Bradley, 2005) have been postulated as:

a. Direct action on nerve. There is evidence from the animal experimental field using excised rat sciatic nerve that 830 nm irradiation with an incident power of 60 mw for 60 seconds (4 Jules per point) and 120 seconds (8 Joules per point) can inhibit the activity of sodium potassium ATP -ase responsible for never depolarization in generation of the action potential (Kudoh et al, 1989). This effect is likely to he maximal for the small diameter C fibers responsible for most chronic pain, due to their lack of a protective myelin sheath.
b. Energization of inactivated enzymes: Enzymes may be inactivated by such factors as hypoxia and acidosis in areas of muscle spasm with ischemia (e.g. trigger points) or in foci of chronic inflammation. There is evidence that laser energy can reactivate these enzymes (Bolognani & Volpi, 1992). Free radicals for example may be a source of pain in dysfunctional muscle where the enzyme super oxide dismutase (SOD) can break down these entities if reactivated.
c. Production of Energy Molecules (ATP) in Dysfunctional Muscle. The interaction of myosin and actin in muscle requires adenosine triphosphate (ATP) and its lack may contribute to painful dysfunction. A characteristic of the response of cells to laser light is the formation of ATP (Krau, 2000).
d. Reduction of prostaglandin levels. There is evidence from the clinical and cell culture work that laser exposure can reduce levels of the algogenic substance PGE2 (Mizutani et al., 2002).

4.5 Contraindication

Absolute contraindications to LPT are not known, but there are several relative contradictions and caveats. Areas of malignancies or suspected malignancies should be avoided at present due to insufficient knowledge. For the same reason irradiation of patients with coagulation disorders and photosensitivity should be avoided. Irradiation over the thyroid has been reported as a contraindication, but current knowledge does not substantiate such risk when irradiation is performed in or close to this area on healthy individuals. However, care is recommended in cases of hyperthyroidism. Pregnancy is reported as a caveat, but this would only apply in case of large doses over the abdomen. As for epilepsy, there are anecdotal reports on seizure attacks triggered by pulsed light, but it would probably have to be in the visible range and observed by the patient. Irradiations over testicles and diabetic wounds have been reported as contraindications for LPT, given the correct diagnosis. Some articles mention patients wearing pacemakers as a contraindication, but this is likely a misunderstanding (Bradley & Tuner, 2007).

4.6 Conclusions

Low level laser therapy has been found to accelerated wound healing and reduce pain, possibly by stimulating oxidative phosphorylation in mitochondria and modulating inflammatory responses. By influencing the biological function of a variety of cell types, it is able to exert a rage of several beneficial effects upon inflammation and healing (Walsh et al,, 2006). LLLT exerts marked effects upon cell in all phases on wound healing, but particularly so during the proliferative phase. There is good evidence that the enhanced cell metabolic functions seen after LLLT are the result of activation of photo-receptors within the electron transport chain of mitochondria. The effects specific for wavelength, and cannot be gained efficiently with normal, non- coherent, non- polarized light sources, such as LEDs(Walsh et al.,2006).

Future trials of new LLLT applications in dentistry should make use of standardized, validated outcomes, and should explore how the effectiveness of the LLLT protocol used may be influenced by wavelength, treatment duration, dosage, and the site of application.

4.7 Photobiomodolation effects of lasers in orthodontics

4.7.1 Pain reduction

Pain or discomfort is a common experience during fixed orthodontic treatment. Pain is usually appears several hours after orthodontic force application and slowly increases until 24 hours, then it returns to the basic level at approximately 5th days. This pain cycle may be repeated after each appointment, although for nearly all patients, it is the most severe after initial arch wire placement. For patients, pain may be the most important side effect of orthodontic treatment and one of the main reasons for their lack of compliance or missing appointments.(Sergl et al., 1998; Turhani et al., 2006; Young et al., 2006; Bird et al., 2007; Polat et al., 2005) Furthermore, nearly all orthodontic patients report pain during chewing and biting and this can oblige them to change diet habits. Finally, it has been demonstrated that pain and discomfort during orthodontic treatment negatively affects the satisfaction of patient from aesthetic results of orthodontic treatment.(Al-Omiri and Abu Alhaija, 2006) If orthodontists are able to prevent or control pain, patients may have a better quality of life and show more tendencies to cooperate with treatment recommendations.

The mechanism through which orthodontic forces produce pain has not well recognized, but there is some evidence indicating that pain is related to the change in blood circulation of periodontal ligament, causing ischemic areas in the PDL. For this reason, a heavier force may cause a greater degree of pain due to the formation of larger ischemic areas in the periodontal ligament. Pain is also dependant to the formation of metabolic products such as prostaglandins and substance P which stimulate pain receptors.

To relieve pain, most orthodontists recommend their patients to use nonsteroidal antiinflammatory drugs (NSAIDs), to inhibit the formation of pain producing agents such as prostaglandins and thus reduce the pain. However, these drugs may have side effects and therefore are contraindicated in some patients. Furthermore, most drugs used for pain control can have negative effects on tooth movement if used chronically, due to their inhibitory effects on prostaglandins.

Considering the side effects of analgesics, researchers have looked for other new, but safer approaches, such as LLLT to reduce pain from orthodontic procedures (Xiaoting 2010). Although only a few studies have dealt with the response of orthodontic patients to LLLT, all concluded that LLLT reduces pain during orthodontic treatment (Lim et al. 1995, Katoh et al. 1997, Harazaki et al. 1997, Harazaki and Isshiki 1998, Turhani et al. 2006, Youssef et al

2008). Lim et al. (1995) observed in orthodontic patients that pain for teeth irradiated with a gallium-arsenic-aluminum diode laser was lower compared with pain when a placebo was used. Harazaki and Isshiki (1998), on irradiating both vestibular and lingual sides of teeth with an orthodontic appliance, using a helium-neon laser with a 632.8-nm wavelength, operated at 6 mW for 30 seconds, reported that the laser therapy not only reduced patient discomfort but also delayed the onset of pain. Data have shown the efficacy of LLLT for pain control after placement of the first archwire (Turhani et al. 2006, Tortamano et al. 2009). In a study by Tortamano et al. (2009) the patients in the experimental group received gallium-arsenic-aluminum diode laser irradiation with a wavelength of 830 nm. The laser beam emitted a constant wave with a mean output of 30 mW. Each tooth received a dose of 2.5 J per square centimenter on each side (buccal and lingual). The patients in the LLLT group had reduced pain duration and a lower intensity of pain. Although these authors couldn't find any effect on the start of pain perception, previous studies showed delayed pain onset in patients who had LLLT (Harazaki 1997, Turhani 2006).

Overall, based on the efficacy of LLLT to control pain in orthodontic treatment, LLLT could be recommended for pain control during fixed orthodontic appliance therapy. The reason for reducing its clinical use seems to be the total time (32–37.5 minutes) for application to both dental arches (Lim et al. 1995, Katoh et al. 1997, Harazaki et al. 1997, Harazaki & Isshiki 1998, Tortamano et al. 2009). Yet many diverse opinions existed concerning the duration of treatment, radiant power, frequency, and energy density.

4.7.2 Tooth movement

The biological control of tooth movement still has not well recognized. The most accepted theory of tooth movement is pressure-tension theory, which is based on stimulating cellular differentiation through chemical mediators. This theory states that force application causes tooth displacement within the PDL, which in turn results in compression in some areas of the PDL, while other parts may be stretched. In the compression side blood circulation is decreased, while in the tension side blood flow is maintained or even increased. The alteration in blood flow creates rapid changes in the proportion of oxygen and other metabolites within the PDL, which in turn can stimulate the release of other biologically active elements. These chemical alterations would stimulate cellular differentiation and cell activity.(Proffit et al., 2007) Prostaglandin E, Interleukin 1α and Interleukin 1β are some of the important mediators released during the process of tooth movement. It is believed that orthodontic tooth movement includes many inflammation like reactions, because it is associated with high vascular activity, release of many leukocytes and macrophages, and involvement of the immune systems. This is important because it implies that the whole cascade of factors involved in an inflammation process may be part of the reactions to orthodontic forces in the tooth-supporting tissues.(Thilander et al., 2005)

Several studies have represented the effects of LLLT on orthodontic tooth movement. In five of nine animal studies about stimulation effects of LLLT on orthodontic tooth movement (Kawasaki and Shimizu 2000, Sun et al. 2001, Goulart et al. 2006, Yamaguchi M et al. 2007, Seifi et al. 2007, Fujita et al. 2008, Yoshida et al. 2009, Yamaguchi et al. 2010, Kim et al. 2010), experiments were performed on albino Wistar rats using the same laser device and the same parameters (Kawasaki and Shimizu 2000, Yamaguchi M et al. 2007, Fujita et al. 2008, Yoshida et al. 2009, Yamaguchi et al. 2010). Even though the energy density used in these studies was considerably higher (54 J, 19.108 J/cm2) than it is thought to be appropriate for biostimulation (2-12 J/cm2), it was concluded in all of the five studies that laser radiation had stimulated tooth movement. When the other animal studies were examined, it was noticed that there were differences about subject type, the energy dose given, and about the results. Seifi et al. (2007) reported the effects of two types of LLL wavelengths (850 nm and 630 nm) on orthodontic tooth movements in rabbits. The total amount of energy in 850 nm and 630 nm laser groups was 8.1 J/cm2 and 27 J/cm2, respectively. The authors showed that the amount of orthodontic tooth movement, after LLL application, was diminished, and there was no significant difference between the laser groups. Cruz et al. (2004), Youssef et al. (2008), and da Silva Sousa et al. (2011) demonstrated clinically that LLLT accelerates the orthodontic movement in humans. Cruz et al. (2004) conducted an experiment on 11 young patients who required tooth movement for extraction space closure. They were irradiated with LLLT of 780 nm wavelength (for 10 s at 20 mW; 5 J/cm2) on one side of the maxilla for 4 days in a month and were not irradiated on the opposite side, which acted as the control. The results showed that the experimental side demonstrated significantly more rapid progression of space closure than the control side. Youssef et al. (2008) evaluate the effect of the GaAlAs diode laser (809 nm, 100 mW) during an orthodontic movement in a group of 15 adult patients. They demonstrated that the velocity of canine movement was significantly greater in the lased group than in the control group. This was confirmed by da Silva Sousa et al. (2011) which used a diode laser (780 nm, 20 mW, 10 sec, 5 J/cm2) for 3 days. However, Limpanichkul et al. (2006) found no difference in tooth movement rate after application of LLL for 3 days in a month. They claimed that the energy capacity of LLL (25 J/cm2) in their study was probably too low to produce stimulatory effects on orthodontic tooth movement. However, their LLL application method for orthodontic tooth movement was different from the others. They used a 0.09 cm2 spectral area to irradiate the alveolar mucosa at some point. This restricted application might be a lack for the whole periodontium surrounding the tooth.

Fujita et al. (2008) and Yamaguchi et al. (2007) reported that LLLT stimulated the velocity of tooth movement via RANK and c-Fms gene expressions *in vitro*. This was confirmed by Yamaguchi et al. (2010) which showed that LLLT accelerates the process of bone remodeling by stimulating MMP-9, cathepsin K, and integrin subunits of a(v)b3 expression during orthodontic tooth movement in rats.

4.7.3 Distraction osteogenesis

Distraction osteogenesis is a method to induce new bone formation and investing soft tissue under the influence of tensional stress at osteotomized sites of a healing bone. Distraction osteogenesis not only induces bone formation but also results in formation of new soft tissue (histogenesis) over the new bone. This method was used successfully by Alizarow in the 1950s to lengthen the bony segments of the limbs, and now is widely used in dentistry for correcting deficient growth of the maxilla and mandible in patients with congenital problems such as cleft lip/palate and hemifacial microsomia. Distraction osteogenesis makes it possible to achieve a greater amount of bone lengthening than that achieved with conventional orthognathic surgery without the need for placing bone grafts. An additional advantage of this technique is that the correction can be performed at an earlier age. However, precise positioning of the jaw is not possible with this method, and consequently orthognathic surgery may be required later to achieve optimal treatment results. Distraction osteogenesis is a suitable option for extensive lengthening of the ramus in patients with moderately severe hemifacial microsomia, and also for advancing the mid face in patients having severe maxillary deficiency such as those with Crouzon syndrome. Furthermore, it is now possible to widen mandibular symphysis through distraction osteogenesis technique, a procedure that cannot be performed with orthognathic surgery due to the lack of soft tissue for covering the bone graft at that area.

Distraction osteogenesis consist of four sequential steps:(Cope and Samchukov, 2005) The first step is osteotomy, which provokes the process of bone repair at surgically created sites. The second stage is called latency, which defines the period between bone fracture and initiation of tensional stress to the bone. In latency period, a reparative callus is allowed to form. In the third stage or distraction phase, a gradual traction is applied to the bone to create new bone at the surgical sites. The bony segments are usually separated at a rate of 0.5-1.5 mm per day during the distraction phase. Consolidation is the fourth step of distraction osteogenesis defining the period between the end of traction application and removal of the distraction device. This stage is necessary to allow complete mineralization of the new bone formed by distraction process. Because of the time required for bone maturation and for removal of the distracter, distraction osteogenesis may generate discomfort, which has led some authors to study solutions to accelerate new bone formation (Hübler et al. 2010).

Miloro et al. (2007) evaluated the effect of LLLT during mandibular distraction osteogenesis and concluded that LLL accelerates the process of bone regeneration during the consolidation phase after distraction osteogenesis. Further, Kreisner et al. (2010) evaluated the action of LLLT on the percentage of newly formed bone in rabbit mandibles that underwent distraction osteogenesis. Infrared GaAlAs LLLT (λ=830 nm, P=40 mW) was applied directly on the bone site that underwent distraction osteogenesis during bone consolidation at 48-hour intervals. The results suggested that the percentage of newly formed bone was greater in the LLLT group than in the control group. Cerqueira et al. (2007) stated that the laser has been more favorable when used in the consolidation period, after bone elongation. The results of a study by Hübler et al. (2010) showed that LLLT had a positive effect on the percentage of newly formed bone, on the chemical composition according to the Ca-to-P ratios, and on the crystallinity and crystalline structure at the distraction osteogenesis sites.

4.7.4 Retention & relapse

Relapse after orthodontic correction of malocclusions is an undesirable but frequent experience for nearly all orthodontists. Teeth that have moved by orthodontic forces tend to return to their original positions, a phenomenon referred to as relapse. Generally, occlusion instability occurs because of the following reasons:

1. Changes related to growth: This type of relapse appears in long time and is usually related to continuation of growth in the original pattern caused malocclusion. An example is deepening of overbite due to growth or uncoordinated growth of maxilla and mandible in orthodontically treated patients. To counteract these changes, active treatment should be continued until growth is essentially complete.
2. Inherent instability of the occlusion due to soft tissue pressure: Alignment of the teeth in the dental arch is in equilibrium between the tongue pressure and labial/buccal soft tissue pressure. If there is any major imbalance between extra and intra oral soft tissue pressures, there would be a relapse tendency. For example widening of the mandibular

arch, particularly in the canine area, is susceptible to relapse. The only solution to counteract relapse in these cases is to use permanent retention.

3. The changes related to fibrous system of PDL and gingival: These fibers may be responsible for most of the short term relapse after orthodontic treatment, for example after correction of rotated teeth and diastema closure. The elastic fibers of the gingival in particular may be stretched and displaced for long times after orthodontic correction, causing tooth movement forces even one year after appliance removal.

After appliance removal, the important stage of retention period is initiated. In this period, the orthodontist aims to retain the corrected tooth position passively, while the alveolar bone and gingival and periodontal fibers are remodeled. During the period of retention, the osteoid is replaced by bundle bone, which is finally changed to lamellated bone with harvesian system, and gingival and periodontal fibers are also reorganized.

LLLT effects on the relapse tendency of orthodontically rotated teeth have not been fully characterized. Kim et al. (2010) investigated the effectiveness of LLLT on orthodontically rotated teeth in beagles. A Ga-Al-As diode laser was used. The biostimulation mode (pulsed wave, 10 Hz, 763 mW, 4.63-6.47 J/cm2) was used for irradiation, with the fiber tip held 2-3 mm away from the gingiva. The coronal and apical thirds of the roots were irradiated every 3 days for 30 seconds each for 4 weeks. They concluded that LLLT of orthodontically rotated teeth without retainers increased the rotational relapse of the teeth compared with the control group.

4.7.5 Growth modification

Maxillary expansion

Maxillary expansion may be required in patients who have deficient maxillary width. This treatment also helps to remove crowding and align the teeth. The mid-palatal suture is separated easily up to age nine or ten, therefore any expansion device is expected to produce a combination of dental and skeletal expansion. However, the midpalatal suture tend to interdigitate more and more with increasing age, and heavy forces are needed to microfracture it in adolescent patients. Usually a fixed type of jackscrew device is used to apply heavy forces to separate the suture, and either slow or rapid expansion protocols can be used for this purpose.

Saito and Shimizu (1997) studied the effects of LLLT on the expansion of midpalatal sutures in rats, comparing the bone regeneration obtained with and without laser treatment. Their results showed that the therapeutic effects of laser are dependent on the total dosage, the frequency, and the duration of the treatment. Their laser-irradiated group showed 20-40% better results when compared to the control group.

Mandibular growth

When mandible is deficient as is seen in most class II patients, growth modification is a suitable treatment option for growing children. To do this, a functional appliance is usually indicated to pull the condyle out of the glenoid fossa a sufficient distance for long durations, enhancing condylar growth amount and creating a more favorable growth direction in mandibular condyle. Growth modification for correcting mandibular deficiency can be performed successfully in late mixed dentition and early permanent dentition patients before the end of the adolescent growth spurt, but the chance of skeletal versus dental correction is reduced as the patient gets older.

It was proposed that if LLLT increases bone and cartilage formation, the treatment might be easier and more stable. In 2010 Seifi et al. investigated the effects of low level GaAs diode laser (λ=904 nm, 2,000 Hz, pulse length 200 ns and output power 4 mW) on chondroblastic and osteoblastic activity of condyles in rats. Laser irradiation was performed either bilaterally or on the right condyle. They showed that LLLT had a significant effect on the increase of mandibular length in rats and might be helpful in the correction of class II malocclusions. However, further studies are required to confirm these results.

5. Conclusion

To have a precise diagnosis and to select a proper and successful laser-assisted treatment modality for a disease, the clinician should have a comprehensive understanding of the principles and fundamentals of laser and its helpful abilities.When considering the use of lasers in clinical dentistry, the practitioner must use clinical experience, receive proper training, and have familiarity with the operating characteristics of each device. Because of the variable composition of human tissue and the differing ways in which laser energies are absorbed, no single laser is appropriate for all dental applications.

6. References

Abalos, C., Herrera, M., Jimenez-Planas, A., & Llamas,R. (2009). Performance of laser fluorescence for detection of occlusal dentinal caries lesions in permanent molars: an in vivo study with total validation of the sample. *Caries Research*, vol. 43, no. 2, pp. 137-141

Abdul-Kader, HM.,& Ibrahim, SA. (1999).A comparative study of CO2 laser debonding of three types of ceramic brackets. *Al-Azhar J Dent Sci*, 2:91-97

Ahrari, F., Heravi, F., Fekrazad, R., Farzanegan F,& Nakhaee S. Does ultra pulse CO2 laser reduce the risk of enamel damage during debonding of ceramic brackets? *Laser Med Sci* ,(In press).

Akarsu, S.,& Koprulu, H. (2006). In vivo comparison of the efficacy of DIAGNOdent by visual inspection and radiographic diagnostic techniques in the diagnosis of occlusal caries. *Journal of Clinical Dentistry*, vol. 17, no. 3, pp. 53-58

Akova, T., Yoldas, O., Toroglu, MS.,& Uysal, H .(2005). Porcelain surface treatment by laser for bracket-porcelain bonding. *Am J Orthod Dentofacial Orthop*, 128(5):630-637

Alcaniz, M., Grau, V., Monserrat, C., Juan, C.,& Albalat, S.(1999). A system for the simulation and planning of orthodontic treatment using a low cost 3D laser scanner for dental anatomy capturing. *Studies in Health Technology and Information*,62:8-14.

Alencar, CJ., Braga, MM., de Oliveira, E., Nicolau, J.,& Mendes, FM. (2009). Dye-enhanced laser fluorescence detection of caries lesions around brackets. *Lasers Med Sci* 24(6):865-70.

Aljehani, A., Bamzahim, M., Yousif, A., & Shi, X. Q. (2006). In vivo reliability of an infrared fluorescence method for quantification of carious lesions in orthodontic patients. *Oral Health & Preventive Dentistry*, vol. 4, no. 2, pp. 145-150

Aljehani, A., Tranaeus, S., Forsberg CM, Angmar-Månsson B, Shi XQ (2004) In vitro quantification of white spot enamel lesions adjacent to fixed orthodontic appliances using quantitative light induced fluorescence and DIAGNOdent. *Acta Odontol Scand* ,62:313-318

Al-Omiri, MK., &Abu Alhaija, ES. (2006). Factors affecting patient satisfaction after orthodontic treatment. *Angle Orthod* ,76(3): 422-431.

Anderson, A., Skold-Larsson, K. , Hallgren, A., Petersson, LG. , & Twetman, S.(2007) .Effect of a dental cream containing amorphous cream phosphate complexes on white spot lesion regression assessed by laser fluorescence. *Oral Health & Preventive Dentistry,* vol. 5, no. 3, pp. 229–233

Anderson, AM., Kao, E., Gladwin, M., Benli, O., Ngan, P.(2002). The effects of argon laser irradiation on enamel decalcification: An in vivo study. *Am J Orthod Dentofacial Orthop*, 122(3), 251-259.

Aoki, A., Sasaki, K. M., Watanabe, H., Ishikawa, I. (2004) .Laser in nonsurgical periodontal therapy. *Periodontal 2000* ,36, 59-97.

Angnes, V., Angnes, G. , Batisttella, M., Grande, RHM., Loguercio, AD.,& Reis, A. (2005). Clinical effectiveness of laser fluorescence, visual inspection and radiography in the detection of occlusal caries.*Caries Research*, vol. 39, no. 6, pp. 490–495

Anic, I., Pavelic, B., Peric, B.,& Matsumoto, K. (1996).In vitro pulp chamber temperature rises associated with the argon laser polymerization of composite resin. *Lasers Surg Med*,19:438-44.

Anttonen, V., Seppa, L., & Hausen, H. A follow-up study of the use of DIAGNOdent for monitoring fissure caries in children. *Community Dentistry and Oral Epidemiology,* vol. 32, no. 4, pp. 312–318, 2004.

Ariyaratnam, MT., Wilson, MA., Blinkhorn, AS. (1999). An analysis of surface roughness, surface morphology and composite/dentin bond strength of human dentin following the application of the Nd:YAG laser. *Dent Mater,* 15:222–228

Ariyaratnam, MT., Wilson, MA., Mackie, IC., Blinkhorn, AS .(1997). A comparison of surface roughness and composite/enamel bond strength of human enamel following the application of the Nd:YAG laser and etching with phosphoric acid. *Dent Mater* ,13:51–55

Arridge, S., Moss, JP., Linney, AD., & James, DR. (1985).Three dimensional digitization of the face and skull. *J Maxillofac Surg,* Jun; 13(3): 136-43.

Artun , J. (1997). A post-treatment evaluation of multibonded ceramic brackets in orthodontics. *Eur J Orthod* ,19(2): 219-228.

Ashmore, JL, Kurland BF, King GJ, Wheeler TT, Ghafari J,& Ramsay DS. (2002).A 3-dimensional analysis of molar movement during headgear treatment. *Am J Orthod Dentofacial Orthop*,121:18–29.

Asquith J, Gillgrass T, Mossey P.(2007)Three-dimensional imaging of orthodontic models: a pilot study. Eur J Orthod. 2007 Oct;29(5):517-22.

Astvaldsdottir A, W. P. Holbrook, and S. Tranaeus, "Consistency of DIAGNOdent instruments for clinical assessment of fissure caries," *Acta Odontologica Scandinavica,* vol. 62, no. 4, pp. 193–198, 2004.

Anusavice, KJ. (2003). *Philips' Science of dental materials.* 11th ed. St. Louis: Saunders Co: 616,617.

Ayoub AF, D. Wray, K.F. Moos, P. Siebert, J. Jin and T.B. Niblett et al., (1996)Three-dimensional modeling for modern diagnosis and planning in maxillofacial surgery, Int J Adult Orthod Orthog Surg vol: 11, pp. 225–233.

Ayoub, AF., Siebert, P., Moos, KF., Wray, D., Urquhart, C., & Niblett, T.B. (1998). A vision-based three-dimensional capture system for maxillofacial assessment and surgical planning, *Br J Oral Maxillofac Surg*, 36: pp. 353–357.

Azzeh, E.,& Feldon, PJ. (2003).Laser debonding of ceramic brackets: a comprehensive review. *Am J Orthod Dentofacial Orthop*, 123:79–83.

Babacan, H., Doruk, C., Bicakci, AA.(2010) .Pulpal blood flow changes due to rapid maxillary expansion. *Angle Orthod*, Nov;80(6):1136-40.

Bader, JD.,& Shugars,DA. (2004).A systematic review of the performance of a laser fluorescence device for detecting caries,*Journal of the American Dental Association*, vol. 135, no. 10, pp. 1413–1426

Baker,SS., Hunnewell JM. Muenzler WS.,&Hunter,GJ. (2002).Laser blepharoplasty: diamond laser scalpel compared to the free beam CO2 laser. Dermatol Surg ,28, pp. 127–131.

Bamzahim, M. ,Aljehani, A.,& Shi XQ., (2005).Clinical performance of DIAGNOdent in the detection of secondary carious lesions, *Acta Odontologica Scandinavica*, vol. 63, no. 1, pp. 26–30

Barghi, N., Berry, T., Hatton, C. (1994). Evaluating intensity output of curing lights in private dental offices. *J Am Dent Assoc* ,125(7): 992-996.

Barwick, PJ.,& Ramsay, DS. (1996).Effect of brief intrusive force on human pulpal blood flow. *Am J Orthod Dentofacial Orthop*,110:273–279.

Basaran, G., Ozer, T., Berk, N.,& Hamamci, O. (2007). Etching enamel for orthodontics with an erbium, chromium:yttrium-scandiumgallium-garnet laser system. *Angle Orthod* , 77:117–124

Benham, AW., Campbell, PM., Buschang, PH .(2009). Effectiveness of pit and fissure sealants in reducing white spot lesions during orthodontic treatment. A pilot study. *Angle Orthod*, 79(2):338-45.

Bertrand, C., le Petitcorps Y, Albing re L, Dupuis V. (2004).Optimization of operator and physical parameters for laser welding of dental materials. *British Dental Journal* ,196:413-418.

Bird, SE., Williams, K,& Kula K.(2007). Preoperative acetaminophen vs ibuprofen for control of pain after orthodontic separator placement. *Am J Orthod Dentofacial Orthop* ,132(4): 504-510.

Bock, JJ., Fraenzel ,W., Bailly J, Gernhardt CR, & Fuhrmann RA. (2008). Influence of different brazing and welding methods on tensile strength and microhardness of orthodontic stainless steel wire. *Eur J Orthod*. Aug;30(4):396-400.

Bihari, J., Mester, A. (1989) The biostimulative effect of low level laser therpy of long standing crural ulcer using helium neon laser, helium neon plus infrared lasers and nocoherent light: Preliminary report of a randomized double- blind comparative study. *Laser Therapy* ,1[2], 97-102.

Biordal, J. M. (2006). Can a Cochrane review in controversial areas be biased? A sensitivity analysis based on the protocol of a systematic Cochrane review low level Laser Therapy in Osteorthritis. Photomed *Laser Surg* ,23(5), 453-458.

Biordal, J, M., Couppe, C., Chow, R.T., Turner, J., Liunggren, A. E. (2003). A systematic review of low level lasertherapy with location – specific doses for pain from chronic joint disorders. *Australian J Physiother*, 49, 107-116.

Bjordal, J. M., Couppe, C., Liunggren, A. (2001) Low level laser therapy for tendinopathies. Evidence of a dose - response pattern. *Physical Therapy Reviews*, 6(2), 91-100.

Bjordal, J.M., Greve, G. (1998) What may alter the conclusions of reviews ? *Physical Therapy Reviews*,3 , 121- 132.

Boloognani, L., Volpi, N.(1992) Low- Power Laser- Enzyme Interaction. *Published Proceedings of the 3rd World Congress of International Soc, for Low Power Laser Application in Medicine and Surgery*. Ed. Galetti, G,. 213-222. Monduzzi Editore.

Bishara, SE., Ostby, AW., Laffoon, J, & Warren, JJ. (2008). Enamel cracks and ceramic bracket failure during debonding in vitro. *Angle Orthod* ,78(6): 1078-1083.

Bishara SE, Trulove TS. 1990a. Comparisons of different debonding techniques for ceramic brackets: an in vitro study. Part II. Findings and clinical implications. Am J Orthod Dentofacial Orthop 98(3): 263-273.

Brouns EM, Schopf PM, Kocjancic B. 1993. Electrothermal debonding of ceramic brackets. An in vitro study. Eur J Orthod 15(2): 115-123.

Bishara SE, Trulove TS. 1990b. Comparisons of different debonding techniques for ceramic brackets: an in vitro study. Part I. Background and methods. Am J Orthod Dentofacial Orthop 98(2): 145-153.

Bradley P, Tuner J.(2007).Laser Phototherapy in Dentistry, In: *Proceedings of the 1st International Workshop of Evidence Based Dentistry on Lasers in Dentistry*, Gutknecht N, pp.(149-171),Quintessence publisher,ISBN:978-1-85097-167-2,Berlin

Bradley, P. (2005) .Abstracts of North American Association of Laser Therapy Conference 4/14.

Brouns, EM., Schopf, PM., & Kocjancic, B. (1993). Electrothermal debonding of ceramic brackets. An in vitro study. *Eur J Orthod* ,15(2): 115-123.

Brodin, P., Linge L,& Aars, H. (1996).Instant assessment of pulpal blood flow after orthodontic force application. *J Orofac Orthop*, 57: 306–309. Cacciafesta, V., Sfondrini, MF., Barina, E., Scribante, A., Garino, F,& Klersy, C.(2005). Effect of different light sources and guides on shear bond strength of brackets bonded with 2 adhesive systems. *Am J Orthod Dentofacial Orthop* ,128(1): 99-102.

Canay, S., Kocadereli ,I., & Ak"ca, E. (2000). The effect of enamel air abrasion on the retention of bonded metallic orthodontic brackets. *Am J Orthod Dentofacial Orthop* ,117(1): 15-19.

Carvalho, Fde A, Almeida RC, Almeida MA, Cevidanes LH, Leite MC.(2010). Efficiency of light-emitting diode and halogen units in reducing residual monomers. *Am J Orthod Dentofacial Orthop* ,138(5): 617-622.

Cerqueira, A., Silveira, RL., Oliveira, MG., Sant'ana Filho, M.,& Heitz, C. (2007).Bone tissue microscopic findings related to the use of diode laser (830nm) in ovine mandible submitted to distraction osteogenesis. *Acta Cir. Bras, Vol 22 (2)*

Cha, BK., Lee, JY., Jost-Brinkmann, PG.,& Yoshida, N.(2007) Analysis of tooth movement in extraction cases using three-dimensional reverse engineering technology. *Eur J Orthod*, 29:325–331.

Chai, T., & Chou, CK. (1998). Mechanical properties of laser-welded cast titanium joints under different conditions . *Journal of Prosthetic Dentistry* , 79 : 477 - 483

Chandra, S., Chandra, S., Chandra, R. (2000). A textbook of dental materials with multiple choice questions. 1st ed. New Delhi: Jaypee brothers medical publishers: 326.

Chen ,HY., Su MZ., Chang HF, Chen YJ, Lan WH, Lin CP.(2007). Effects of different debonding techniques on the debonding forces and failure modes of ceramic brackets in simulated clinical set-ups. *Am J Orthod Dentofacial Orthop* ,132(5): 680-686.

Chu, CH., Lo, ECM., & You, DSH.(2009) Clinical diagnosis of fissure caries with conventional and laser-induced fluorescence techniques. *Lasers in Medical Science*, pp. 1–8

Cilesiz ,I. (2004).Laser-Tissue Interaction. *Marcel Dekker, Inc.*, ISBN: 0-8247-4258-3, New York, NY, USA

Cobb, DS., Dederich, DN., & Gardner TV. (2000) In vitro temperature change at the dentin/pulpal interface by using conventional visible light versus argon laser. *Lasers Surg Med*, 26:386-97.

Combe, EC. (1981). Notes on dental materials. 4th ed. Edinburgh: Churchill Livingstone: 271.

Cook, PA., Youngson, CC. (1988). An in vitro study of the bond strength of a glass ionomer cement in the direct bonding of orthodontic brackets. Br J Orthod 15(4): 247-253.

Cope, JB.,& Samchukov, ML. Craniofacial distraction osteogenesis: Basic principles and clinical applications. In: Graber TM, Vanarsdall RL, Vig KWL. Orthodontics: Current principles & techniques. 4th ed. St. Louis: Mosby: 1058-1061.

Cruz, DR., Kohara, EK., Ribeiro, MS., &Wetter NU. (2004). Effects of low-intensity laser therapy on the orthodontic movement velocity of human teeth: a preliminary study. *Lasers Surg Med* ,35: 117–120

Da Silva Sousa, MV., Scanavini, MA., Sannomiya, EK., Velasco, LG.,& Angelieri, F. (2011) Influence of low-level laser on the speed of orthodontic movement. *Photomed Laser Surg*, Mar;29(3):191-6. Epub Jan 23.

Dubroc, GC., Jr., Mayo JA, Rankine CA.(1994). Reduction of caries and of demineralization around orthodontic brackets: effect of a fluoride-releasing resin in the rat model. *Am J Orthod Dentofacial Orthop* ,106(6): 583-587.

Duncan, Y., Powell GL, Higuchi WI, Fox J. (1993)Enhancement of argon laser effect on dissolution and loss of human enamel. *J Clin Laser Med Surg*; 11: 259–261.

Dunn ,WJ., & Taloumis LJ. (2002). Polymerization of orthodontic resin cement with light-emitting diode curing units. *Am J Orthod Dentofacial Orthop* ,122(3): 236-241.

Dyson, M. (2005). Abstracts of North American Association of Laser Therapy Conference 14.

Einstein ,A.(1905). Uber einen die Erzeugung und Verwandlung des Lichtes betreffenden heuristischen Gesichtspunkt. *Annalen der physik* 17:132

Einstein, A. (1917).Zur quantentheorie der strahlung. *Physikalische* Z 18:121-128,1917

Elaut, J., & Wehrbein, H. (2004).The effects of argon laser curing of a resin adhesive on bracket retention and enamel decalcification: a prospective clinical trial. *Eur J Orthod*;26:553-60.

Eliades, T. (2007). Orthodontic materials research and applications: part 2. Current status and projected future developments in materials and biocompatibility. *Am J Orthod Dentofacial Orthop* ,131(2): 253-262.

Elvebak, BS., Rossouw, PE., Miller, BH., Buschang, P.,& Ceen, R. (2006). Orthodontic bonding with varying curing time and light power using an argon laser. *Angle Orthod* ,76:837–844

Emshoff, R., Kranewitter R., Brunold S, Laimer K, &Norer, B. (2008) Characteristics of pulpal blood flow levels associated with non-segmented and segmented Le Fort I osteotomy. *Oral Surg Oral Med Oral Pathol Oral Radiol Endod,* 105: 379–384.

Emshoff, R., Kranewitter, R., Gerhard S, Norer B, Hell, B. (2000). Effect of segmental Le Fort I osteotomy on maxillary tooth type related pulpal blood flow characteristics. *Oral Surg Oral Med Oral Pathol Oral Radiol Endod,* 89: 749–752.

Ferracane, JL. (2001). Materials in dentistry: principles and applications. 2nd ed. Philadelphia: Lippincott Williams & Wilkins: 288.

Firestone, AR., Wheatley AM,& Thu¨er, UW. (1997).Measurement of blood perfusion in the dental pulp with laser Doppler flowmetry. *Int J Microcirc,*17: 298–304.

Flaitz, CM., Hicks, MJ.,& Westerman, GH. (1995).Argon laser irradiation and acidulated phosphate fluoride treatment in caries-like lesion formation in enamel: an in-vitro study. *Pediatr Dent,* 17: 31-39.

Fornaini, C., Passaretti, F., Villa, E., Rocca, JP., Merigo, E,& Vescovi, P. (2010). Intraoral laser welding: ultrastructural and mechanical analysis to compare laboratory laser and dental laser. *Lasers Med Sci.*

Fox, JL., Duncan, Y.,& Otsuka, M. (1992).Initial dissolution rate studies on dental enamel after CO_2 laser irradiation. *J Dent Res* ,71: 1390-1398.

Fox, NA., McCabe, JF.,& Gordon, PH. (1991). Bond strengths of orthodontic bonding materials: an in-vitro study. *Br J Orthod* ,18(2): 125-130.

Fuhrmann, R., Gutknecht, N., Magunski, A.,Lampert, F.,& Diedrich, P. (2001). Conditioning of enamel with Nd:YAG and CO2 dental laser systems and with phosphoric acid. An in-vitro comparison of the tensile bond strength and the morphology of the enamel surface. *J Orofac Orthop.*Sep;62(5):375-86.

Fujita, S., Yamaguchi, M., Utsunomiya T, Yamamoto, H.,& Kasai, K.(2008). Low-energy laser stimulates tooth movement velocity via expression of RANK and RANKL. *Orthod Craniofac Res* ,11:143–155

Gazelius, B., Olgart, L., Edwall, B.,& Edwall, L. (1986).Non-invasive recording of blood flow in human dental pulp. *Endod Dent Traumatol* ,2:219-21.

Geiger ,AM., Gorelick, L., Gwinnett, AJ.,& Benson, BJ.(1992). Reducing white spot lesions in orthodontic populations with fluoride rinsing. *Am J Orthod Dentofacial Orthop,* 101(5): 403-407

Geusic, J.E. (1966) The continuous Nd: YAG laser . *IEEE J Quant Electron* ,2(4), 105

Geusic, J. E., Marcos, H.M., & Van Uitert, L. G. (1964). Laser Dscillations in Nd- doped yttrium alum aluminium, yttrium gallium and gadolinium garnets. *Appl Phys Lett* ,4 (101), 182-184.

Goldman, L., Ingelman, JM., & Richfield, DF. (1964).Impact of the laser on nevi and melanomas. *Arch Dermatol* , 90: 71–75.

Gomi, A., Kamiya, K., Yamashita, H., Ban Y., Senda. A., Hara, G., Yamaguchi, M., Narita. Te.,& Hasegaw, J. (1989). A clinical study on the soft laser 632 a He Ne Low energy medical laser . 2 nd laser. 2 nd report: The effect in relieving the pain of hypersensitive dentin and the pain during seating an inlay. *Aichi Gakuin Daigaku Shigakkai Shi,* 24 (3), 890-399.

Goodman, BD., & Kaufman, HW.(1977).Effects of an argon laser on the crystalline properties and rate of dissolution in acid of tooth enamel in the presence of sodium fluoride. *J Dent Res*; 56: 1201-1207.

Gordon, E. I., Labuda, E.F., & Bridges, W.B. (1964). Continuous visible laser action in singly ionized argon, Krypton and exenon. *Appl Opt Lett* ,4(10) , 178.

Gorelick, L., Geiger, AM., & Gwinnett, AJ. (1982). Incidence of white spot formation after bonding and banding. *Am J Orthod* ,81(2): 93-98.

Gostanian, HV., Z. Shey C. ,Kasinathan, J. Caceda, & Janal, M. N. (2006). An in vitro evaluation of the effect of sealant characteristics on laser fluorescence for caries detection, *Pediatric Dentistry*, vol. 28, no. 5, pp. 445–450

Goulart, CS., Nouer, PRA, Mouramartins, L., Garbin, IU.,& Lizarelli RDZ .(2006). Photoradiation and orthodontic movement: experimental study with canines. *Photomed Laser Surg*, 242:192–196

Hall, A., & Girkin, J. M. (2004). A review of potential new diagnostic modalities for caries lesions. *J Dent Res*, 83 (Spec Iss C), C89-C94.

Hall, R. N., Fenner, G.E., Kingsley, J.D., Soltys, T.J.,& Carlson, R. O. (1962) Coherent light emission from GaAs junctions. *Phys Rev Lett* ,9(9). 366.

Hamblin, MR.,& Demidova, T.(2006).Mechanisms for Low Level Light Therapy, *Proc. of the SPIE* ,Vol.6140-614001.PP:1-12

Harada, K., Sato, M.,& Omura, K. (2004) Bloodflow and neurosensory changes in the maxillary dental pulp after differing Le Fort I osteotomies. *Oral Surg Oral Med Oral Pathol Oral Radiol Endod* ,97: 12–17

Harazaki, M.,& Isshiki Y. (1998). Soft laser irradiation effects on pain reduction in orthodontic treatment. *Bull Tokyo Dent Coll*, 39: 95-101.

Harazaki M, Takahashi H, Isshiki Y. (1997). Soft laser irradiation induced pain reduction in orthodontic treatment. *Bull Tokyo Dent Coll*,38:291-5.

Hayakawa, K. (2005). Nd:YAG laser for debonding ceramic orthodontic brackets. *Am J Orthod Dentofacial Orthop* ,128:638–647

Hayashi, K., Araki, Y., Uechi, J., Ohno, H., & Mizoguchi, I. .(2002).A novel method for the three-dimensional (3-D) analysis of orthodontic tooth movement-calculation of rotation about and translation along the finite helical axis. *J Biomech*, 35(1):45-51.

Hayashi, K., Uechi, J., Murata, M.,& Mizoguchi, I. (2004).Comparison of maxillary canine retraction with sliding mechanics and a retraction spring: a three-dimensional analysis based on a midpalatal orthodontic implant. *Eur J Orthod*, 26:585–589.

Haytac, MC.& Ozcelik, O.(2006). Evaluation of patient perceptions after frenectomy operations: a comparison of carbon dioxide laser and scalpel techniques. J Periodontol, 77(11), pp. 1815–1819.

Hibst, R.,& Gall,R. (1998). Development of a diode laser-based fluorescence caries detector. *Caries Research*, vol. 32, no. 4, article 294

Hibst ,R.,& Keller, U.(1989). Experimental studies of the application of the Er YAG laser on dental hard substances: 1. Measurement of ablation rate. *Lasers Surg Med* , 9: 338-344.

Hicks, MJ., Flaitz, CM.,& Westerman GH. (1994) Argon laser irradiation in root surface caries: in vitro study examines laser's effects. *J Am Dent Assoc*, 125: 401-407.

Hicks, MJ., Flaitz, CM., &Westerman, GH. (1993) Caries-like lesion initiation and progression in sound enamel following argon laser irradiation: an in-vitro study.*ASDC J Dent Child*, 60(3): 201-206.

Hicks, MJ., Flaitz, CM.,& Westerman, GH. .(1995).Enamel caries initiation and progression following low fluence (energy) argon laser and fluoride treatment. *J Clin Pediatr Dent*, 20: 9-13.

Hicks MJ, Flaitz CM,& Westerman GH. (1997).Roots caries in-vitro after low fluence argon laser and fluoride treatment. *Compend contin educ dent,* 18: 543-552.

Hicks, J., Winn, D.II, Flaitz, C., & Powell , L. (2004). In vivo caries formation in enamel following argon laser irradiation and combined fluoride and argon laser treatment: A clinical pilot study. *Quintessence Int*,35(1), 15-20.

Hildebrand ,NK., Raboud, DW., Heo G, Nelson AE,& Major, PW. (2007).Argon laser vs conventional visible light-cured orthodontic bracket bonding: an in-vivo and in-vitro study. *Am J Orthod Dentofacial Orthop.* Apr;131(4):530-6.

Hirogaki, Y., Sohmura, T., Satoh, H., Takahashi, J., & Takada, K.(2001).Complete 3-D reconstruction of dental cast shape using perceptual grouping. *IEEE Trans Med Imaging, 20:1093-1101.*

Hodgson, N., & Weber, H. (1997). Optical resonators. Ch. 3/3 1.1., P.102. *Springer- Verlag,* New York.

Holonyak Jr., N.,& Bevacqua. S. F. (1962). Coherent (visible) light emission form Ga (As_{1-x} P_x) junctions. *Appl Phys Lett,* 1(4), 82-83.

Hossain M, Kimura Y, Nakamura Y, Yamada Y, Kinoshita JI, & Matsumoto K. (2001).A study on acquired acid resistance of enamel and dentin irradiated by Er,Cr:YSGG laser. *J Clin Laser Med Surg*;19:159-63.

Hossain M, Nakamura Y, Yamada Y, Kimura Y, Matsumoto N, & Matsumoto K. (1999). Effects of Er,Cr:YSGG laser irradiation in human enamel and dentin: ablation and morphological studies. *J Clin Laser Med Surg.* ,17(4):155-9.

Huang, YY., Chen, AC., Carroll JD, & Hamblin, MR.(2009). Biphasic dose response in low level light therapy, Dose Response. Sep 1;7(4):358-83

Hübler, R., Blando, E., Gaião, L., Kreisner, PE., Post, LK., Xavier, CB.,& de Oliveira MG.(2010). Effects of low-level laser therapy on bone formed after distraction osteogenesis. *Lasers Med Sci.* Mar;25(2):213-9.

Huth, KC., Neuhaus,KW., Gygax,M. Clinical performance of a new laser fluorescence device for detection of occlusal caries lesions in permanent molars. *Journal of Dentistry*, vol. 36, no. 12, pp. 1033–1040, 2008.

Gwinnett, AJ.(1988). A comparison of shear bond strengths of metal and ceramic brackets. *Am J Orthod Dentofacial Orthop* ,93(4): 346-348.

Iijima, M., Yasuda, Y., Muguruma, T., Mizoguchi ,I.(2010). Effects of CO2 laser debonding of a ceramic bracket on the mechanical properties of enamel. *Angle Orthod,*Nov;80(6):1029-35.

Ikawa M, Fujiwara M, Horiuchi H, Shimauchi H. (2001).The effect of short-term tooth intrusion on human pulpal blood flow measured by laser Doppler flowmetry. *Arch Oral Biol*, 46: 781–787.

Inberg ,A., Oksman, M., Ben-David M,& Croitoru N. (1998).Hollow waveguide for mid and thermal infrared radiation. *J Clin Laser Med Surg* ,16: 127–133.

Ip, TB., &Rock, WP.(2004). A comparison of three light curing units for bonding adhesive pre-coated brackets. *J Orthod* ,31(3): 243-247; discussion 202-243.

Ismail SF, J.P. Moss and R. Hennessy. (2002). Three-dimensional assessment of the effects of extraction and nonextraction orthodontic treatment on the face. Am J Orthod Dentofacial Orthop ,121: 244–256.

Iwasaki K , Ohkawa S , Rosca I D , Uo M , Akasaka T , Watari F (2004) Distortion of laser welded titanium plates . *Dental Materials Journal*, 23 : 593 - 599

Jaberi ansari Z, Fekrazad R, Younessian F, AM Kalhori K, Gutknecht N. The effect of Er,Cr:YSGG laser on microshear bond strength of composite to enamel and dentin of human permanent teeth. *Lasers Med Sci ,(in press)*

James JW, Miller BH, English JD, Tadlock LP, Buschang PH.(2003) Effects of high-speed curing devices on shearbond strength and microleakage of orthodontic brackets. *Am J Orthod Dentofacial Orthop*, 123:555-61.

Jang, I., Tanaka, M., Koga, Y., Iijima, S., Yozgatian JH, Cha, BK.& Yoshida, N. (2009). A novel method for the assessment of three-dimensional tooth movement during orthodontic treatment. *Angle Orthod* , May;79(3):447-53.

Javan, A., Bennett Jr., W.R.,& Herriott, D.R. (1961). Population inversion and continuous optical maser oscillation in a gas discharge containing a He-Ne mixture. *Phys Rev Let* ,6(3). 106- 110.

Ji Y, Zhang F, Schwartz J, Stile F, Lineaweaver WC. (2002).Assessment of facial tissue expansion with three dimensional digitizer scanning. *J Craniofac Surg*, 13: 687-92.

Jones, SP., Gledhill, JR.,& Davies, EH. (1999). The crystal growth technique--a laboratory evaluation of bond strengths. *Eur J Orthod* ,21(1): 89-93.

Jost-Brinkmann, PG., Stein H, Miethke RR, &Nakata, M. (1992). Histologic investigation of the human pulp after thermodebonding of metal and ceramic brackets. *Am J Orthod Dentofacial Orthop* ,102(5): 410-417.

Kafas, P., Stavrianos, C., Jerjes, W., Upile, T., Vourvachis, M., Theodoridis, M.& Stavrianou, I. (2009). Upper-lip laser frenectomy without infiltrated anaesthesia in a paediatric patient: a case report. *Cases J*. May 20;2:7138.

Kara, C. (2008).Evaluation of patient perceptions of frenectomy: a comparison of Nd:YAG laser and conventional techniques. *Photomed Laser Surg*.Apr;26(2):147-52.

Karu, T. (2003) Low power laser therapy . In: *Biomedical Photonics Handbook*. Chapter 48 and references therein. CRC Press- Taylor & Francis.

Karu, T.(2000) Mechanisms of Low Power Laser Action on a Cellular. Level .*Lasers in Medicine and Dentistry*, Ed. Simunovic, Z, 97-125.

Karu, T. (2007). Ten Lectures on Basic Science of Laser Phototherapy . Prima Books, Grangesberg.

Kato, J., Wijeyeweera, RL.(2007) The effect of CO2 laser irradiation on oral soft tissue problems in children in Sri Lanka. Photomed Laser Surg. 25:264–268.

Katoh, H., Chen, RC., Chai, CT., Saito S, Yamasaki K,& Shibasaki, Y. (1997)Effect of far infrared rays radiation on pain reaction associated with orthodontic tooth movement. *J Japan Orthod* ,Soc 56: 17-25.

Kau, CH.(2005) . Reliability of measuring facial morphology with a 3-dimensional laser scanning system. *American Journal of Orthodontics and Dentofacial Orthopedics* ,128: 424-430.

Kau, CH., Knox, J., Zhurov, AI.,& Richmond, S.(2004)Validity and reliability of a portable 3D optical scanning device for field studies. In: Proceedings of the 7th European

Craniofacial Congress. Bologna: Monduzzi Editore-International Proceedings Division, (in press).

Kawasaki, K.,& Shimizu, N. (2000). Effects of low-energy laser irradiation on bone remodeling during experimental tooth movement in rats. *Lasers in Surgery and Medicine* ,26: 282–291

Kelsey, WP., Blankenau, RJ., Powell, GL., Barkmeier, WW., Cavel, WT.,& Whisenant BK.(1989) Enhancement of physical properties of resin restorative materials by laser polymerization. *Lasers Surg Med* ,9:623-7.

Khalife, MA, J. R. Boynton, J. B. Dennison, Yaman,P. & Hamilton,JC.(2009).In vivo evaluation of DIAGNOdent for the occlusal dental caries.*Operative Dentistry,* 34(2), pp. 136–141.

Khambay, B., Nebel, JC. Bowman, J. , Walker, F.,Hadley DM. & Ayoub. (2002) 3D stereophotogrammetric image superimposition onto 3D CT scan images: the future of orthognathic surgery. A pilot study, Int J Adult Orthod Orthog Surg 17: 331–341.

Kim, JH., Kwon OW, Kim HI, Kwon YH.(2006). Acid resistance of erbium-doped yttrium aluminum garnet laser–treated and phosphoric acid–etched enamels. *Angle Orthod* , 76: 441-445.

Kim JH, Kwon OW, Kim HI, Kwon YH.(2005). Effectiveness of an Er:YAG laser in etching the enamel surface for orthodontic bracket retention. *Dent Mater J.* Dec;24(4):596-602.

Kim JT, Cho SA .(2009). The effects of laser etching on shear bond strength at the titaniumceramic interface. *J ProsthetDent* 101:101–106

Kim SJ, Paek JH, Park KH, Kang SG, Park YG. Laser-aided circumferential supracrestal fiberotomy and low-level laser therapy effects on relapse of rotated teeth in beagles. Angle Orthod. 2010 Mar;80(2):385-90.

Kim SJ, Paek JH, Park KH, Kang SG, Park YG.(2010). Laser-aided circumferential supracrestal fiberotomy and low-level laser therapy effects on relapse of rotated teeth in beagles. *Angle Orthod,*Mar;80(2):385-90.

Kim YD, Kim SS, Kim SJ, Kwon DW, Jeon ES, Son WS .(2010). Low-level laser irradiation facilitates fibronectin and collagen type I turnover during tooth movement in rats. *Lasers Med Sci* ,25: 25–31

Kim YO, Park SB, Son WS, Ko CC, García-Godoy F, Kim HI,& Kwon YH.(2010)Diode-pumped solid-state laser for bonding orthodontic brackets: effect of light intensity and light-curing time. *Lasers Med Sci.* Jun 8. [Epub ahead of print]

Kimura, Y., Wilder-Smith, P., & Matsumoto, K. (2000) Lasers in endodontics: A review. *Int Endod J*;33:173-85.

Klein, AL., Rodrigues LK, Eduardo CP, Nobre dos Santos M,& Cury, JA. (2005).Caries inhibition around composite restorations by pulsed carbon dioxide laser application. Eur J Oral Sci;113: 239-44.

Klockowski, R., Davis, EL., Joynt RB, Wieczkowski G, Jr., &MacDonald, A. (1989). Bond strength and durability of glass ionomer cements used as bonding agents in the placement of orthodontic brackets. *Am J Orthod Dentofacial Orthop* ,96(1): 60-64.

Kobayashi Y, Takagi H, Sakay H, Hashimoto F, Mataki S, Kobayashi K, Kato Y (1998). Effects of local administration of osteocalcin on experimental tooth movement. *Angle Orthod* 68: 259–266.

Konig, K., Flemming G,& Hibst R. (1998) .Laser-induced autofluorescence spectroscopy of dental caries. *Cell Mol Biol (Noisy-legrand)*, 44:1293–1300

Konorov, S O., Mitrokhin, V P., Fedotov, A.(2004) .Hollow-core photonic-crystal fibres for laser dentistry. *Phys Med Biol* , 49: 1359–1368.

Konno, Y., Daimaruya T, Iikubo M, Kanzaki R, Takahashi I, Sugawara J,& Sasano, T. (2007).Morphologic and hemodynamic analysis of dental pulp in dogs after molar intrusion with the skeletal anchorage system. *Am J Orthod Dentofacial Orthop.* 132: 199–207.

Kreisner PE, Blaya DS, Gaião L, Maciel-Santos ME, Etges A, Santana-Filho M, de Oliveira MG. (2010).Histological evaluation of the effect of low-level laser on distraction osteogenesis in rabbit mandibles. *Med Oral Patol Oral Cir Bucal.*2010 Jul 1;15(4):e616-8.

Krishnan V, Kumar K J. 2004 Weld characteristics of orthodontic archwire materials. Angle Orthodontist 74 : 533 - 538

Kronenberg O, A. Lussi, and S. Ruf, "Preventive effect of ozone on the development of white spot lesions during multibracket appliance therapy," *Angle Orthodontist*, vol. 79, no. 1, pp. 64–69, 2009.

Kudoh, C., Inomata, K., Okayami, K., Motegi, M.,Ohshiro T. (1989). Low Level Laser Therapy Pain Attention Mechanisms. *Laser Therapy* ,1(1), 3-6.

Lalani N, Foley TF, Voth R, Banting D, Mamandras A. Polymerization with the argon laser: curing time and shear bond strength. Angle Orthod 2000;70:28-33.

Lee BS, Hsieh TT, Lee YL, Lan WH, Hsu YJ, Wen PH, Lin CP (2003) Bond strength of orthodontic bracket after acid-etched, Er:YAG laser-irradiated and combined treatment on enamel surface. Angle Orthod 73:565–570

Lenz P, Glide H, Walz R. Studies on enamel sealing with the CO2 laser. Dtsch Zahnarztl Z 1982;37: 469-78.

Li R, Ren Y, Han J (2000) Effects of pulsed Nd:YAG laser irradiation on shear bond strength of composite resin bonded to porcelain. Hua Xi Kou Qiang Yi Xue Za Zhi 18:377–379

LI, Lu P, Zhongke Wang Y, Chen J, Zhao J. The research and development of noncontact 3-D laser dental model measuring and analyzing system. Chinese Journal of Dental Research 2000;3:7-14.

Lim HM, Lew KKK, Tay DKL. A clinical investigation of the efficacy of low level laser therapy in reducing orthodontic post adjustment pain. Am J Orthod Dentofacial Orthop 1995;108:614-22.

Limpanichkul W, Godfrey K, Srisuk N, Rattanayatikul C (2006) Effects of low-level laser therapy on the rate of orthodontic tooth movement. Orthod Craniofac Res 9:38–43

Limpanichkul W, Godfrey K, Srisuk N, Rattanayatikul C. Effects of low-level laser therapy on the rate of orthodontic tooth movement. Orthod Craniofac Res. 2006; 9: 38–43.

Lioubavina-Hack N. Lasers in dentistry. 5. The use of lasers in periodontology. Ned Tijdschr Tandheelkd. 2002;109:286–292.

Lioubavina-Hack N. Lasers in dentistry. 5. The use of lasers in periodontology. Ned Tijdschr Tandheelkd. 2002;109:286–292.

Liu, J. , Watanabe, I., Yoshida, K ,& Atsuta M.(2002). Joint strength of laser-welded titanium . Dental Materials 18 : 143 - 148

Lovrov, S., Hertrich, K., Hirschfelder U. (2007). Enamel Demineralization during Fixed Orthodontic Treatment - Incidence and Correlation to Various Oral-hygiene Parameters. *J Orofac Orthop* ,68(5): 353-363.

Lussi, A., E. Hellwig, "Performance of a new laser fluorescence device for the detection of occlusal caries in vitro," *Journal of Dentistry*, vol. 34, no. 7, pp. 467–471, 2006.

Lussi A, Hack A, Hug I, Heckenberger H, Megert B, Stich H (2006) Detection of approximal caries with a new laser fluorescence device. Caries Res 40:97–103

Lussi A, R. Hibst, & Paulus,R. (2004).DIAGNOdent: an optical method for caries detection,*Journal of Dental Research*, vol. 83, supplement 1, pp. C80–C83

Maijer, R., Smith DC. (1979). A new surface treatment for bonding. *J Biomed Mater Res* ,13(6): 975-985.

Maiman, TH.(1960). Stimulated optical radiation in ruby masers. Nature 187: 493–494.

Marcusson, A., Norevall LI, Persson M. (1997). White spot reduction when using glass ionomer cement for bonding in orthodontics: a longitudinal and comparative study. *Eur J Orthod* ,19(3): 233-242.

Ma, T., Marangoni., RD,& Flint W .(1997) .In vitro comparison of debonding force and intrapulpal temperature changes during ceramic orthodontic bracket removal using carbon dioxide laser. *Am J Orthod Dentofacial Orthop* ,111:203–210

Marmulla, R., Hassfeld S, Luth, T,& Muhling, J. (2003).Laser-scan-based navigation in cranio-maxillofacial surgery. *J Craniomaxillofac Surg* , 31: 267–77.

Martinez-Insua, A., Da Silva, Dominguez, L., Rivera FG, Santana-Penin UA. 2000. Differences in bonding to acid-etched or Er:YAG-laser-treated enamel and dentin surfaces. *J Prosthet Dent* ,84(3): 280-288.

Mattson, J. S., Blankenau. R., Keene, J.J. (1998) Use of an argon laser to treat drug-induced gingival over growth. *JADA*, 129, 78-89.

McCance AM, J.P. Moss, W.R. Fright, A.D. Linney and D.R. James, Three-dimensional analysis techniques—Part 1: three-dimensional soft-tissue analysis of 24 adult cleft palate patients following Le Fort I maxillary advancement: a preliminary report, Cleft Palate Craniofac J 34 (1997): 36–45.

McCance, AM., Moss, JP. W.R. Wright, A.D. Linney & James, DR. (1992). A three-dimensional soft tissue analysis of 16 skeletal Class III patients following bimaxillary surgery. *Br J Oral Maxillofac Surg* ,30: 221–232.

McDonagh S., J.P. Moss, P. Goodwin and R.T. Lee, .(2001). A prospective optical surface scanning and cephalometric assessment of the effect of functional appliances on the soft tissues, *Eur J Orthod* ,23: 115–126.

McCartney ,JW.,& Doud R.(1993).Passive adaptation of the prosthesis-implant interface by soldering gold cylinders to the framework casting. *Journal of Prosthetic Dentistry* , 70:17-20.

McDonald F, Pitt Ford TR. (1994).Blood flow changes in permanent maxillary canines during retraction. *Eur J Orthod*,16: 1–9.

McGuinness, NJ., Stephens CD. (1992). Storage of orthodontic study models in hospital units in the U.K. *British Journal of Orthodontics* ,19:227-232.

Meister, J.(2007).Basic Research, In: *Proceedings of the 1st International Workshop of Evidence Based Dentistry on Lasers in Dentistry*, Gutknecht N, pp.(3-27),Quintessence publisher,ISBN:978-1-85097-167-2,Berlin

Merberg G N.(1993). Current status of infrared fiber optics for medical laser power delivery. *Lasers Surg Med* , 13: 572–576.

Meserendino, LJ., Pick ,RM. (1995), *Lasers in Dentistry, Chicago, Ill: Quintessence*

Mester,E., Szende, B. & Gartner,P.(1968). The effect of laser beams on the growth of hair in mice, Radiobiol Radiother (Berl) 9 621-6.

Moulton, P. F. (1982) Ti-doped sapphire tunable solid state lasers. Optics News 8,9.

Mills, RW. (19950. Blue light emitting diodes--another method of light curing? *Br Dent J* ,178(5): 169.

Miloro M, Miller JJ, Stoner JA.(2007). Low-level laser effect on mandibular distraction osteogenesis.*J Oral Maxillofac Surg*.Feb;65(2):168-76.

Mimura, H., Deguchi, T., Obata, A., Yamagishi T, Ito M (1995) Comparison of different bonding materials for laser debonding. *Am J Orthod Dentofacial Orthop* ,108:267–273

Mizutani, K., Musha, Y., Tobe, M. (2002). Clinical study on prostaglandin E2 with diode laser therapy. *Proc. 4th Congr World Assoc for Laser Therapy,*. Tsukuba, Japan, 82.

Moritz, A. (2006).Oral Laser Application. *Chicago, Ill*: Quintessence.

Moslemi, M., Fekrazad, R., Tadayon, N., Ghorbani, M., Torabzadeh, H.,& Shadkar, MM. (2009) .Effects of ER,Cr:YSGG laser irradiation and fluoride treatment on acid resistance of the enamel. *Pediatr Dent*, Sep-Oct;31(5):409-13.

Moss, JP., Grindrod, SR., Linney AD, Arridge SR,& James D. (1988).A computer system for the interactive planning and prediction of maxillofacial surgery. *Am J Orthod Dentofacial Orthop,* Dec; 94(6): 469-75.

Moss, JP., Linney, AD., Grindrod SR, Arridge SR, Clifto,JS.(1987).Three-dimensional visualization of the face and skull using computerized tomography and laser scanning techniques. *Eur J Orthod,*Nov;9(4):247-53.

Moss JP, S.F. Ismail and R.J. Hennessy, (2003). Three-dimensional assessment of treatment outcomes on the face, Orthod Craniofac Res 6 (Suppl 1), pp. 126–131; 179-82.

Myers, TD., Myers, WD., & Stone, RM. (1989).First soft tissue study utilising a pulsed Nd YAG dental laser. *Northwest Dent*; 68: 14–17

Nalbantgil D, Oztoprak MO, Tozlu M, Arun T (2010). Effects of different application durations of ER:YAG laser on intrapulpal temperature change during debonding. *Lasers Med Sci,*

Nathan, M. l., Dumke, W. P., Burns, G., Dill Jr., F. H., Lasher, G. (1962) Stimulated emission of radiation from GaAs p-n junctions. *Appl Phys Lett* ,1(3), 62-64.

Niemz, MH. (2002) *Laser-Tissue Interactions: Fundamentals and Applications*. Berlin, Germany: *Springer Verlag*: 45-80.

Nelson, DG., Shariati M, Glena R, Shields CP, Featherstone JD. (1986).Effect of pulsed low energy infrared laser irradiation on artificial caries-like lesion formation. *Caries Res* , 20:289-99.

Nelson, DG., Wefel JS, Jongebloed WL, Featherstone JD.(1987). Morphology, histology, and crystallography of human dental enamel treated with pulsed low-energy infrared laser radiation. *Caries Res*,21:411-26.

Nute SJ, Moss JP. (2000). Three-dimensional facial facial growth studied by optical surface scanning.J Orthod, 27: 31–38.

Obata A, Tsumura T, Niwa K, Ashizawa Y, Deguchi T, Ito, M .(1999) .Super pulse CO2 laser for bracket bonding and debonding. *Eur J Orthod* , 21:193–198

O'brien, WJ. (1997). Dental materials and their selection. 2nd ed. Chicago: Quintescence Publishing Co: 308,309.

Odegaard J, Segner D. 1988. Shear bond strength of metal brackets compared with a new ceramic bracket. Am J Orthod Dentofacial Orthop 94(3): 201-206.

Tocchio RM, Williams PT, Mayer FJ, Standing KG. 1993. Laser debonding of ceramic orthodontic brackets. *Am J Orthod Dentofacial Orthop* 103(2): 155-162.

Odor TM, Pitt Ford TR, McDonald F. Effect of wavelength and bandwidth on the clinical reliability of laser Doppler recordings. Endod Dent Traumatol 1996;12:9-15.

Oho T, Morioka T. A possible mechanism of acquired acid resistance of human dental enamel by laser irradiation. Caries Res 1990;24:86-92.

Olivi G, Chaumanet G, Genovese MD, Beneduce C, Andreana S.(2010). Er,Cr:YSGG laser labial frenectomy: a clinical retrospective evaluation of 156 consecutive cases. *Gen Dent.* May-Jun;58(3):e126-33.

Ogaard B, Rolla G, Arends J. (1988)a. Orthodontic appliances and enamel demineralization. Part 1. Lesion development. Am J Orthod Dentofacial Orthop 94(1): 68-73.

Ogaard B, Rolla G, Arends J, ten Cate JM. (1988)b. Orthodontic appliances and enamel demineralization. Part 2. Prevention and treatment of lesions. *Am J Orthod Dentofacial Orthop*, 94(2): 123-128.

Orthod Dentofacial Orthop 128(5):630–637

Ozer, T., Başaran G, Berk N.(2008). Laser etching of enamel for orthodontic bonding. *Am J Orthod Dentofacial Orthop.* Aug;134(2):193-7.

Oztoprak MO, Nalbantgil D, Erdem S, Tozlu M, Arun T. (2010) .Debonding of ceramic brackets by a new scanning laser method. *Am J Orthod Dentofacial Orthop,* Aug;138(2):195-200.

Paghdiwala, A. F. (1988) Application of the erbim: YAG laser on hard dental tissues: measurement of the termperature changes and depth of cut. In: *Laser research in medicine, surgery and dentistry,* ed. Profio, A. E., ICA-LEO '88. Vol. 64, 192-201.

Parker, s.(2007) .Verifiable CPD paper: introduction, history of lasers and laser light production, Br Dent J , January 202, 21 - 31

Patel, C. K. N. (1964 a) Continuos-wave laser action on vibrational - rotational transitions of CO2. *Phys Rev* Lett,136(5A), A1187-A1193.

Patel, C.K. N. (1964 b) Interpretation of CO2 optical maser experiments. *Phys Rev Lett* ,12(21), 588-590.

Polat, O., Karaman, AI.,& Durmus, E. (2005). Effects of preoperative ibuprofen and naproxen sodium on orthodontic pain. *Angle Orthod* ,75(5): 791-796.

Poosti, M., Jahanbin, A., Mahdavi, P., Mehrnoush, S. (2011).Porcelain conditioning with Nd:YAG and Er:YAG laser for bracket bonding in orthodontics. *Lasers Med Sci,* Jan 18.

Powell, GL., Anderson, JR.,& Blankenau, RJ. Laser and curing light induced in vitro pulpal temperature changes. *J Clin Laser Med Surg* 1999;17:3-5.

Powell, G.L., Ellis, R., Blankenau, R. J., Schouten, J.R. (1995). Evaluation of argon laser and conventional light cured composites. *J Clin Laser Med Surg* ,13(5), 315- 317.

Proffit, WR., Fields, HW.,& Sarver, DM .(2007). Contemporary orthodontics. 4th ed. St. Louis: Mosby: 335

Qiao, LY., Yu JT.,& Jia XY. (2005).A study on acquired acid resistance of enamel and dentin irradiated by Er,Cr:YSGG laser in vitro. *Zhonghua Kou Qiang Yi Xue Za Zhi* ,40:34-7

Quimby, ML., Vig, KWL., Rashid, RG.,& Firestone, AR. (2004). The accuracy and reliability of measurements made on computer-based digital models. *Angle Orthodontist* ,74:298-303.

Quist, T.M., Rediker, R.H., Keyes, R. J., Krag, W. E., Lax, B., McWhorter, A. L., Zeigler, H. J. (1962) Semiconductor master of GaAs. *App Phys Lett* ,1(4), 91-92.

Reis, A., F. M. Mendes, V. Angnes, G. Angnes, R. Grande, HM., & Loguercio, AD.(2006). Performance of methods of occlusal caries detection in permanent teeth under clinical and laboratory conditions. *Journal of Dentistry*, vol. 34, no. 2, pp. 89–96

Rickabaugh, JL., Marangoni, RD., McCaffrey KK (1996).Ceramic bracket debonding with the carbon dioxide laser. *Am J Orthod Dentofacial Orthop* , 110:388–393

Rocha,R., Ardenghi,TM., Oliveira,LB., Rodrigues,CRMD., & Ciamponi,AL. (2003).In vivo effectiveness of laser fluorescence compared to visual Inspection and radiography for the detection of occlusal caries in primary teeth. *Caries Research*, vol. 37, no. 6, pp. 437–441

Rocha, R., Pinheiro, AL., &Villaverde AB.(2006) Flexural strength of pure Ti, Ni-Cr and Co-Cr alloys submitted to Nd:YAG laser or TIG welding. *Brazilian Dental Journal* , 17:20-23.

Roelandts, R.(2002).The history of phototherapy: something new under the sun, *J Am Acad Dermatol* ,46 :926-30.

Rose, RK. (2000)a. Binding characteristics of Streptococcus mutans for calcium and casein phosphopeptide. *Caries Res* ,34(5): 427-431.

Rose, RK. 2000b. Effects of an anticariogenic casein phosphopeptide on calcium diffusion in streptococcal model dental plaques. *Arch Oral Biol*, 45(7): 569-575.

Rossman, JA., & Cobb, CM. (1995).Lasers in periodontal therapy. *Periodontol 2000* , oct; 9, pp. 150–164.

Rueggeberg, FA., Caughman, WF., Curtis, JW. (1994). Effect of light intensity and exposure duration on cure of resin composite. *Oper Dent* ,19(1): 26-32.

Saito, S., & Shimizu ,N .(1997). Stimulatory effects of low-power laser irradiation on bone regeneration in midpalatal suture during expansion in the rat. *Am J Orthod Dentofacial Orthop* , 111(5):525–532

Sano, Y., Ikawa, M., Sugawara, J., Horiuchi, H., &Mitani, H. (2002). The effect of continuous intrusive force on human pulpal blood flow. *Eur J Orthod*,24:159–166.

Santoro, M., Galkin ,S., Teredesai, M., Nicolay ,OF.,& Cangialosi TJ.(2003). Comparison of measurements made on digital and plaster models. *American Journal of Orthodontics and Dentofacial Orthopedics* ,124:101-105.

Saperia, D., Glassberg, E., Lyons, R. F., Abergel. R. P., Baneux, P., Castel, J. C., Dwyer, R.M., Uitto, J. (1986) Demonstration of elevated type I and type III procollagen m RNA levels in cutaneous wounds treated with helium - neon laser. *Biochem Biophys Res Commun* ,3 (138), 1123- 1128.

Sarver, DM.(2006). Use of the 810 nm diode laser: soft tissue management and orthodontic applications of innovative technology. Practice Proced Aesthet Dent ,18 (suppl), pp. 7-13.

Sarver, DM.,& Yanosky M.(2005). Principles of cosmetic dentistry in orthodontics: part 2. Soft tissue laser technology and cosmetic gingival contouring. *Am J Orthod Dentofacial Orthop*, 127:85–90.

Sasano, T. (1998). Neural regulation of pulpal blood flow and pulp diagnosis. *Tohoku Univ Dent J*, 17:1-21.

Schawlow, AL. ,Townes, CH.(1940,1949,1958).Infrared and Optical Masers . *Phys*, Rev 112.

Seifi, M., Shafeei, HA., Daneshdoost, S. (2007). Effects of two types of low-level laser wave lengths (850 and 630 nm) on the orthodontic tooth movements in rabbits. *Lasers Med Sci* ,22:261-264

Sergl, HG., Klages, U.,& Zentner A. (1998). Pain and discomfort during orthodontic treatment: causative factors and effects on compliance. *Am J Orthod Dentofacial Orthop* ,114(6): 684-691.

Sestini, S., Notarantonio, L., Cerboni B, Alessandrini C, Fimiani M, Nannelli P, Pelagalli A, & Giorgetti, R.(2006). In vitro toxicity evaluation of silver soldering, electrical resistance, and laser welding of orthodontic wires. *Eur J Orthod.* Dec;28(6):567-72.

Sholts, SB., Wa¨rmla¨nder SKTS., Flores,LM., Miller,KWP., Walker, PL. (2010). Variation in the measurements of cranial volume and surface area using 3D laser scanning technology. *J. Forensic Sci,*(April 8) (Epub ahead of print).

Silta, YT., Dunn, WJ,& Peters, CB.(2005). Effect of shorter polymerization times when using the latest generation of light-emitting diodes. *Am J Orthod Dentofacial Orthop* ,128(6): 744-748.

Skold-Larsson K., Fornell,AC., Lussi,A. & Twetman,S. (2004).Effect of topical applications of a chlorhexidine/thymol-containing varnish on fissure caries assessed by laser fluorescence," *Acta Odontologica Scandinavica*, vol. 62, no. 6, pp. 339–342

Sognnaes, RF., & Stern, RH. (1965). Laser effect on resistance of human dental enamel to demineralization in-vitro. *J S Calif Dent Assoc* ,33: 328–329.

Solmi, R. ,Martini, D., Zanarini, M., Isaza Penco S, Rimondini, L., Carinci, P., Borea, G.,& Ruggeri ,A.. (2004). Interactions of fibroblasts with soldered and laser welded joints. *Biomaterials*, 25: 735–740

Srimaneepong, V., Yoneyama, T., Kobayashi, E., Doi, H., Hanawa,T. (2005). Mechanical strength and microstructure of laser-welded Ti-6Al-7Nb alloy castings . *Dental Materials Journal* ,24 : 541 - 549

Staudt ,CB., Lussi, A., Jacquet, J., & Kiliaridis, S. (2004).White spot lesions around brackets: in vitro detection by laser fluorescence. *Eur J Oral Sci* ,112:237–243

Strobl, K., Bahns, TL., Willham, L., Bishara SE, Stwalley WC .(1992). Laser-aided debonding of orthodontic ceramic brackets. *Am J Orthod Dentofacial Orthop* ,101:152–158

Sun, X., Zhu, X., Xu, C., Ye, N.,& Zhu, H .(2001). Effects of low energy laser on tooth movement and remodeling of alveolar bone in rabbits. *Hua Xi Kou Qiang Yi Xue Za Zhi* 19(5):290–293

Talbot, TQ., Blankenau RJ, Zobitz, ME., Weaver, AL., Lohse, CM., & Rebellato J.(2000). Effect of argon laser irradiation on shear bond strength of orthodontic brackets: an in vitro study. *Am J Orthod Dentofacial Orthop* ,118:274-9.

Taylor JC. , Hondrum SO. , Prasad, A. , Brodersen, CA. (1998). Effects of joint configuration for the arc welding of cast Ti-6Al-4V alloy rods in argon . *Journal of Prosthetic Dentistry* 79 : 291 - 297

Tehranchi, A., Fekrazad, R., Zafar, M., Eslami, B., Kalhori, KA., & Gutknecht, N. (2010). Evaluation of the effects of CO2 laser on debonding of orthodontics porcelain brackets vs. the conventional method. *Lasers Med Sci,* Aug 20. [Epub ahead of print]

Theodorakopoulou, LP., Sadowsky, PL., Jacobson, A., Lacefield W, Jr. 2004. Evaluation of the debonding characteristics of 2 ceramic brackets: an in vitro study. *Am J Orthod Dentofacial Orthop* ,125(3): 329-336.

Thilander, B., Rygh, P., & Reitan K. Tissue reactions in orthodontics. In: Graber TM, Vanarsdall RL, Vig KWL. Orthodontics: Current principles & techniques. 4th ed. St. Louis: Mosby: 168,169.

Turhani, D., Scheriau M, Kapral D, Benesch T, Jonke E,& Bantleon, HP. (2006). Pain relief by single low-level laser irradiation in orthodontic patients undergoing fixed appliance therapy. *Am J Orthod Dentofacial Orthop* ,130(3): 371-377.

Tocchio, RM., Williams, PT., Mayer, FS, & Standing KG. (1993). Laser debonding of ceramic orthodontic brackets. *Am J Orthod Dentofacial Orthop*, 103:155–162

Tortamano, A., Lenzi, DC., Haddad, AC., Bottino, MC., Dominguez, GC., Vigorito, JW.(2009). Low-level laser therapy for pain caused by placement of the first orthodontic archwire: a randomized clinical trial. *Am J Orthod Dentofacial Orthop*, 136: 662–667.

Townes, CH.(1994). Making waves. New York: Springer-Verlag,

Tranaeus, S., Lindgren,LE., Karlsson, L.& Angmar-Mansson,B. (2004).In vivo validity and reliability of IR fluorescence measurements for caries detection and quantification. *Swedish Dental Journal*, vol. 28, no. 4, pp. 173–182

Tronstad, L.(1992). Recent development in endodontic research. *Scand J Dent Res* ,100:52-9.

Tufekci, E., Dixon, JS., Gunsolley, JC., Lindauer SJ. 2011. Prevalence of white spot lesions during orthodontic treatment with fixed appliances. Angle Orthod 81(2): 206-210.

Turhani, D., Scheriau, M., Kapral, D., Benesch, T., Jonke E, &Bantleon, HP.(2006). Pain relief by single low-level laser irradiation in orthodontic patients undergoing fixed appliance therapy. *Am J Orthod Dentofacial Orthop*,130: 371–377.

Usumez, S., Buyukyilmaz, T.,& Karaman, AI. (2003). Effects of fast halogen and plasma arc curing lights on the surface hardness of orthodontic adhesives for lingual retainers. *Am J Orthod Dentofacial Orthop* ,123(6): 641-648.

Usümez, S., Orhan, M., Usümez, A. (2002).Laser etching of enamel for direct bonding with an Er,Cr:YSGG hydrokinetic laser system. *Am J Orthod Dentofacial Orthop*;122:649-56.

Vanarsdall, RL.,& Secchi, AG. Periodontal orthodontic interrelationships. In: Graber TM, Vanarsdall RL, Vig KWL. Orthodontics: Current principles & techniques. 4th ed. St. Louis: Mosby: 919.

Van Noort, R. (2002). Introduction to dental materials. 2nd ed. Edinburgh: Mosby: 284

Visuri, SR., Gilbert, JL., Wright, DD., Wigdor ,HA., Walsh, JT Jr. Shear strength of composite bonded to Er:YAG laser-prepared dentin. J Dent Res 1996;75:599-605.

Vongsavan N, Matthews B. Some aspects of the use of laser Doppler flow meters for recording tissue blood flow. Exp Physiol 1993;78:1-14.

Vukovich ,ME., Wood, DP.,& Daley ,TD.(1991). Heat generated by grinding during removal of ceramic brackets. *Am J Orthod Dentofacial Orthop* ,99(6): 505-512.

Walsh LJ, Goharkhay K, Verheyen P, Moritz A.(2006).Low Level Laser Therapy, In: *Oral Laser Application,* Mortiz A, PP.(521-539),Quintessenz Publisher,ISBN:1-85097-150-1,Berlin,Germany

Watanabe I , Baba N , Chang J , Chiu Y 2006 Nd:YAG laser penetration into cast titanium and gold alloy with different surface preparations . *Journal of Oral Rehabilitation*, 33 : 443 - 446

Watanabe, I., Liu, J.,& Atsuta, M.(2001). Effects of heat treatments on mechanical strength of laser-welded equi-atomic AuCu-6at%Ga alloy. *Journal of Dental Research ,80:1813-1817.*

Watanabe, I., Liu, J., Atsuta M, Okabe T.(2003). Effect of welding method on joint strength of laser-welded gold alloy. *American Journal of Dentistry* , 16:231-234.

Watanabe, I., Liu, J., Baba N, Atsuta M,& Okabe T. (2004).Optimizing mechanical properties of laser-welded gold alloy through heat treatment. *Dental Materials*, 20:630-634.

Watanabe I , Topham D S (2004) Tensile strength and elongation of laserwelded Ti and Ti-6AL-7NB . *Journal of Biomedical Materials Research Part B, Applied Biomaterials* 71 : 46 - 51

Watanabe, I. ,& Topham, DS.(2006). Laser welding of cast titanium and dental alloys using argon shielding . *Journal of Prosthodontics* ,15 : 102 - 107

Wendl, B., & Droschl, H. (2004). A comparative in vitro study of the strength of directly bonded brackets using different curing techniques. *Eur J Orthod* ,26(5): 535-544.

Wigdor, H., Abt ,E., Ashrafi, S.,& Walsh, JT . (1993). The effect of lasers on dental hard tissues. *J Am Dent Assoc,* 124(2):65–70

Wigdor, HA., Walsh, JT., Featherstone, JDB., Visuri, SR., Fried, D., &Waldvogel JL. (1995).Lasers in dentistry. *Laser Surg Med* ,16:103-33.

Xianglong ,H., Xiaolin, L., Ding, B., Yao, M., &Lan, H. (2008) Nd: YAG laser-aided ceramic brackets debonding: effects on shear bond strength and enamel surface. *Appl Surf Sci* , 255(2):613–615

Xiaoting, L., Yin, T., & Yangxi, C.(2010). Interventions for pain during fixed orthodontic appliance therapy. *Angle Orthodontist,* 80: 925-32.

Yamada, T., Mori, Y., Katsuhiro, M., Katsuaki, M., &Tsukamoto Y. (2002).Three-dimensional analysis of facial morphology in normal Japanese children as control data for cleft surgery, Cleft Palate .Craniofac J ,39: 517–526.

Yamagishi, T., Ito, M.,&Fujimura, Y.,(1993) Mechanical properties of laser welds of titanium in dentistry by pulsed Nd:YAG laser apparatus . *Journal of Prosthetic Dentistry* ,70 : 264 - 273

Yamaguchi, M. (2007). Low-energy laser irradiation stimulates the tooth movement velocity via expression of M-CSF and c-fms. *Orthodontic Waves* 66: 139–148

Yamaguchi, M., Hayashi ,M., Fujita, S., Yoshida, T., Utsunomiya ,T., Yamamoto, H., &Kasai, K. (2010). Low-energy laser irradiation facilitates the velocity of tooth movement and the expressions of matrix metalloproteinase-9, cathepsin K, and alpha(v) beta(3) integrin in rats.*European J Orthodont* ,32(2): 131–139.

Yamamoto, HY., &Sato, K.(1980). Prevention of dental caries by Nd:YAG laser irradiation. *J Dent Res* , 59: 2171–2177.

Yan, XJ., Yang, DZ.(2006). Corrosion resistance of a laser spot-welded joint of NiTi wire in simulated human body fluids. *Journal of Biomedical Materials Research Part A*, *77:97-*102.

Yao, CC., Lee ,JJ., Chen, HY., Chang, ZC., Chang ,HF.,& Chen YJ.(2005). Maxillary molar intrusion with fixed appliances and miniimplant anchorage studied in three dimensions. *Angle Orthod*, 75:754–760.

Yoshida, S., Kazuhiko, O., & Kazuo, T. (1996).Biological responses of the pulp to single-tooth dento-osseous osteotomy. *Oral Surg Oral Med Oral Pathol Oral Radiol Endod* , 82: 152–160.

Yoshida, T., Yamaguchi, M., Utsunomiya, T., Kato, M., Arai, Y., Kaneda ,T., Yamamoto, H., &Kasai, K. (2009) .Low-energy laser irradiation accelerates the velocity of tooth movement via stimulation of the alveolar bone remodeling. *Orthod Craniofac Res* ,12(4):289–298

Youssef, M., Ashkar,S., Hamade, E., Gutknecht, N., Lampert, F.,& Mir, M. (2008) .The effect of low-level laser therapy during orthodontic movement: a preliminary study. *Lasers Med Sci* 23(1):27–33

Young, AN., Taylor, RW., Taylor SE, Linnebur SA,& Buschang PH.(2006). Evaluation of preemptive valdecoxib therapy on initial archwire placement discomfort in adults. *Angle Orthod* ,76(2): 251-259.

Zachrisson, BU., Buyukyilmaz, T .(2005). Bonding in orthodontics. In: Graber TM, Vanarsdall RL, Vig KWL. Orthodontics: *Current principles & techniques*, 4th ed. St. Louis: Mosby: 596-600.

Zang, DY., Millerd ,JE., Wilder-Smith, PB., Arrastia, AM.(1996). A novel laser Doppler flowmeter for pulpal blood flow measurements. *Proceedings of the International Society for Optical Engineering* , 2672:21-6.

Zharikov, E. V., Osiko, V. V., Prokhorov. A. M., Scherbakov, I. A. (1984) Crystals of rare - earth gallium garnets with chromium as active media for solid - state lasers . *Inorg Aat* ,48, 81-94.

Zharikov, E.V.,Zhekov, V. I., Kulevskii, L. A., Murina, T. M., Oslko, V.V., Prokhorov, A. M., Savel'ev , A. D., Smirnov, V.V., Starikov, B.P., Timoshechkin, M.I. (1975) Stimulated emission from Er3- ions in yttrium aluminium garnet crystals at λ = 2.94 µm. *Sov J Quant Electron* ,4(8), 1039-1040.

Zupancic, R., Legat, A., & Funduk, N.(2006). Tensile strength and corrosion resistance of brazed and laser-welded cobalt-chromium alloy joints. *Journal of Prosthetic Dentistry* ,96:273-282.

8

Modern Etching and Bonding Materials in Orthodontics

Güvenç Başaran and İlknur Veli
Dicle University
Turkey

1. Introduction

Esthetics has been an indispensable element in human life for centuries. The elimination of esthetic problems substantially aids in confident self-expression. In addition to the different departments dealing with esthetics in medicine, orthodontists also make arrangements to eliminate various esthetic and functional concerns. These arrangements include the correction of skeletal and dental anomalies. Dental arrangements mostly involve the use of fixed orthodontic attachments. Previously, orthodontic treatments with fixed attachments had been performed by soldering brackets onto bands. In 1907, gold clamp bands were used by Angle as part of his edgewise philosophy. (Angle,1907) In later years, pitch-fit bands were used in full-mouth banding techniques, followed by the use of prefabricated stainless steel bands for orthodontic treatment. However, full-mouth banding techniques had some disadvantages, including increased chair-time, diastemata resulting from the removal of bands at the end of the treatment, unaesthetic appearances and soft tissue irritation.

In 1955, Buonocore applied 85% phosphoric acid to enamel and became a pioneer in science by providing a method for bonding acrylic structures by etching on enamel.(Buonocore, 1955) However, Newman (Newman,1965) and Retief (Retief,1970) started to use phosphoric acid with modification in percentage and application time in the 1960s. The preliminary results of the studies began to be shared in the 1970s(Silverman& Cohen, 1972), and the most extensive follow-up results were reported in 1977.(Zacrisson BU, 1977) In contemporary practice, 37% orthophosphoric acid gel or solution is applied to enamel for 30 seconds, and the minerals on the enamel surface are dissolved. The appearance of retention sites on enamel are as follows: the enamel prism walls remain stable while the cores are removed, the prism walls are removed while the cores remain stable or both structures are removed. (Type 1and 2 etching pattern) (Silverstone & Saxton, 1975; Galil & Wright, 1979) These demineralized areas, which are present after water rinsing and air drying, do not have uniform depths, and fixed attachments are bonded to the enamel surface by bonding adhesive materials to the gaps on the walls or in the center of the hexagonal enamel prisms.

Advances in etching and bonding materials took place over time with new developments in technology and clinician demands. In this chapter, information about the preliminary preparation for direct bonding and the development of etching, bonding and adhesive materials and their application guidelines will be given.

2. Surface and bonding preparation

2.1 Cleaning procedure

Organic pellicle layers on the enamel surface cannot be totally removed by brushing. This organic pellicle layer has been reported to reduce the bond strength between the adhesive resin on the base of the bracket and the tooth. (Ireland & Sherriff, 2002; Lew & Chew, 1991; Swartz, 1994) To prevent this, polishing is recommended before performing the bonding procedure. (Lew & Chew , 1991; Swartz ML, 1994) For the polishing procedure, using polishing brushes or rubber cups disposable or sterilization avaible (Fig. 1) with low-speed (lower than 20000 rpm) micromotors and non-fluoride pastes for 10 seconds is recommended. (Reisner &, Levitt, 1997; Burgess & Sherriff, 2006) Enamel loss of 5-14 µm in depth was reported as a result of the type and application time of the rubber cups or polishing brushes.(Pus& Way, 1980)
Another effective method for removing the pellicle layer is effective tooth brushing by the patient. Effective tooth brushing may be taught by enabling patients to see plaque layers over tooth surfaces by means of plaque disclosing tablets.(Fig. 2) No negative effects of fluoride- containing toothpastes on bracket failures have been reported. Furthermore, fluoride-containing toothpastes have been reported to be beneficial in preventing cariogenic factors.(Øgaard & Bishara, 2004)

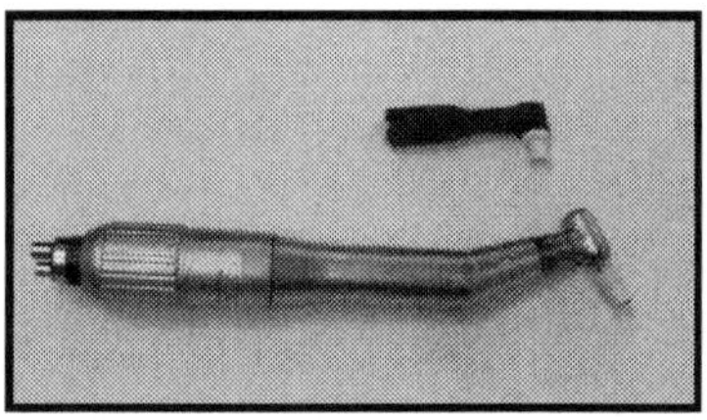

Fig. 1. Low speed handpieces for polishing that can be sterilized which are disposable.

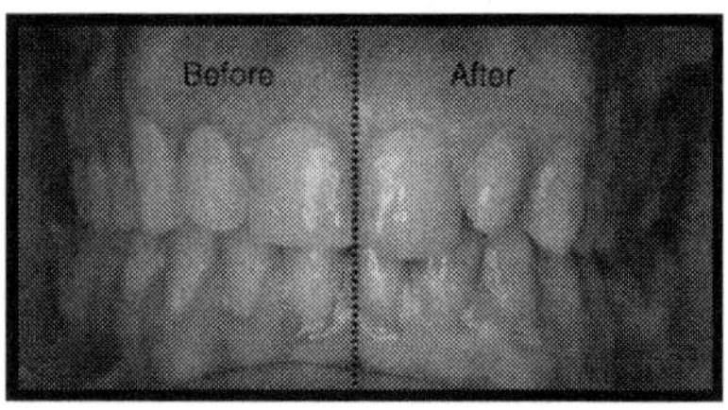

Fig. 2. Intraoral application of plaque staining solution.

The next step after intraoral preliminary preparation is controlling moisture contamination before etching because the available acid, primer and adhesive depend on a hydrophobic system. To enhance bond strength and reduce bonding failure, it is necessary to control saliva flow and provide a dry working field. For this, lip expanders, cheek retractors, vacuum systems and cotton pellets may be used. To eliminate difficulties in the supply and maintenance of dry surfaces before bracketing the posterior teeth, prefabricated cotton pellets can be used at the output of the parotid duct. (Fig. 3) Additionally, an appropriate working field for clinicians can be obtained by using antisialagogue tablets (Carter, 1981;

Zachrisson & Büyükyılmaz, 2005), such as atropine sulfate or injectable solutions (Brandt &, Servoss, 1981; White, 1975), in patients whose saliva flow control is difficult to achieve. However, in the literature, there is no consensus regarding the evaluation of success after clinical use of these premedical agents.(Ponduri & Turnbull, 2007)

3. Etching procedures

3.1 Phosphoric acid application

Phosphoric acid is used to eliminate oxidation of metal surfaces and enhance adhesion of dyes to metal surfaces in the metal and dye industry.(Rossouw, 2010) In light of this information, Buonocore used phosphoric acid to obtain as effective an adhesion on enamel surface as on metal surfaces. The concentration of the first phosphoric acid solution used by Buonocore was 85% (Buonocore, 1955), and it was applied for 30 seconds. Buonocore adhered acrylic materials onto the non-etched teeth surfaces and etched surfaces. Although acrylic materials adhered onto the etched surfaces were bonded with enough strength that they needed debonding procedures, failures were observed on non-etched surfaces. (Rossouw, 2010) This technique was an important advance in directly bonding orthodontic attachments to the tooth surface by means of micro-retention. However, honeycombed structures were not obtained in enamel prisms after etching with 85% phosphoric acid, and successful results in terms of retention were not achieved. Retief (Retief & Dreyer, 1970) investigated the use of 50% phosphoric acid and achieved successful bond strength results. Chow and Brown (Chow & Brown, 1973) reported easy removal of "monocalcium phosphate monohydrate," which can be soluble in use of concentrations higher than 27%, by washing. In concentrations phosphoric acid lower than 27%, there was production of "dicalcium phosphate dihydrate," which presented difficulties in removal by washing and thus negatively affected bond strength. Many researchers (Øgaard & Fjeld, 2010; Zacrisson & Büyükyılmaz, 2005, Üşümez & Erverdi, 2010) reported that a 35-38% concentration of phosphoric acid is effective in terms of optimum bond strength; however, 5-10% concentration changes did not have negative effects on bond strength.(Reynolds, 1979; Carstensen,1995; Bhad & Hazarey, 1995) Today, 35-38% orthophosphoric acid is effectively used to change enamel surface characteristics and to provide micromechanic bond strength by means of an opaque appearance where micromechanic retention areas occur. (Buonocore & Matsui, 1968; Gwinnett &, Buonocore, 1965; Gwinnett & Matsui, 1967)

An etching time of 15-30 seconds is accepted as the optimum working time by manufacturers and clinic. (Brännström & Malmgren, 1982; Brännström & Nordenvall, 1978, Newman, 1978; Nordenvall & Brännström, 1980; Wang & Lu, 1991;. Barkmeier &, Gwinnett, 1987; Sadowsky & Retief, 1990; Carstensen, 1995; Powers &, Kim, 1997; Sheen & Wang, 1993; Abdullah & Rock, 1996) It has been previously reported that etching times of less than 10 seconds and more than 60 seconds do not produce enough shear bond strength. (Üşümez & Erverdi, 2010; Olsen & Bishara, 1996) Ten seconds of etching time does not produce enough tagged areas on the enamel, and etching times of 60 seconds or more than 60 seconds impair the integrity of honeycombed prismatic structures on the enamel, which negatively affects bond strength. (Wang & Lu, 1991) For the protection of dental structures, a topical fluoride application is generally preferred. It is reported that no additional etching time is required for fluoride applied teeth before treatment. (Ng'anga & Øgaard, 1992; Büyükyilmaz & Øgaard, 1995; Garcia-Godoy & Hubbard, 1991; Meng & Wang, 1997)

Phosphoric acid is produced in a liquid or gel form, (Fig. 4) and neither form demonstrated any negative effects on bond strength. (Brännström & Malmgren, 1982) However, only the intended area is etched when using a gel. (Fig. 5) by means of this, opaque enamel surface is gained only in the wanted region. (Fig 6) A more extended area beyond the bracket base is etched by the liquid form due to displacement of the acid by gravitational force. Therefore, redundant demineralized areas are produced in the enamel surface, which can cause plaque and bacterial retention areas. Additionally, gingival structures should be carefully protected during etching with liquid form because ulceration (Øgaard & Field, 2010) on gingival structures and unwanted bleeding (Øgaard & Field, 2010) can occur during application. However, when using bonding brackets or an eruption appliance on partially erupted or impacted teeth, procedures such as protective liquid polishing must be applied before contamination occurs to prevent negative effects on bond strength. (Sayınsu & Işık, 2007)

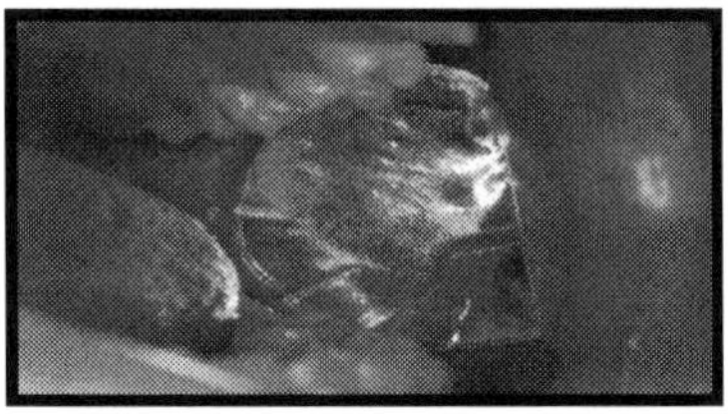

Fig. 3. Application of cotton to the cheek for restricting salive flow.

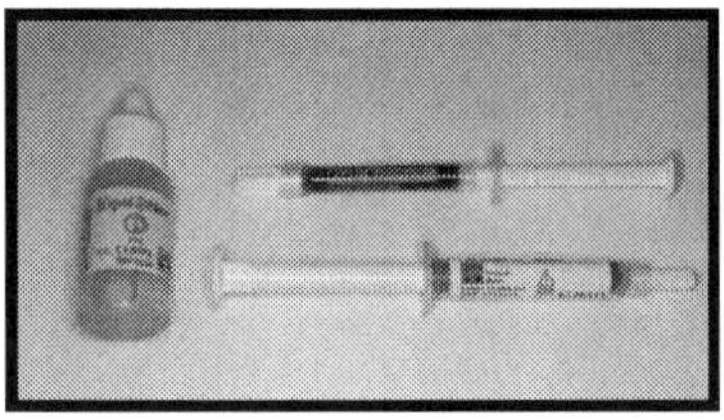

Fig. 4. Liquid and gel phosphoric acids.Likid ve jel fosforik asitler

The presence of prismatic and aprismatic enamel affects the efficacy of phosphoric acid. While a more uniform surface appearance is achieved by etching in the presence of prismatic enamel, bond strength is reduced in the presence of aprismatic enamel. Due to moisture contamination during respiration and the presence of aprismatic enamel, more bracket failures are observed in the lower second premolars of patients in permanent dentition. (Mattick & Hobson, 2000) Uniform prism structures on the outer enamel layer of deciduous teeth are not observed. Therefore, phosphoric acid application after sandblasting with 50-µm aluminum oxide is needed for deciduous teeth. (Zachrisson & Büyükyılmaz, 2005)

Etching procedures with phosphoric acid differ in terms of microtopographic etching patterns over enamel surfaces. (Mattick & Hobson, 2000; Hosein & Sherriff, 2004) The intended etching pattern was only observed in 1/20 of enamel etched with phosphoric acid. This was attributed to the presence of aprismatic enamel and partial contact between phosphoric acid and the enamel surface. (Mattick & Hobson, 2000) Microtopographic evaluation depending on the etching procedure revealed a non-uniform depth. It was reported that a depth of 3-15 µm or more is necessary to provide optimum shear bond strength and penetration.(Hosein & Sherriff, 2004) However, in literature, surface depths between 10 µm and 175 µm were presented. (Diedrich, 1981; Gwinnett, 1973; Silverstone, 1977) The difference in the depth (Hobson & McCabe, 2002; Daronch & DeGoes, 2003) are thought to be caused by aprismatic enamel and remineralization of Ca-P to enamel surface. (Chow & Brown, 1973)

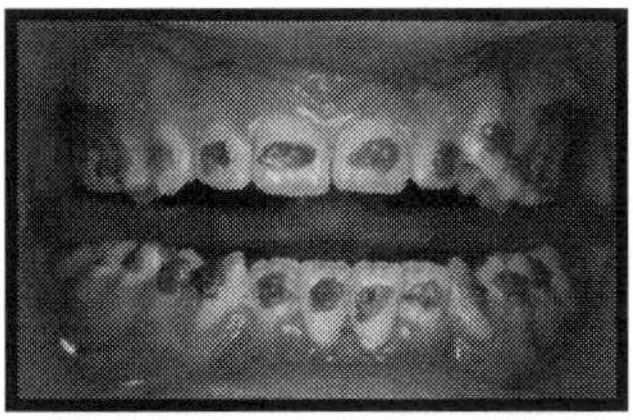

Fig. 5. 37 %Phosphoric acid gel application to the places that the brackets will be positioned.

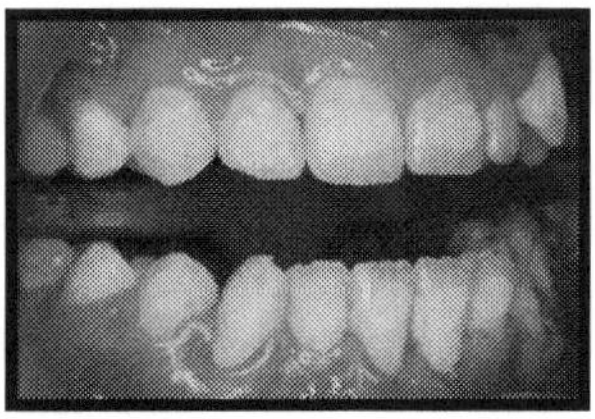

Fig. 6. The micromechanical bonding places of the enamel after etching with phosphoric acid

Another alternative to phosphoric acid is maleic acid. Ten percent maleic acid is used by orthodontists. When the scanning electron microscopy (SEM) examination of enamel surfaces exposed to either phosphoric acid or maleic acid was evaluated, similar morphologic patterns were observed. (Baş-Kalkan & Orhan, 2007; Olsen & Bishara, 1997; Hermsen & Vrijhoef, 1993) However, in the topographic evaluation of surface depth, retention areas with less depth were observed. (Triolo & Swift, 1993) When compared with 37% orthophosphoric acid, some researchers found lower bond strength (Smith & Cartz, 1973; Årtun & Bergland, 1984; Maijer & Smith, 1986); however, other researchers found similar strengths. (Triolo & Swift, 1993) In any case, maleic acid has never been as popular as orthophosphoric acid worldwide. Gottlieb et al. (Gottlieb & Nelson, 1996) reported that 95.6% of orthodontists in the USA have never used maleic acid and only 0.5% have routinely used maleic acid.

3.2 Self-etching application

Advances in adhesive technology lead orthodontists to use new adhesives, composite resins and bonding techniques in their clinical practices. Self-etching primers (SEP), which combine acid and primer, carry out bonding procedures by simultaneously etching and infiltrating the enamel surface. They ease the bonding procedure by reducing chair time and eliminating side-effects of etching. (Chigira & Koike, 1989; Nishida &, Yamauchi, 1993) Two-step SEPs and new single-step self-etching adhesive systems are new additives to a clinician's adhesive toolbox. (Pashley & Tay, 2001; Bishara & Adam, 2008; Amra &, Samsodien, 2007)

Advances in the next generation of bonding systems extends from etching enamel to dentine conditioning, treatment of smear layers and different application procedures of adhesive systems. (Schaneveldt & Foley, 2002) Fourth generation bonding systems consist of a 3-step application: etching, primers (which provide maximum adhesion by increasing monomer penetration to the etched enamel and hydrophilic dentine and increasing the wettability of tooth surfaces) and an adhesive resin agent. This system is also known as the total etch technique.

A new SEP (5th generation dentin bonding system) which combines the etching and priming steps to affect both enamel and dentine simultaneously has been developed to ease the dentin/enamel bonding systems. (Miyazaki & Hirohata, 1999) However, a reduction in bond strength by manufacturers as a way of easing clinical applications is a concern to clinicians. (Miyazaki & Hirohata, 1999) Studies regarding the development of SEPs have progressed with the presentation (Amra & Samsodien, 2007) of new single-step bonding systems. The current system is the 6th generation of bonding systems.

However, because it is difficult to form compounds with chemically evident concentrations (acid, primer and adhesive), 6th generation bonding systems are designed to be preserved separately in 2 compartments until mixing for clinical applications. This separation procedure prevents possible changes in initializers due to increases in sensitivity against acidity. (Van Meerbeek, 2003)

The main feature of single step acid/primer bonding systems is that no separate acid-etching of the enamel and rinsing with water and air drying are necessary. The liquid has a component that conditions the enamel surface. The active component of the SEPs is the methacrylated phosphoric acid ester that dissolves calcium from hydroxyapatite. The removed calcium forms a complex when the primer polymerizes. Etching and monomer penetration to the exposed enamel rods are simultaneous, and the depth of penetration is equal.

Three mechanisms stop the etching process. First, acid groups attached to monomers are neutralized by forming a complex with calcium from hydroxyapatite. Second, as the solvent evaporates from the primer during the air drying, the viscosity increases, and the transport of acid groups to the enamel interface slows down. Finally, as the primer monomers are polymerized with light curing, transport of acid groups to the interface is stopped. (Jost-Brinkmann & Schiffer, 1992; Cinader, 2001) The acid component of a self-etching primer is reported to cause as much demineralization on enamel surface as 30-50% phosphoric acid. However, dissolved calcium is not removed from the tooth surface, and it produces a complex with a phosphate group. The primer unites with this complex during polymerization to neutralize the acid. Most of the bonds in minimal etching obtained with SEPs occur by binding to the calcium in the enamel with chemical bond, which differs from the mechanical bond obtained with the conventional phosphoric acid application. (Swartz ML, 2004)

There are studies presenting the importance of enamel topography in terms of bond strength. The thickness of the resin-infiltrated layer after enamel treatment with SEP agents compared with a conventional method was evaluated by Hannig et al. (Hannig &, Bock, 2002) who observed 1.5–3.2 µm wide netlike, resinous structures with SEPs. A similar pattern, but a greater depth (6.9 µm) of enamel surface hybridization, was found with phosphoric acid. (Hannig &, Bock, 2002) The hybrid layer was measured at 4 µm for SEPs and 8 µm for phosphoric acid by Pashley and Tay (Pashley &, Tay, 2001) Despite being less distinct, a similar etch pattern was observed when using SEPs with nanoretentive interlocking between enamel crystallites and resin when compared with a phosphoric acid etch. (Hannig & Bock, 2002) These similar etch patterns, in addition to nanoretentive interlocking, could explain the potential of the SEP systems. (Hannig & Bock, 2002)

In dentistry, there are many self-etching systems, such as Clearfil SE Bond (Kuraray ,Japan), Clearfil S3 Bond (Kuraray, Japan), One Step (Bisco, USA), Adper Prompt L-Pop (3M Espe, USA), Futurabond NR (Voco, Germany). However, Transbond Plus Self-Etching Primer (3M/Unitek,) is the most commonly used system in orthodontics. The single-use package consists of three compartments. (Fig. 7) The first one contains methacrylated phosphoric acid esters, photosensitizers and stabilizers. The second compartment contains water and soluble fluoride, and the third compartment contains an applicator microbrush. Squeezing and folding the first compartment over to the second compartment activates the system. (Fig. 8 a) The mixed component is passed to the third compartment to wet the applicator tip. (Fig. 8 b,c) To prevent gingival irritation, the application only occurs on the tooth surface. (Fig. 8 d) Transbond Plus Self-Etching Primer is applied by rubbing for at least 3 seconds. To ensure monomer penetration, the surface must be always wet with new solution. The presence of water in the chemical composition of Transbond Plus SEP may necessitate air drying during the procedure; however, the solvent evaporates and drying is no longer necessary. Today, etching patterns (Kawasaki & Hayakawa, 2003) and bond strengths similar to those from phosphoric acid etching are obtained by using the technologically advanced self-etching systems. (Erhardt & Cavalcante, 2004; Lührs & Guhr, 2008; Lalani & Foley, 2000)

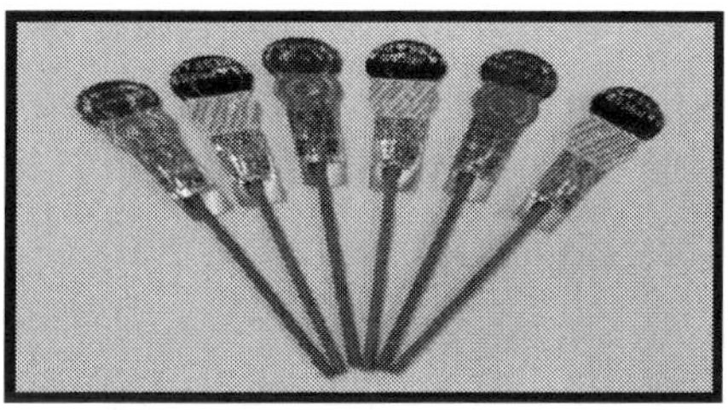

Fig. 7. Self etching primer examples that are used in orthodontic bonding

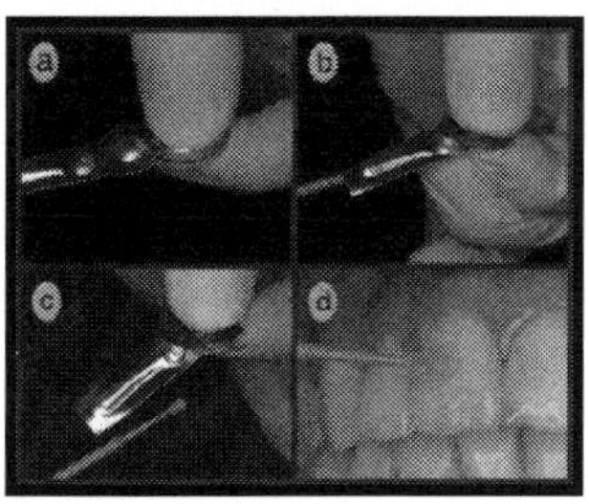

Fig. 8. a-c a) Mixing first and second compartments, b) Mixing second and third compartments, c) The image of primer, d) Application of self etching primer on tooth surface.

3.3 Laser etching application

Use of light for diagnosis and treatment has continued since ancient history. The ancient Greeks and Romans used sunbath and solarium. (Katzir, 1993) The ancient Egyptians, Chinese and Indians treated rickets, psoriasis, skin cancer and even psychological disorders by taking advantage of the treatment effects of light. (Daniell & Hill, 1991)

Gordon and Towness invented **M**icrowave **A**mplification by **S**timulated **E**mission of **R**adiation (MASER) by microwave simulation during their military research in Bell labs in 1958 and, and they also published theoretical calculations related to LASER. (Miserendino & Levy, 1995) In 1960, the Massachusetts Institute of Technology (MIT) made a laser device to strengthen radio waves for use as a sensitive detector in space research. The Ruby laser (694 nm) was first used in medicine by Theodore Maiman. (Maiman, 1966)The first dental laser applications were conducted by Dr. Leon Goldman in 1962.

Laser light has some differences when compared to visible light. These differences arise from the features of coherence, monochromacy and columniation in laser light. Coherence is a particular phase relationship of electromagnetic field and direction. Columniation is the observation of progress in a laser light source without disintegration in the same direction. During the observation of light, there is disintegration due to different wavelengths of visible light. Monochromacy is the generation of single color laser light in a specific frequency band.

Electrons moving in a particular orbit are the basis of laser light. Electrons release energy in the form of radiation called emissions when electrons from a particular spin move to a higher energy orbit. (Fig. 9 a) Electrons spontaneously return to low-energy orbit when they move out to a higher orbit and release a photon as energy. This ensures the atomic structure remains stable while spontaneous emissions also remain stable. An atom with the appropriate energy level forces an electron at the same level to enter a lower energy level while it enters the electromagnetic field of an excited atom. (Fig 9 b) The difference between the two levels manifests itself as another photon. (Fig. 9 c) If there are a collection of atoms in a stimulated environment, the excitation process will continue exponentially as a result of the energy release of each atom and the stimulation of others. (Fig. 10)

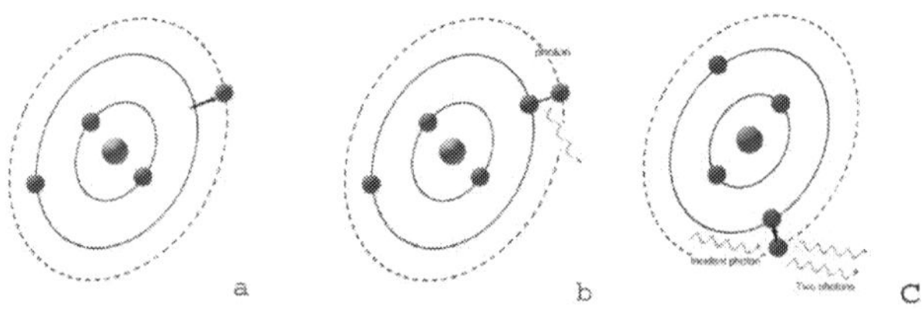

Fig. 9. a-c, a) Moving to a higher energy orbit of an atom after stimulation, b) Releasing of energy when returning to a lower energy orbit, c) Manifesting itself as another photon before returning to the old level.

Laser beam-producing devices are composed of an optical cavity, an energy source and cooling systems. The stimulation of the photon chain reaction takes place in an optical cavity. There are two parallel mirror systems in the optical cavity design. (Fig. 11) While a mirror in one direction provides 100% reflection, the mirror in the other surface has some permeability. Light reflection continues by photon emission from the surface of the mirror with 100% reflection, and more photon energy is stimulated with the emitted energy. Thus, the motion of photons toward each other with constant energy transfer from an energy source achieves continuity. Because of the coherence, monochromacy and columniation properties of the semi-permeable surface structures, the photons move out and form laser light. An amount of energy is converted into heat during this formation. To neutralize this thermal effect, intra-device cooling units are used.

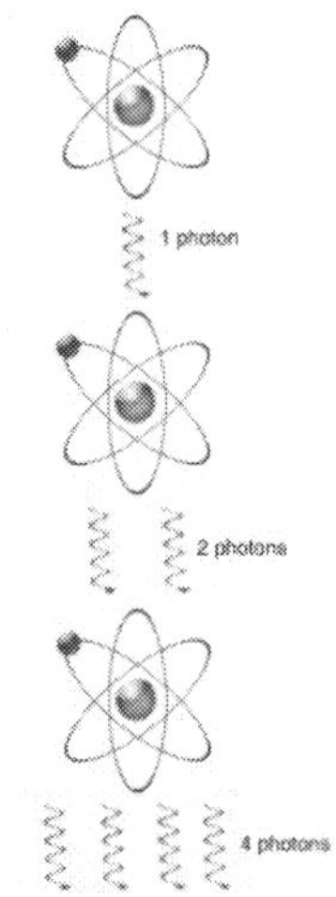

Fig. 10. Forming process of LASER light.

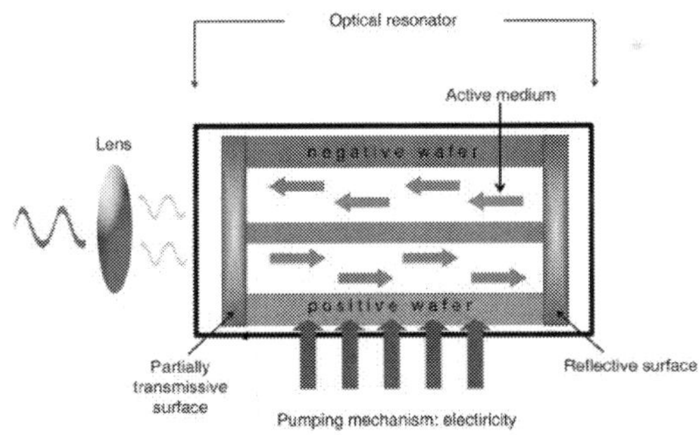

Fig. 11.The study mechanism of laser device

When the laser light hits the tissue surface, a layer of heated gas called "plasma" is generated. This layer allows the passage of decreased energy by absorbing the excess beams. However, this layer causes ablation and extreme warming by transferring the heat to the tissue surface. To minimize thermal effects on live tissue, air-water cooling systems are used in the current erbium laser systems.

The wavelength (λ) of light is the most important parameter in the effect of light on the tissue. The wavelength of light is the electromagnetic form of light produced by laser energy. This structure is determined as the distance between any two points. Light is divided into two parts, including visible and invisible wavelengths in the electromagnetic spectrum. The invisible wavelengths are divided into two parts: thermal and ionized. (Fig12)

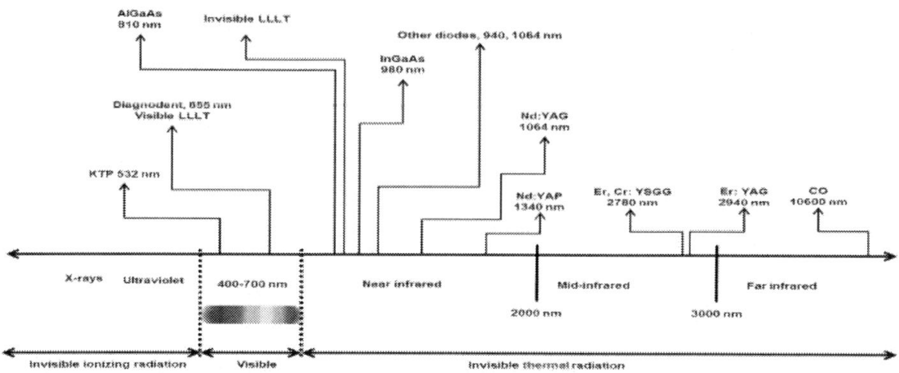

Fig. 12. Dental lasers in electromagnetic spectrum.

Dental laser devices are comprised of visible and invisible thermal energy wavelengths (Manni, 2004; Coluzzi & Convissar, 2007). The wavelengths of dental lasers are quite small and, therefore, are indicated as nanometers (nm) or micrometers (µm). While wavelengths of light determine the relationship between the laser and the tissue as well as the type of reaction, the amount of energy and texture characteristics of the tissue determine the depth of effect and the amount of the reaction.

In hard tissues of the tooth, pulsated lasers are used due to their thermo-mechanical effects. Micro-explosions can occur depending on increased propulsion as a result of pulsations at the nanosecond level, which prevents the formation of plasma and the occurrence of microscopic mechanical ruptures. In millisecond-level explosions, while micromechanical effects decrease, thermal effects increase, and dehydration and cracks can occur as a result. If a pulsation period between 100-350 µs is used in conjunction with a cooling system, a sufficient mechanical effect can be obtained. (Akkurt, 2008) When light moves as a wavelength, it exhibits a motion around the zero axis known as the oscillation during each second. This structure is the frequency, which is measured in hertz (Hz).

Based on this basic information about lasers, the relationship between a laser device and tissue should be determined because a large number of laser devices with different wavelengths are available in dentistry. (Fig. 10) Certain laser devices should be preferred depending on the wavelength of laser beam, the energy density, and the optical properties of tissue because these determine the thermal and mechanical effects. Protective glasses in accordance with the wavelength should be worn. Laser light shows interactions in 4 different manners on tissue surfaces. The interactions are defined as reflection, absorption, scattering and transmission. (Miserendino & Levy, 1995)

During these movements, the physician, staff and patients need effective protection against reflected and scattered laser light. For example, while carbon dioxide (CO_2) and Erbium lasers affect the cornea and lens of the eye, retinal areas are affected by Neodymium: YAG (Nd: YAG) and Diode lasers. (Niemz, 2007) However, these effects are prevented by protective glasses, which are manufactured according to suitable wavelength.

Argon, Diode, Nd: YAG, CO_2 and Erbium lasers are commonly used in dentistry. While Argon, Diode and Nd: YAG laser systems are efficiently used in the soft tissues, Erbium: YAG (Er: YAG) with a wavelength of 2940 nm and Erbium, Yttrium-Scandium-Gallium-Garnet Chromium-doped (ErCr: YSGG) lasers with a wavelength of 2780 nm are used in dental hard tissues.

Laser use in etching has increased in recent years. However, there are conflicting results in terms of effects on the enamel surface before bonding. This situation depends on different power outputs and designs of the planned study. However, many researchers agree that there is heat increase in pulpal level as a result of laser energy applied to the enamel surface. (Wigdor & Walsh, 1995; Aoki & Sasaki, 2000; Berk & Başaran, 2008) This increase in temperature is especially noted in differences in depth when using Nd: YAG lasers. Reversible pulpal hyperemia occurs at temperatures between 43 and 49 °C. Temperatures above 49 °C cause pulpal necrosis. Reversible changes occur in the heat exchanges below 16 °C. (Miserendino & Levy, 1995; Miserendino & Neiburger, 1989; Powel &, Morton, 1989) Reversible injuries occur in dentin near the pulp as a result of Erbium lasers, and these injuries are self-tolerated by secondary dentin formation in 2 weeks. (Akkurt, 2008) In addition, a better recovery capacity is detected in the regeneration of perforated pulpal tissue when using cavitation studies rather than rotary instruments. Optimal micromechanic retention is provided in procedures at the enamel level with active cooling by means of air and water rates.

Researchers reported honeycomb-like fields similar to type 1 etching pattern on the surface of enamel. However, to obtain this pattern, appropriate power, frequency and time setting planning should be performed. Otherwise, although the amount of water and organic matrix in the enamel tissue are less than those in dentin, vaporization will occur in the hydroxyapatite matrix, and irregular heterogeneous micro-etching patterns will be observed due to the irreversible damage from microexplosions. (Rechmann & Goldin, 1998)(Fig 13) To minimize these effects, lasers should be used with appropriate power output and air-water rates.

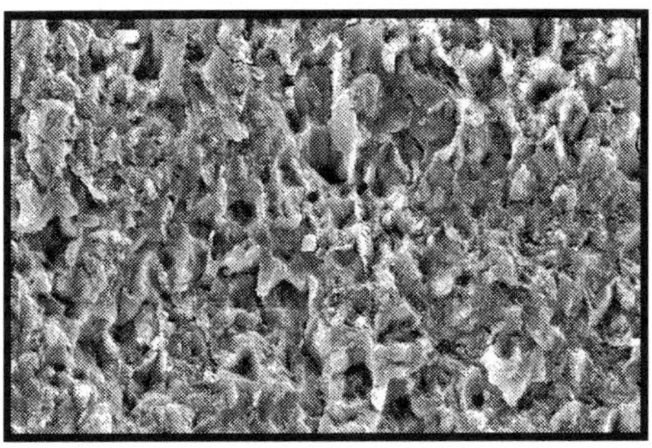

Fig. 13. The view of microcracks after laser application on the enamel surface.

Laser use is recommended at a non-contact mode or a distance of 1 mm by researchers. (Özer & Başaran, 2008) Bond strength is reported to be negatively affected by increasing distance between the tooth surface and laser output. (Başaran & Hamamcı, 2011) However, there is insufficient data about etching depth. Micro-cracks were sometimes observed in nearly ideal etched areas on the surface of enamel. (Akkurt, 2008) This constitutes a negative effect for the preservation of the integrity of the enamel after the treatment period.

3.4 Sandblasting (air-abrasive) application

The diameter of aluminum oxide powder used for pumicing dental surfaces is 50 µm. (Fig. 14) Reisner et al. (Reisner & Levitt, 1997) examined the effects of sandblasting techniques in comparison to conventional acid etching by using 50 µm aluminum oxide powder with 65-70 psi pressure for a period of 2-3 sec in their study. They observed decreased bond strength on the enamel surface. However, this situation is attributed to the exposure of enamel surface to less sandblasting time in comparison to the acid-etching procedure. Berk et al. (Berk & Başaran, 2008) observed a similar effect in their study on molar tubes in the posterior region. Sandblasting etching procedures alone are reported to be insufficient generators of bond strength in clinical studies. (Hogervorst & Feilzer, 2000; Olsen & Bishara, 1997; Reisner & Levitt, 1997) An inconsistent etching pattern was observed on enamel surfaces by SEM visualization. (Fig. 15) There are studies presenting additional retention areas when using the sandblasting method following orthophosphoric acid in terms of bond strength when compared with phosphoric acid (Black, 1950; Black, 1955; Goldstein & Parkins, 1994). Additionally, there are reports of reduced clinical bond strength when using resin modified glass ionomer cement instead of a splint mount design. (Özer & Arıcı, 2005)

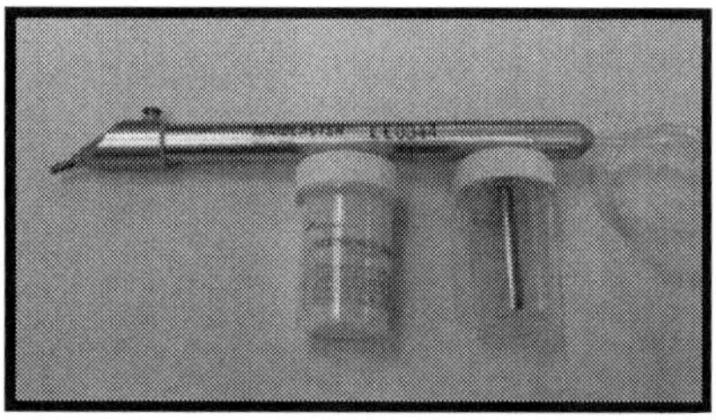

Fig. 14. Microetcher system

Fig. 15. The enamel surface view after 50µm Al_2O_3 application

3.5 Porcelain, amalgam and composite surface etching applications

Today, orthodontic treatment is frequently preferred by adults to overcome esthetic considerations. However, different types of restorations, such as porcelain prosthesis or laminate veneers, are encountered in an adult's mouth. A mechanical or chemical method different from etching procedures on the enamel surface must be followed in individuals thought to be treated with fixed orthodontic appliances to support these restorations. One point to be considered is the type of porcelain used in the restoration and the type of bracket.

A sufficient bond strength could not be obtained when using a mechanical etching procedure with diamond stone burs (Barbosa & Almedia, 1995 ; Cochran & O'Keefe, 1997), sandblasting (Andreasen & Stieg, 1998; Kocadereli & Canay, 2001; Cochran & O'Keefe, 1997; Zachrisson & Zachrisson, 1996), or sandpaper discs. (Barbosa & Almedia, 1995 ; Cochran & O'Keefe, 1997) To ensure an adequate bond strength, removal of the glaze layer on a porcelain surface and a suitable mechanical retention area are needed. Therefore, bonding to glazed ceramic with a coupling agent (silane) and a chemical preparation of the ceramic with acids, such as hydrofluoric acid (HFA) or acidulated phosphate fluoride, are used. (Major & Koehler, 1995; Hayakawa & Horie, 1992; Bourke & Rock, 1999) Silane coupling agents enhance bond strength by increasing the chemical bond between the resin composite and the ceramic material. (Tylka & Stewart, 1994; Nebbe & Stein, 1996; Aida & Hayakawa, 1995; Wood & Bubb, 1997; Gillis & Redlich, 1998) The silica of the ceramic is chemically joined with the acrylic group of the composite resin through silanization (Bowen & Rodriguez, 1962). Silane enhances the bonding of brackets to glazed ceramic surfaces, but the bond strengths achieved through this process may not be adequate for clinical use. Generally, a silane coupling agent is applied with chemical and mechanical roughening procedures. (Schmage & Nergiz, 2003; Özcan & Vallittu, 2004; Harari & Shapira-Davis, 2003; Huang & Kao, 2001) (Fig. 16)

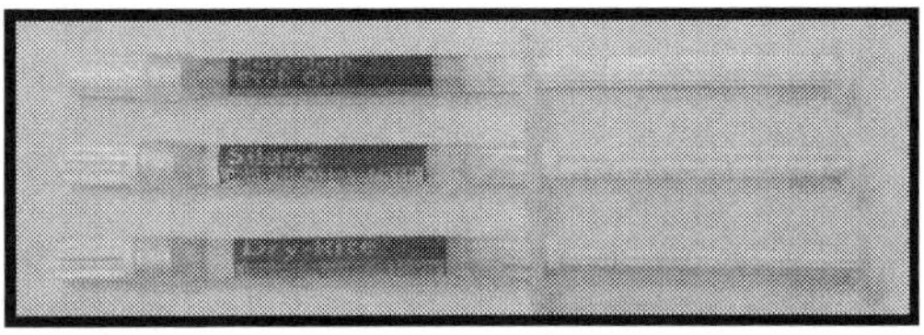

Fig. 16. Hydroflouric acid, silane and ethyl alcohol that are used for porcelain surface treatments.

HFA is applied at concentrations of 5-9.6%. However, gingival barriers should be used to eliminate the negative effects of HFA in gingival tissues before application. In addition to studies indicating that a 5% concentration is sufficient (Trakyalı & Malkondu, 2009), the use of 9.6% HFA for a period of 120 sec is recommended to ensure optimal bond strength. (Al Edris & al Jabr, 1990; Simonsen & Calamia, 1983; Zacrisson & Büyükyılmaz, 2005)

Etching procedure on amalgam restorations varies depending on the size of amalgam restoration. If amalgam restorations are present in a limited area, enamel around the restoration can be conditioned with 37% orthophosphoric acid following by sandblasting with 50 µm aluminum oxide powder for 3 seconds. If there are large amalgam restorations covering the area to be bonded, a metal primer is applied onto the amalgam restoration following sandblasting with 50 µm aluminum oxide powder for 3 seconds and a 30 second waiting period. (Zacrisson & Büyükyılmaz, 2005; Zacrisson & Büyükyılmaz, 1993; Zacrisson & Büyükyılmaz, 1995)

Previous composite restoration is removed with the help of a rotary instrument, and sealant application onto a dry composite surface is completed with single bonding procedure. Clinical failures in these restorations are not frequently observed. (Jost-Brinkmann & Can, 1996; Klocke & Shi, 2003)

4. Sealant and primer applications

Depending on the type of primer used for orthodontics, the tooth surface can be either completely dry or slightly damp. If the primer is moisture sensitive, the enamel surface should be completely dried. Following the appearance of an opaque enamel surface, primer is applied in a thin layer onto the etched tooth surface with the help of a microbrush. Then, a quick application of the bracket and dental adhesive material onto the teeth is performed. To prevent bracket failures occurring from the difficulty of application, especially in the posterior region, primers with hydrophilic features were produced. Although the bond strength in hydrophobic primer applications onto dry surfaces is higher than the bond strength in wet surfaces, these hydrophilic primers provide significant convenience for clinicians in cases with partially impacted teeth and bonding to the second molar teeth.

5. Adhesive applications

5.1 Composite resins

Dental composites are the materials produced by the homogeneous dissolution of inorganic fillers. Monomers, such as the organic matrix Bis-Glycidyl methacrylate (BisGMA) ; Urethane Dimethacrylate (UDMA), which provides good adhesion and is resistant to discoloration; and Triethylene glycol Dimethacrylate (TEGDMA), which is used to reduce viscosity, are used in commercially available dental composites. Good physical bonding between composite resins and metal brackets used in orthodontic treatments is especially provided by BisGMA. (Buzitta & Hallgren, 1982; Jost-Brinkman & Schiffer, 1992; Zachrisson & Brobakken, 1978)

Inorganic structures are composed of filler particles scattered into a matrix such as quartz, borosilicate glass, lithium aluminum silicate, strontium, barium, zinc, yttrium glass or barium aluminum silicate of various shapes and sizes. These materials give some properties to the composite resin materials. Strontium, barium, zinc and yttrium provide radiopacity for resins. Silica particles strengthen the mechanical properties. Pure silica is available in crystalline and non-crystalline forms. Because crystalline forms are hard, finishing and polishing of composite resins are difficult. For this reason, composite resins are produced using non-crystalline forms of silica. In addition, camphorquinone (CQ) is used as polymerization initiator for photopolymerization, and benzoyl peroxide is used for chemical polymerization. Close binding is necessary between the organic polymer matrix phase and the inorganic phase in composite resins. This binding is provided with an intermediate phase. This phase consists of silane, which is an organic silicon compound. In modern composite resins, surface silica particles are pre-coated with silane binding agents, and a thin layer is formed with single- molecule and dual-function molecules on the surface of the silica particles. One end of the molecules in this layer is bound with hydroxyl groups on the surface of silica particles, and the other end is bound with polymer in an organic matrix. Silane binding agents develop the physical and mechanical properties of resin, provide the hydrolytic balance by preventing the passage of water along the resin-particle interface and reduce the resolution and the water absorption of resin.

Hybrid and NanoFil composites are widely used in modern dentistry. In hybrid composite resins, inorganic filler particles of different sizes, including small particles (0.6 to 5 microns) and micro-fillers (0.04 m), are combined and added to the organic matrix (Duke, 2003; Davis, 2003). In this type of composite resins, a mixture of colloidal silica (0.04 m) and heavy metals containing glass particles (1 to 3.6 microns) are used as inorganic filler. (Oduncu, 2009) The ratio of inorganic particles is 75-80%. The fact that hybrid composites do not negatively affect bond strength under brackets is a result of less polymerization shrinkage than microfilm composites and a decreased need for technical sensitivity (Powers & Kim, 1997).

Composites used in orthodontics are divided into either no-mix (Fig 17) or light-cured (Fig 18) composites based on the polymerization form. Following the application of a thin layer of liquid primer and no-mix composites to the bracket base, brackets are placed onto etched and dry tooth surfaces. Because polymerization begins immediately, even minimal revision of bracket positioning causes micro-fractures in the composite material, and thus, bond strength will be negatively affected. Optimal polymerization of the system occurs after 60 min. There are some disadvantages to this system. They include the fact that polymerized liquid activators and polymerization occur. Additionally, there is an increased waiting period for polymerization, and there are toxic and allergic effects in direct proportion to the amount of non-polymerized residual monomers and liquid activators present in the system. (Fredericks, 1981; Thompson & Miller, 1982)

Light-curing adhesive systems began to be used clinically in the early 1970s and are widely preferred today by orthodontists because of their advantages in working time and comfort. Light-curing adhesives enable bracket placement on impacted canine teeth after surgical uncovering, bracket repositioning of single tooth bracket loss, ease of applicability in areas with risk of bleeding and the possibility to check bracket position on premolar teeth. (Zacrisson & Büyükyılmaz, 2005) While ultraviolet light was used for polymerization in the first years of use, polymerization now takes place with visible light sources. Today, orthodontists perform direct bonding procedures by using halogen, plasma arc and light-emitting diode (LED) sources.

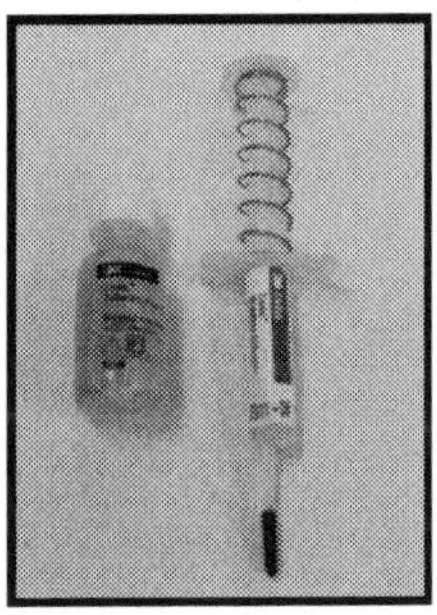

Fig. 17. No-mix composite system

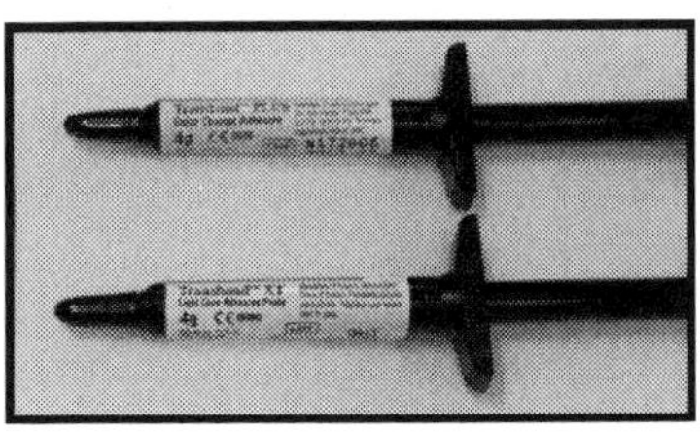

Fig. 18. Light curing composites

6. Light-curing devices and orthodontic adhesive applications

6.1 Quartz-tungsten halogen

Quartz-tungsten halogen light (QTH) is produced by an electric current passing through a tungsten filament, and this process takes place at very high heat levels. Halogen lights should be filtered to infiltrate unwanted waves and keep the 400-500 nm light (blue light). Thus, only a small amount of energy from this source is used for polymerization and a large amount of energy is converted into heat. In QTH light sources, 70% of the energy is converted into heat. Only 10% is visible light. In fact, 90% of visible light is lost due to the use of filters. Because of this result, blue light output is only 1% of the total energy input. More heat may shorten the life of light filters, bulbs and halogen light devices over time. The operating life of halogen bulbs is around 100 hours, on average. (Mills & Jandt, 1999; Jandt & Mills, 2000) In the polymerization process, a 20 second irradiation time for composite resin and 40 second irradiation time for light-cured resin modified glass ionomer cement (RM-GIC) with a halogen light source are proposed for every bracket. (Zacrisson & Büyükyılmaz, 2005; Sfondrini & Cacciafesta, 2001) Light intensity of 500 mW/cm^2 from a halogen light source was increased up to 900mW/cm^2 to reduce working time by "turbo tips". Approximately 50% of the polymerization time is saved with these fast halogen devices. Plasma arc carbon (PAC) lamps have a tungsten anode and cathode in a quartz tube filled with xenon gas. The gas becomes ionized and forms a plasma that consists of negatively and positively charged particles and generates an intense white light when an electrical current is passed through the xenon. Plasma arc lights are contained in base units rather than in "guns" because of the high voltage used and heat generated. (Zacrisson & Büyükyılmaz, 2005; Büyükyılmaz & Üşümez, 2003)

6.2 Plasma arc light sources

Plasma arc light sources do not emit distinct frequencies but instead give continuous-frequency bands that are much narrower than those of conventional lights. Consequently, less radiation needs to be filtered to remove undesired frequencies. Plasma arc lights provide light intensity of 1500 mW/cm^2 and a wavelength range of 380-490 nm. Due to the intensity of the light source, manufacturers reported that a 1-3 seconds irradiation time would be sufficient for polymerization of composite restorations in restorative dentistry. In direct bonding, it is reported that a polymerization period of 3-5 sec for metal bracket and less time for ceramic brackets is sufficient. Similar results were obtained with 20 seconds polymerization using a halogen light source. (Hotz & McLean, 1977) However, prior to polymerization, the harmony between the adhesive material and light source should be evaluated. Hotz & McLean, 1977, Üşümez & Büyükyılmaz,2008) A common problem related to the use of plasma arcs is the high pulpal temperature increase generated during polymerization. When the temperature in the pulp reaches 42.5 ° C, irreversible hyperemic pulp tissue reactions begin. While the heat increase in a halogen light source is 1.8 ° C, the heat increase in the plasma arc light source can reach almost 3 times that level. (Özturk & Üşümez, 2004)

6.3 Light-emitting diode light source

Today, another widely used light source is a light-emitting diode (LED). Mills et al. (Mills & Jandt, 1999) proposed solid-state LED devices for dental adhesive polymerization to eliminate some of the disadvantages of conventional halogen systems. There are two separate semi-conductors that transfer electrons from one another. When electricity is given by combination of these two separate semi-conductors, light with a specific wavelength (430-490 nm) is emitted from an LED lamp. The most important distinctive feature is the production of blue light. Approximately 95% of the produced light has the necessary qualification for polymerization. This situation gives the opportunity to work with less electricity and have up to 10,000 hours of bulb life. (Zacrisson &Büyükyılmaz, 2005) LEDs are resistant to shock and vibration during the production of blue light because of the absence of any filtration process. Very high rates of light-cured composite resins contain camphorquinone as photo-initiator in their composition. Camphorquinone is a material which is activated with visible blue light at a wavelength of 400-500 nm (peak level 468 nm). The main feature of the LED light sources is the production of visible blue light in this wavelength. Active spectra are reported to be 430-490 nm. However, LED light sources are effective on camphorquinone-containing dental materials. Therefore, the structures of materials used for polymerization should be well-known.

Light sources can be deleterious for orthodontists during long-term use because light sources can produce a wide range of light, ranging between ultraviolet and infrared ray beams. Light production in available wavelengths can cause irreversible changes in the retinal region depending on the wavelength of light used over time. As a result of this interaction in the retinal region, photochemical processes may cause a loss of vision, also known as a cataract, which is characterized by a loss of elasticity and quality of the lens in the long term. (Üşümez &Erverdi, 2010) In addition, loss of the receptor that provides nutrition for the cells in the retinal region may lead to retinal degeneration due to nutritional disorders. Clinicians should use protective eye glasses that have filtration effects of wavelengths of light to minimize these negative effects.

7. Bonding procedure

Bonding procedures in orthodontics are divided into direct and indirect bonding procedures. Direct bonding procedures involve bonding brackets onto the teeth in the dental arch during the same session; in the indirect technique, first implemented by Silverman and Cohen in 1972 (Silverman & Cohen, 1972), brackets are bonded following certain laboratory procedures.

7.1 Direct bonding procedure

There are some procedures to be followed for success of direct bonding technique. Bonding procedures begin following isolation and etching of the tooth surfaces (normal tooth surfaces or restored tooth surfaces). First, the mesiodistal and occlusogingival positions of teeth to be bonded should be determined separately for each tooth with the help of the guide. Thus, possible repositioning of brackets depending on the position differences will be eliminated. Second, the bracket is gripped with reverse action tweezers and the adhesive is applied to the bracket base. (Fig 19) It is important that the adhesive be evenly distributed on the bracket base without any gaps in the adhesive. (Fig20) The presence of a gap may act as a weak point and lead to premature failure. After the adhesive is added, the bracket is then placed on the tooth immediately.

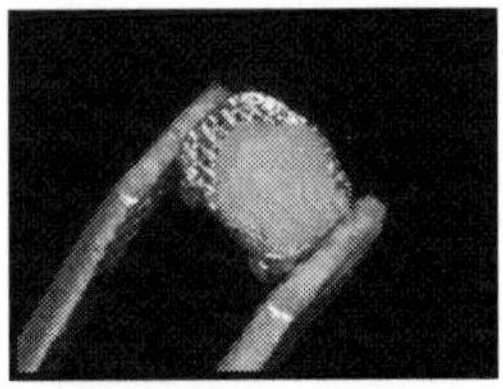

Fig. 19. Application of composite to the bracket base

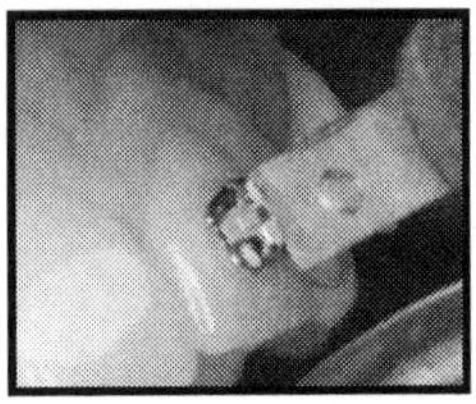

Fig. 20. Force application the the bracket in order not to leave any empty spaces.

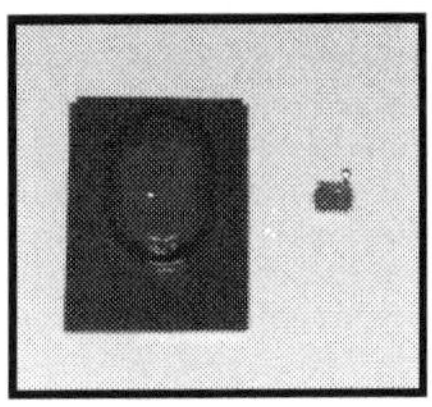

Fig. 21. APC system that is marketed for orthodontists

A scaler or round probe is used to position brackets on tooth surfaces in occlusogingival and mesiodistal directions. Positioning errors should be eliminated by making use of intraoral mirrors and retractors due to the difficulty in imaging of posterior region. Proper positioning of the bracket on the enamel should be provided during bracketing, and excess adhesive resin overflowing around the bracket must be cleaned before polymerization by a probe or scaler. Polymerization is completed by an equal amount of irradiation from all surfaces, followed by the removal of excess adhesive resin. This excess adhesive resin can allow for bacterial colonization. Today, pre-colored adhesive material (Transbond XT, 3M Unitek)(Fig. 18) or bracket systems including colored adhesives placed on the bracket base (APC Plus, 3 M Unitek) are used for the comfort of clinicians. (Fig 21) Unwanted movements occur due to improper fitting, and rotation movement is generally observed as a result. Therefore, each bracket should be checked carefully, and brackets in non-appropriate positions should be removed and rebonded immediately. If this procedure is not performed immediately, position errors will occur in other sessions and treatment times will be longer.

6.2 Indirect bonding procedure

Silverman and Cohen (Silverman & Cohen1972; Silverman & Cohen, 1976) became pioneers of the indirect bonding technique. Today, this technique is preferred due to advantages that

include reduced chair time, higher comfort of patients during bonding procedures, elimination of equipment such as separators or bands, good vertical control of teeth, successful implementation of the bracket positions, good supply of proper oral hygiene, good adaptation of lingual brackets, and minimization of the need for staff. (Thomas, 1979; Klange, 2004; Klange, 2007) However, time lost during removal of excess adhesive on bracket bases due to lack of clinician experience, unwanted formation of lesions in interproximal areas (e.g., caries, decalcification, gingival irritation) and predisposition to poor oral hygiene are among the disadvantages. (Zacrisson & Büyükyılmaz, 2005)
Indirect bonding systems are used with carrier systems such as the full-arch, sectioned full arch, single tooth and double tray systems. The working procedure of this technique includes the transfer of brackets, which are exactly positioned in cast models with a temporary resin or sealant to a silicone carrier and removal of the resin located in silicone with the sandblast method. This is followed by a thorough cleaning of the base of the bracket with a solvent. Then, intra-oral adaptation via thermal, chemical or a light-curing adhesion occurs following the implementation of A and B resins to the tooth and bracket surfaces. Finally, the resins are removed following the 2 min suppression period.

7. Debonding applications

The debonding process is of great importance in orthodontics. Debonding procedures may lead to serious fractures due to the differences in bond strength between the enamel and the metal and ceramic bracket structures. Spending sufficient time for the debonding procedures and independent implementation of debonding procedures on each tooth (without the arch wire) are among the simple measures taken to minimize failure.

7.1 The removal of steel brackets

To prevent damage to the enamel during removal of stainless steel brackets, failure at the bracket-adhesive interface is preferred. Zachrisson and Büyükyılmaz (Zachrisson & Büyükyılmaz, 2005) recommended using peeling type forces, which allow for a recycling process without deformation of bracket during the removal. In this technique, the debonding procedure is easily performed by eliminating the peripheral stresses with low force (Øilo, 1993) In this manner, failure will occur between the bracket and adhesive and the remaining adhesive on the enamel surface. Additionally, this method will prevent the formation of cracks and fractures. (Zacrisson & Büyükyılmaz, 2005)

7.2 Ceramic bracket removal

Debonding procedures is easily and reliably performed in metal brackets with peripheral forces. However, substnatial damage is observed to both enamel surfaces and brackets when debonding of ceramic brackets is performed by adding peripheral forces because ceramic brackets adhere strongly to enamel surfaces and do not show flexibility during implementation of the debonding pliers. (Redd & Shivapuja, 1991; Artun, 1997) Ceramic brackets behave differently during the debonding procedure depending on the differences in bracket structure and bonding mechanisms. For instance, fewer problems occur in ceramic brackets with mechanical retention than those with chemical retention. (Redd & Shivapuja, 1991, Viazis & Cavanaugh, 1990; Winchester, 1991) Squeezing brackets with twin-beaked pliers oriented mesiodistally is not recommended because it may cause horizontal enamel cracks. However, possible fractures may be minimized by the development of bracket designs. For example, a vertical debonding slot was added to minimize fracture during debonding (Clarity bracket, 3M Unitek), and fracture risks were significantly eliminated in porcelain brackets designed with a ball-band reduction (Inspri Ice Bracket, Ormco Corp., Calif.) (Chen & Su, 2007; Bishara & Olsen, 1997) Grinding ceramic brackets with low speed and no water coolant may cause irreversible damage or dental pulp necrosis. Therefore, water cooling is necessary. Finally, thermal debonding (Stratmann & Schaarschmidt, 1996; Bishara & Fehr, 1997; Crooks & Hood, 1997; Rueggeberg & Lockwood, 1990) and the use of lasers(Ma & Marangoni, 1997; Rickabaugh & Marangoni, 1996; Tocchio & Williams, 1993) have the potential to be less traumatic, less risky for enamel damage and more easily applicable due to the its effect on water in composite. However, these techniques are still at an introductory stage.

7.3 Removal of residual adhesive

Bond strength of resin materials on enamel increased considerably due to technological advances. Therefore, complete removal of adhesive resin from enamel is sometimes not achieved during clinical use, and colored and plaque retention sites are observed over time. (Brobakken & Zachrisson, 1981; Hong & Lew, 1995)

In addition to low-speed applications with tungsten carbide burs, which are commonly used and diamond burs (Zachrisson & Årtun, 1979; Krell & Courey, 1993; Oliver & Griffiths, 1992) and laser devices (Thomas & Hook, 1996; Alexsander & Xie, 2002) can be utilized depending on the demands of clinicians and patients. About 30,000 rpm is reported to be the optimal speed for rapid adhesive removal without enamel damage. (Zachrisson & Årtun, 1979) The bur is moved in one direction as the resin layers are removed. (Cambell, 1995)Water cooling should not be used during the removal of last remnants because water lessens the contrast with enamel. Fine fluted tungsten carbide burs with speeds higher than 30,000 rpm may be useful for bulk removal but are not indicated closer to the enamel. (Zacrisson & Büyükyılmaz, 2005) Slower speeds (10,000 rpm and less) are ineffective, and the jiggling vibration of the bur may disturb the patient. (Hong & Lew, 1995) Following the removal of all adhesive, the enamel surface must be cleaned with soft discs and cups and polished with pumice (Campbell, 1995) (or a commercial prophylaxis paste).

Clinicians and staff are exposed to aerosol particles via inhalation during all of these applications. In addition to calcium, phosphor, silica, aluminum and iron particles (Price & Sandy, 2008), hepatitis B virus (HBV) has been observed to be transmitted depending on blood contamination. (Toroğlu & Bayramoğlu, 2003) In studies on the use of chlorhexidine gluconate during the debonding procedure, no positive impacts on infectious agents were detected. (Toroğlu & Bayramoğlu, 2003) In use of masks that do not have appropriate filtration mechanisms, terminal lung diseases were observed over time. (Toroğlu & Haytaç, 2001) However, aerosol contamination can be prevented when using masks with appropriate filtration mechanisms.

8. Problem encountered after orthodontic treatment

The formation of white spot lesions.(WSL) is a frustrating occurrence after orthodontic treatment. WSLs frequently occur due to lack of effective tooth brushing and cleaning during treatment. To eliminate this problem, the clinicians should provide hygiene control during treatment sessions. A high incidence at the 5-year follow-up of patients receiving orthodontic treatment was determined.(Ǿgaard, 1989) Much evidence exists from in vivo and in vitro studies to support the claim that small carious lesions can heal, a process usually referred as remineralization.(Siverstone, 1982; Artun& Thylstrup, 1986; Øgaard & Rolla, 1988) To prevent WSL formation, topical fluoride containing mouth rinse and tooth pastes are recommended for patients and orthodontists may take precaution such as the use of fluoride-releasing adhesive materials and elastics. Daily routine use of casein phosphopeptide-amorphous calcium phosphate (CPP-ACP) containing tooth pastes (Wiltshire, 1999; Fraizer & Southard, 1996; Lefeuvre & Amjaad, 2005; Uysal & Baysal, 2011) or fluoride containing mouth rinses (Gorelick & Geiger, 1982; Jordan, 1998) have been reported to significantly inhibit the formation of WSLs. However during all of these applications, the effective use has vital importance.

Microorganisms such as Streptococcus Mutans (SM) in microflora, which penetrate the flat surfaces better and effective in WSL formation leads to an acidic environment due to the digestion of nutrients and increase in the number of microorganisms. This situation increases the formation of decalcification by causing the dissolution of componenets on enamel. (Alves& Alviano, 2008; Başaran& Hamamcı, 2007, Başaran & Başaran, 2006) However the use of chlorhexidine gluconate containing mouth washes significantly impedes the formation of WSL. The use of fluoride releasing eleastic ligatures is one of the methods for the prevention of microorganism reproduction in retention areas around the brackets.(Cacascia & Gomes, 2007) However, the formation of effective sites for microorganism reproduction due to water absorbtion over time is a disadvantage of fluoride releasing eleastic ligatures.(Li & Hobson, 2007, Başaran & Hamamcı, 2007) If the use of glass-ionomer cement is planned for the bonding of brackets or bands in the posterior region, the use of high fluoride releasing adhesives such as Fuji Orto LC (GC International Corp., Itabashiku,Tokyo, Japan) will affect the incidence of WSL formation.(Marcusson & Norevall, 1997; Pascotto & Novarro, 2004) Another effective method for the prevention of SM is the use of Cervitec vanish. This application leads to a significant decrease in the number of SM between treatment sessions while the bond strength is not negatively effected. (Ǿgaard & Rolla, 1993; Eronat & Alpöz, 1994)

With technological advances such as the use of prebiotic bacteria, efficiency of harmful bacteria is reduced and and effective protection can be achieved (Çağlar & Sandallı, 2005; Meurman & Antila, 1995)

In patients with WSLs, effective fluoride applications in early period have been reported to inhibit the superficial appearence of demineralized areas. (Årtun & Thylstrup, 1986)

Another method for WSL treatment is a microabrasion method proposed by Gelgör and Büyükyılmaz. (Gelgör & Büyükyılmaz, 2003) In this method a custom-made abrasive gel is prepared with 18% hydrochloric acid, fine powdered pumice, and glycerin. The active mixture is applied using an electric toothbrush for 3 to 5 minutes following the isolation of gingiva by block-out resin or rubber dam. (Zacrisson & Büyükyılmaz, 2005) For best results, and depending on the severity of lesions, the repetition of the procedure monthly for 2 to 3 times is suggested and in 3-month follow-up period, WSL disappears gradually.

A new method recently came into use in the treatment of WSL is a technique called the micro-invasive infiltration technolgy (Icon-Etch-DMG, Chemische-Pharma. Fabrik GmbH, Hamburg) (www.drilling-no-thanks.com) The aim of this technique is to delay the drilling or filling in cases which does not require cavitation according to Gorelick's classification (Stage 2 or 3) but may need drilling due to improper oral hygiene and to preserve the available structure without no harm to the patient. The patients are controlled annually.

9. Conclusion

Todays orthodontists have a vast variety of adhesive and bonding materials. However, contemporary techniques that produce materials with nanotechnology lead to revolutionary developments in orthodontics as in other sciences and as a result of this, more effective materials could be produced. In the future, studies that would be in the area of biocompatible materials with genes would be interest of researchers.

10. Acknowledgement

Authors thank to Dr Celal GENÇ for the photos and illustrations shown in this chapter.

11. References

Abdullah, MSB.& Rock, WP. (1996) The effect of etch time and debond interval upon the shear bond strength of metallic orthodontic brackets *British Journal of Orthodontics Vol:*23 pp.121-124

Aida, M.;, Hayakawa, T. &, Mizukawa, K. (1995) Adhesion of composite to porcelain with various surface conditions *Journal of Prosthetic Dentistry Vol:*73 pp.464 - 470

Al Edris, A.; al Jabr, A.; Cooley, RL & et al. (1990) SEM evaluation of etch pattern by three etchants on three porcelains *Journal of Prosthetic Dentistry Vol:*64 pp.734

Alexsander, R.; Xie, J. & Fried, D. (2002) Selective removal of residual composite from dental enamel surface using the third harmonic of a Q-switched Nd:YAG laser *Laser Surgery Medicine Vol:*30 pp.240-245

Alves, PV.; Alviano, WS.; Bolognese, AM. & Nojima, LI. (2008) Treatment protocol to control Streptecocus Mutans level in an orthodontic patient with high caries risk *American Journal of Orthodontics and Dentofacial Orthopedics Vol:133 pp. 91-94*

Akkurt A. (2008) In vitro evaluation of shear bond strength of bonded premolar brackets with using erbium laser, self etching primer and ortofosforic acid etching systems vie SEM. Doctoral Thesis, Diyarbakır

Amra, I.; Samsodien, G.; Shaikh, A. & Lalloo, R. (2007) Xeno III self-etching adhesive in orthodontic bonding: the next generation. *American Journal of Orthodontics and Dentofacial Orthopedics Vol:*131 pp. 160–165

Aoki, A.; Sasaki, KM.; Watanabe, H. & et al. (2000) Lasers in nonsurgical periodontal therapy. Periodontology *Vol:*36 pp.59-97

Årtun, J. & Berglandi S. (1984) Clinical trials with crystal growth conditioning as an alternative to acid-etch pretreatment *American Journal of Orthodontics Vol:*85 pp.333

Artun, J. (1997) A post-treatment evaluation of multobonded ceramic brackets in orthodontics *European Journal of Orthoodntics Vol:*19 pp.219-228

Årtun, J. & Thylstrup, A. (1986) Clinical and scanning electron microscopic study of surface changes of incipient caries lesions after debonding *Scandinavia Journal of Dental Research* Vol: 94 pp.193

Andreasen, G F. & Stieg, M A. (1998) Bonding and debonding brackets to porcelain and gold *American Journal of Orthodontics and Dentofacia Orthopedics Vol:*93 pp.341 - 345

Angle AH. (1907) *The Malocclusion of the Teeth*, SS White Dental Manufacturing Philadelphia, 1907

Barbosa, V L.; Almedia, M A,; Chevitarese, O. &, Keith, O. (1995) Direct bonding to porcelain . *American Journal of Orthodontics and Dentofacial Orthopedics Vol:*107 pp.159–164

Barkmeier, WW.; Gwinnett, AJ. & Shaffer, SE. (1987) Effect of reduced acid concentration and etching time on bond strength and enamel morphology. *Journal of Clinical Orthodontics Vol:*21 pp.395- 398

Baş-Kalkan, A.; Orhan, M. & Üşümez, S. (2007) The effect of enamel etching with different acids on the bond strength of metallic brackets. *Turkish Journal of Orthodontics Vol:*20 pp.35-42

Başaran, G.; Hamamcı, N. & Akkurt, A.(2011) Shear bond strength of bonding to enamel with different laser irradiation distances. *Lasers in Medical Science Vol:*26 pp.149-156

Başaran, G. & Hamamcı O. (2007) Evaluation of the effect of different ligature system on microbial attack *Balkan Journal of Stamatology* Vol: 11 pp. 201-203

Başaran, G.; Başaran E. & Hamamcı, O. (2006) effects of orthodontic adhesive materials on S. Mutans and Lactobacilli levels in human saliva Biotechnolog & Biotechnological Equipment Vol: 20 pp. 156-159.

Berk, N.; Basaran, G. & Özer, T. (2008) Comparison of sandblasting, laser irradiation, and conventional acid etching for orthodontic bonding of molar tubes *European Journal of Orthoodntics Vol:*30 pp.183-189

Bhad, WA. & Hazarey, PV. (1995) Scanning electron microscopic study and shear bond strength measurement with 5% and 37% phosphoric acid. *American Journal of Orthodontics Dentofacial Orthopedics Vol:*108 pp.410-414

Bishara, S E.; Adam, W.; Otsby, AW.; Ajlouni, R.; Laffoon, JF. & Warren, JJ. (2008) A new premixed self-etch adhesive for bonding orthodontic brackets *Angle Orthodontist Vol:*78 pp.1101–1104

Bishara, SE.; Olsen, ME. & VonWald, L. (1997) Evaluation of debonding characteristics of a new collapsible ceramic brackets *American Journal of Orthodontics Vol:*112 pp.552

Bishara, SE. & Fehr, DE. (1997) Ceramic brackets: something old, something new—a review *Seminers in Orthodontist Vol:*3 pp.17

Black, RB. (1950) Airbrasive some fundementals *Journal of american Dental Associatation Vol:*11 pp.701-710

Black RB. (1955) Application and evaluation of air abrasive technique. *Journal of American Dental Associatation Vol:*50 pp.408-414

Brandt, S.; Servoss, JM. & Persily, KB. (1981) Atropine sulphate: an effective antisialogogue *Journal of Clinical Orthodontics Vol:*15 pp.629

Brännström, M.; Malmgren, O. & Nordenvall, KJ. (1982) Etching of young permanent teeth with an acid gel, *American Journal of Orthodontics Vol:*82 pp.379

Brännström, M.; Nordenvall, KJ. & Malmgren, O. (1978) The effect of various pretreatment methods of the enamel in bonding procedures, *American Journal of Orthodontics Vol:*74 pp.134

Bourke, BM. & Rock, WP. (1999) Factors affecting the shear bond strength of metal orthodontic brackets to porcelain *British Journal of Orthodontics Vol:*26 pp.285–290

Bowen, RL. & Rodriguez, MS. (1962) Tensile strength and modulus of elasticity of tooth structure and several restorative materials *Journal of the American Dental Association Vol:*64 pp.378–387

Brobakken, BO. & Zachrisson, BU. (1981) Abrasive wear of bonding adhesives: studies during treatment and after bracket removal, *American Journal of Orthodontics Vol:*79 pp.134

Buonocore, MG.; Matsui, A. & Gwinnett, AJ. (1968) Penetration of resin dental materials into enamel surfaces with reference to bonding *Archive of Oral Biology Vol:*13 pp.61–70

Buonocore, MG. (1955) A simple method of increasing the adhesion of acrylic filling material to enamel surfaces *Journal of Dental Research Vol:*34 pp. 849–853

Burgess, AM.; Sherriff, M. & Ireland, AJ. (2006) Self etching primers: is prophylactic pumicing necessery? A randomized clinical trial *Angle Orthodontist Vol:*29 pp.114-118

Buzitta, VAJ.; Hallgren, SE. & Powers, JM. (1982) Bond strength of orthodontic direct-bonding cement-bracket systems as studied in vitro *American Journal of Orthodontics Vol:*81 pp.87

Büyükyilmaz, T.; Øgaard, B. & Dahm, S. (1995) The effect on the tensile bond strength of orthodontic brackets of titanium tetrafluoride (TiF4) application after acid etching, *American Journal of Orthodontics Vol:*108 pp.256

Cambell, PM. (1995) Enamel surfaces after orthodontic bracket debonding *Angle Orthodontist Vol:*65 pp.103-110

Carter, RN. (1981) Salivary control *Journal of Clinical Orthodontics Vol:*15 pp.562

Carstensen, W. (1995) Effect of reduction of phosphoric acid concentration on the shear bond strength of brackets. *American Journal of Orthodontics and Dentofacial Orthopedics Vol:*108 pp.274-277

Chen, HY.; Su, MZ.; Chang, HF.; Chen, YJ.; Lan, WH. & Lin, CP. (2007) Effects of different debonding techniques on the debonding forces and failure modes of ceramic brackets in simulated clinical set ups *American Journal of Orthodontics Dentafacial orthopedics Vol:*132 pp.680-686

Chigira, H.; Koike, T.; Hasegawa, T.; Itoh, K.; Wakumoto, S. & Hayakawa, T. (1989) Effect of the self etching dentin primers on the bonding efficacy of dentin adhesive *Dental materials Vol:*8 pp.86-92

Chow, LC. & Brown, WE. (1973) Phosphoric acid condition of teeth for pit and fissure sealeants *Journal of Dental Research Vol:*52 pp.1158

Cinader, D. (2001) Chemical processes and performance comparisons of Transbond Plus self etching primer, Orthodontic Perspective *Vol:*8 pp.5-6

Cochran, D.;, O'Keefe, KL.;, Turner, DT. &, Powers, JM. (1997) Bond strength of orthodontic composite cement to treated porcelain . *American Journal of Orthodontics and Dentofacial Orthopedics Vol:*111 pp.297 - 300

Coluzzi, DL. & Convissar, RA. (2007) *Atlas of laser applications in dentistry*, Quintessentence, Hanover Park III

Crooks, M.; Hood, J. & Harkness, M. (1997) Thermal debonding of ceramic brackets: an in vitro study, *American Journal of Orthodontics Vol:*111 pp.163

Çağlar, E. & Sandallı N. (2005) Probiotics and their effect on dental health *Turkish Journal of Orthodontics* Vol:18 pp. 287-292

D Price, R.; Sandy, JR. & Ireland, AJ. (2008) Inhalation aerosol produced during the removal of fixed orthodontic appliances: a comparasion of 4 enamel clean up methods *American Journal of Orthodontics Dentofacial Orthopedics Vol:*133 pp.11-17

Daniell, MD. & Hill, JS. (1991) A history of photodynamic therapy *The Australian and New Zelland Journal of Surgery Vol:*61 pp.340-348

Daronch, M.; DeGoes, MF.; Garrilho, MR.; Chan, DC.; Darochi, M.& Sinhoreti, MA. (2003) Antebacterial and conventional self etching primer sytem: morphological evaluation of intact primary enamel *Journal of Clinical Pediatric Dentistry Vol:*27 pp.251-256

Davis, NA, (2003, "Nanotechnology Composite", *Compendium Vol:* 24 pp.662-667

Diedrich, P. (1981) Enamel alterations from bracket bonding and debonding a study with the scanning electron microscope *American Journal of Orthodontics Vol:*79 pp.:500-522

Duke, ES. (2003) "Has Dentistry Moved into The Nanotechnology Era?" *Compendium Vol:*24 pp.380-382

Erhardt, MC.; Cavalcante, LM. & Pimenta, LA. (2004) Influence of phosphoric acid pretreatment on self-etching bond strengths *Journal of Esthetic and Restorative Dentistry Vol:*16 pp.33–40

Eronat, C. & Alpöz, AR. (1994) Effect of cervitec varnish on the salivary streptecocus mutans levels in patients with fixed orthodontic appliances *Journal of Dental Research* Vol:73 pp.425 (abstract)

Forsberg, CM.; Brattström, V.; Malmberg, E. & Nord, CE. (1991) Ligature wires and elastomeric rings: two methods of ligation and their association with microbial colonization of Streptococcus mutans and lactobacilli *European Journal of Orthodontics* Vol:13 pp.416

Fraizer, MC.; Southard, TC. & Doster, PM. (1996) Prevention of enamel demineralization during orthodontic treatment: an in vitro study using pit and fissure sealent. *American Journal of Orthodontics Dentafacial Orthopedics Vol:110 pp. 459-465*

Fredericks, HE. (1981) Mutagenic potential of orthodontic bonding materials *American Journal of Orthodontics Vol:* 80 pp.316

Galil, KA. & Wright, GZ. (1979) Acid etching patterns on buccal surfaces of permanenet teeth *Pediatric Dentistry Vol:*1 pp.230-234

Garcia-Godoy, F.; Hubbard, GW. & Storey, AT. Effect of a fluoridated etching gel on enamel morphology and shear bond strength of orthodontic brackets *American Journal of Orthodontics Vol:*100 pp.163

Gelgör, IE. & Buyukyilmaz, T. (2003) A practical approach to white spot lesion removal, World Journal of Orthodontics Vol: 4 pp.152-156

Gillis, I. & Redlich, M. (1998) The effect of different porcelain conditioning techniques on shear bond strength of stainless steel brackets . *American Journal of Orthodontics* and Dentofacial Orthopedics *Vol:*114 pp.387 - 392

Goldstein, RE. & Parkins, FM. (1994) Air-abrasive technology: its new role in restorative dentistry *Journal of american Dental Associatation Vol:*125 pp.551-557

Gottlieb, EL.; Nelson, AH. & Vogels, DS. (1996) Study of orthodontic diagnosis and treatment procedures. Part I. Results and Trend *Journal of Clinical Orthodontics Vol:*30 pp.615-630

Gorelick, L; Geiger, AM. &, Gwinnett, AJ. (1982) Incidence of white spot formation after bonding and banding, *American Journal of Orthodontics* Vol:81 pp.93

Gwinnett, AJ. & Buonocore, MG. (1965) Adhesion and caries prevention. A preliminary report. *British Dental Journal Vol:*119 pp.77–80

Gwinnett, AJ. & Matsui, AA. (1967) Study of enamel adhesives. The physical relationship between enamel and adhesive *Archive of Oral Biology Vol:*12 pp.1615–1620

Gwinnett, AJ. (1973) The bonding of sealants to enamel *The Journal of the American Society for Preventive Dentistry Vol:*3 pp.21

Hannig, M.; Bock, H.; Bott, B. & Hoth-Hannig, W. (2002) Inter-crystallite nanoretention of self-etching adhesives at enamel imaged by transmission electron microscopy *European Journal of Oral Science Vol:*110 pp.464–470

Harari, D.; Shapira-Davis, S.; Gillis, I.; Roman, I. & Redlich, M. (2003) Tensile bond strength of ceramic brackets bonded to porcelain facets. *American Journal of Orthodontics Dentofacial Orthopedics Vol:*123 pp.551- 554

Hayakawa, T.; Horie, K.; Aida, M.; Kanaya, H.; Kobayashi, T. & Murata, Y. (1992) The influence of surface conditions and silane agents on the bond of resin to dental porcelain *Dental Materials Vol:*8 pp.238 - 240

Hermsen, RJ. & Vrijhoef, MMA. (1993) Loos of enamel due to etching with phosphoric or maleic acid *Dental Materials Vol:*9 pp.332-336

Hogervorst, WW.; Feilzer, AJ. & Prahl-Andersen, B. (2000) The air abrasion technique versus the conventional acid-etching technique: a quantification of surface enamel loss and a comparision of shear bond strength. *American Journal of Orthodontics Dentafacial Orthopedics Vol:*117 pp.20-26

Hosein, I.; Sherriff, M. & Ireland, AJ. (2004) Enamel loss during bonding, debonding and cleanup with use of self etching primer *American Journal of Orthodontics Dentofacial Orthopedics Vol:*126 pp.17-724

Hobson, RS. & McCabe, JF. (2002) Relationship between enamel etch characteristic and resin-enamel bond strength *British Dental Journal Vol:*192 pp.163-68

Hong, YH. & Lew, KK. (1995) Quantative and qualative assesment of enamel surface fallowing five composite removal methods after bracket debonding *European Journal of Orthodontics Vol:*17 pp.121-128

Hotz, P.; McLean, JW.; Seed, I. & Wilson, AD. (1977) The bonding of glass ionomer cements to metal and tooth substrates *British Dental Journal Vol:*142 pp.41-47

Huang, TH. & Kao, CT. (2001) The shear bond strength of composite brackets on porcelain teeth *Eurpean Journal of Orthodontics Vol:*23 pp.433–439

http://www.drilling-no-thanks.com/us/landing.html

Ireland, AJ. & Sherriff, M. (2002) The effect of pumicing on the in vivo use of rezin modified glass poly(alkenoate) cement and a conventional no-mix composite for bonding orthodontic brackets *Journal of orthodontics Vol:*29 pp.217-220

Jandt, KD.; Mills, RW.; Blackwell, GB. & Ashworth, SH. (2000) Depth of cure and compressive strength of dental composites cured with blue light emitting diodes(LEDs) *Dental Materials Vol:*16 pp.41-47

Jordan C. (1998) prevention of white spot enamel formation during orthodontic treatment *General Dentistry* Vol:46 pp. 498-502

Jost-Brinkmann, PG.; Schiffer, A. & Miethke, RR. (1992) The effect of adhesive layer thickness on bond strength *Journal of Clinical Orthodontics Vol:* 26 pp.718-720

Jost-Brinkmann, PG. & Can S, Drost C. (1996) In-vitro study of the adhesive strengths of brackets on metals, ceramic and composite. 2. Bonding to porcelain and composite resin *Journal of Orafacial Orthopedics Vol:* 57 pp.132

Katzir, A. (1993) Lasers and optical fibers in medicine, Academic press, San Diego, ,

Kawasaki, M.; Hayakawa, T.; Takizawa, T.; Sirirungrojying, S.; Saitoh, K. & Kasai, K. (2003) Assessing the performance of a methyl methacrylatebased resin cement with self-etching primer for bonding orthodontic brackets *Angle Orthodontist Vol:*73 pp.702–709

Klange, JT. (2004) Indirect bonding: a comprehensive review of the advantages *World Journal of Orthodontist Vol:*4 pp.301-307

Klange, JT. (2007) Indirect bonding: a comprehensive review of the literature *Seminers in Orthodontist Vol:*13 pp.3-10

Klocke, A.; Shi, J.; Kahl-Nieke, B. & Bismayer, U. (2003) Bond strength with custom base indirect bonding technique *Angle Orthodontist Vol:*73 pp.176-180

Kocadereli, İ.; Canay, Ş. & Akça, K. (2001) Tensile bond strength of ceramic orthodontic brackets bonded to porcelain surfaces . *American Journal of Orthodontics and Dentofacial Orthopedics Vol:*119 pp.616 - 620

Krell, KV.; Courey, JM. & Bishara, SE. (1993) Orthodontic bracket removal using conventional and ultrasonic debonding technique: enamel loss and time requirements *American Journal of Orthodontics Dentofacial Orthopedics Vol:*103 pp.258-266

Lalani, N.; Foley, TF.; Voth, R.; Banting, D. & Mamandras, A. (2000) Polymerization with the argon laser: curing time and shear bond strength *Angle Orthodontist Vol:*70 pp.28–33

Lefeuvre, M.; Amjaad, W.; Goldberg, M. & Stanislawski, L. (2005) TEGDMA induces miticindrial denage and oxidative stress in human gingival fibroblasts *Biomaterials* Vol: 26 pp. 5130-5137.

Lew, KK.; Chew, CL. & Lee, KW. (1991) A comparison of shear bond strengths between new and recycled ceramic brackets *European Journal of Orthoodntics* Vol:13 pp.306

Li, S.; Hobson, RS.; Bai, Y.;Yan, Z.; Carrick, TM. & McCabe JF. (2007) Method for producing controlled fluoride release from an orthodontic bracket *European Journal of orthodontics* Vol:29 pp. 550-554

Lührs, AK.; Guhr, S.; Schilke, R.; Borchers, L.; Guertsen, W. & Günay, H. (2008) Shear bond strength of self-etch adhesives to enamel with additional phosphoric acid etching *Operative Dentistry* Vol:33 pp.155–162

Ma, T.; Marangoni, RD. & Flint, W. In vitro comparison of debonding force and intrapulpal temperature changes during ceramic orthodontic bracket removal using a carbon dioxide laser *American Journal of Orthodontics and Dentafacial Orthopedics Vol:*111 pp.203

Maijer, R. & Smith, DC. (1986) Crystal growth on the outer enamel surface an alternative to acid etching. *American Journal of Orthodontics Dentofacial Orthopedics* Vol:89 pp.183-193

Maiman, TH. (1966) A look at things to come: biomedical lasers evolve toward clinical application, hosp Manage Vol:101 pp.39-41

Major, PW.; Koehler, JR. & Maning. KE. (1995) 24-hour shear bond strength ofmetal orthodontic brackets bonded to porcelain using various adhesion promoters *American Journal of Orthodontics Dentofacial Orthopedics* Vol:108 pp.322–329

Manni, JG. (2004) Dental applications of advanced lasers. Burlington,

Marcusson, A.; Norevall, LI. & Person M. (1997) White spot reduction when using glass ionomer cement for bonding in orthodontics: a longitudinal and comperative study *Eurpean Journal of Orthodontics* Vol:19 pp. 133-242

Mattick, CR. & Hobson, RS. (2000) A comperative micro-topographic study of the buccal enamel of different tooth types *Journal of Orthodontist* Vol:27 pp.143-148

Meng, CL.; Wang, WN. & Yeh, IS. (1997) Fluoridated etching on orthodontic bonding, *American Journal of Orthodontics* Vol:112 pp.259

Meurman, JH.; Antila, H.; Korhanen, A. & Salminen, E. (1995) Effect of lactobacillus rhamnosus strain GG (ATCC 53103) on the growth of streptococcus sobrinus in vitro, *European Journal of Oral Science* Vol: 103 pp. 253-258

Mills, RW.; Jandt, KD. & Ashworth SH. (1999) Dental composite depth of cure with halogen and blue light emitting diode technology *British Dental Journal* Vol:186 pp.88-91

Miserendino, LJ.; Levy, G. & Miserendino, CA. (1995) In: *Laser interaction with biologic tissues*. Miserendino LJ, Pick RM, editors: Lasers in dentistry, Quintessence Chigaco

Miserendino, LJ.; Neiburger, EJ.; Waila, H.; Luebke, N. & Brantley, W. (1989) Thermal effects of continuous wave CO_2 laser exposure on human teeth: an in vitro study *Journal of Endodontics* Vol:15 pp.302-305

Miyazaki, M.; Hirohata, N.; Takagaki, K.; Onose, H. & Moore, BK. (1999) Influence of self-etching primer drying time on enamel bond strength of resin composites *Journal of Dentistry* Vol:27 pp.203–207

Nebbe, B. & Stein, E. (1996) Orthodontic brackets bonded to glazed and deglazed porcelain surfaces . *American Journal of Orthodontics and Dentofacial Orthopedics* Vol:109 pp.431–436

Newman, GV. (1978) A posttreatment survey of direct bonding of metal brackets *American Journal of Orthodontics* Vol:74 pp.197

Newman, GV. (1965) Epoxy adhesives for orthodontic attachments *American Journal of Orthodontics* Vol:51 pp. 901–912.

Ng'anga, P.; Øgaard, B.; Cruz, R.;, et al. (1992) Tensile bond strength of orthodontic brackets bonded directly to fluorotic and non-fluorotic teeth. *American Journal of Orthodontics and Dentofacial Orthopedics* Vol:102 pp.244-250

Niemz, MH. (2007) *Laser tissue interaction: fundementals and applications*, Springer ed 3, Berlin

Nishida, K.; Yamauchi, J.; Wada, T. & Hosoda, H. (1993) Development of a new bonding system *Journal of Dental Research Vol:*:72 pp.137(abstract)

Nordenvall, KJ.; Brännström, M. & Malmgren, O. (1980) Etching of deciduous teeth and young and old permanent teeth: a comparison between 15 and 60 seconds of etching, *American Journal of Orthodontics* vol:78 pp.99

Olsen, ME.; Bishara, SE.; Boyer, DB. & Jakobsen, JR. Effect of varying etching times on the bond strength of ceramic brackets. *American Journal of Orthodontics Dentofacial Orthopedics* 1996;109:403-9.

Olsen, ME.; Bishara. SE.; Damon, P. & Jakobsen, JR. (1997) Evaluation of scotchbond multipurpose and maleic acid as alternative methods of bonding orthodontic brackets *American Journal of Orthodontics Dentofacial Orthopedics* Vol:111 pp.498-501

Özcan, M.; Vallittu, PK.; Peltomaki, T.; Huysmans, M. & Kalk, W. (2004) Bonding polycarbonate brackets to ceramic: effects of substrate treatment on bond strength. *American Journal of Orthodontics Dentofacial Orthopedics* Vol:126 pp.220–227

Oduncu. BS. (2009) Investigation Of Polymerization Shrinkage Of Dental Composites Prepared With Different Fillers During Photopolymerization Biongineering, M.S. Thesis, Istanbul

Oliver, RG. & Griffiths, J. (1992) Different technique of residual composite removal following debonding: time taken and surface enamel appreance *British Journal of Orthodontist* Vol:19 pp.131-137

Özer, T.; Başaran, G. & Berk, N. (2008) Laser etching of enamel for orthodontic bonding *American Journal of Orthodontics and Dentofacial Orthopedics* Vol:134 pp.193-197

Özer, M. & Arıcı, S. (2005) Sandblasted metal brackets bonded with rezin modified glass ionomer cement in vivo *Angle Orthodontist* Vol:75 pp.406-409

Özturk, B.; Üşümez, A. & Üşümez, S. (2004) Temperature rise during adhesiveand rezin composite polymerization with various light curing sources *Operative Dentistry* Vol:29 pp.325-332

Pascotto, RC.; Navorro, MF.; Capelozza. FL. & Cury, JA. (2004) In vivo effect of rezin modified glass ionomer cement on enamel demineralization around orthodontic brackets *American Journal of Orthodontics Dentofacial Orthopedics* Vol:125 pp.36-41

Pashley, DH. & Tay, FR. (2001) Aggressiveness of contemporary self-etching adhesives. Part II: etching effects on unground enamel *Dental Materials* Vol:17 pp.430–444

Ponduri, S.; Turnbull, N.; Birnie, D.; et al. (2007) Does atropine sulphate improve orthodontic bond survival? A randomized clinical trial. *American Journal of Orthodontics Dentofacial Orthopedics* Vol:132 pp.663-670

Powers, JM.; Kim, HB. & Turner, DS. (1997) Orthodontic adhesives and bond strength *Seminers in Orthodontist* Vol:3: pp.47-156

Powel, GL.; Morton, TH. & Larsen, AE. (1989) Pulpal response to irridation of enamel with continuous wave CO2 laser *Journal of Endodontics* Vol:15 pp.581-583

Pus, MD. & Way, DC. (1980) Enamel loss due to orthodontic bonding with filled and unfilled resins using various clean-up techniques. *American Journal of Orthodontics* Vol:79 pp.269-283

Rechmann, P.& Henning, T. (2001) Lasers in periodontology today and tomorrow *Medical Laser Application* Vol:15 pp. 223-230

Redd, TB. & Shivapuja, PK. (1991) Debonding ceramic brackets: effects on enamel *Journal of Clinical Orthodontics Vol:*25 pp.475-481

Reisner, KR.; Levitt, HL. & Mante, F. (1997) Enamel preparation for orthodontic bonding: a comparison between the use of a sandblaster and current techniques *American Journal of Orthodontics* Vol:111 pp.366

Casaccia, RG.; Gomes, JC.; Alviano, D.; Ruellas OC. & Sant'Anna EF. (2007) Microbial evaluation of elastomeric chains. *The Angle Orthodontist* Vol: 77 pp. 890-893

Retief, DH.; Retief, CJ.; Dreyer. & Gavron G. (1970) The direct bonding of orthodontic attachments to teeth by means of an epoxy resin adhesive *American Journal of Orthodontics* Vol:58 pp. 21–40

Rickabaugh, JL. Marangoni, RD. & McCaffrey, KK. (1996) Ceramic bracket debonding with the carbon dioxide laser *American Journal of Orthodontics* Vol:110 pp.388

Rossouw, PE. (2010) A Historical Overview of the Development of the Acid-Etch Bonding System in Orthodontics *Seminers in Orthodontist* Vol:16 pp.2-23

Rueggeberg ,FA. & Lockwood, P. (1990) Thermal debracketing of orthodontic resins, *American Journal of Orthodontics* Vol:98 pp.56

Sadowsky, PL.; Retief, DH.; Cox, PR.; Hernandez, R.; Rape, WG. & Bradley EL. (1990) Effects of etchant concentration and duration on the retention of orthodontic brackets: an in vivo study. *American Journal of Orthodontics Dentofacial Orthopedics* Vol:98 pp.417-421

Sayınsu, K.; Işık, F.; Sezen, S. & Aydemir, B. (2007) The effect of blood and saliva contamination on bond strength of brackets bonded with a protective liquid polish and a light-cured adhesive. *American Journal of Orthodontics Dentofacial Orthopedics* Vol:131 pp.391-394

Schaneveldt, S. & Foley, TF. (2002) Bond strength comparison of moisture-insensitive primers. *American Journal of Orthodontics and Dentofacial Orthopedics* Vol:122 pp.267-273

Schmage, P.; Nergiz, I.; Herrman, W. & Özcan, M. (2003) Influence of various surface-conditioning methods on the bond strength of metal brackets to ceramic surfaces. *American Journal of Orthodontics Dentofacial Orthopedics* Vol:123 pp.540-546

Sheen, DH.; Wang, WN. & Tarng, TH. (1993) Bond strength of younger and older permanent teeth with various etching times *Angle Orthodontist* Vol:63 pp.225-230

Silverman, E. Cohen, M.; Gianelly, AA. & Dietz, VS. (1972) A univesal direct bonding system for both metal and plastic brackets. *American Journal of Orthodontics* Vol:62 pp.236

Silverman, E. & Cohen, ML. The twenty minute full strap up *Journal of Clinical Orthodontics* vol:10 pp.764

Silverstone, LM.; Saxton, CA.; Dogon, IL. 81975) Variation in the pattern of acid etching of human dental enamel examinated by scanning electron microscopy *Caries Research* 1Vol:9 pp.373-87

Silverstone, LM. (1977) Remineralization phenomena *Caries Research* Vol:11 pp.59

Silverstone, LM. (1982) The effect of fluoride in the remineralization of enamel caries and caries-like lesions in vitro *Journal of Public Health Dentistry* Vol: 42 pp.42

Sfondrini, MF.; Cacciafesta, V.; Pistorio, A.;et al. (2001) Effects of conventional and high-intensity light curing on enamel shear bond strength of composite resin and resin modified glass ionomer *American Journal of Orthodontics Dentofacial Orthopedics Vol:*119 pp.30-35

Smith, DC. & Cartz, L. (1973) Crystalline interface formed by polyacrilic acid tooth enamel *Journal of Dental Research* Vol:52 pp.1155

Simonsen, RJ. & Calamia, JP. (1983) Tensile bond strength of etched porcelain *Journal of Dental Research* Vol:61 pp.279

Stratmann, U.; Schaarschmidt, K.; Wegener, H.; et al. (1996) The extent of enamel surface fractures: a quantitative comparison of thermally debonded ceramic and mechanically debonded metal brackets by energy dispersive micro- and image-analysis *European Journal of Orthoodntics Vol: 18* pp.655

Swartz, ML. (1994) Why prophy prior to bracket bonding? *Clinical Impressions* Vol:3 pp.11

Swartz, ML. (2004) Orthodontic bonding Orthodontist Select Vol:16 pp.1-4

Thompson, IR.; Miller, EG. & Bowles, WH. (1982) Leaching of unpolymerized materials from orthodontic bonding resin *Journal of Dental Research Vol:61 pp.989*

Thomas, RG. (1979) Indirect bonding: simplicity in action *Journal of Clinical Orthodontics Vol:*13 pp.93-104

Thomas, BV.; Hook, CR. & Draughn, RA. (1996) Laser-aided degradation of composite resin *Angle Orthodontist* Vol:66 pp.281-286

Tocchio, RM.; Williams, PT.; Mayer, FJ.; et al. (1993) Laser debonding of ceramic orthodontic brackets, *American Journal of Orthodontics Dentofacial Orthopedics* Vol:103 pp.155

Toroğlu, MS.; Bayramoğlu, O.; Yarkın, F. & Tuli, A. (2003) Possibility of blood and hepatit B contamination throught aerosol generated during debonding procedures *Angle Orthodontist* Vol:73 pp.571-578

Toroğlu, MS.; Haytaç, MC. & Köksal, F. (2001) Evaluation of aerosol contamination during debonding procedures *Angle Orthodontist* Vol:71 pp.229-306

Trakyalı, G.; Malkondu, Ö.; Kazazoğlu, E. & Arun, T. (2009) Effects of different silanes and acid concentrations on bond strength of brackets to porcelain surfaces *European journal of orthodontics* Vol:31 pp.402-406

Triolo, PT. Jr; Swift, EJ. Jr; Mudgil, A. & Levine, A. (1993) Effects of etching time on enamel bond strengths *American Journal of Dentistry* Vol:6 pp.302-304

Tylka, DF. & Stewart, GP. (1994) Comparison of acidulated phosphate fluoride gel and hydrofluoric acid etchants for porcelain-composite repair *Journal of Prosthetic Dentistry* Vol:72 pp.121-127

Øgaard, B.; Bishara, S. & Duschner, H. (2004) Enamel effects during bonding-debonding and treatment with fixed appliances, in: *Risk Management in Orthodontics: Experts' Guide to Malpractice* Graber T, Eliades T editors, pp. 19-46:. Quintessence, Chicago

Øgaard, B. & Fjeld, M. (2010) The enamel surface and bonding in orthodontics *Seminers in Orthodontist Vol:*16 pp.37-48

Øgaard, B.; Rølla, G., Arends J, et al: (1988) Orthodontic appliances and enamel demineralization. 2. Prevention and treatment of lesions, *American Journal of Orthodontics Dentafacial Orthopedics Vol:* 94 pp.123

Ǿgaard B. (1989) Prevalance of white spot lesion in 19 year olds: a study on untreated and ortodontically treated person 5 years after treatment *American Journal of Orthodontics Dentafacial Orthopedics Vo:76 pp.423-427*

Øgaard, B.; Rølla G. (1993) Cariological aspects of treatment with fixed orthodontic appliances. Part II. New concept on cariostatic mechanism of topical fluoride *Kieferorthop Mitterlung* Vol:6 pp. 45-51

Øilo, G. (1993) Bond strength testing: What doesit mean? *International Dental Journal* Vol:43 pp.492-498

Uysal, T.; Baysal, A.; Uysal, B.; Aydınbelged, M. & Al-Qunaian T. (2011) Do fluoride and casein phosphopeptide-amorphous calcium phosphate affect shear bond strength of orthodontic brackets bonded to a demineralized enamel surface? *Angle Orthodontist* Vol:81 pp.490–495

Üşümez, S. & Erverdi, N. (2008) *Adhesive and bonding in orthodontics.* pp. 45-67, Elsevier.

Üşümez, S.; Büyükyılmaz, T. &, Karaman, AI. (2003) Effects of fast halogen and plasma arc curing lights on the surface hardness of orthodontic adhesivesfor lingual retainer *American Journal of Orthodontics Dentafacial Orthopedics Vol: 123 pp. 641-648*

Van Meerbeek, B.; De Munck, J.; Mattar, D.; Van Landuyt, K. & Lambrechts, P. (2003) Adhesion to enamel and dentin: current status and future challenges. Operative Dentistry Vol:28 pp.215–235

Viazis, AD.; Cavanaugh, G. & Bevis, RR. (1990) Bond strength of ceramic brackets under shear stress: an in vitro report *American Journal of Orthodontics* Vol:98 pp.214

Wang, WN. & Lu, TC. (1991) Bond strength with various etching times on young permanent teeth, *American Journal of Orthodontics* Vol:100 pp.72-79

White, LW. (1975) Effective saliva control for orthodontic patients *Journal of Clinical Orthodontics Vol:9* pp.648

Wigdor, HA.; Walsh, JT.; Featherstone, JD.; Visuri, SR.; Fried, D. & Waldvogel LJ. (1995) Lasers in dentistry *Lasers Sureryg Medicine* Vol:16 pp.103-108

Wiltshire, WA. (1999) In vitro and in vivo fluoride release from orthodontic elastomeric ligature ties. *American Journal of Orthodontics Dentafacial Orthopedics* Vol:115 pp. *288-292*

Winchester, LJ. (1991) Bond strength of five different ceramic brackets: an in vitro study *European Journal of Orthoodntics* Vol:13 pp. 293-305

Wood, DJ.; Bubb, NL.; Millar, BJ. & Dunne SM. (1997) Preliminary investigation of a novel retentive system for hydrofl uoric acid etch-resistant dental ceramics *Journal of Prosthetic Dentistry* Vol:78 pp.275–280

Zacrisson, BU. (1977) A posttreatment evaluation of direct bonding in orthodontics *American Journal of Orthodontics* Vol: 71pp.173

Zachrisson, BU. & Årtun, J. (1979) Enamel surface appearance after various debonding techniques *American Journal of Orthodontics* Vol:75 pp.121

Zachrisson, BU. & Büyükyılmaz, T. (2005) Bonding in Orthodontics. In: *Orthodontics: current principles and techniques* , Graber TM, Vanarsdall RL, Vig KW of editors: pp.579-659, Elsevier Healt Sciences, St Louis

Zachrisson, YO.; Zachrisson, BU. & Büyükyilmaz, T. (1996) Surface preparation for orthodontic bonding to porcelain . *American Journal of Orthodontics and Dentofacial Orthopedics* Vol:109 pp.420 - 430

Zacrisson, BU. & Büyükyılmaz, T. (1993) Recent advences in bonding to gold, amalgam and porcelain *Journal of Clinical Orthodontics* Vol:27 pp.661

Zacrisson, BU.; Büyükyılmaz, T. & Zacrisson, YØ. (1995) Improving orthodontic bonding to silver amalgam *Angle Orthodontist* Vol:65 pp.35

Zachrisson, BU. & Brobakken, BO. (1978) Clinical comparison of direct versus indirect bonding with different bracket types and adhesives *American Journal of Orthodontics* Vol:74 pp.

Part 3

Methodology

9

An Overview of Selected Orthodontic Treatment Need Indices[1]

Ali Borzabadi-Farahani
Craniofacial Orthodontics, Children's Hospital Los Angeles, University of Southern California, Los Angeles, CA USA

1. Introduction

Dentistry is unique in utilizing objective indices to measure the deviation of oral health components from ideal. Examples include various plaque, caries experience, tooth wear and periodontal indices (Quigley & Hein, 1962; Silness & Löe, 1964; Acharya, 2006; Hooper et al., 2004; Ainamo et al., 1982; Croxson, 1984). However, objective assessment of malocclusion has been different since malocclusion is a developmental condition and deviation from normal. Malocclusion is not an acute condition, and therefore, treatment of malocclusion has been associated with a great degree of subjectivity and distorted perceptions of treatment need. The main traditional reasons to justify providing orthodontic treatment are (I) improvement in the functioning of the dentition, (II) improvement in oral or dental health and (III) improvement in facial or dental aesthetic. In the era of evidence-based orthodontics; however, it is hard to justify the treatment based on improvement in oral or dental health for the majority of orthodontic patients (Burden, 2007; Bollen, 2008). Occlusal indices were used initially as epidemiological tools to rank or classify the occlusion. A large number of occlusal indices started to appear in the 1950s and 1960s to assist epidemiological studies. The orthodontic treatment need index is a form of occlusal index used to prioritize the need for treatment. Their use minimizes the subjectivity related to the diagnosis, outcome and complexity assessment of orthodontic treatment.

A well-developed occlusal index should be reliable (indicate reproducibility) and valid. Validity means whether an index measures what it claims to measure (e.g. determination of treatment need) (Carlos, 1970). Indices should be able to identify people not needing treatment (specificity) and those in need of treatment (sensitivity). An index should be quick and easy to use, acceptable to cultural norms, and finally be adaptable to available resources. Dr William Shaw and co-workers divided occlusal indices into five different categories (Shaw et al., 1995). These are the diagnostic, epidemiologic, orthodontic treatment need, treatment outcome, and Orthodontic treatment complexity indices (Table 1).

The purpose of this chapter is to provide an overview on the most commonly used American and European orthodontic treatment need indices. The modifications, advantages, and limitations of these orthodontic treatment need indices are discussed briefly.

---

[1] This chapter is the longer and more detailed version of an article that has previously been published in a peer-reviewed journal: Borzabadi-Farahani A. An insight into four orthodontic treatment need indices, Progress in Orthodontics, 2011;12(2):132-142.

Occlusal indices	
Diagnostic indices	Angle classification system (Angle, 1899) Incisal categories of Ballard and Wayman (Ballard & Wayman, 1964) Five-point system of Ackerman and Proffit (Ackerman & Proffit, 1969)
Epidemiologic indices	Index of Tooth Position (Massler & Frankel, 1951) Mal-alignment Index (Van Kirk & Pennel, 1959) Occlusal Feature Index (Poulton & Aaronson, 1961) The Bjork method (Bjork et al., 1964) Summer's occlusal index (Summers, 1971) The FDI method (Baume et al., 1973) Little's irregularity index (Little, 1975)
Orthodontic treatment need indices	Handicapping Labio-lingual Deviation Index (HLD) (Draker, 1960, 1967) Swedish Medical Board Index (SMBI) (Swedish Medical Health Board, 1966; Linder-Aronson, 1974, 1976). Dental Aesthetic index (DAI) (Cons et al., 1986) Index of Orthodontic Treatment Need (IOTN) (Brook & Shaw, 1989) Index of Complexity, Outcome and Need (ICON) (Daniels & Richmond, 2000)
Orthodontic treatment outcome indices	Peer Assessment Rating index (PAR) (Richmond et al., 1992a) ICON
Orthodontic treatment complexity indices	Index of Orthodontic Treatment Complexity (IOTC) (Llewellyn et al., 2007) ICON

Table 1. Different types of occlusal indices.

2. Orthodontic treatment need indices

These types of occlusal indices categorize the malocclusion based on treatment need. It is estimated that at least one-third of the population has a clear need for orthodontic treatment (Richmond et al., 1992b); however, this estimation varies depending on the population and/or the perception of need in that population. An orthodontic treatment need index identifies patients in need of orthodontic treatment and prioritizes their treatment needs (Carlos, 1970; Tang & Wei, 1993). There is usually a cut-off point for each index and the lowest index score that allows treatment determines the cut-off point. Exploring the ideas and conventions that made up the ranking systems and cut-off points for orthodontic treatment need indices is beyond the scopes of this chapter, but briefly, this was the opinion of experts in the field, the orthodontists, that initially determined the cut-off points (Järvinen, 2001). These cut-off points are adjustable depending on available resources and the perception of need in the country which index is used. Clearly, the perception of treatment need can be different among various cultures, and that is why index validation in different countries is advisable. Orthodontic treatment need indices have been used to plan the provision of orthodontic treatment in the Northern Europe. In these countries, government subsidizes the dental health services either as part of the National Health

Service or national health insurance. Some authors also used these indices to determine the prevalence and severity of malocclusions in epidemiological studies.

Several orthodontic treatment need indices have been introduced to quantify the malocclusion. Examples can include, but not limited to, the Salzmann's Handicapping Malocclusion Assessment Record (Salzmann, 1968), the Draker's HLD index (Draker, 1960, 1967) and its modifications [HLD (CalMod) (Parker, 1998), HLD (Md) (Code of Maryland Regulations, 1982; Han & Davidson, 2001), and the Washington modification (Theis et al., 2005)], the Orthodontic Treatment Priority Index (Grainger, 1961), the Summer's occlusal index (Summers, 1971), the Swedish national board for health and welfare index or 'the Swedish Medical Board Index (SMBI)' (Swedish Medical Health Board, 1966; Linder-Aronson, 1974, 1976), the Indication Index (Lundstrom, 1977), the DAI (Cons et al., 1986), the Norwegian index of orthodontic treatment need (Espeland et al., 1992), the SCAN index (the Standardized Continuum of Aesthetic Need) (Evans & Shaw, 1987), the IOTN (Brook & Shaw, 1989), and the ICON (Daniels & Richmond, 2000). Some orthodontic treatment need indices are non-parametric, such as the first version of the SMBI (Linder-Aronson, 1974) and the Norwegian index of orthodontic treatment need (Espeland et al., 1992). For instance, the Norwegian index of orthodontic treatment need and the first version of the SMBI use 4 categories of need: very great, great, obvious, and little/no need. Alternatively, there are other indices that employ scales to rate malocclusion such as, the DAI (Cons et al., 1986) and the ICON (Daniels & Richmond, 2000).

The scoring or rating system that indices employ reflects the opinion of index developer (s) about the health risks (e.g. dental or physiological) of malocclusion and the potential benefits of orthodontic treatment (Burden, 2007). These indices consider the psycho-social gain and oral health-related benefits of orthodontic treatment. However, based on the existing research evidence there is only a weak association between occlusal abnormalities and dental health (Burden, 2007). With the exception of severe conditions, such as cleft lip and palate, the contemporary orthodontics does not claim to prevent caries, periodontal disease, and temporo-mandibular dysfunction (Burden, 2007; Bollen, 2008). This is perhaps a reason for general agreement among orthodontists that orthodontic treatment indices cannot be completely validated (SBU, 2005; Mockbil & Huggare, 2009). The American Association of Orthodontists (AAO) does not recognize any index as a scientifically valid measure of need for orthodontic treatment (AAO, 2001). The use of orthodontic treatment need indices reduces the subjectivity associated with orthodontic diagnosis and assessments (Richmond & Daniels, 1998a), and despite the lack of evidence and clinical trials to support the ranking systems in orthodontic treatment need indices, they are widely used in the Northern Europe and are part of the daily practice in some countries such as the United Kingdom (Shaw et al., 1995). In the United States public health planners in 15 states have adopted several orthodontic treatment need indices with cut-off points to determine eligibility for orthodontic treatment with state funds (Younis et al., 1997). However, because of the AAO view on orthodontic indices (AAO, 2001), the use of occlusal indices in the United States is not encouraged and is limited (Han & Davidson, 2001).

3. The Swedish Medical Board Index (SMBI) and the Index of Orthodontic Treatment Need (IOTN)

The SMBI and the IOTN have some similarities. Peter Brook and William Shaw developed the IOTN and initially called it the Index of Orthodontic Treatment Priority (Brook & Shaw,

1989). Later, it was renamed to the Index of Orthodontic Treatment Need (IOTN). The IOTN is one of the most commonly used occlusal indices that assesses the orthodontic treatment need among children and adults. The IOTN has two separate components, a clinical component called the Dental Health Component (DHC) and an Aesthetic Component (AC). There was no attempt to combine these two components and both are recorded separately (Brook & Shaw, 1989). The DHC of IOTN is similar to an index used by the Swedish Medical Health Board 'the Swedish Medical Board Index (SMBI) ' (Swedish Medical Health Board, 1966; Linder-Aronson, 1974, 1976). The original form of this Swedish index was developed having 4 categories of need (grade 1 to 4). Later on, Linder-Aronson and co-workers (1976) revised the index and added a fifth category, the grade zero, describing subjects with no need for treatment (Table 2). This revised SMBI index is very similar to the DHC of IOTN; however, the DHC in IOTN is graded from 1 to 5. The SMBI calls for the subjective views and patient's wishes to be considered when deciding on the treatment need (Mockbil & Huggare, 2009). It has been suggested the arbitrary grading system in the SMBI leads to low level of reproducibility, particularly when the index is used by non-professionals (Danyluk, 1998).

Grade		
4	Very urgent need	Aesthetically and/or functionally handicapping anomalies, such as deft lip and palate, extreme post-normal or pre-normal occlusion, retained upper incisors, extensive aplasia.
3	Urgent need	Pre-normal forced bite, deep bite with gingival irritation not only on papilla incisiva, large overjet with lower lip behind upper centrals, extremely open bite, crossbite causing transverse forced bite, scissors bite interfering with articulation, severe frontal crowding or spacing, retained canines, aesthetically and/or functionally disturbing rotations.
2	Moderate need	Aesthetically and/or functionally disturbing proclined or retroclined incisors, deep bite with gingival contact but without gingival irritation, severe crowding or spacing, infra-occlusion of deciduous molars and permanent teeth, moderate frontal rotations.
1	Little need	Mild deviations from normal (ideal) occlusion, such as pre-normal occlusion with little negative overjet, post-normal occlusion without other anomalies, deep bite without gingival contact, open bite with little frontal opening, crossbite without a forced bite, mild crowding or spacing, mild rotations of only little aesthetic and/or functional significance.
0	No need	Normal (ideal) occlusion without deviations.

Table 2. The modified 5-grade index (ISMHB) for orthodontic treatment need (Swedish Medical Health Board, 1966; Linder-Aronson, 1974, 1976).

As it can be seen in Table 3, the DHC has five grades ranging from grade one, 'no need', to grade five, 'very great need'. A grade is allocated according to the severity of the worst single occlusal trait and describes the priority for treatment. In recording the worst trait following hierarchical scale is used (in a descending order), Missing teeth, Overjet, Crossbites, Displacement of contact points, and **O**verbite (including open bite). To remember the hierarchical scale, the acronym of 'MOCDO' can be constructed and used

Grade 5	Very great need
5i	Impeded eruption of teeth (with the exception of third molars) due to crowding, displacement, the presence of supernumerary teeth, retained deciduous teeth and any pathological cause.
5h	Extensive hypodontia with restorative implications (more than one tooth missing in any quadrant) requiring pre-restorative orthodontics.
5a	Increased overjet > 9 mm.
5m	Reverse overjet greater than 3.5 mm with reported masticatory and speech difficulties.
5p	Defect of cleft lip and palate/craniofacial anomalies.
5s	Submerged deciduous teeth.
Grade 4	Great need
4h	Less extensive hypodontia requiring pre-restorative orthodontics or orthodontic space closure to obviate the need for a prosthesis.
4a	Increased overjet > 6 mm but ≤ 9 mm.
4b	Reverse overjet > 3.5 mm with no masticatory or speech difficulties.
4m	Reverse overjet greater than 1 mm but ≤ 3.5 mm with recorded masticatory and speech difficulties.
4c	Anterior or posterior crossbites with > 2 mm discrepancy between retruded contact position and intercuspal position.
4l	Posterior lingual crossbite (scissors bite) with no functional occlusal contact in one or both buccal segments.
4d	Severe contact point displacements of teeth > 4 mm.
4e	Extreme lateral or anterior open bites > 4 mm.
4f	Increased and complete overbite with gingival or palatal trauma.
4t	Partially erupted teeth, tipped and impacted against adjacent teeth.
4x	Presence of supernumerary (e.g. Supplemental teeth).
Grade 3	Borderline need
3a	Increased overjet > 3.5 mm but ≤ 6 mm with incompetent lips.
3b	Reverse overjet greater than 1 mm but ≤ 3.5 mm.
3c	Anterior or posterior crossbites with >1 mm but ≤ 2 mm discrepancy between retruded contact position and intercuspal position.
3d	Contact point displacement of teeth > 2 mm but ≤ 4 mm.
3e	Lateral or anterior open bite greater than 2 mm but ≤ 4 mm.
3f	Increased and complete overbite without gingival or palatal trauma.
Grade 2	Little need
2a	Increased overjet > 3.5 mm ≤ 6mm with competent lips.
2b	Reverse overjet > 0 mm but ≤ 1mm.
2c	Anterior or posterior crossbite with ≤ 1 mm discrepancy between retruded contact position and intercuspal position.
2d	Contact point displacement of teeth >1 mm but ≤ 2 mm.
2e	Anterior or posterior open bite > 1 mm but ≤ 2mm.
2f	Increased overbite ≥ 3.5 mm without gingival contact.
2g	Pre-normal or post-normal occlusions with no other anomalies. Includes up to half a unit discrepancy.
Grade 1	No need, Extremely minor malocclusions including displacements ≤ 1 mm.

Table 3. Dental Health Components of the IOTN (Brook & Shaw,1989)

(Richmond et al., 1992b). For instance, if two or more occlusal anomalies achieve the same DHC grade, the hierarchical scale is used to determine which dental anomaly should be recorded (i.e. dental anomaly with higher rank in the hierarchical scale is recorded). In recording the DHC, only in recording the DHC only the worst occlusal feature/anomaly is recorded.

The Aesthetic Component (AC) consists of a 10-point scale illustrated by a series of photographs that were rated for attractiveness by a panel of lay judges and were selected as being equidistantly spaced through the range of grades (Evans & Shaw, 1987). The AC, as Figure 1 shows, is based on the SCAN scale (Evans & Shaw, 1987). The SCAN scale, as described by Ruth Evans and William Shaw (Evans & Shaw, 1987), is arranged from the least to the most attractive dentition, while the AC scale is arranged from the most to the least attractive. The photographs for this study were taken from 12-year-olds during a large multi-disciplinary survey (Evans & Shaw, 1987). Orthodontists rarely use the SCAN scale nowadays. The recording of the IOTN components should take between 1 to 3 minutes (Shaw et al., 1995). The DHC and AC can be applied clinically and on study casts (Richmond et al., 1992b). Without clinical information, *the dental cast protocol* is used when recording the DHC on study casts (Richmond et al., 1992b). This protocol always assumes the worst case scenario. For instance, if crossbite is present on study cast, the protocol assumes that a discrepancy between retruded contact position and the intercuspal position of more than 2 mm is present, and therefore, the DHC recording will be 4a. The details and conventions for the IOTN can be found in the literature (Richmond et al., 1992b).

The validity and reliability of the IOTN have been verified previously (Richmond et al., 1993; Burden & Holmes 1994; Burden et al., 1994). In order to assess the validity of the Aesthetic Component of IOTN, a validation exercise involving 74 dentists (44 orthodontist and 30 non-orthodontist) was carried out (Richmond, 1990). This was aimed at determining cut-off points that represent different levels of orthodontic treatment need. A scale of 10 colour photographs showing different levels of dental attractiveness was used, grade 1 representing the most attractive and grade 10 the least attractive dentitions. The validation panel judged grades 1-4 to represent 'no or little need', grades 5, 6, and 7 as 'borderline need', and grades 8, 9, and 10 to represent a clear need for treatment on aesthetic grounds. However, different cut-off points and major changes in the Aesthetic and Dental Health Components of the IOTN has been suggested (Lunn et al., 1993; Beglin et al., 2001). An improved reliability has been reported for the IOTN if both Dental Health and Aesthetic Components were reduced to three grades (Lunn et al., 1993). In an interesting study, Beglin and co-workers (Beglin et al., 2001) assessed the validity of DHC and the AC of the IOTN by a group of American orthodontists and suggested the optimized cut-off points of 3 and 5, respectively.

Sometimes, there is a discrepancy between the DHC and AC grades and they can be contradictory. Some occlusal anomalies such as ectopic teeth, hypodontia, deep traumatic overbites or crossbites have dental health implications; however, they do not necessarily attract a high Aesthetic Component grade. When using AC, the use of frontal photographs of dentition limits overjet and lip-incisor evaluations (Fields et al., 1982). A recent study showed there is only a moderate diagnostic agreement between AC and DHC (Borzabadi-Farahani & Borzabadi-Farahani, 2011a). This difference between the DHC and AC reflects that AC assesses the aesthetic aspects of the malocclusion, only in frontal view, and highlights the subjective nature of it. Therefore, any clinician who is interested in using the IOTN should receive proper training and undergoes the calibration process (Richmond et al., 1995).

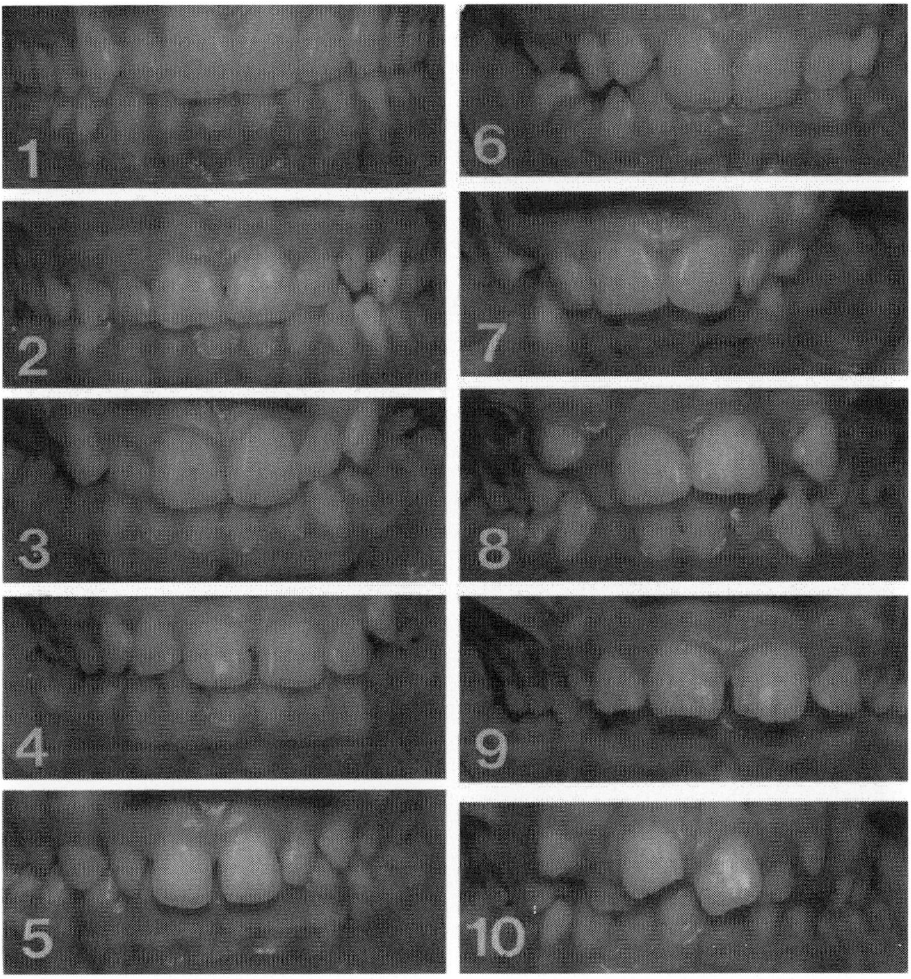

Fig. 1. The Aesthetic Component of the IOTN. The Aesthetic Component was originally described as "SCAN", Evans R and Shaw WC (1987). A preliminary evaluation of an illustrated scale for rating dental attractiveness European Journal of Orthodontics 9:314-18. By kind permission of Oxford University Press.

4. The modified IOTN

The modified IOTN is a two-grade scale (need/no definite need), instead of 5 grade scale with 30 sub-categories. The modified IOTN is based on idea that the IOTN is not an index to measure the complexity; and therefore, there is no benefit in recording the occlusal anomaly that placed the child in treatment need category (Burden et al., 2001. The modified IOTN simplifies identifying people in need of treatment and improves the reliability and validity of the index (Burden et al., 2001). By using the modified IOTN, every case with IOTN DHC ≥ 4 and/or IOTN AC ≥ 8 is classified as being in need of treatment. Since its introduction, few epidemiological studies used the modified IOTN (Chestnutt et al., 2006; Puertes-Fernandez et al., 2010). Briefly by using the modified IOTN, the index has been simplified to two categories: Definite Need for Treatment and No Definite Need for Treatment.

5. Dental Aesthetic Index (DAI)

The Dental Aesthetic Index (DAI) (Cons et al., 1986) looks into the aesthetic aspects of occlusion. The DAI links clinical and aesthetic components, mathematically, to produce a single score. This score reflects the malocclusion severity (Cons et al., 1986). By using cut-off points, index was subsequently used to determine the need for orthodontic treatment. The DAI is based on a social acceptability scale of occlusal conditions (Jenny et al, 1980). Dr. Naham C. Cons, a public health dentist, and co-workers used the opinions of the lay public to find out what constituted unacceptable dental arrangements from the aesthetic standpoint (Cons et al., 1986). Contrary to the European indices such as IOTN (Brook & Shaw, 1989), the DAI reflects the North American culture, aesthetic, and psychosocial values. The DAI highlights the importance of physical attractiveness and by considering societally defined norms for dental appearance, it recognizes conditions that are potentially psycho-socially handicapping.

The regression procedures used a sample of 200 photographs of occlusal configurations during development of DAI. These were selected by a disproportionate, stratified, random sampling procedure. This sample was selected from a larger sample of 1337 study models (collected from high school students in the New York state, with age range of 15 -18 years) (Ast et al., 1965; Cons et al., 1978). The regression procedures provided the statistical basis for regression coefficient weightings to be used against the 10 occlusal traits chosen by regression procedures (Proshek et al., 1979) (Table 4). The DAI used a regression equation that called for the measured components of DAI to be multiplied by their regression coefficients (weights), addition of their products and a constant number (n=13) to the total. The resulting sum was the DAI score. The World Health Organization Oral Health Survey Methods recognized the DAI as a cross-cultural index (1997). Table 4 shows the DAI components and the adopted weights. The DAI was designed to be used in permanent dentition and a modified version of the index has been suggested for the mixed dentition (Johnson et al, 2000). Nonetheless, the DAI index has also been used in the mixed dentition (Johnson & Harkness, 2000). The study by Keay and co-workers (Keay et al., 1993) revealed performance of the DAI in the mixed dentition group was slightly lower than the permanent dentition group. A longitudinal study of 150 children in New Zealand also revealed a fall in orthodontic treatment need which was attributed to over-sensitivity of Index in the mixed dentition period (Chi et al., 2000).

Several studies showed the DAI is a valid (Beglin et al., 2001; Spencer et al., 1992; Jenny et al., 1993; Jenny & Cons, 1996a) and reliable index (Jenny et al., 1993). An advantage of the

DAI is the use of threshold scores (i.e. 31 or higher) to equate with the need for orthodontic services. This threshold limits changes based on available resources and funding. Different cut-off points for the DAI have been proposed to prioritize orthodontic care needs. Jenny and co-workers (Jenny et al., 1993) initially suggested cut-off point of 36 to identify handicapping malocclusions. However, they later proposed a cut-off point of 31 to determine the number of individuals who require treatment (Jenny & Cons, 1996b). Similarly, Keay and Freer (Keay & Freer, 1993; Bernabé et al., 2006) and Beglin and co-workers (Beglin et al., 2001; Bernabé et al., 2006) suggested revised cut-off points of 32.5 and 28, respectively. Table 5 shows the current treatment need categories used for the DAI.

DAI	Component	Calculated weights	Rounded weights
1	No. of visibly missing teeth: incisors, canines, and premolars in the maxillary and mandibular arches	5.76	6
2	Assessment of incisal segment crowding (0,1, or 2): 0= no segment crowded; 1=1 segment crowded; 2=2 segments crowded	1.15	1
3	Assessment of incisal segment spacing (0,1, or 2): 0=no segment spaced; 1=1 segment spaced; 2=2 segments spaced	1.31	1
4	Diastema (mm) $	3.13	3
5	Largest anterior maxillary irregularity (mm) *	1.34	1
6	Largest anterior mandibular irregularity (mm) *	0.75	1
7	Anterior maxillary overjet (mm) ^	1.62	2
8	Anterior mandibular overjet (mm) ^	3.68	4
9	Vertical anterior open bite (mm) ^	3.69	4
10	Assessment of antero-posterior molar relation: largest deviation from normal either left or right: 0= normal; 1= ½ cusp either mesial or distal; 2= full cusp or more either mesial or distal ^	2.69	3
11	Constant	13.36	13
	Total	DAI Score	

$ Largest measurement
* Site of greatest rotations or displacement from normal arch alignment
^ Measured with teeth in centric occlusion

Table 4. DAI components, their calculated, and final rounded weights

DAI score	Malocclusion severity	Treatment need category
=< 25	Normal / minor	No treatment need / slight need
26-30	Definite	Treatment elective
31-35	Severe	Treatment highly desirable
>= 36	Very severe / handicapping	Treatment mandatory

Table 5. The DAI treatment need categories

There are possible limitations with using the DAI. The lack of assessment of occlusal anomalies such as buccal crossbite, impacted teeth, centre-line discrepancy, and deep overbite weakens the index (Otuyemi & Noar 1996a, 1996b; Danyluk et al., 1999). The DAI also does not account for missing molars. Although deviations for crowding and spacing components are scored as present or absent, there is no distinction between varying degrees of arch length discrepancy. These limitations should be considered when using the DAI for epidemiological studies or in studies assessing relationship between malocclusion and other variables. There are inherent differences between the DAI and other orthodontic treatment need indices. For instance, the DAI and the modified IOTN (Burden et al., 2001) showed only a moderate agreement in estimating the treatment need (Kappa statistics=0.47) (Manzanera et al., 2010). Correspondingly, the observed percentage agreement between them was 83 percent, showing a difference of 17 percent in treatment need estimates of these indices (Manzanera et al., 2010). This highlights the different mechanisms these indices use to rank the malocclusion.

6. Handicapping Labio-lingual Deviation index (HLD)

The intent of the HLD index is to measure the degree of handicap caused by the different components of malocclusion. The Medicaid statutes in the early 1960s recognized there was a need for a method to identify those with a medically handicapping malocclusion. Dr Harry L. Draker developed the Handicapping Labio-lingual Deviation index (HLD) (Draker, 1960, 1967) which was one of the first indices used in the United States to identify those with handicapping malocclusions (Theis et al., 2005). The HLD selects deviations from ideal and these are scored and weighted. The HLD index has been modified by some states to determine and prioritize eligibility for the state-funded orthodontic treatment. The original cut-off point of 13 selected for the HLD index. The Maryland's version of HLD, the HLD (Md) index (Code of Maryland Regulations, 1982; Han & Davidson, 2001), modified the HLD's original scoring formula for overjet and overbite. The Maryland's index, the HLD (Md), changed the cut-off from 13 to 15 points and modified the Draker's scoring formula by subtracting 2 mm from overjet and 3 mm from overbite measurements (Code of Maryland Regulations, 1982; Cooke et al., 2010). The state of Washington HLD modification has five qualifying conditions and the cut-off point has changed to 30 (Theis et al., 2005).

The original form of the HLD index is not a reliable index to assess the orthodontic treatment need. This is because it does not record missing, impacted teeth, spacing between teeth, and transverse discrepancies such as midline deviations and crossbites. The HLD index was modified in the state of California, the HLD (CalMod) index (Parker, 1998), and used the cut-off point of 26. The HLD (CalMod) index (Parker, 1998) has been created because of the settlements originating from two lawsuits against the state of California claiming the state of California failed to comply with the orthodontic provisions of the Medicaid statutes (Brown V. Kizer, 1989; Duran V. Belshe, 1994). As a result of these lawsuits, two qualifying exceptions that cause tissue damage were added to the original HLD index, namely the deep impinging bites and crossbites of individual anterior teeth with tissue destruction (Parker, 1998). In addition, overjets greater than 9 mm and reverse overjets more than 3.5 mm were added as additional qualifying exceptions. The ectopic eruption and unilateral posterior crossbite were also added as weighted factors (Parker, 1998). Table 6 shows the components of the HLD (CalMod) index that is currently used in the state of California.

No	Condition	Score
1	Cleft palate deformity	
2	Cranio-facial anomaly	
3	Deep impinging overbite When the lower incisors are destroying the soft tissue of the palate. Tissue laceration and/or clinical attachment loss must be present.	
4	Crossbite of individual anterior teeth When clinical attachment loss and recession of the gingival margin are present.	
5	Severe traumatic deviations Attach a description of condition, i.e. loss of a premaxilla by burn, trauma or pathology.	
6	Overjet greater than 9 mm Reverse overjet greater than 3.5 mm	
7	Overjet (=<9 mm)	(mm)
8	Overbite including the reverse overbite	(mm)
9	Mandibular protrusion (reverse overjet =< 3.5 mm)	(mm) * 5
10	Open bite	(mm) * 4
11	Ectopic eruption: Count each tooth, excluding third molars	(count) * 3
12	Anterior crowding: Score one point for the maxilla, and/or one point for mandible; two points maximum for anterior crowding.	(0, 1, or 2) * 5
13	Labio-Lingual spread, Arch length insufficiency must exceed 3.5 mm excluding mild rotations that may react favorably to stripping or mild expansion procedures.	(mm)
14	Posterior unilateral crossbite Must involve 2 or more adjacent teeth, one of which must be a molar and not including the posterior bilateral crossbite	4
		Total Score

Table 6. The California Modification of the Handicapping Labio-lingual Deviation Index, the HLD (CalMod) index (Parker, 1998). Conditions 1 to 6 are the qualifying conditions and if present further scoring is not needed. Otherwise, the sum of other conditions (7-14) must be 26 or above to be considered as a handicapping malocclusion. All measurements are recorded in the order given and rounded off to the nearest millimeter (mm). If both anterior crowding and ectopic eruption are present in the anterior portion of the mouth, the most severe condition will be scored, not both conditions. Overjet is recorded with the patient's teeth in centric occlusion and measured from the labial portion of the lower incisors to the labial of the upper incisors.

The HLD (CalMod) index records twelve factors and occlusal traits to produce the final score. These factors are: Overjet, overbite, open bite, cleft lip-palate, anterior crowding, mandibular protrusion, labio-lingual spread, deep impinging overbite, severe traumatic deviations, crossbite of individual anterior teeth, ectopic eruption of anterior teeth, and posterior unilateral crossbite. Dr. William S. Parker who was involved in developing the HLD (CalMod) index recommended using the index on individuals of 13 years of age and older (Parker, 1998). The different criteria's that were added to the HLD (CalMod) and HLD (Md) indices resulted in different treatment need thresholds and cut-off points. Han and Davidson compared the HLD (CalMod) and HLD (Md) indices using a sample of 313 patients (Han & Davidson, 2001). The HLD (CalMod) index showed a lower treatment need threshold compared to the HLD (Md) index (Han & Davidson, 2001). Cooke and co-workers assessed the validity of the HLD (CalMod) index with a panel of 13 practicing orthodontists (Cooke et al., 2010). They assessed the validity of the index using two cut-off points of 26 and 18.5. With the recommended cut-off point of 26, index failed to identify a considerable percentage of handicapping malocclusions (Cooke et al., 2010). According to their findings, with the cut-off point of 26, index showed a low sensitivity (25.9%) and high specificity (96.8%). Using the cut-off point of 18.5, specificity decreased to 55.6%; however, the sensitivity increased considerably to 92.9%. Similarly, Beglin and co-workers suggested the optimized cut-off point of 12 for the HLD (CalMod) index (Beglin et al., 2001). Despite these findings, the HLD (CalMod) index is still used in the state of California.

7. Index of Complexity, Outcome and Need (ICON)

The Index of Complexity, Outcome and Need (ICON) was developed by Drs Charles Daniels and Stephen Richmond of Cardiff University (Daniels & Richmond, 2000). This was based on the average opinion of 97 practicing specialist orthodontists from eight European countries and the United States (Richmond & Daniels, 1998a, 1998b). In this exercise, the degree of need in 240 sets of pre-treatment study casts and the treatment outcome for 98 paired pre- and post-treatment records were subjectively assessed. The multiple regression analysis was then used and different occlusal traits were given weightings according to their relative importance. The sum of these weighted scores formed the final ICON score The ICON is a single assessment method to measure the orthodontic treatment complexity, outcome and need. The ICON is unique in incorporating an aesthetic score as an integral part of the treatment need evaluation. The ICON is a multifunctional index; it is both an index of treatment need and treatment outcome assessment. The ICON also assesses the malocclusion complexity, and therefore, it offers significant advantages over the other indices of treatment need. The need for treatment does not necessarily equate to the complexity of treatment (Richmond et al., 1997), and there is a need to assess the complexity of treatment. Assessing the complexity of malocclusion helps to: (I) to identify the most proper setting in which the patient receives treatment (i.e. general practice, hospital or specialized practices), (II) to inform the patient of treatment likely success, and finally (III) to identify cases that are more difficult and are likely to take longer to treat.

The ICON has been shown to be a reliable and valid index for assessing orthodontic treatment need (Koochek et al., 2001; Firestone et al., 2002). A relatively high sensitivity (being able to detect treatment need in an individual) and specificity (the ability to identify correctly those individuals who do not need treatment) have been reported for the ICON (Koochek et al., 2001; Firestone et al., 2002). The ICON was also found to be valid for assessing the complexity and outcome of orthodontic cases (Savastano et al., 2003). However, the perception of treatment need can be different in various countries. This leads to recommending different cut-off points. For instance, Dutch orthodontists suggested changing the cut-off point to 52, instead of the recommended cut-off point of 43, to increase the validity of the index (Louwerse et al., 2006).

	Components:	Score						Weight
		0	1	2	3	4	5	
1	Aesthetic assessment	Score 1 to 10						7
2$	Upper arch crowding	< 2mm	2.1-5mm	5.1-9mm	9.1-13mm	13.1-17mm	> 17mm	5
	Upper arch spacing	< 2mm	2.1-5mm	5.1-9mm	> 9mm		Impacted teeth	5
3	Crossbite	No crossbite	Crossbite present					5
4*	Incisor open bite	Edge to edge	< 1mm	1.1-2mm	2.1-4mm	> 4mm		4
	Incisor overbite	<1/3 lower incisor coverage	1/3 to 2/3 coverage	2/3 up to fully covered	Fully covered			4
5^	Buccal segment A-P	Cusp to embrasure only, Class I,II or III	Any cusp relation up to but not including cusp to cusp	Cusp to cusp				3

$ The difference between the sum of the mesio-distal tooth diameters and the available arch circumference in the upper arch is recorded on a 5 point score. Impacted teeth (score 5) must be un-erupted and either ectopic or have less than 4 mm of space between adjacent permanent teeth. Retained deciduous teeth (without permanent successor), erupted supernumerary teeth or lost teeth due to trauma are counted as space, unless they are to be maintained and obviate the need for prosthetic replacement or space is maintained for a prosthetic replacement (i.e. tooth lost in trauma).
* If both anterior open bite and deep bite are present only the highest score is counted.
^ Quality of buccal segment interdigitation, not the Angle Classification, is measured on both sides then added together

Table 7. The ICON scoring method and its components (Daniels & Richmond, 2000).

The ICON consists of five components: The Aesthetic Component (AC) which is similar to the Aesthetic Component of the IOTN (Brook & Shaw, 1989) (Figure 1), upper and lower crowding / spacing assessment, the presence of a crossbite, degree of incisor open bite/overbite, and the fit of the teeth in the buccal segment in terms of the anterior-posterior relationship (Table 7). Each component can be measured on the study cast as well as on the patient. The practical application of the index is simple and takes approximately one minute for each case (Daniels & Richmond, 2000). The various occlusal anomalies are scored and then weighted scores are summed to produce the final ICON score. A score of 44 or greater indicates the individual needs treatment. In assessing the treatment outcome, a score of 30 or less indicates the end treatment occlusion is acceptable. Table 7 shows the ICON scoring method and its components. The threshold for treatment need in ICON is lower compared to the IOTN (DHC and AC) (Daniels & Richmond, 2000; Borzabadi-Farahani et al., 2010). Similarly, the study by Theis and co-workers (Theis et al., 2005) revealed the ICON found significantly more treatment need compared to the HLD index. Table 8 shows the complexity grades for the ICON. As previously mentioned ICON is unique in ability to assess the orthodontic outcome. The ICON uses the following formula to assess the orthodontic treatment outcome:

Improvement grade = Pre-Treatment Score - 4 x Post-Treatment Score

ICON Complexity Grade	Score Range
Easy	< 29
Mild	29 to 50
Moderate	51 to 63
Difficult	64 to 77
Very Difficult	> 77

Table 8. ICON complexity grade score ranges

Using the formula and the Table 9, the outcome of orthodontic treatment can be assessed. The ICON is a good substitute for the Dental Health Component (DHC) of IOTN (36) and showed high correlation with the DHC of the IOTN (Borzabadi-Farahani et al., 2010). The ICON and the DHC (IOTN) showed a good agreement in estimating the treatment need (Kappa statistics=0.78) (Borzabadi-Farahani & Borzabadi-Farahani, 2011a). The observed percentage agreement between them was 89.5 percent, indicating a difference of 10.5 percent in treatment need estimates between these indices (ICON and DHC of IOTN) (Borzabadi-Farahani & Borzabadi-Farahani, 2011a). The ICON offers several advantages over IOTN, including the ability to assess the complexity of malocclusion and assessing the treatment outcome. In comparison to the DAI (Cons et al., 1986), the ICON does not suffer from similar deficiencies (Otuyemi & Noar 1996a, 1996b; Danyluk et al., 1999). This is the lack of assessment of some occlusal anomalies such as posterior crossbites, impacted teeth, and deep overbite (Otuyemi & Noar 1996a, 1996b; Danyluk et al., 1999). Compared to the DAI, recording of the ICON is significantly easier, takes less time to calculate the final score (Daniels & Richmond, 2000), and ICON has been suggested as a good substitute for DAI in assessment of treatment need (Onyeaso & Begole, 2007).

Similar to other orthodontic treatment need indices there are possible limitations with using ICON. The index is heavily weighted for aesthetics (weighting of seven), which relies on subjective opinion of clinician. This reduces the objectivity of the index and potentially affects the intra or inter-examiner agreements for different functions of the ICON (Savastano et al., 2003; Koochek et al., 2001). Overall, ICON is simple to use, measures relatively few traits, does not need hierarchy and can be used on patients or study casts without protocol modification.

Improvement Grade	Score Range
Greatly improved	> -1
Substantially improved	-25 to -1
Moderately improved	-53 to -26
Minimally improved	-85 to -54
Not improved or worse	< -85

Table 9. Assessment of the orthodontic treatment improvement (outcome assessment) using the ICON

8. Possible applications of orthodontic treatment need indices

The ranking system that orthodontic treatment need indices employ helps the orthodontic profession in many ways. These are discussed briefly in the following.

Giving confidence to the orthodontic speciality. The use of orthodontic treatment indices by properly trained general dentist and dental specialists helps with identification and referral of potential orthodontic patients. This reduces the subjectivity of orthodontic referrals and gives confidence to the orthodontic speciality.

Resource allocation and manpower planning. Setting the cut-off points in different orthodontic treatment need indices helps the governments and dental bodies in resource allocation and future manpower planning.

Assessing the relationship between malocclusion and other medical or dental conditions. Assessing the link between malocclusion and other medical and dental conditions is important. Within this context, indices that have a scale provide more information (e.g. ICON). Examples of these links can include, but not limited to, periodontal status (Ngom et al., 2007a), masticatory function (Ngom et al., 2007b), dental trauma (Borzabadi-Farahani & Borzabadi-Farahani, 2011b), and caries experience (Borzabadi-Farahani et al., 2011).

Assessing the orthodontic treatment outcome and clinical performance. The aim of orthodontic treatment is to deliver a high standard of care and this should be at the individual, institutional and national level. Therefore, it is important to find out the outcome of treatment and evaluate the outcome acceptability. In comparison to the PAR index (Richmond et al., 1992a), the ICON (Daniels & Richmond, 2000) has been shown to be more critical and suggested to be more valid in detecting the treatment failure (Fox & Chapple, 2004). This function is particularly helpful in orthodontic litigation cases.

Assessing the malocclusion complexity. Difficulty in achieving an ideal occlusion might arise from, but not limited to, the pre-treatment occlusion (e.g. complex or simple malocclusion), patient associated factors (compliance), and treatment related factors. The orthodontic treatment complexity has been defined as an entity that reduces post-treatment success (Richmond et al., 1997; Llewellyn et al., 2007). According to Richmond et al. (2001) difficulty and complexity in orthodontics are synonymous. They are measurement of effort and skill, while severity is a measurement of how far a malocclusion deviates from normal (Richmond et al., 2001; Llewellyn et al., 2007). Orthodontic indices that assess the complexity identify the individual that should be treated in hospital setting and need a different competency for their treatment (e.g. need surgical interventions) or those who have milder problems and can be treated by general dentists or specialist practices.

Assessing the cost-effectiveness of orthodontic treatment. In publicly funded or insurance-based services, the cost-effectiveness is of interest to health care providers. This is particularly important when patient pays the cost of treatment as it is of interest to both patients and practitioner. Improved cost-effectiveness results in lower patient costs, increased practitioner profit, and provides treatment for more patients in publicly funded orthodontic services (Deans et al., 2009). In order to perform a cost-effectiveness study, a well-defined treatment outcome is required (Deans et al., 2009, Richmond et al., 2005). An orthodontic index provides a valid and reliable method of measuring treatment outcomes (Shaw et al., 1991). The ICON (Daniels & Richmond, 2000) allows quality assurance assessments to be carried out and compared between different operators and clinics. A simple way of comparing the cost-effectiveness between practitioners is to calculate the cost per ICON point reduction that is an average cost-effectiveness ratio (Shaw et al., 1991).

9. Conclusion

Despite the shortcomings of orthodontic treatment need indices they are used in many European countries and some states in the United States. The use of contemporary , multifunctional orthodontic indices, based on international consensus, that provides information on the need/complexity and treatment outcome is recommended. As mentioned earlier orthodontic treatment need indices are based on consensus opinion of their developer (s) and are not entirely based on the research evidence. Future studies should be aimed at creating an evidence-based scoring system for the orthodontic treatment need indices.

10. References

Acharya, S. (2006). Specific caries index: A new system for describing untreated dental caries experience in developing countries. Journal of Public Health Dentistry, Vol. 66, pp. 285-287.

Ackerman, JL; Proffit, WR. (1969). The characteristics of malocclusion: a modern approach to classification and diagnosis. American Journal of Orthodontics, Vol.56, pp.443-454.

Ainamo, J; Barmes, D; Beagrie, G; Cutress, T; Martin, J; Sardo-Infirri, J. (1982). Development of the World Health Organization (WHO) community periodontal index of treatment needs (CPITN). International Dental Journal, Vol.32, pp. 281-291.

AAO. (2001). American Association of Orthodontists, Bulletin 2001, Fall 2001.

Angle, H. (1899). Classification of malocclusion. Dental Cosmos, Vol.41, pp. 248-264.

Ast, DB; Carlos, JP; Cons, NC. (1965). The prevalence and characteristics of malocclusion among senior high school students in upstate New York. American Journal of Orthodontics, Vol.51, pp. 437-445.

Ballard, CF; Wayman, JB. (1964). A report on a survey of the orthodontic requirements of 310 army apprentices. Transactions of the British Society for the Study of Orthodontics, Vol.86, pp. 81-86.

Baume, LJ; Horowitz, HS; Summers, CJ; Dirks, BO; Brown, WAB; Carlos, JP; et al. (1973). A method for measuring occlusal traits. International Dental Journal, Vol.23, pp. 530-537.

Beglin, FM; Firestone, AR; Vig, KW; Beck, FM; Kuthy, RA; Wade D. (2001). A comparison of the reliability and validity of 3 occlusal indexes of orthodontic treatment need. American Journal of Orthodontics and Dentofacial Orthopedics, Vol.120, pp. 240-246.

Bernabé, E; Flores-Mir, C. (2006). Orthodontic treatment need in Peruvian young adults evaluated through dental aesthetic index. Angle Orthodontist, Vol.76, pp. 417-421.

Bjork, A; Krebs, A; Solow, B. (1964). A method for the epidemiological registration of malocclusion. Acta Odontologica Scandinavica, Vol.22, pp. 27-41.

Bollen, AM. (2008). Effects of malocclusions and orthodontics on periodontal health: evidence from a systematic review. Journal of Dental Education, Vol.72, pp. 912-918.

Borzabadi-Farahani, A; Borzabadi-Farahani, A; Eslamipour, F. (2010). The relationship between ICON index and Dental and Aesthetic components of IOTN index. World Journal Orthodontics, Vol.11, pp. 43-48.

Borzabadi-Farahani, A; Borzabadi-Farahani, A. (2011a). Agreement between the index of complexity, outcome, and need and the dental and aesthetic components of the index of orthodontic treatment need. American Journal of Orthodontics and Dentofacial Orthopaedics, Vol. 140, pp. 233-238.

Borzabadi-Farahani, A; Borzabadi-Farahani, A. (2011b). The association between orthodontic treatment need and maxillary incisor trauma, a retrospective clinical study. Oral Surgery, Oral Medicine, Oral Pathology, Oral Radiology, and Endodontology, In Press.

Borzabadi-Farahani, A; Eslamipour, F; Asgari, I. (2011). Association between orthodontic treatment need and caries experience, Acta Odontologica Scandinavica, Vol.69, pp. 2-11.

Brook, PH; Shaw, WC. (1989) The development of an index of orthodontic treatment priority. European Journal of Orthodontics, Vol.20, pp. 309-320.

Burden, DJ; Holmes, A. (1994). The need for orthodontic treatment in the child population of the United Kingdom. European Journal of Orthodontics, Vol.16, pp. 395-399.

Burden, DJ; Mitropoulos, CM; Shaw, WC. (1994). Residual orthodontic treatment need in a sample of 15- and 16-year-olds. British Dental Journal, Vol.176, pp. 220-224.

Burden, DJ; Pine, CM; Burnside, G. (2001). Modified IOTN: an orthodontic treatment need index for use in oral health surveys. Community Dentistry and Oral Epidemiology, Vol.29, pp. 220-225.

Burden, DJ. (2007). Oral Health-Related Benefits of OrthodonticTreatment. Seminars in Orthodontics, Vol.13, pp. 76-80.

Carlos, JP. (1970). Evaluation of indices of malocclusion. International Dental Journal, Vol.20, pp. 606-617.

Chestnutt, IG; Burden, DJ; Steele, JG; Pitts, NB; Nuttall, NM; Morris, AJ. (2006). The orthodontic condition of children in the United Kingdom, 2003. British Dental Journal, Vol.10, pp. 609-612.

Chi, J; Johnson, M; Harkness, M. (2000). Age changes in orthodontic treatment need: a longitudinal study of 10- and 13-year-old children, using the Dental Aesthetic Index. Australian Orthodontic Journal, Vol.16, pp. 150-156.

Code of Maryland Regulations. (1982). Attachment No 1, EPSDT Services Regulation. Baltimore, Maryland, USA.

Cons, NC; Mruthyunjay, YC; Pollard, ST. (1978). Distribution of occlusal traits in a sample of 1,337 children aged 15-18 residing in upstate New York. International Dental Journal, Vol.28, pp. 154-164.

Cons, NC; Jenny, J; Kohout, FJ. (1986). DAI: The dental aesthetic index. College of Dentistry, Iowa City, IA: University of Iowa.

Cooke, M; Gerbert, B; Gansky, S; Miller, A; Nelson, G; Orellana, M. (2010). Assessment of the validity of HLD (CalMod) in identifying orthodontic treatment need. Community Dentistry and Oral Epidemiology, Vol.38, pp.50-57.

Croxson, LJ. (1984). A simplified periodontal screening examination: the Community Periodontal Index of Treatment Needs (WHO) in general practice. International Dental Journal, Vol.34, pp.28-34.

Daniels, C; Richmond, S. (2000). The development of the index of complexity, outcome and need (ICON). Journal of Orthodontics, Vol.27, pp. 149-162.

Danyluk, K. (1998). The development of an objective orthodontic treatment-need index. MSc thesis, University of Manitoba. p.29.

Danyluk, K; Lavelle, C; Hassard, T. (1999). Potential application of the dental aesthetic index to prioritize the orthodontic service needs in a publicly funded dental program. American Journal of Orthodontics and Dentofacial Orthopedics, Vol.116, pp. 279-286.

Deans, J; Playle, R; Durning, P; Richmond, S. (2009). An exploratory study of the cost effectiveness of orthodontic care in seven European countries. European Journal of Orthodontics, Vol.31, pp. 90-94.

Draker, HL. (1960). Handicapping labio-lingual deviations: a proposed index for public health purposes. American Journal of Orthodontics, Vol.46, pp. 295-305.

Draker, HL. (1967). American association of orthodontists approval of the assessment record form and the definition of handicapping malocclusion, Journal of American Dental Association, Vol. 75, pp. 1441-1442.

Espeland, LV; Ivarsson, K; Stenvik, A. (1992). A new Norwegian index of orthodontic treatment need related to orthodontic concern among 11-year-olds and their parents. Community Dentistry and Oral Epidemiology, Vol.20, pp. 274-279.

Evans, R; Shaw, WC. (1987). Preliminary evaluation of an illustrated scale for rating dental attractiveness. European Journal of Orthodontics, Vol.9, pp. 314-318.

Fields, HW; Vann, WF and Vig, KWL. (1982): Reliability of Soft Tissue Profile Analysis in Children, Angle Orthodontist, Vol.52, pp. 159-165.

Firestone, AR; Beck, FM; Beglin, FM; Vig, KW. (2002). Validity of the Index of Complexity, Outcome, and Need (ICON) in determining orthodontic treatment need. Angle Orthodontist, Vol.72, pp. 15-20.

Fox, NA; Chapple, JR. (2004). Measuring failure of orthodontic treatment: a comparison of outcome indicators. Journal of Orthodontics, Vol.31, pp. 319-322.

Grainger, RM. (1961). Burlington Orthodontic Research Center progress report. Series 6. University of Toronto, Division of Dental Research, pp. 9-11.

Han, H; Davidson, WM. (2001). A useful insight into 2 occlusal indexes: HLD (Md) and HLD (CalMod). American Journal of Orthodontics and Dentofacial Orthopedics, Vol.120, pp. 247-253.

Hooper, SM; Meredith, N; Jagger, DC. (2004). The development of a new index for measurement of incisal/occlusal tooth wear. Journal of Oral Rehabilitation, Vol.31, pp.206-212.

Järvinen, S. (2001). Indexes for orthodontic treatment need. American Journal of Orthodontics and Dentofacial Orthopedics, Vol.120, pp. 237-9.

Jenny, J; Cons, NC. (1996a). Comparing and contrasting two orthodontic indices, the index of orthodontic treatment need and the dental aesthetic index. American Journal of Orthodontics and Dentofacial Orthopedics, Vol.110, pp. 410-416.

Jenny, J; Cons, NC. (1996b). Establishing malocclusion severity levels on the Dental Aesthetic Index (DAI) scale. Australian Dental Journal, Vol.41, pp. 43-46.

Jenny, J; Cons, NC; Kohout, FJ; Frazier, PJ. (1980). Test of a method to determine socially acceptable occlusal conditions. Community Dentistry and Oral Epidemiology, Vol.8, pp. 424-433.

Jenny, J; Cons, NC; Kohout, FJ; Jakobsen, J. (1993). Predicting handicapping malocclusion using the Dental Aesthetic Index (DAI). International Dental Journal, Vol.43, pp. 128-132.

Johnson, M; Harkness, M. (2000). Prevalence of malocclusion and orthodontic treatment need in 10-year-old New Zealand children. Australian Orthodontic Journal, Vol.16, pp. 1-8.

Johnson, M; Harkness, M; Crowther, P; Herbison, P. (2000). A comparison of two methods of assessing orthodontic treatment need in the mixed dentition: DAI and IOTN. Australian Orthodontic Journal, Vol.16, pp. 82-87.

Keay, PA; Freer, TJ. (1993). Orthodontic treatment need and the dental aesthetic index. Australian Orthodontic Journal, Vol.13, pp. 4-7.

Keay, PA; Freer, TJ; Basford, KE. (1993). Orthodontic treatment need and the dental aesthetic index. Australian Orthodontic Journal, Vol.13, pp. 4-7.

Koochek, AR; Yeh, MS; Rolfe, B; Richmond, S. (2001). The relationship between Index of Complexity, Outcome and Need, and patients' perceptions of malocclusion: a study in general dental practice. British Dental Journal, Vol.191, pp. 325-329.

Llewellyn, SK; Hamdan, AM; Rock, WP. (2007). An index of orthodontic treatment complexity. European Journal of Orthodontics, Vol.29, pp.186-92.

Linder-Aronson, S. (1974). Orthodontics in the Swedish public dental health service. Transactions of the European Orthodontic Society, pp. 233-240.

Linder-Aronson, S; Fridh, G; Jensen, R. (1976). Need of orthodontic treatment and orthodontic specialists in Sweden. Swedish Dental Journal, Vol.68, pp. 383-402.

Little, RM. (1975). The irregularity index. American Journal of Orthodontics, Vol.68, pp. 554-563.

Louwerse, TJ; Aartman, IH; Kramer, GJ; Prahl-Andersen, B. (2006). The reliability and validity of the Index of Complexity, Outcome and Need for determining treatment need in Dutch orthodontic practice. European Journal of Orthodontics, Vol.28, pp. 58-64.

Lundstrom, A. (1977). Need for treatment in cases of malocclusion. Transactions of the European Orthodontic Society, pp. 111-123.

Lunn, H; Richmond, S; Mitropoulos, C. (1993). The use of the Index of Orthodontic Treatment Need (IOTN) as a public health tool: a pilot study. Community Dental Health, Vol.10, pp. 111-121.

Manzanera, D; Montiel-Company, JM; Almerich-Silla, JM; Gandía, JL. (2010). Diagnostic agreement in the assessment of orthodontic treatment need using the Dental Aesthetic Index and the Index of Orthodontic Treatment Need. European Journal of Orthodontics, Vol.32, pp. 193-198.

Massler, M; Frankel, JM. (195 1): Prevalence of Malocclusion in Children Aged 14 to 18 Years, American Journal of Orthodontics, Vol. 37, pp. 751-768.

Mockbil, N; Huggare, J. (2009). Uniformity in selection for subsidized orthodontic care--focus on borderline treatment need. Swedish Dental Journal, Vol.33, pp.19-25.

Ngom, PI; Benoist, HM; Thiam, F; Diagne, F; Diallo, PD. (2007a). Influence of orthodontic anomalies on periodontal condition, Odonto-stomatologie tropicale, Vol.30, pp. 9-16.

Ngom, PI; Diagne, F; Aïdara-Tamba, AW; Sene, A. (2007b). Relationship between orthodontic anomalies and masticatory function in adults. American Journal of Orthodontics and Dentofacial Orthopedics, Vol.131, pp. 216-222.

Onyeaso, CO; Begole, EA. (2007). Relationship between index of complexity, outcome and need, dental aesthetic index, peer assessment rating index, and American Board of Orthodontics objective grading system. American Journal of Orthodontics and Dentofacial Orthopedics, Vol.131, pp. 248-252.

Otuyemi, OD; Noar, JH. (1996a). A comparison between DAI and SCAN in estimating orthodontic treatment need. International Dental Journal, Vol.46, pp. 35-40.

Otuyemi, OD; Noar, JH. (1996b). Variability in recording and grading the need for orthodontic treatment using the HMAR, OI and DAI. Community Dentistry and Oral Epidemiology, Vol.24, pp. 222-224.

Parker, WS. (1998). The HLD (CalMod) index and the index question. American Journal of Orthodontics and Dentofacial Orthopedics, Vol.114, pp. 134-141.

Poulton, DR; Aaronson, SA. (1961): The relationship between occlusion and periodontal Status. American Journal of Orthodontics, Vol.47, pp. 690-699

Proshek, JM; Jenny, J; Cons, NC; Summers, CJ; Mruthyunjaya, YC. (1979). A factor analysis of traits measured by COCSTOC-MOT to identify occlusal trait combinations. Community Dentistry and Oral Epidemiology, Vol.7, pp. 274-282.

Puertes-Fernández, N; Montiel-Company, JM; Almerich-Silla, JM; Manzanera, D. (2010). Orthodontic treatment need in a 12-year-old population in the Western Sahara. European Journal of Orthodontics, 2010 Oct 6.

Quigley GA, Hein JW. (1962). Comparative cleansing efficiency of manual and power brushing. Journal of American Dental Associan, Vol.65, pp. 26-9.

Richmond, S. (1990). A critical evaluation of orthodontic treatment in the General Dental Services of England and Wales, PhD thesis. University of Manchester 1990.

Richmond, S; Shaw, WC; O'Brien. KD; Buchanan, IB; Jones, R; Stephens, CD; Roberts, CT; Andrews, M. (1992a). The development of the PAR Index (Peer Assessment Rating): reliability and validity. European Journal of Orthodontics, Vol.14, pp. 125-139.

Richmond, S; O'Brien, K; Buchanan, I; Burden, D. (1992b). An Introduction to occlusal indices, Mandent Press, Victoria University of Manchester, Manchester, UK.

Richmond, S; Shaw, WC; Stephens, CD; Webb, WG; Roberts, CT; Andrews, M. (1993). Orthodontics in the General Dental Service of England and Wales: A critical assessment of standards. British Dental Journal, Vol.174, pp. 315-329.

Richmond, S; Buchanan, IB; Burden, DJ; O'Brien, KD; Andrews, M; Roberts, CT; Turbill, EA. (1995). Calibration of dentists in the use of occlusal indices. Community Dentistry and Oral Epidemiology, Vol.23, pp. 173-176.

Richmond, S; O'Brien, K. (1996). Health gain in orthodontics: a comparison of the general dental services and the hospital service in England and Wales. Community Dental Health, Vol.13, pp. 128-132.

Richmond, S; Daniels, CP; Fox, NA; Wright, J. (1997). The professional perception of orthodontic treatment complexity. British Dental Journal, Vol.183, pp. 365-370.

Richmond, S; Daniels, CP. (1998a). International comparisons of professional assessments in orthodontics: Part 1--Treatment need. American Journal of Orthodontics and Dentofacial Orthopedics, Vol.113, pp. 180-185.

Richmond, S; Daniels, CP. (1998b). International comparisons of professional assessments in orthodontics: Part 2--treatment outcome. American Journal of Orthodontics and Dentofacial Orthopedics, Vol.113, pp. 324-328.

Richmond, S; Aylott, NAS; Panahei, ME ; Rolfe, B ; Harzer, W ; Tausche, E. (2001). A 2-centre comparison of orthodontists' perceptions of orthodontic treatment difficulty. Angle Orthodontist, Vol.71, pp. 404-410

Richmond, S; Dunstan, F; Daniels, C; Durning, P; Leahy, F. (2005). Measuring the cost, effectiveness and cost effectiveness of orthodontic care. World Journal of Orthodontics, Vol.6, pp. 161-170.

Salzmann, JA. (1968). Handicapping malocclusion assessment to establish treatment priority. American Journal of Orthodontics, Vol.54, pp. 749-765.

Savastano, NJ Jr; Firestone, AR; Beck, FM; Vig, KW. (2003). Validation of the complexity and treatment outcome components of the index of complexity, outcome, and need (ICON). American Journal of Orthodontics and Dentofacial Orthopedics, Vol.124, pp. 244-248.

SBU. (2005) The Swedish council on technology assessment in health care. malocclusions and orthodontic treatment in a health perspective.

Shaw, W; Richmond, S; O'Brien, K; Brook, P; Stephens, C. (1991). Quality control in orthodontics: indices of treatment need and treatment standards. British Dental Journal, Vol.170, pp. 107-112.

Shaw, WC; Richmond, S.; O'Brien, KD (1995). The use of occlusal indices: a European perspective. American Journal of Orthodontics and Dentofacial Orthopedics, Vol.107, pp.1-10.

Silness, J; Löe, H. (1964). Periodontal Disease in Pregnancy II. Correlation between Oral Hygiene and Periodontal Condition. Acta Odontologica Scandinavica, Vol.22, pp.121-135.

Spencer, AJ; Allister, JH; Brennan, DS. (1992). Utility of the Dental Aesthetic Index as an Orthodontic Screening Tool in Australia. Adelaide, University of Adelaide, Australia.

Summers, CJ. (1971). The occlusal index: a system for identifying and scoring occlusal disorders. American Journal of Orthodontics, Vol.59, pp. 552-567.

Swedish Medical Health Board. (1966). Socialstyrelsen Kungl Medicinalstyrelsens circular den 21 februari 1966 angående anvisningarna för journalföring inom folktandvårdens tandregleringsvård. Stockholm.

Tang, EL; Wei, SH. (1993). Recording and measuring malocclusion: a review of the literature. American Journal of Orthodontics and Dentofacial Orthopedics, Vol.103, pp. 344-351.

Theis, JE; Huang, GJ; King, GJ; Omnell, ML. (2005). Eligibility for publicly funded orthodontic treatment determined by the handicapping labiolingual deviation index. American Journal of Orthodontics and Dentofacial Orthopedics, Vol.128, pp. 708-715.

Van Kirk, LK and Pennell, EH. (1959). Assessment of malocclusion in population groups. American Journal of Orthodontics, Vol. 45, pp. 752-758.

Younis, JW; Vig, KW; Rinchuse, DJ; Weyant, RJ. (1997). A validation study of three indexes of orthodontic treatment need in the United States. Community Dentistry and Oral Epidemiology, Vol.25, pp. 358-362.

10

Orthodontic Retreatment: Dental Trauma and Root Resorption

Pedro Marcelo Tondelli, Fabiana Akemy Kay,
Osmar Aparecido Cuoghi and Marcos Rogério de Mendonça
Dental School of Araçatuba, UNESP – Universidade Estadual Paulista
Brazil

1. Introduction

This chapter describes aspects related to orthodontic retreatment, care and control of root resorption. A clinical case is presented to illustrate the control forces on the teeth allows to perform orthodontic treatment in cases where a large root resorption for tooth movement associated with dental trauma.

Even though both Dentistry and Orthodontics have presented continuous improvement, when one or more teeth are submitted to a dental trauma, the treatment of malocclusion can be completely altered (Malmgren & Malmgren, 2007). Previous detailed evaluation of the root morphology, at the beginning of the orthodontic treatment, is a requirement emphasized by Levander & Malmgren (1988). These authors advised a through examination of the root outline, observing the occurrence of any root resorptions, surface concavities and malformations, since teeth with these characteristics may be severely reabsorbed during treatment. When facing evident root resorptions, the treatment purposes must be reviewed (Malmgren et al., 1982).

However, dental movement on traumatized teeth still receives inadequate attention by the specialized literature. Examining the related literature, many different publications about the topic can be found which do not contribute to the development of a safe protocol for clinical procedures. Kindelan et al., 2008, published a review about dental trauma and its influence on the management of orthodontic treatment, contributing with the currently best evidence on the topic. Recently, a research with questionnaires showed that about 40% of orthodontists were not acquainted with the recommendations for the orthodontic movement of traumatized teeth (Tondelli et al., 2010).

2. Dental trauma and orthodontics

Dentoalveolar trauma represents an emerging public health problem. Traumatic injuries to one or more teeth can alter remarkably an ongoing or planned orthodontic treatment. The clinical protocols for traumatized teeth are still uncertain, which increases the risks associated to orthodontic mechanics and influences directly the prognosis. In patients with trauma to the oral region, an appropriate treatment plan after the injury is mandatory for a good prognosis. For dentists and health care providers, knowledge and skills to manage cases of dentoalveolar trauma allied to a sound clinical judgment dictated by the conditions of a given traumatic situation are key factors for delivering the best care possible with more predictable outcomes (Andreasen, Andreasen & Andersson, 2007).

People of all ages and types of malocclusions can suffer traumatic dental injuries, but children and preadolescents are the most frequently affected groups. Increased overjet is a risk factor for dentoalveolar trauma. This risk is 2-fold higher in individuals with 3 to 6 mm overjet and 3-fold higher in individuals with >6 mm overjet (Andreasen, Andreasen & Andersson, 2007).

Maxillary incisor exposure and lack of lip seal predispose to traumatic injuries to the anterior oral region, with boys being affected twice as often as girls (Andreasen, Andreasen & Andersson, 2007). These characteristics are present in most patients that seek for orthodontic treatment. Information collected from clinical interview, clinical examination and radiographs are of great value for establishing an accurate diagnosis and case prognosis. In some cases, history of dentoalveolar trauma is not reported by patients or parents/caregivers, evolving to sequelae, such as root resorption or ankylosis, which may alter completely the treatment plan or even result in major damage to the patient, leading to legal proceedings or lawsuit.

It is imperative that all patients be questioned about any previous dental trauma prior to commencing on a course of orthodontic treatment. This will allow the orthodontist to anticipate any potential complications which may occur and to carefully monitor the traumatized tooth during orthodontic movement (Kindelan et al., 2008).

The relevance of this topic increases when the professional faces a traumatized tooth during the orthodontic treatment, a fact which may change the initial planning completely. Based on literature data, before undergoing orthodontic movement, a repairing period of 3 to 5 months is recommended for slight dental traumas such as concussion and subluxation, to repair the cement layer affected (Kindelan et al., 2008; Malmgren & Malmgren, 2007).

In a severe trauma such as luxation, a period of 6 months to 1 year is recommended. In root fractured teeth, the recommended period is of 1 to 2 years and in reimplanted teeth at least 1 year (Kindelan et al., 2008; Malmgren & Malmgren, 2007).

When a root fracture is detected, the repairing may be provided through a fusion of the fractured segment, and the tooth remains in its original size, or through interposition of conjunctive tissue between the fragments. In both cases, the teeth could be moved after a repairing period of 1 to 2 years, though, with the fragment separation, the movement would occur upon a tooth with a shorter root (Kindelan et al., 2008; Malmgren & Malmgren, 2007).

A trimestrial radiographic control of the traumatized teeth was suggested, analyzing root resorptions, the root outline and surface concavity. When a minimal root resorption is detected during the orthodontic treatment, there is low risk of severe resorption in these teeth, however, in greater resorption, treatment should be interrupted and the possibility of discontinuity or limitation of procedures taken into account. Inflammatory root resorption may be radiographically detected within 3 weeks after its initial and ankylosis within the period of 2 months to 1 year (Brezniak & Wasserstein, 1993a; 1993b; Malmgren & Malmgren, 2007).

One of the protocols for intrusive luxation treatment includes the extrusive orthodontic movement to traumatic tooth repositioning (Turley, Joiner & Hellstrom, 1984; Turley, Crawford & Carrington, 1987). In cases of intrusive luxations of about 3mm and the teeth present open apexes, it is possible to await spontaneous eruption, in case this does not happen, orthodontic repositioning is indicated, observing the pulp vitality (Kinirons, 1998). In teeth with complete root formation, the surgical or orthodontic repositioning must be adopted as soon as possible, together with the endodontic treatment with calcium hydroxide, otherwise the dental pulp will become necrotic (Malmgren & Malmgren, 2007). When traumatically intruded teeth don't present mobility, surgical luxation, previously to orthodontic extrusion, would be helpful to enable the movement, without compromising anchorage units, and promote their intrusion (Turley, Joiner & Hellstrom, 1984; Turley, Crawford & Carrington, 1987).

The ankylosis results from severe periodontal injuries, mainly as a result of an intrusion or avulsion. It can also develop following inflammatory resorption where the damage to the cementum has resulted in a defect beyond the critical size for healing by favourable healing. In these situations the root will slowly be replaced by bone, governed by the age of the patient and speed of bone turnover, and eventually lost (Day et al., 2008; Malmgren & Malmgren, 2007). There are different treatment options like periodontal regeneration, surgical repositioning, distraction osteogenesis, build-up to the incisal level, extraction and decoronation (Day et al., 2008).

Bauss et al. (2008) have conclude that previously traumatized maxillary incisors, and especially lateral incisors, with severe periodontal injuries have higher susceptibility to pulp necrosis during orthodontic intrusion than nontraumatized teeth.

Some of the sequels which may occur due to dental trauma are: ankylosis, external root resorption, pulp necrosis, pulp obliteration, marginal bone loss, alveolar fracture, crown fracture, root fracture, concussion, subluxation, luxation, avulsion (Kindelan et al., 2008; Malmgren & Malmgren, 2007; Turley, Joiner & Hellstrom, 1984; Turley, Crawford & Carrington, 1987)

According to Malmgren et al. (2007), there is no single explanation for the reasons that lead to the occurrence of root resorption, but dentoalveolar trauma is always implicated as an etiological factor. The authors refer to dental trauma as a predisposing condition to root resorption, which may be exacerbated by the orthodontic treatment.

A literature review was not the scope of this paper, but to focus the current clinical evidence. A practical guide has been prepared summarizing the clinical and orthodontic protocols to be adopted by general dentists and orthodontists dealing with cases of dentoalveolar trauma in patients undergoing orthodontic care and patients with indication for further orthodontic therapy (Table 1).

Type of trauma	Clinical and radiographic findings	Clinical protocol	Orthodontic protocol	Source of information (#Reference)
Concussion	The tooth has increased sensitivity to percussion without increased mobility or displacement. No radiographic abnormalities are observed	Monitoring of pulpal condition for at least 1 year	Wait 3-5 months to start orthodontic movement, maintaining radiographic control during 1 year after trauma. Use of mild and intermittent forces	Brezniak & Wasserstein, 1993a; 1993b; Kindelan et al., 2008; Malmgren & Malmgren, 2007

Type of trauma	Clinical and radiographic findings	Clinical protocol	Orthodontic protocol	Source of information (#Reference)
Subluxation	The tooth has increased sensitivity to percussion with increased mobility. Bleeding from gingival crevice may be noted. No radiographic abnormalities are observed	Stabilization of the tooth with a flexible splint for 2 weeks. Monitoring of pulpal condition for at least 1 year	Wait 3-5 months to start the orthodontic movement, maintaining radiographic control during 1 year after trauma. Use of mild and intermittent forces	Brezniak & Wasserstein, 1993a; 1993b; Kindelan et al., 2008; Malmgren & Malmgren, 2007
Extrusive luxation	The tooth appears elongated and is excessively mobile. Pulp revascularization may occur, especially in immature teeth. Radiographic examination reveals increased periodontal ligament space apically	Gentle repositioning of the tooth into its socket, stabilization of the tooth for 2 weeks using a flexible splint, monitoring of pulpal condition and radiographic control for 5 years.	Wait at least 6 months to start the orthodontic movement. Radiographic control should be performed every 3 months throughout the orthodontic treatment. Use of mild and intermittent forces. The orthodontic treatment should be simplified if necessary.	Brezniak & Wasserstein, 1993a; 1993b; Kindelan et al., 2008; Malmgren & Malmgren, 2007
Lateral Luxation	The tooth is buccally or lingually/palatally displaced, is immobile, and percussion gives a metallic sound. Pulp revascularization may occur, especially in immature teeth. The periodontal ligament space is widened in an occlusal radiographic view.	Gentle repositioning of the tooth, stabilization of the tooth for 4 weeks using a flexible splint, monitoring of pulpal condition and radiographic control for 5 years.	Wait at least 6 months to start the orthodontic movement. Radiographic control should be performed every 3 months throughout the orthodontic treatment. Use of mild and intermittent forces. The orthodontic treatment should be simplified if necessary.	Brezniak & Wasserstein, 1993a; 1993b; Kindelan et al., 2008; Malmgren & Malmgren, 2007

Type of trauma	Clinical and radiographic findings	Clinical protocol	Orthodontic protocol	Source of information (#Reference)
Intrusive Luxation	The tooth is displaced axially into the alveolar bone, is immobile, and percussion gives a metallic sound. Pulp revascularization may occur in immature teeth, while pulp necrosis is expected in teeth with fully developed roots. Radiographically, the periodontal ligament space may be either completely or partially absent	Watchful waiting for spontaneous re-eruption during 3 weeks is indicated only for immature teeth with intrusion ≤3 mm. Cases of intrusion >3mm and ≤ 6 mm may be treated by orthodontic repositioning, while surgical repositioning is recommended for teeth with intrusion >6 mm. Monitoring of pulpal condition and radiographic control should be performed for at least 5 years.	After spontaneous eruption, orthodontic repositioning or surgical repositioning, wait at least 6 months to start orthodontic movement. Radiographic control should be performed every 3 months throughout the orthodontic treatment. Use of mild and intermittent forces. The orthodontic treatment should be simplified if necessary.	Brezniak & Wasserstein, 1993a; 1993b; Day et al., 2008; Kindelan et al., 2008; Kinirons, 1998; Malmgren & Malmgren, 2007
Avulsion	Complete displacement of the tooth from its socket	Tooth replantation is the treatment of choice, but the prognosis depends on the measures taken at the site of accident, tooth storage conditions, alveolar wound care and extra-alveolar time elapsed before replantation. Immobilization for 2 weeks, monitoring of the pulpal conditions and radiographic control for 5 years. Prescription of de antibiotics and anti-tetanic vaccination	If normal periodontal conditions are observed, wait at least 1 year to start the orthodontic movement. Radiographic control should be performed every 3 months throughout the orthodontic treatment. Use of mild and intermittent forces. The orthodontic treatment should be simplified if necessary.	Brezniak & Wasserstein, 1993a; 1993b; Kindelan et al., 2008; Malmgren & Malmgren, 2007

Table 1. Clinical and orthodontic protocols face dentoalveolar trauma

3. Clinical considerations about orthodontic retreatment, root resorption and force control

When the objectives of orthodontic treatment are not met, or if recidivism occurs, orthodontic retreatment can be indicated since the teeth, bone tissues and periodontium are healthy. So, a previous detailed evaluation of the root morphology is recommended, examination of the root outline, observing the occurrence of any root resorptions, surface concavities and malformations, since teeth with these characteristics may be severely reabsorbed during treatment (Levander & Malmgren, 1988).

The presence of limited resorption at the root apex does not contra-indicate orthodontic retreatment. However, care must be taken such that there is no continuation of the resorption and, consequently, commitment to long-term support for the tooth. The literature shows that resorptions larger than 4mm are considered severe and require greater control and care. This "severity" may reflect the degree of root structure loss, compared with other cases of apical root resorption, but cannot be termed "severe" in terms of threatening tooth longevity. The apical root resorption is less critical in terms of periodontal support than is crestal bone loss (Vlaskalic, Boyd & Baumrind, 1998).

After detecting resorption, a three-month period of radiographic control is indicated for repair of the tissues. The control of stress, or even of the forces acting on the teeth, becomes fundamental to avoid or reduce the continuation of root resorption. In orthodontic treatment, this control can be achieved through the amount of force applied, by the type of movement, and by the type of force.

The amount of force must be smooth, and induce movement of the teeth. More important than the amount is the distribution of force in the periodontal ligament and in the root surfaces. This must avoid concentrating the force in small areas of the ligament, as occurs in the inclined movements in the cervical and apical regions. Alignment and leveling of the teeth must be done in a controlled way, observing the periods recognized as favorable for cellular reorganization. It should be noted that the installation of rectangular wires to control torque provides a distribution of force or stress over a larger area of the periodontal ligament and root surface.

During the movement of the teeth, interruption of the force, for dissipation of stress in the ligament and recovery of the tissues, is important for maintaining the vitality of the tissues and preventing root resorption. One study about types of forces - continuous, continuous-interrupted and intermittent - during the movement of the teeth, showed this to be more important than the intensity of the force. (Van Leeuwen, Malta & Kuijipers-Jagtman, 1999). The interruption or removal of force permits repair of the periodontal ligament and faster elimination of hyaline areas (Proffit & Fields, 1993). In 2003, Weiland found that by using super-elastic wires that apply continuous force and, thus, without interrupting the stress, the possibility of root resorption is 140% greater than with steel wires that permit interruption of force, thus making tissue repair possible. It was concluded that magnitude of force, as a single factor, is probably not decisive for root resorption. The combination of magnitude of force and duration of application, however, appears to be a key factor (Weiland, 2006).

Independent of the type of alloy that constitutes the various types of wires or springs used to move the teeth, what is important is to promote an interruption of the force to obtain better tissue repair. Figures 1 and 2 show that continuous force has a greater potential for forming hyaline areas when compared with continuous-interrupted force, after 5 days of

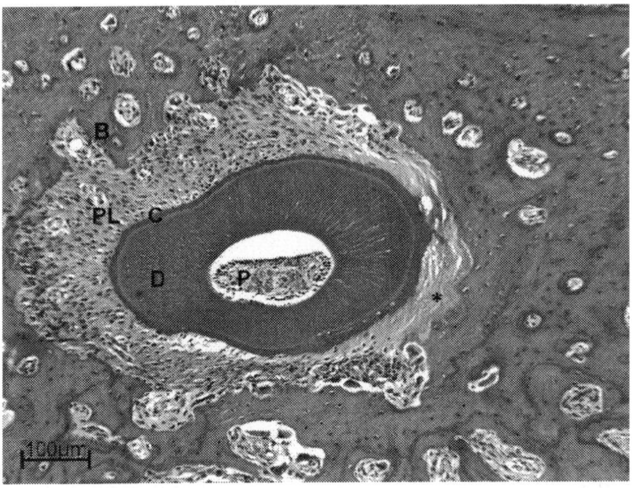

Fig. 1. Intermediate root of the 1st superior molar of the wistar rat, submitted to movement of the teeth for 5 days with continuous force, showing extensive hyaline area (*). Alveolar bone (B), periodontal ligament (PL), cementum (C) and dentin (D)

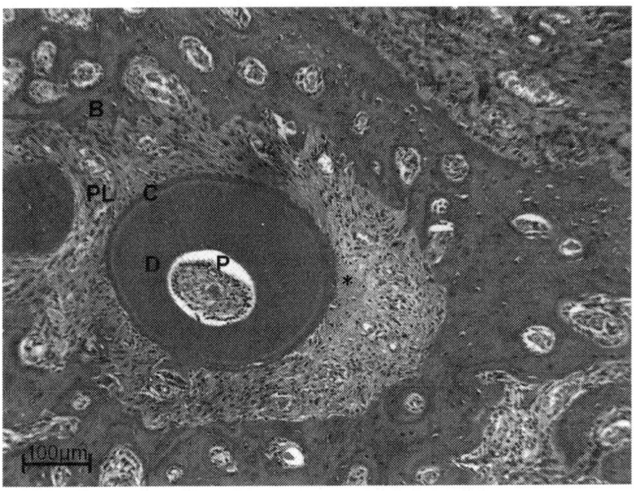

Fig. 2. Intermediate root of the 1st superior molar of the wistar rat, submitted to movement of the teeth for 5 days with continuous-interrupted force, showing moderate hyaline areas (*). Alveolar bone (B), periodontal ligament (PL), cementum (C) and dentin (D)

movement in the teeth of rats (Tondelli, 2011). The presence of smaller hyaline areas, through the use of continuous-interrupted force, shows that the repair period supports the more satisfactory elimination of hyaline areas. Additionally, the greater number of hyaline areas, using continuous force without interruption, confirms the occurrence of a greater period of stress in the periodontal ligament, resulting in greater potential for root resorption. In this way, the interruption of force could be recommended to reduce or prevent the continuation of resorptions.

4. Case report

A female patient presented a malocclusion of angle's class II division 2 subdivision left, agenesis of upper lateral incisors and second premolars. The patient had had prior orthodontic treatment, but was dissatisfied with the outcome which had been interrupted by the large root resorption of the incisors.
The radiographic analysis and clinical examination showed ankylosis in the lower left first molar and root resorption of the anterior teeth (Fig.3).

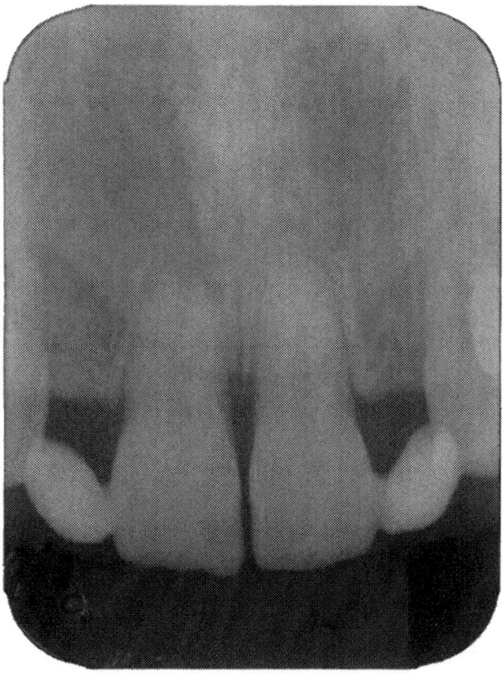

Fig. 3. Inicial radiographic

The space of the upper lateral incisors was not sufficient to place implants, but the space of the second lower right premolar was good for implant placement. The space of the second left premolar was closed (Fig. 4).
The patient reported that during treatment she suffered a trauma to the anterior teeth; she was hit by volleyball, and did not report it to the orthodontist. Also, she reported that the teeth were very sensitive for several days, sometimes for more than one week, after activation of the device. Therefore, root resorption may be due to excessive force, with or without dental trauma.

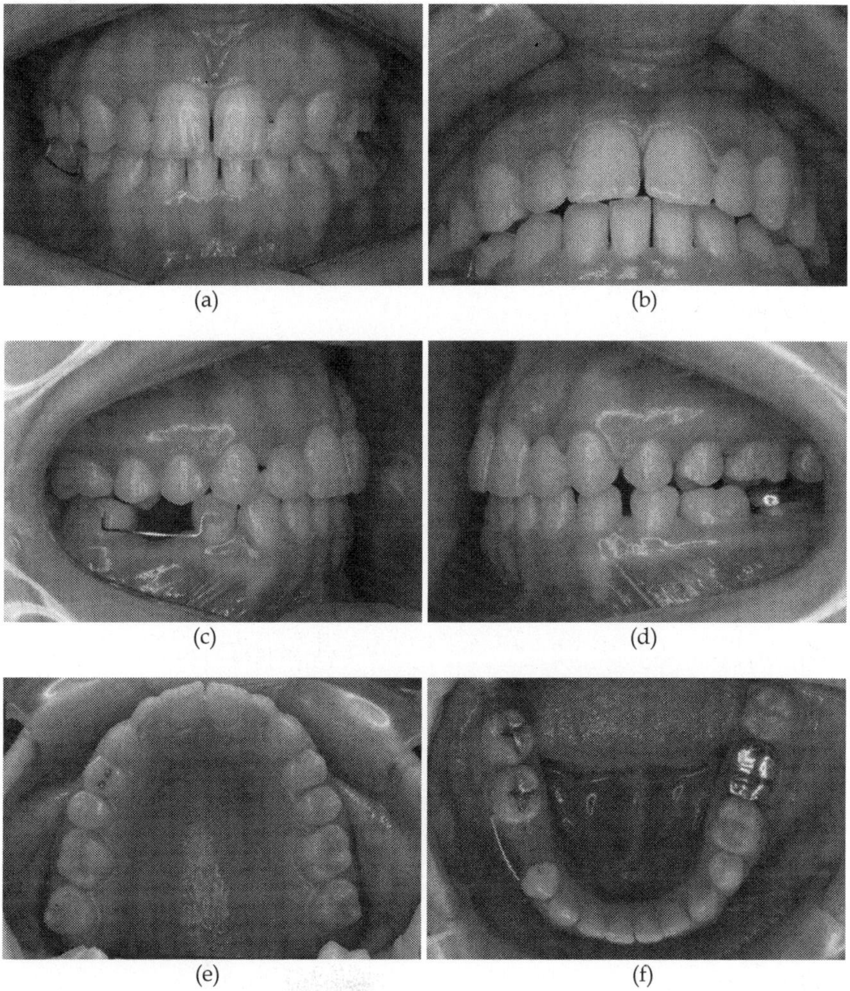

Fig. 4. Inicial photographics (a-f)

This way, to get a normal relationship of the canines, good occlusion, and to make space for installation of implants in maxillary lateral incisors, it was proposed that the first left upper premolar be extracted.

With straight-wire brackets we followed the alignment and leveling, with light force, until the steel wire "019x025". The first left upper premolar was extracted and distalization of the upper left canine was initiated.

Interrupted light forces were used to enable the repair of tissues, thus reducing the chances of root resorption by concentrating stress on the periodontal ligament. For this, the steel wires were replaced only when they were passive, when they could be inserted or removed easily, without pressure in the slots.

The elastic chain was measured to produce a maximum 100cN of force on the upper left canine. The elastic chain has the characteristic of losing strength after a few days, allowing the periodontal repair. NiTi springs were used to move the maxillary incisors and to establish the correct space for the implants. The springs were cut only 0.5mm greater in length than the spaces between the brackets. Thus, the teeth were moved 0.5mm and stopped, thus allowing periodontal repair until the next activation, which was an average of every 30 days. One implant was installed on the second lower right premolar (Fig.5).

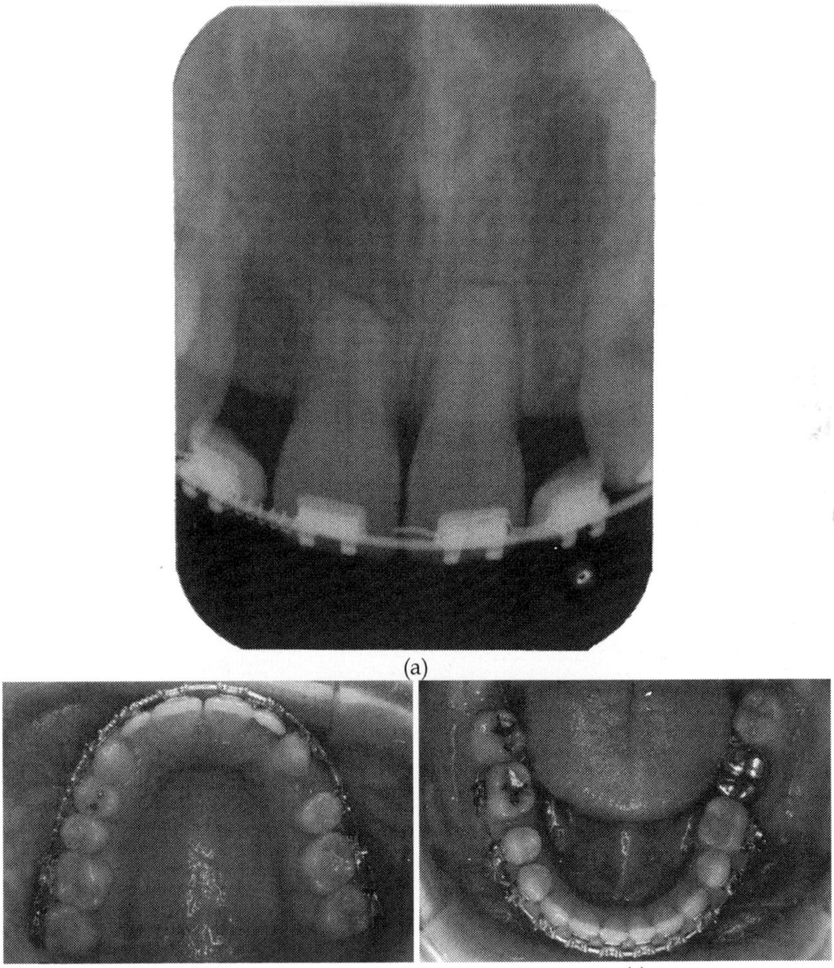

(a)

(b) (c)

Fig. 5. Radiographic image (a). Occlusal photographs showing the movement of upper incisors and left canine (b). Lower alignment with implant on second lower right premolar (c)

The implants on the lateral upper incisors were installed after the establishment of the spaces, with the aid of guides for correct positioning. The incision in the gum preserved the papillae to obtain a cosmetically better gum (Fig. 6).

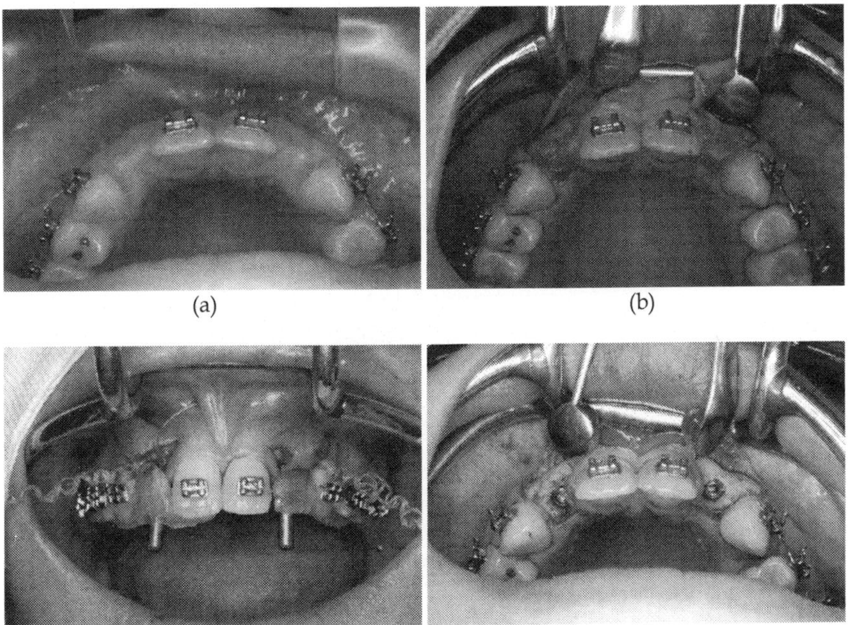

(a) (b) (c) (d)

Fig. 6. Established spaces (a). Opening of the gingival flap (b). Positioning of the guides for the installation of the implants (c). Installed implants (d)

After 5 months to allow osseointegration, the reopening of the implants was done with "H" incisions, to preserve the papillae and to achieve a better gingival contour (Fig. 7).

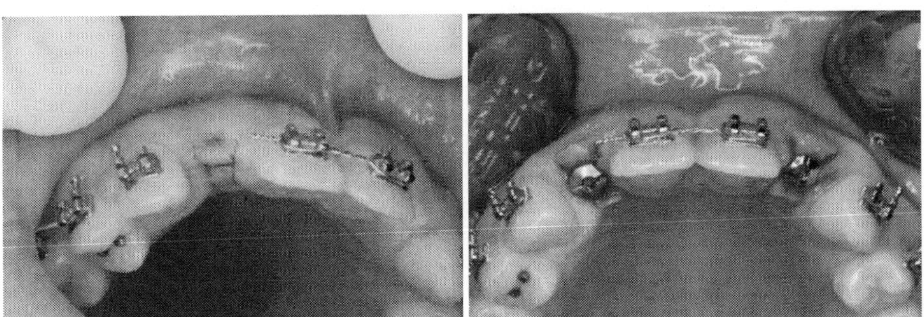

(a) (b)

Fig. 7. Reopening of the implants, preserving the papillae for better gingival esthetics (a, b)

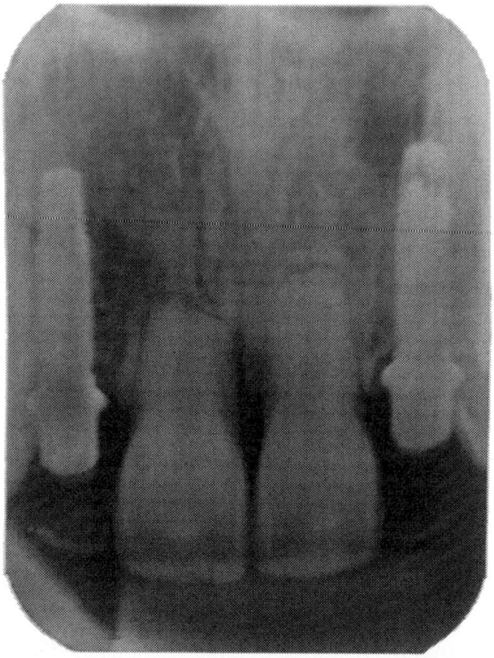

(a)

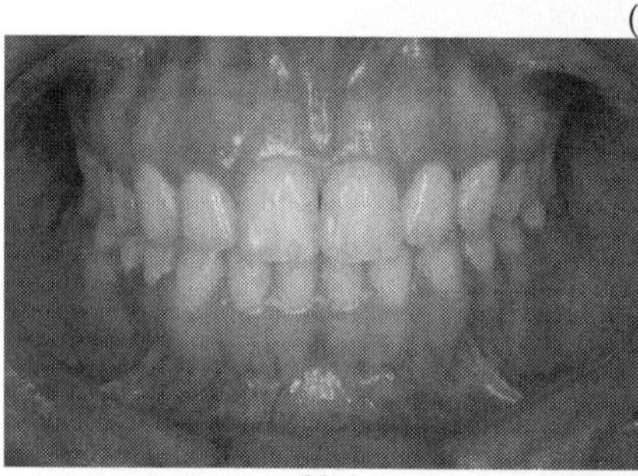

(b)

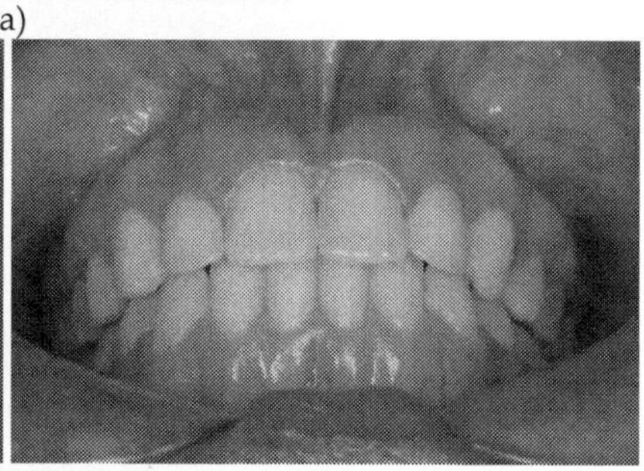

(c)

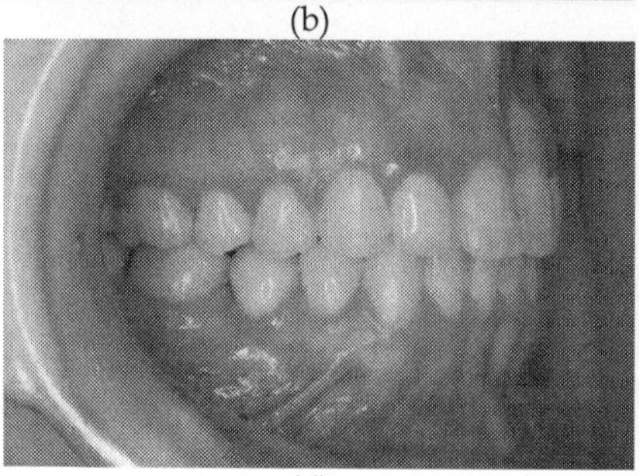

(d)

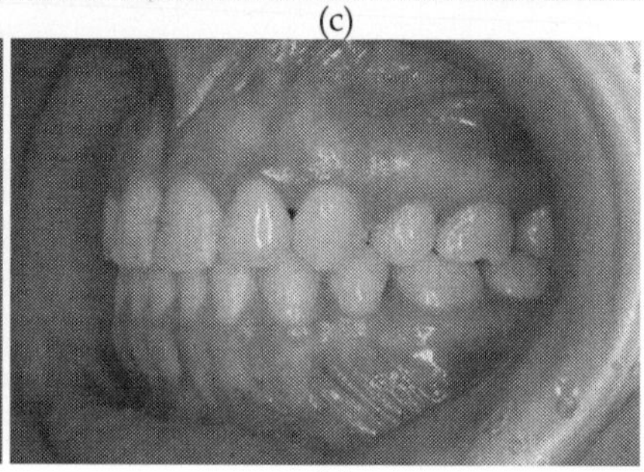

(e)

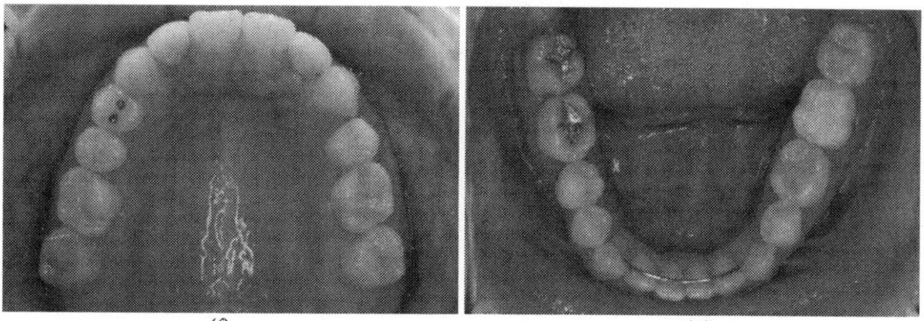

(f) (g)

Fig. 8. Final radiographic (a).Orthodontic retreatment with esthetic, stable and functional occlusion (b-g)

After 30 months of orthodontic retreatment, a stable and functional occlusion was obtained. The root resorption was controlled. The lower premolars were resized with light-cured resin (Fig. 8). Figure 9 shows the smile and facial harmony.

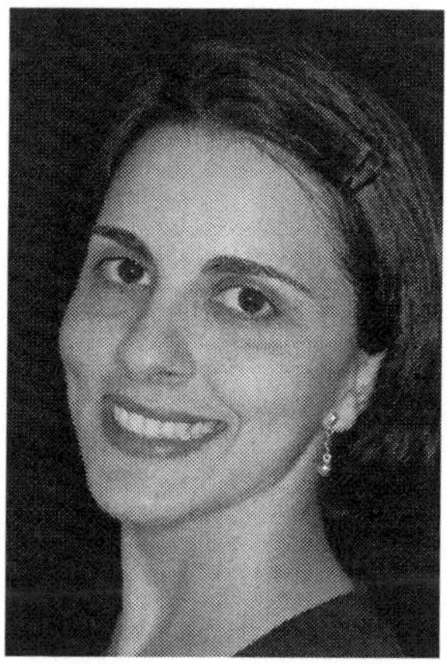

Fig. 9. Final facial photograph

5. Conclusion

In patients with trauma to the oral region, an appropriate treatment plan after the injury is mandatory for a good prognosis. The knowledge and skills to manage cases of dentoalveolar trauma, supplemented by sound clinical judgment, and guided by the conditions of a given traumatic situation, are key factors for delivering the best care possible with more predictable outcomes.

A period of repair or rest for the tissues is advised, after finding root resorptions or dental traumas. Movement of the teeth also requires these periods of repair for the complete dissipation of stress in the ligament, and the recovery of the tissues. This allows movement of the teeth with root resorption by trauma or previous orthodontic treatment.

6. References

Andreasen, J.O., Andreasen, F.M. & Andersson L. (2007). *Textbook and Color Atlas of Traumatic Injuries to the Teeth*, 4th ed. Oxford: Blackwell Munksgaard.

Bauss, O., Röhling, J., Sadat-Khonsari, R. & Kiliaridisd, S. (2008). Influence of orthodontic intrusion on pulpal vitality of previously traumatized maxillary permanent incisors. *Am J Orthod Dentofacial Orthop* 134:12-7.

Brezniak, N. & Wasserstein, A. (1993). Root resorption after orthodontic treatment: Part 1. Literature review. *Am J Orthod Dentofacial Orthop* 103:62-6 (a).

Brezniak, N. & Wasserstein, A. (1993). Root resorption after orthodontic treatment: Part 2. Literature review. *Am J Orthod Dentofacial Orthop* 103:138-46 (b).

Day, P.F., Kindelan, S.A., Spencer, J.R., Kindelan, J.D. & Duggal, M.S. (2008). Dental trauma: Part 2. Managing poor prognosis anterior teeth - treatment options for the subsequent space in a growing patient. *J Orthod* 35:144-55.

Kindelan, S.A., Day, P.F., Kindelan, J.D., Spencer, J.R. & Duggal, M.S. (2008). Dental trauma: an overview of its influence on the management of orthodontic treatment. Part 1. *J Orthod* 35:68–78.

Kinirons, M.J. (1998). Treatment of traumatically intruded permanent incisor teeth in children. *Int J Paediat Dent* 8:165-8.

Levander, E. & Malmgren, O. (1988). Evaluation of the risk of root resorption during orthodontic treatment: a study of upper incisors. *Eur J Orthod* 10(1):30-8.

Malmgren, O., Goldson, L., Hill, C., Orwin, A., Petrini, L. & Lundberg, M. (1982). Root resorption after orthodontic treatment of traumatized teeth. *Am J Orthod* 82(6):487-91.

Malmgren, O. & Malmgren, B. (2007). Orthodontic management of the traumatized teeth. *In*: Andreasen, J.O., Andreasen, F.M. & Andersson, L., editors. *Textbook and color atlas of traumatic injuries to the teeth*. 4th ed. Oxford: Blackwell Munksgaard; 2007. pp. 699-715.

Proffit, R.W. & Fields, H.W.J. (1993). *Contemporary Orthodontics*. 2 ed. St. Louis: Ed. Mosby.

Tondelli, P.M., Mendonça, M.R., Cuoghi, O.A., Pereira, A.L.P. & Busato, M.C.A. (2010). Knowledge on dental trauma and orthodontic tooth movement held by a group of orthodontists. *Braz Oral Res* 24(1):76-82.

Tondelli, P.M. (2011). *Avaliação histomorfométrica da movimentação dentária induzida em ratos com força contínua, contínua interrompida e intermitente*. [Tese]. Araçatuba: Univesidade Estadual Paulista - UNESP.

Turley, P.K., Joiner, M.W. & Hellstrom, S. (1984). The effect of orthodontic extrusion on traumatically intruded teeth. *Am J Orthod* 85:47-56.

Turley, P.K., Crawford, L.B. & Carrington, K.W. (1987). Traumatically intruded teeth. *Angle Orthod* 57:234-44.

Van Leeuwen, E.J., Malta, J.C. & Kuijipers-Jagtman, A.M. (1999). Tooth movement with light continuous and discontinuous forces in beagle dogs. *Eur J Oral Scien* 107;468-74.

Vlaskalic, V., Boyd, R.L. & Baumrind, S. (1998). Etiology and Sequelae of Root Resorption. *Semin Orthod* 4(2):124-131

Weiland, F. (2003). Constant versus dissipating forces in orthodontics: the effect on initial tooth movement and root resorption. *Eur J Orthod* 25;335-42.

Weiland, F. (2006). External root resorptions and orthodontic forces: correlations and clinical consequences. *Prog Orthod* 7(2):156-63.

11

Early Treatments in Orthodontics

Ousehal Lahcen and Lazrak Laila
Department of Orthodontics, Faculty of Dentistry, Casablanca
Morocco

1. Introduction

It is said that Chinese physicians were paid only so long as their patients were in good health. Such an approach to healthcare lent physicians an incentive to develop preventive therapy to ensure their patients remained healthy.

Medicine in the 21st century strives to be preventive first and foremost, and so preventive and interceptive treatments hold once more an important place in the armamentarium of modern medicine. Dentistry and orthodontics are no exception to this rule.

Even so, current orthodontic practice still comprises two schools: some orthodontists favour early treatment before the permanent teeth have erupted, while others refuse this approach, to which they are radically opposed.

We consider that initiating early treatment is reasonable and eminently logical, because is allows partial or even total correction of an evolving orthodontic anomaly in a growing child. Such early therapy is often brief, uses simple means, elicits little cooperation from patients and their parents and prevents the anomaly from worsening. In defence of this approach GUGINO (1998) pointed out that the earlier the treatment was applied, the better the face adapted to it, whereas the longer it was deferred, the more it would have to adapt to the face.

Since then the orthodontic literature has abounded with reports on early orthodontic treatment: major orthodonticians who have advocated early orthodontic treatment include RICKETTS, GUGINO, MCNAMARA, DALE, FRANKEL, DELAIRE, GRABER, PHILLIPE, LANGLADE and BENCH.

However, we stress that early treatment is no simpler: on the contrary, it has to be based an overall analysis of the patient's condition, and so requires thorough knowledge of human growth, the physiology of the orofacial functions, the morphogenesis of the dental arches and child psychology. These basic considerations will help the practitioner choose the right therapy at the right time, thereby avoiding prolonged therapeutic efforts that are tiring for both children and their parents and discouraging for the practitioner.

Early treatments often fail to remedy anomalies entirely, but they greatly simplify subsequent orthodontic treatment. Children and their parents can thus expect a two-stage treatment.

The purpose of this chapter is to describe the early interceptive approach to different orthodontic anomalies. We will deal with the early treatment of dentomaxillary disharmonies, anterior open bites, Class II abnormalities and skeletal Class III abnormalities. We will illustrate our presentation with clinical examples.

2. Definitions and terminology

McNamara defines early treatments in orthodontics as therapeutic procedures undertaken on deciduous or mixed dentition for the purpose of preventing, intercepting or correcting a specific orthodontic problem.
Some define early treatment in orthodontics as removable or fixed appliance intervention in the primary, early mixed (permanent first molars and incisors present), or midmixed(inter-transitional period, before, before the emergence of first premolars and permanent mandibular canines).
Others define them as late-mixed dentition stage treatment (before the emergence of second premolars and permanent maxillary canines). (Ghafari and al 1998)
The American Association of Orthodontists' Council of Orthodontic Education defines *interceptive orthodontics* as "that phase of the science and art of orthodontics employed to recognize and eliminate potential irregularities and malpositions in the developing dentofacial complex." Orthodontics: Council on Orthodontic Education. St Louis;AAO:1971.

3. Objectives of early orthodontic treatment

Early orthodontic treatment aims to:

- Establish correct occlusion in both deciduous and permanent dentition (interceptive guidance of occlusion);
- Correct or reduce vertical or anteroposterior skeletal discrepancies ;
- Correct transverse asymmetry ;
- Favour the child's psychosocial integration;
- Forestall risk of tooth damage due to malocclusion (trauma, periodontal problems, etc.).

4. Advantages and disadvantages of early treatment

The workshop discussions on early orthodontic treatment, held by the american board of orthodontics in 1977, indicated that most participants considered early interventions as viable option in many malocclusions cases. Early treatment is suggested to bring about many benefits including better use of the patient growth potential, reduced need of extractions and orthognathic surgery, less risk for adverse iatrogenic effects, better patient compliance, and better and more stable results (KESKI-NISULA and al 2003)
The disadvantages of this approach are increased cost and duration of overall patient care, increased risk of caries and fatigue in both child and parents.

5. Early interceptive therapy

5.1 Early treatment of dental crowding

Crowding is often a sign of dentomaxillary disharmony (DMD).
This is defined as a misfit of the arch perimeter and the dental volume, which can be due to relative microdontia, with arch diastemas, or by relative macrodontia, causing arch crowding.
The early treatment of DMD due to relative macrodontia can be either preventive or interceptive. The preventive approach consists in ensuring that no arch space is lost. The deciduous dentition must thus be conserved, and if a milk tooth is lost, the space must be kept open by a fixed or removable device (Cases 1 and 2). If several deciduous teeth are lost,

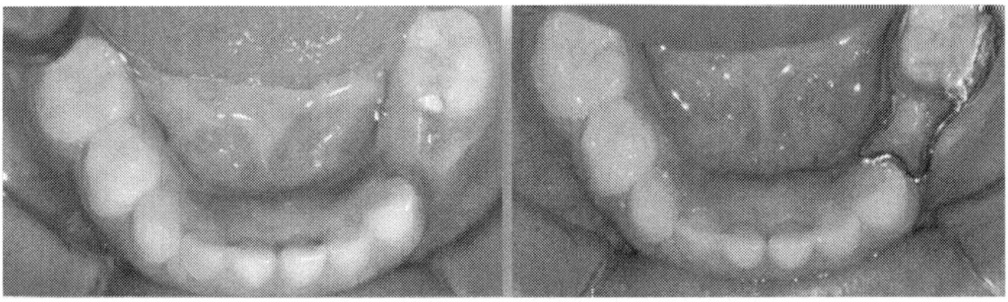

Case 1. Unilatéral space maintainer

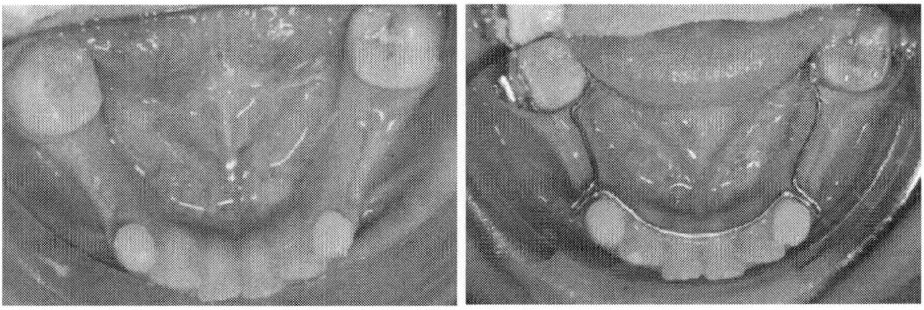

Case 2. Bilateral space maintainer

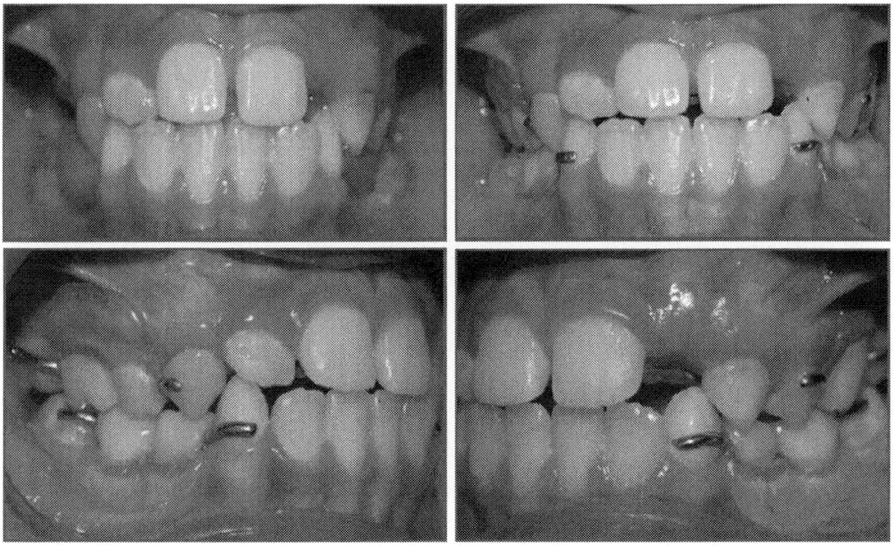

Case 3. Maintaining space by a removable paedodontic appliance

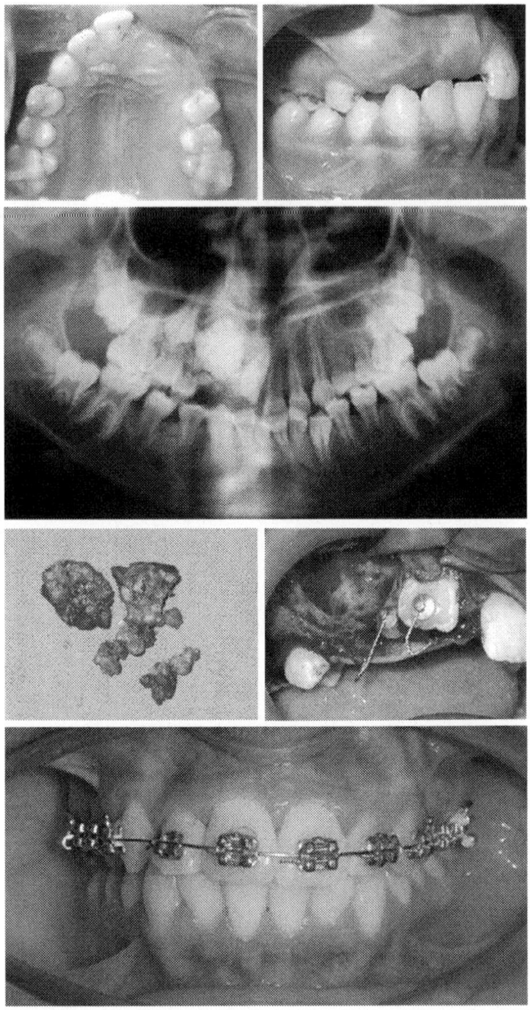

Case 4. Early treatment of the inclusion of teeth 11,12 and 13 due to dontoid formations

a paedodontic appliance will restore appearance and masticatory function, while retaining the space for the permanent teeth (Case 3)

If supernumerary teeth or odontoid formations are present, blocking the eruption of permanent teeth, they can be removed surgically as a preventive measure against crowding of permanent dentition (Case 4 and 5).

The interceptive approach will depend on the degree of crowding.

If the crowding is less than 6 mm, a transverse or anterioposterior arch expansion is indicated, to increase the arch perimeter and so prepare enough space to accommodate the permanent teeth (Case 6).

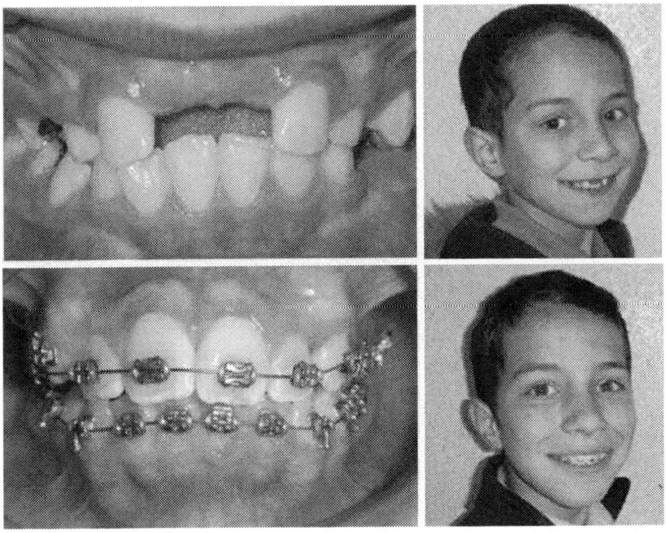

Case 5. Early treatment of the inclusion of 11 and 21

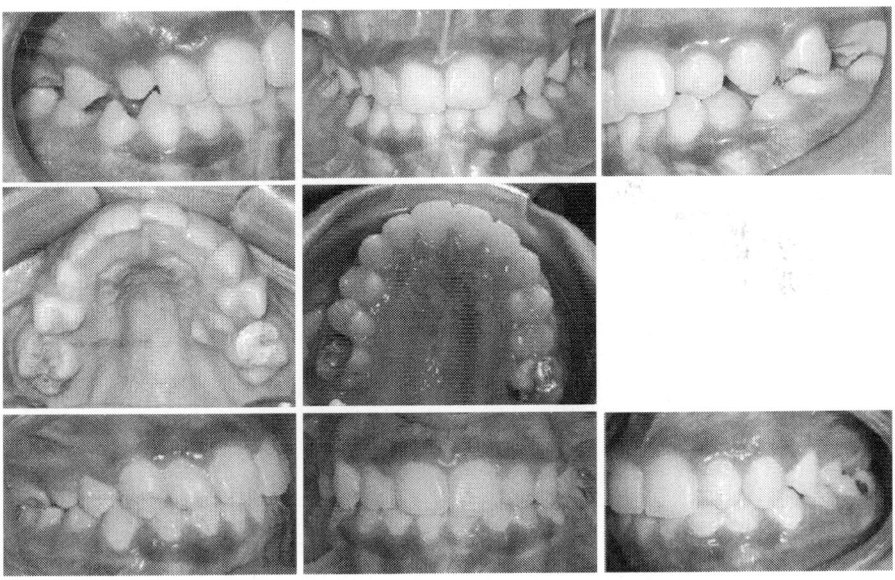

Case 6. Early treatment of lateral DMD bydistalization of maxillary molars

If the DMD exceeds 7 mm, the interceptive approach of choice remains programmed extraction, also still called serial extractions or interceptive guidance of occlusion (J DALE) (Cases 7 and 8)

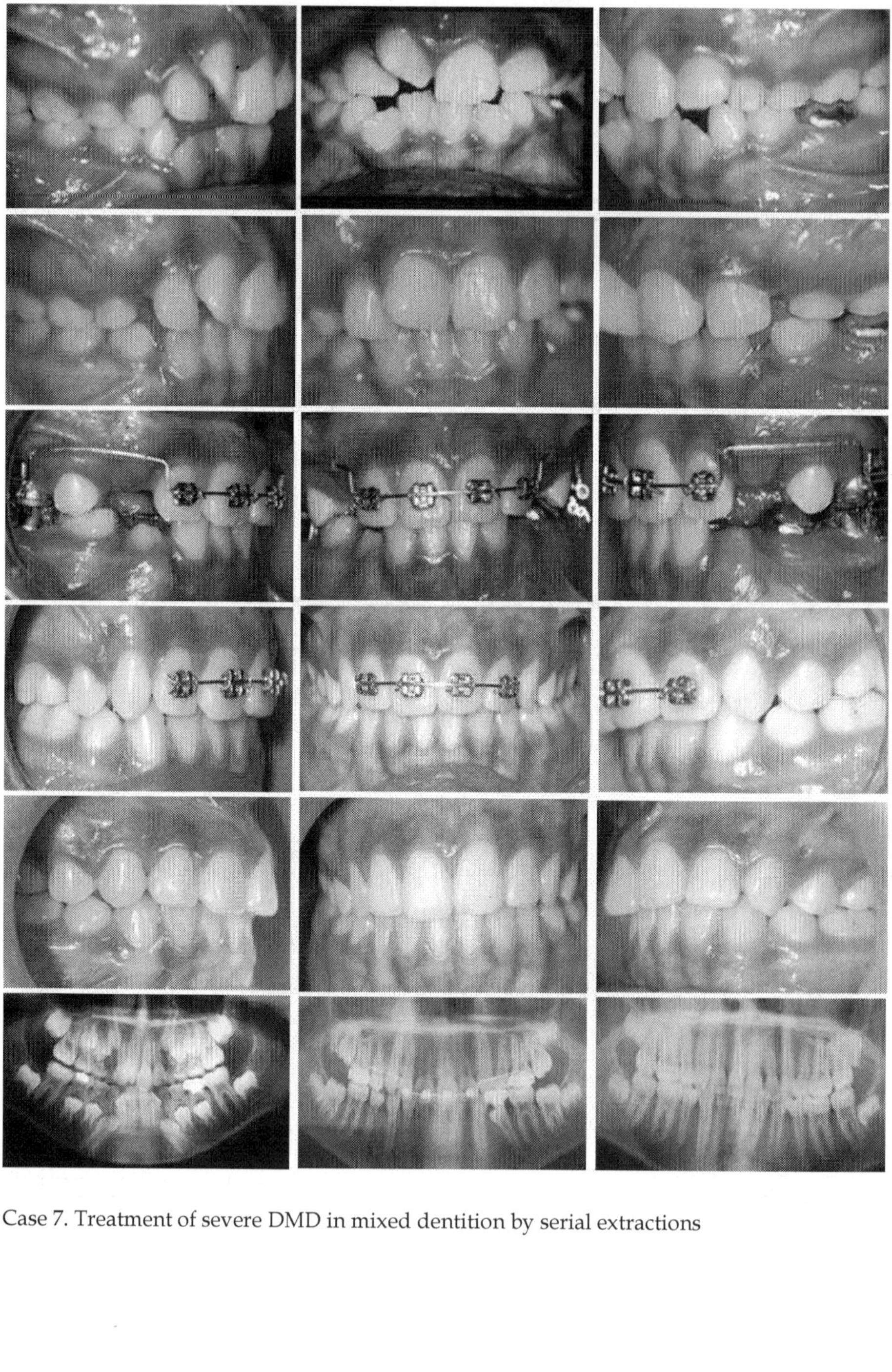

Case 7. Treatment of severe DMD in mixed dentition by serial extractions

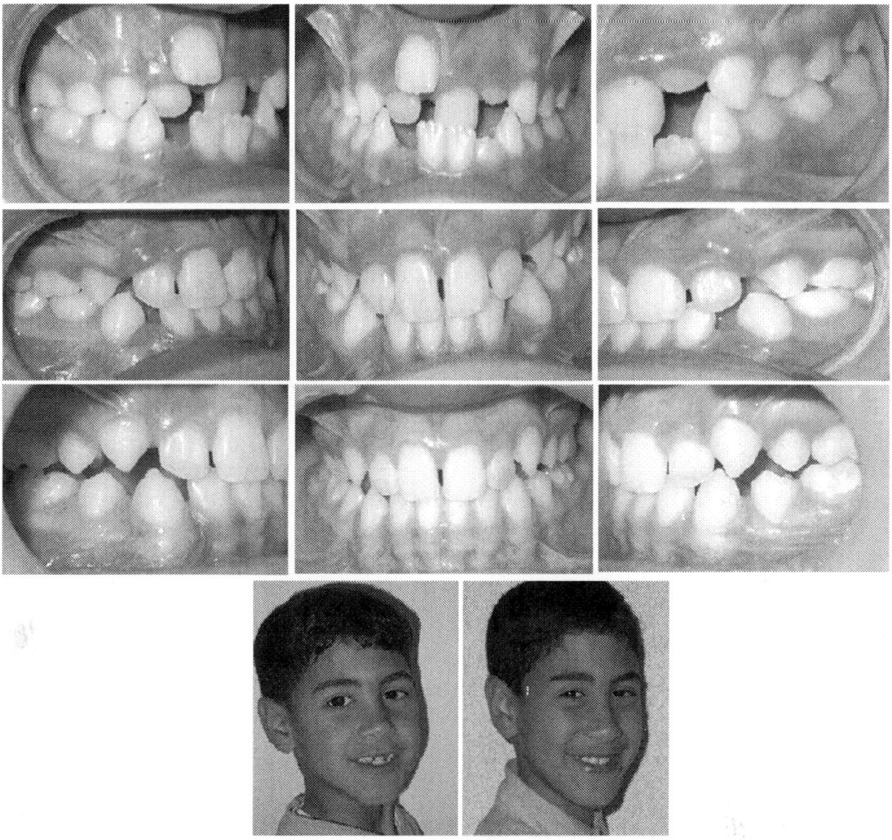

Case 8. Treatment of severe DMD in mixed dentition by serial extractions

ROBERT BUNON in "Essay on the Diseases of the Teeth," published as long ago as 1743 (1 in serial 13) was the first to describe these, but it was HOTZ (18 in serial 8) and KELLEGREEN (19 in serial 8) who first published the protocol, defined by DALE as interceptive guidance of occlusion.

Thus HOTZ, in a case of severe crowding in mixed dentition in a child with a favourable facial pattern, advocated extracting the deciduous canines at age 8 years, the first deciduous molars 6 months later, and then extracting the first premolars which have erupted. The aim is to make room for the permanent canines.

GRABER (1971) emphasised the fact that serial extractions are an orthodontic act and so must result from a precise diagnosis of the abnormality, which implies sound scientific knowledge and adequate clinical experience.

On programmed extractions, Dale (2000) wrote:

"Serial extraction ... nobody does that anymore! That was the comment that was made to me recently by an orthodontic educator. General practitioners are doing it, paediatric dentists are doing it, and if orthodontists are not doing it they are missing out, their patients are missing out, and ... so is orthodontics. Serial extraction is an excellent treatment procedure! It can reduce appliance treatment time, the cost of treatment, discomfort to patients, and time lost by both the patients and their parents. It is logical to intercept a malocclusion as early as possible, and to reduce, or in rare instances, to avoid multibanded, multibracket mechanotherapy at the sensitive teenage period".

The protocol often requires a multibracket treatment to complete it, but this is greatly simplified and of greatly shortened duration. This argues in favour of serial extractions, which thus reduce the overall cost of orthodontic treatment in children.

LITTLE et al. (1990) showed that cases treated by serial extraction were more stable in the long term as regards incisor alignment than cases treated later with extraction of four premolars and a conventional full brace treatment.

Similarly, PERSON et al. (1989) studied the stability of incisor alignment 30 years after treatment by comparing a sample of 42 cases treated by serial extraction and another sample of 29 untreated cases. He found no significant difference between the two groups.

5.2 Early therapy for transverse abnormalities

These abnormalities are the result of in sufficient or excessive transverse development of the basal bone or the alveolar arch. They can be maxillary or mandibular. Special attention must be paid to the mandibular lateral deviation caused by the maxillary transverse deficit (EGERMARK-ERIKSSON et al. 1990, KUROL & BERGLUND 1992).

This functional lateral deviation will be responsible for craniomandibular disorders: electromyographic studies have shown that the activity of temporal and masseter muscles is disturbed in children with a posterior crossbite (TROESTRUP B &MÖLLER 1970, INGERVALL & THILANDER 1975).

Other studies have shown that adolescents and adults presenting a posterior crossbite are more likely to develop cranio-mandibulaire disorders. If untreated, this lateral deviation can evolve with growth into a true laterognathy. This orthodontic abnormality is difficult to treat, often requiring orthognathic surgery in adulthood (PROFFIT 2002, McNAMARA 2002), whence the utility of treating such abnormalites early on. We take the view that addressing these abnormalities is a true orthodontic emergency. Transverse abnormalities are most often secondary to some orofacial dysfunction, such as atypical swallowing, buccal resorption or thumbsucking (LARSSON 1968, LINDER-ARONSON 1970, BEHLFELT 1989). The first early act to be undertaken will be to re-educate these functions.

Maxillary expansion will thus be initiated as early as possible to re-centre the mandible and so rebalance facial growth (KUTIN & HAWES 1969, PROFFIT 2000, CLIFFORD 1971). This expansion can be achieved using a median screw expander (Case 10) or fixed appliances, of which the quad helix is the device of choice (Case 11 and 12). This expander is used specifically for basal maxillary insufficiency (endognathy). The purpose of the device is to expand the median palatine suture. One type can be inserted into attachments bonded or welded to molar or premolar bands. Once the disjunction is achieved the appliance must be held in place for several months until the median palatine suture has grown in.

The quad helix was designed by Ricketts. As its name suggests, it is a transpalatine arc made of .032 Blue Elgiloy with four loops to increase its elasticity. It can produce both an alveolar expansion and a slow maxillary disjunction.

Maxillary expansion frees the condyles of all strain due to a non-physiological occlusion in the maximum contact position secondary to a functional lateral mandibular deviation. It also allows improvement of breathing and correction of a Class 2 malocclusion by correcting the rotation of the maxillary molars.

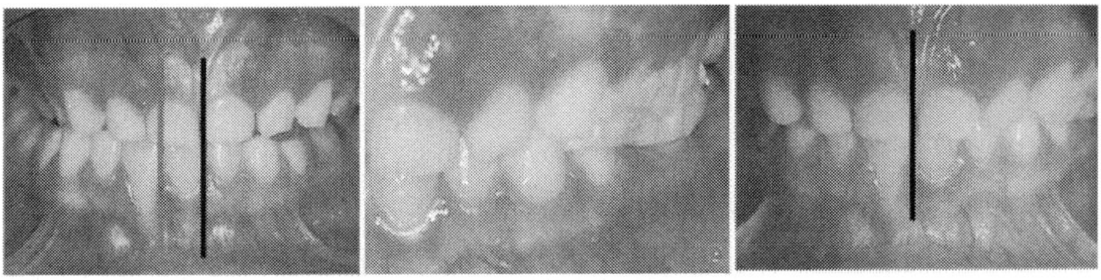

Case 9. Interceptive treatment of a right mandibular lateral deviation by resin direct tracks

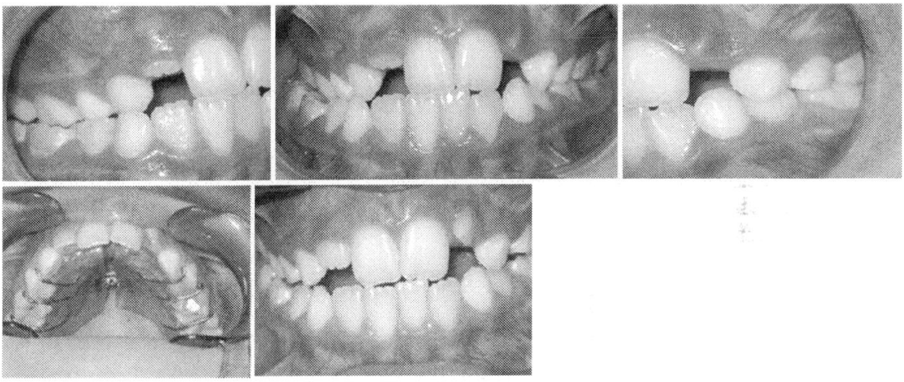

Case 10. Interceptive treatment of a mandibular lateral right deviation following a bilateral maxillary endoalveolitis by maxillary expansion using a median screw expander

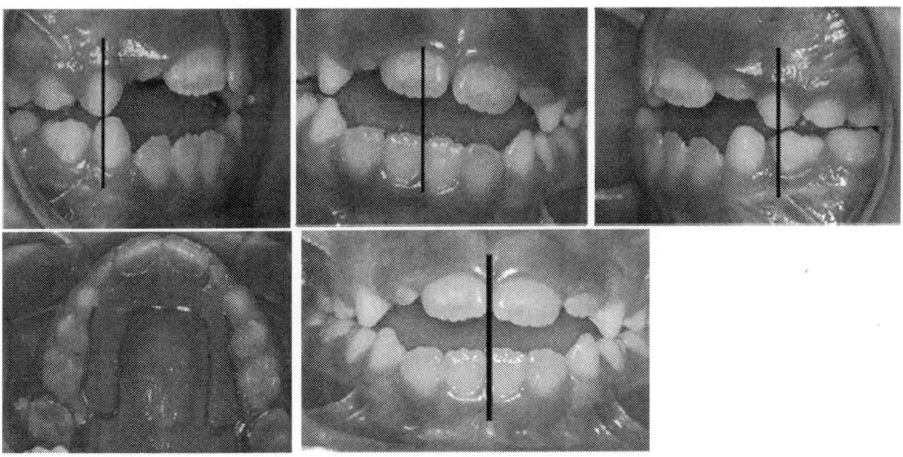

Case 11. Interceptive treatment of a mandibular lateral right deviation following a bilateral maxillary endoalveolitis by maxillary expansion using a quad helix

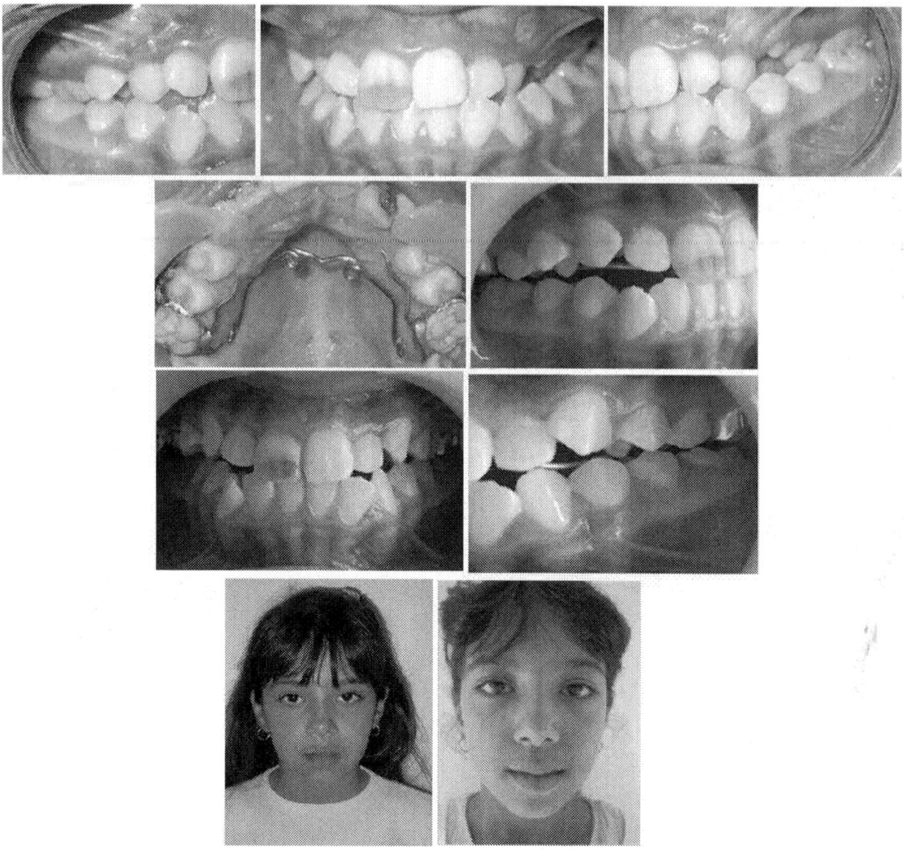

Case 12. Interceptive treatment of a mandibular lateral right deviation following a bilateral maxillary endoalveolitis by maxillary expansion using a quad helix

5.3 Early treatment of anterior open bites

These disorders are defined as an insufficient vertical development of the anterior alveolar processes (SUBTENLY & SAKUDA 1964). KELLY et al. (1973) have reported a prevalence of 3.5% in Caucasian American children and 16.5% among Afro-Americans. PROFFIT et al. (1988) report a prevalence of approximately 3.5% in patients aged 8 to 17 years. Anterior open bites can be of skeletal origin, linked to a hyperdivergent facial typology (TOLLARO 1983, RICHARDSON 1981), but are often functional in origin. Mouth breathing, atypical swallowing by tongue-thrusting and thumbsucking are the main aetiologies (SASSOUNI 1969, NGAN 1997, TULLEY 1972, STRAUB 1962). Hence it is mandatory to correct these dysfunctions as early as possible to remove the obstacle to vertical alveolar growth: this sometimes leads to spontaneous correction of the gap (BASCIFTCI 2002). Lingual re-education will be both active, through swallowing exercises that the child will be asked to perform regularly, and passive, by the fitting of a tongue repositioning appliance

such as the nocturnal tongue envelope of BRUNO BONNET (Case 14) or a thumb guard to prevent thumbsucking (Case 15).
The planned outcome will be achieved in 4-8 months if the child cooperates.
A systematic review by PARLA COZZA et al. (2005) shows that early treatment of anterior gaps intercepts the malocclusion and reduces the need for treatment during adolescence (Case 13).

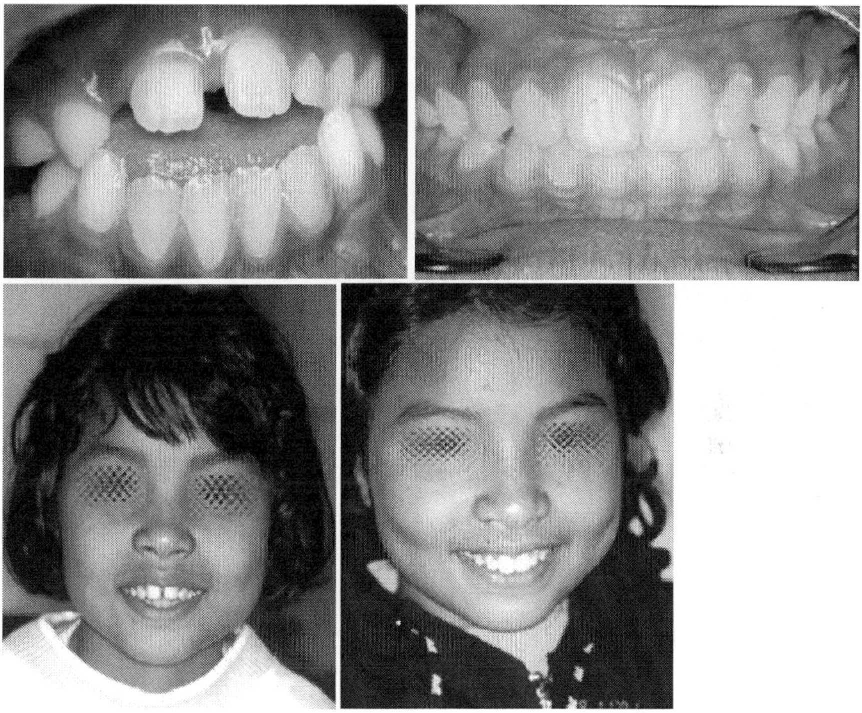

Case 13. Functional treatment of anterior open bite

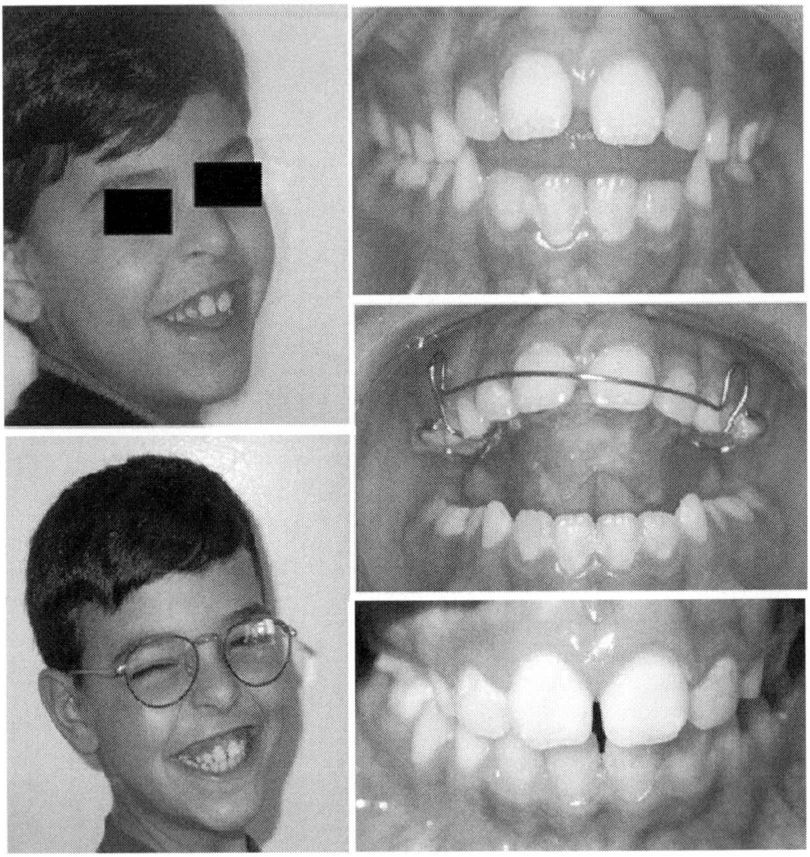

Case 14. Functional treatment of anterior open bite by the nocturnal tongue envelope

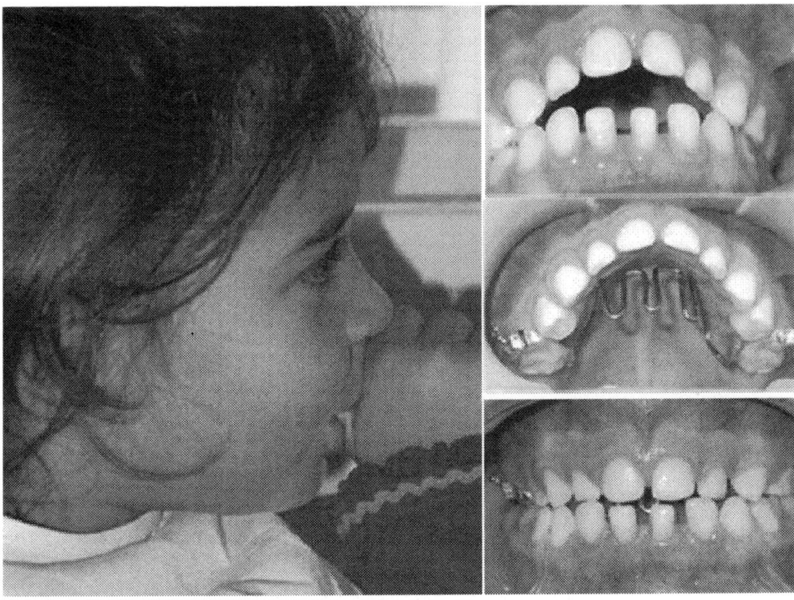

Case 15. Functional treatment of anterior open bite secondary to thumb sucking by a thumb guard

5.4 Early treatment of class II abnormalities

Skeletal Class II abnormalities are defined as those in which the maxilla is overhung relative to the mandible. They can be of maxillary, mandibular or mixed origin.

In children, Class II abnormalities are often due to locked mandibular growth. GUGINO describes three types of lock: functional, mechanical and psychological. Incisor overjet, a transverse deficit of the maxillary arch, and a distopalatine rotation of the maxillary molars are examples of mechanical locks that give the mandible a permanent retroposition.

It is thus important to remove these locks early on to permit free mandibular growth. This is the concept of unlocking developed by the bioprogressive school of Ricketts.

To address hereditary forms (maxillary overjet or mandibular underjet), early treatment consists is fitting an activator of mandibular growth sometimes associated with an extraoral force.

Two facts justify early care for Class II abnormalities. The first is that the tissues of the craniofacial complex tend to respond more readily in young subjects. The second is that young patients cooperate better than older ones (KING, 1989). Several studies have shown that the best age for patient cooperation is preadolescence (ELDER 1974, DROSCHL 1973).

For mixed dentition the correction of molar rotations will be performed using a quad helix or a palatine rod.

Incisor overbite can be reduced by a Ricketts basal arch. This is a device made of .016 × .016 Blue Elgiloy wire fixed to bands fitted on the first permanent molars and on brackets cemented to incisors (Cases 16 and 17).

There are several types of mandibular growth activators, e.g. ROBIN's monobloc, FRANKEL's function regulator, BALTERS' Bionator and the HERBST apparatus. All place the mandible in a propulsive position by activating the mandibular propulsors, and in particular the lateral pterygoid muscle. These form the functional matrix of the condylar cartilage, itself the main centre of mandibular growth, as shown by the work of MOSS and PETROVIC (Case 18).

However, this mandibular response secondary to the activators remains controversial: some see an orthopaedic effect, while others find merely an alveolodental effect. Animal trials have shown that extraoral forces (ELDER 1974, DROSCHL1973) and functional orthopaedic appliances (McNAMARA 1973, STOCKLI 1971) cause significant modifications to craniofacial growth. These findings are supported by others on humans using activators (DEMISCH 1972, FREUNTHALLER 1967) or FRANKEL's functional regulator (RIGHELLIS 1983, McNAMARA 1985), which have shown a significant increase in mandibular growth. Other clinical studies (BAUMRIND 1983, KING 1957) have shown that extraoral forces applied to the maxilla cause a slowing of maxillary forward growth. Other authors have even found extraoral forces to cause a rearward, downward repositioning of the maxillary complex (WATSON 1972,WIESLANDER 1963, POULTON 1967).

AMSTRONG (1971) has described a rapid correction of Class II abnormalities par light extraoral forces parallel to the occlusion plane in growing children. However, we must bear in mind that these skeletal effects are always accompanied by alveolodental effects. GIANELLY (38 in 5) concluded that the main alveolodental effect of Class II orthopaedic procedures was egression and distalisation of the maxillary molars and mesialisation of the mandibular dentition.

The benefits of early treatment of Class II abnormalities are numerous: e.g. the prevention of trauma to the maxillary incisors by overcorrection of overhang (KREIT 1968, O'MULLANE 1973), the interception of worsening malocclusion, and better psychological and social integration of the child. It has also been reported that the correction of Class II malocclusions improves orofacial functions (JANSON & HASUND 1981, WIGDOROWICS-MAKOWEROWA 1979).

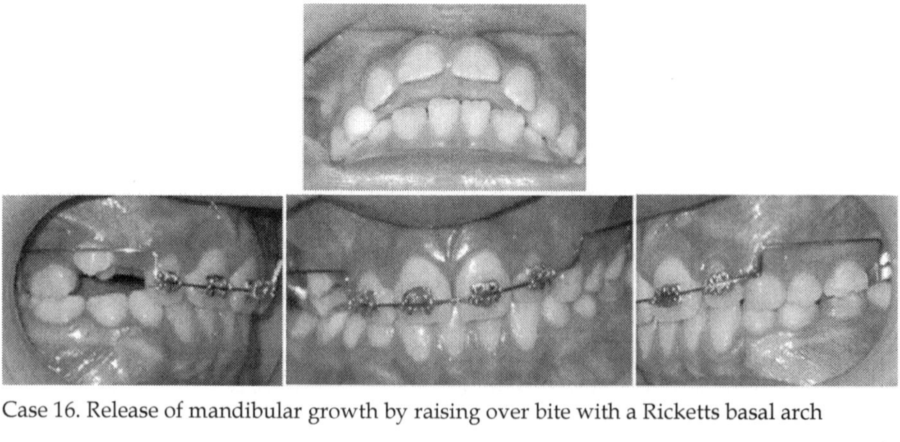

Case 16. Release of mandibular growth by raising over bite with a Ricketts basal arch

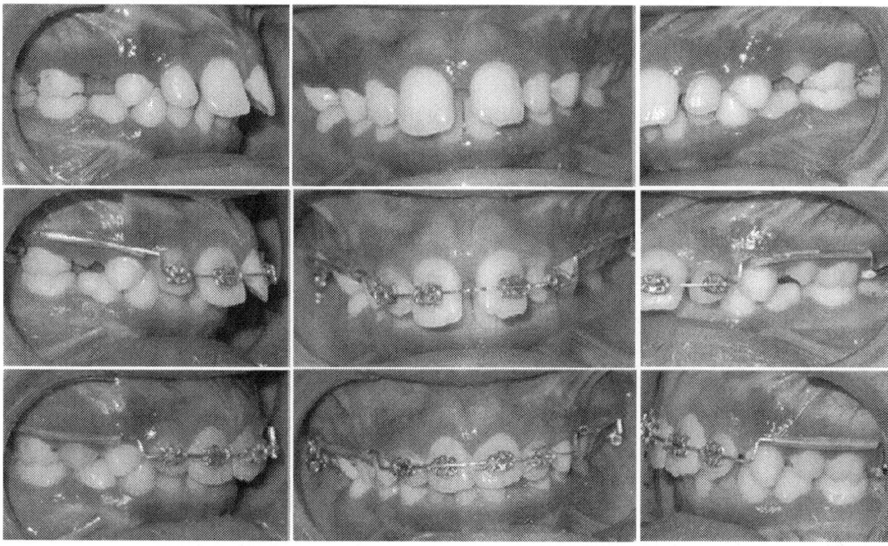

Case17. Ricketts basal arch as interceptive treatment of overbite

5.5 Early treatment of skeletal class III abnormalities

Class III malocclusions are syndromic: the discrepancy between the maxilla and the mandible has many anatomical expressions. The most frequent abnormality is maxillary retrognathy and not, as often thought, mandibular prognathy. There seems to be a consensus concerning the utility of early treatment of skeletal Class III disorders.

The treatment of Class III abnormalities is straightforward, and is more efficacious if applied early, on deciduous dentition before age 6 years. This therapy undertaken early induces a new maxillary growth. The maxilla, repositioned correctly, grows together with the mandible (KAPSUT 1998, MACNAMARA 1987, NGAN1998, TORRES 2000)

The work of DELAIRE and co-workers, initiated 30 years ago, has allowed great strides in the treatment of Class III malocclusions, in particular through the use of a facial mask. Today it is generally acknowledged that the treatment of Class III malocclusions should preferably be orthopaedic and early. The interceptive treatment should be applied as early as possible; the rate of mandibular growth is the factor that guides the choice of therapeutic procedures.

These early treatments are useful for the forward shift of the mandible through the elimination of its aetiology, which can be functional or occlusal. The correction of the anterior or lateral crossbite lies within the scope of interceptive treatment of mandibular forward shift. They are also useful for Class III malocclusions due to maxillary underjet. DELAIRE's face mask is the main appliance used.

5.5.1 Justification for early treatment of class III abnormalities

We know that one of the most important factors in maxillary growth is the mandibular stroke: it is this hammer and anvil movement that causes the maxilla to develop. If there is a

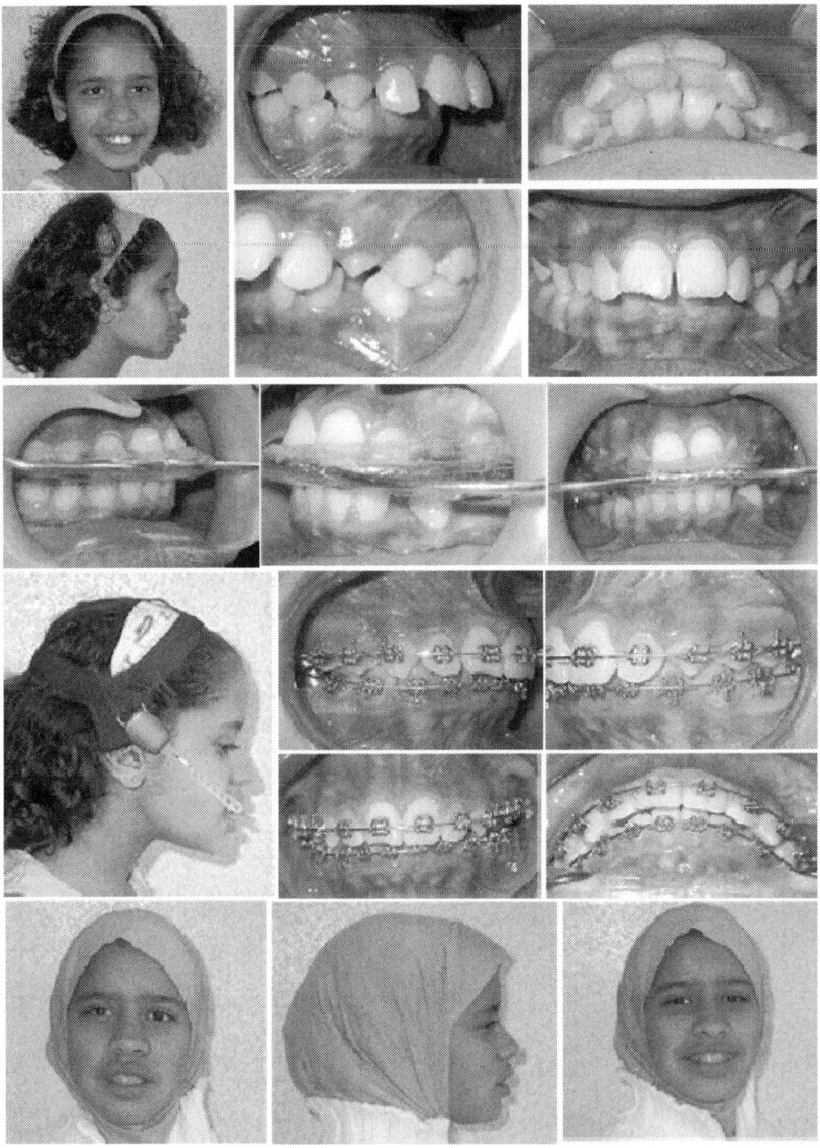

Case 18. Treatment in two phases of a skeletal Class II malocclusion

reversed incisor occlusion, then the maxillary growth is insufficiently elicited; the maxilla will stop growing while the mandible continues to develop regardless of the maxilla.

It is thus necessary to establish the secant function of the incisors. This normalisation enables lateral movements that restore masticatory function. In addition, the early intervention of the practitioner induces a change in the angulation of the base of the skull, increasing the sphenoid angle and developing the anterior frontal part. It is possible to bring forward the implantation of the upper end of the maxilla to some extent. This was demonstrated by both DELAIRE and DESHAYES.

MCNAMARA (1987) found the result to be "engrammed in the new growth". We believe this to be true insofar as the treatment is applied early. LOREILLE confirmed this, finding that it was clearly possible to act on the causes of a great many facial dysmorphisms, provided early treatment could act on the causes of impaired growth.

In the literature, all the authors who have shown an interest in the treatment of Class III disorders emphasise the importance of early treatment (SAKAMOTO 1981, SUGWARA 1990, GRABER & PROFITT 2007). MCNAMARA (1993) justifies early intervention with the orthopaedic mask by pointing out that as the patient is young, the results of the treatment by facial mask are subsequently incorporated in future growth. BACETTI (1998) et al. claim that early treatment is more efficacious when applied to deciduous than to mixed dentition. For DESHAYES, the best time to apply an orthopaedic treatment, with lasting results and no relapse, is while the telencephalon is still very actively growing (i.e. before age 6 years).

5.5.2 Preventive treatment

Functional re-education is the first interceptive preventive component of Class III malocclusions. It is necessary to re-educate breathing and tongue posture through active and passive re-education.

The tongue is not the only factor responsible for maxillary hypodevelopment, and re-habilitation of bilateral mastication has also to be integrated into the therapy. Professor Planas must have been the first to demonstrate that the narrowness of the maxilla, which favours unilateral mastication, has an influence not only on the maxilla but also on mandibular symmetry. Accordingly, selective impressions are made from the deciduous dentition: these impressions are used for selective guidance and unlocking, and give excellent results. For Planas, they form the basis of a neuro-occlusal rehabilitation therapy.

In Class III abnormalities of maxillary origin, maxillary retrognathy is often accompanied by endognathy. To address this, several appliances can be used such as the quad helix and the palatine expander. Disjunction in the transverse direction allows a widening of the bone base and the floor of the nasal cavity. It thus favours mouth breathing and pushes out the insertions the buccinator. In the anteroposterior direction the SNA angle is increased by 0-25°. In the vertical direction there is an upward movement of point N and a downward movement of points A and ENA.

The anteroposterior relations of the dental arches can also be corrected using Planas direct tracks, which allow an end-to-end occlusion to be obtained and all occlusal obstacles to be removed so that the mandible resumes it usual normal low amplitude excursions. Their action is based on the 'minimum height laws'. The tracks are inclined planes 4 mm wide located just on the lingual face of the dental arches, thus preventing tongue interposition.

A removable Hawley plate fitted with a simple cantilever spring made of 0.6 mm wire can be used to vestibulate the upper incisors. (Cases 19 and 21)

The anterior inclined plane: here is a resin or composite brace cemented to the lower incisors with a tooled inclined plane opposite the teeth in a reversed bite translating the muscle forces into mechanical forces to correct the bite. (Case 20)

Elastic bands for crossbite occlusion: they are used to displace the bite from one tooth or group of teeth. Multiband treatment can also be applied to vestibulate the upper incisors and so correct the incisor bite. (Case 22)

Two-band device: this is a bihelix acting on the sagittal plane to vestibulate the upper incisors, with two lateral loops. The opening of the loops causes a vestibular tilting of the upper incisors.
Occlusal elevator wedges: these are bonded onto the occlusal surfaces of the deciduous maxillary molars. The height of the composites is adjusted for centred occlusion and set so as to obtain an anterior occlusion of about 1 mm. The tongue, by centrifugal pressure, brings the incisors naturally into the correct position.

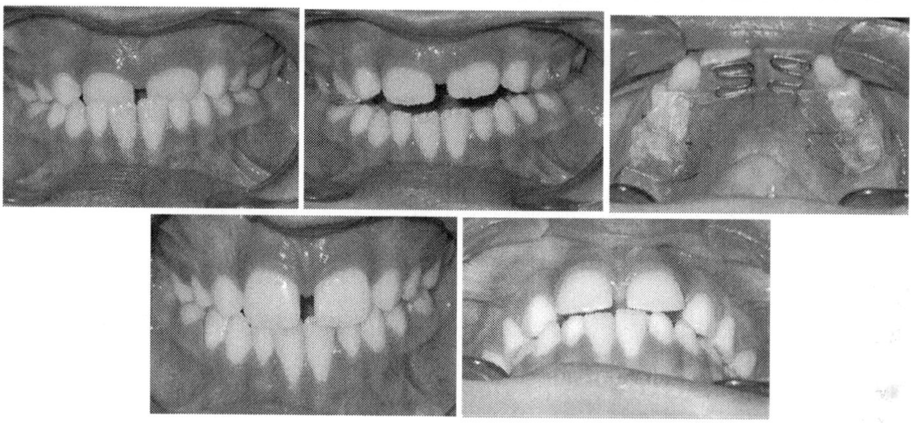

Case 19. Early correction of anterior crossbite with a removable Hawley plate fitted with a simple cantilever spring

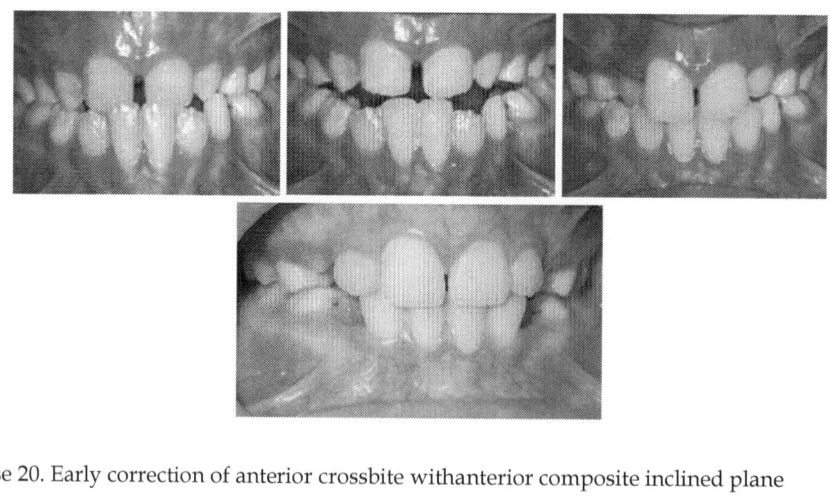

Case 20. Early correction of anterior crossbite withanterior composite inclined plane

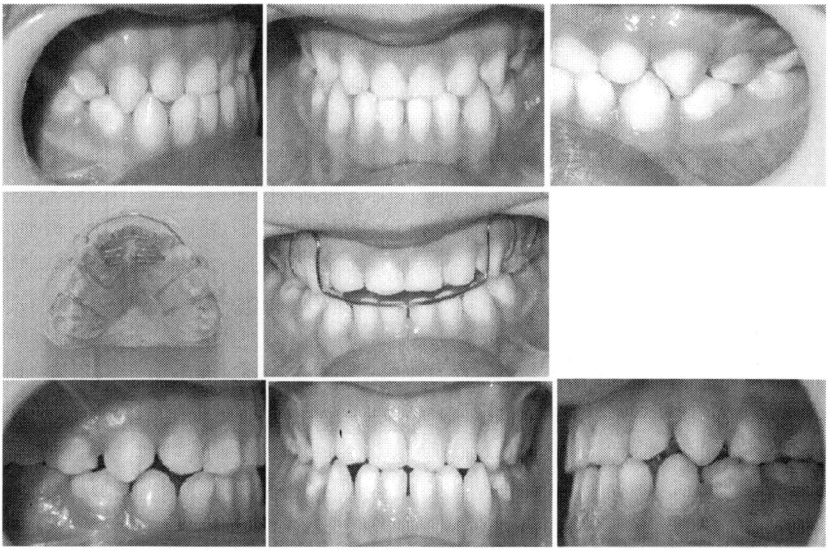

Case 21. Early correction of anterior crossbite with a removable Hawley plate fitted with a simple cantilever spring

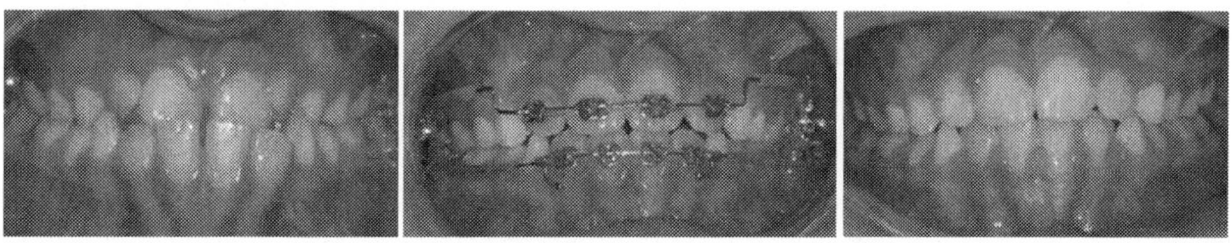

Case 22. Multiband treatment to vestibulate the upper incisors and to correct the incisor bite

5.5.3 Orthopaedic treatment of class III abnormalities

In the presence of a sagittal skeletal disharmony, only the orthopaedic approach will yield a satisfactory result that is stable in the long term. Successful use of maxillary protraction appliances in the treatment of skeletal Class III cases attributable to maxillary retrognathy has been reported in many studies.

DELAIRE's face mask (1971)

In most cases this is the therapy of choice for Class III disorders. The method was described by DELAIRE (1971) and thoroughly codified by Verdon and SALAGNAK.

A review of the different orthodontic textbooks: CHATEAU, BASSIGNY, MCNAMARA , PROFITT, GRABER, etc. confirms the utility of this therapy, while at the same time detailing the different indications.

The treatment consists in applying a posteroanterior orthopaedic force on an anterior facial location through elastic bands connected to an intrabuccal appliance (Cases 23, 24 and 25)

DELAIRE's face mask is composed of an external appliance and an intrabuccal device. There are several types of orthopaedic mask: the most classical type has a forehead support connected to a chincap by metal rods. At the level of the commissural line is welded a hoop to attach the elastic bands. If necessary, the forehead support can be custom-shaped to the child's forehead. Adolescents seem to prefer another type of protraction mask, the Petit model, which is less bulky with a mid-positioned bar, which replaces the support frame. The intrabuccal device can be either of the following:

- A double arch: this is made of two very stiff 10/10 arches welded onto two molar bands. The palatine arch is adjusted to the tooth necks. The vestibular arch must be placed at least 1 mm in front of the vestibular surface of the teeth to allow the premaxilla to expand.
- Plate or cemented brace: the cemented brace method described by Amoric has the advantage being rapid, given the removal of the occlusal interference, but also the disadvantage of cementing, with attendant risk for dental tissue.

Elastic bands are stretched on each side to balance the forces. Traction must always be oblique, downwards and forwards.

The maxillary shift must always be overcorrected by a few millimetres.

The modifications observed using this type of appliance reported by BACCETTI, 1998 comprise:

- Maxilla: a change in the orientation of the maxilla relative to the base of the skull, an increase in the length of the upper alveolar area and an average increase in the ENA-ENP distance of 3 mm.
- Mandible: a rearward and downward shift of the mandible, and closing of the goniac angle.
- Occlusion: a modification of the tooth contact and of the orientation of the occlusal plane, which is rotated anteriorly.
- Profile: an improved interlabial contact.

These immediate modifications have an impact on the labial, lingual, masticatory and occlusal functions, etc., which in turn progressively and favourably modify the facial skeleton.

We also point out that the association of the facial mask with maxillary disjunction proves more efficacious (GUYER 1986, NARTALLO-TURLEY 1992).

Activators

An activator is a removable device that uses intrinsic forces (orofacial muscles) to correct sagittal discrepancies. Class III abnormalities that are chiefly due to functional problems enjoy a favourable prognosis when such activators are used provided they are associated with functional re-education of the tongue and respiratory functions.

The mandible is brought into a more rearward position, as the appliance is fixed to the maxillary arch; the mandible pushes the maxilla forward. The anterior guide is thereby modified; we generally see a mandibular plicature and a closing of the goniac angle, together with a 'verticalisation' of growth and a slight overall posterior rotation.

To conclude, we can assert that early orthodontic treatment is the key to successful, straightforward treatment of Class II malocclusion. It must be undertaken as early as possible, as soon as the child is seen in consultation.

This will ensure that it gives best results, which are most often spectacular.

There is much theory here, although it is backed by large amounts of practice. However, the child's developing personality and capabilities must once more become central: early treatment of Class III abnormalities will ensure the child enjoys a better social integration.

We can sum up by quoting the judicious advice of Dr Marc Vesse: 'Opt for early treatment: your young patientswill thank you and so will their parents'.

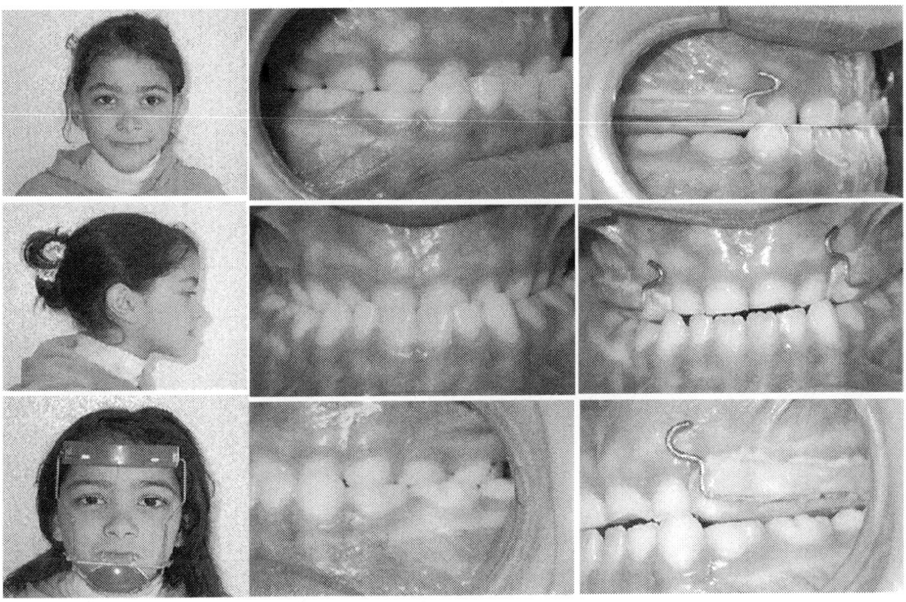

Case 23. Early treatment of skeletal Class III cases attributable to maxillary retrognathy with a DELAIRE's face mask

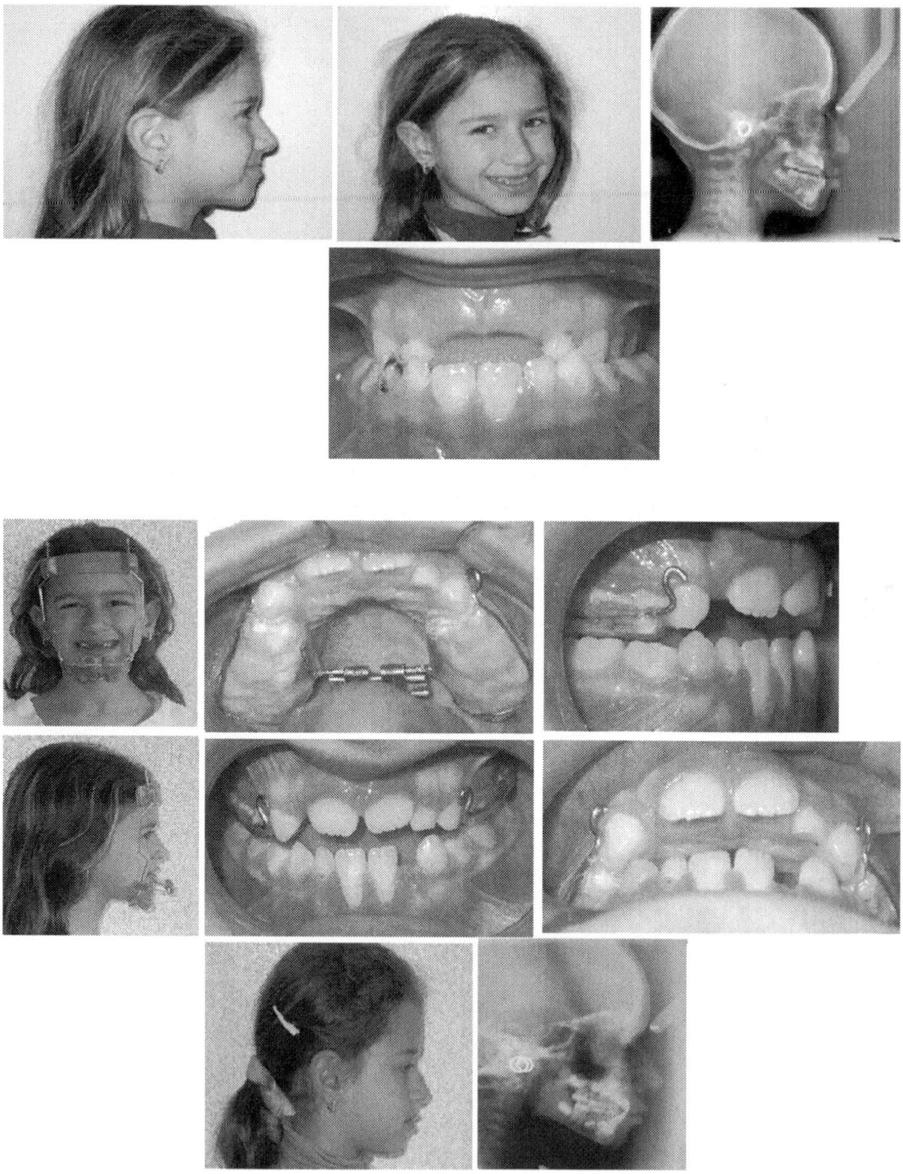

Case 24. Early treatment of skeletal Class III with a DELAIRE's face mask

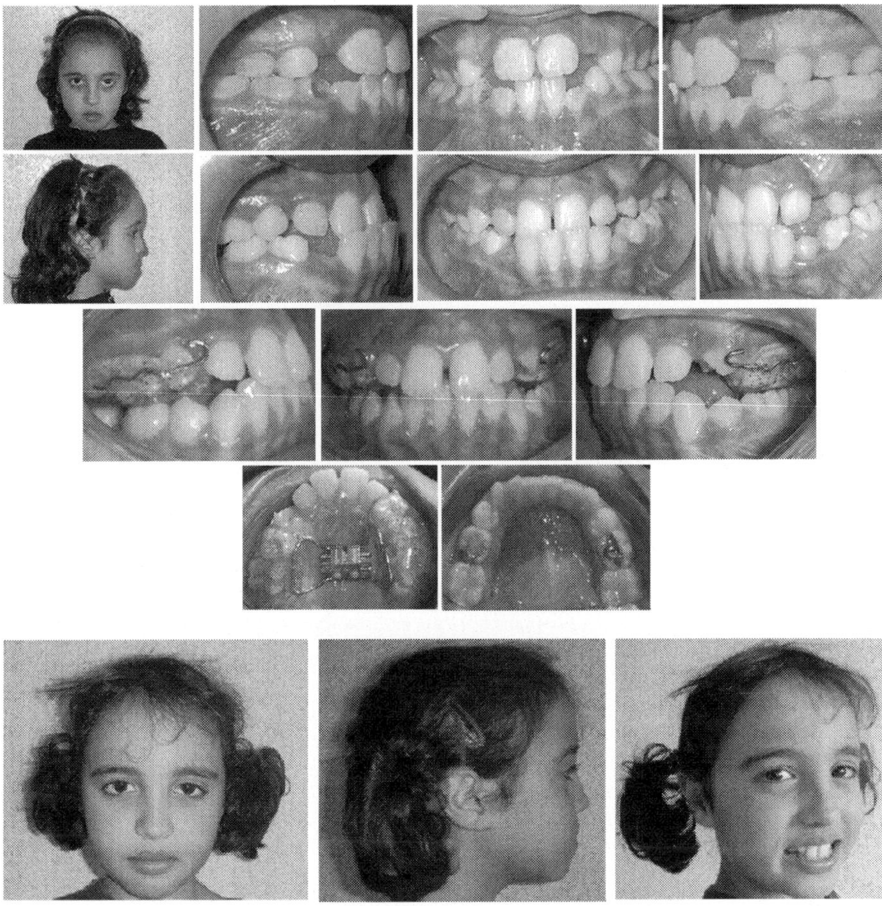

Case 25. DELAIRE's face mask to treat a skeletal Cl III

6. Conclusion

Early treatment orthodontic procedures are relatively simple and inexpensive treatment approaches that target developing malocclusions during the mixed or deciduous dention. Orthodontists perceive these as useful ways to reduce the severity of malocclusions, improve a patient's self image, eliminate destructive habits, facilitate normal tooth eruption, and improve some growth patterns. (GREGORY KING 2010)

Early treatments in orthodontics do not produce finished orthodontic results without a second phase of treatment in the permanent dentition. But several studies have suggested that systematically planned interceptive treatment in the mixed dentition might contribute to a significant reduction in treatment need between the ages of 8 and 12 years, often producing results so that further need can be categorized as elective.

7. References

Armstrong MM.(1971) : Controlling the magnitude, direction, and duration of extraoral force. *Am J Orthod.*,Vol.59, N°3, pp:217-43.

Baccetti T,and al.(1998) : Skeletal effects of early treatment of Class III malocclusion with maxillary expansion and face-mask therapy. *Am J Orthod Dentofacial Orthop.* Vol.113, N°3, pp:333-43.

Basciftci FA, Karaman AI.(2002) :Effects of a modified acrylic bonded rapid maxillary expansion appliance and vertical chin cap on dentofacial structures. *Angle Orthod.*Vol.72, N°1, p:61-71.

Baumrind S, and al. (1983) :Superimpositional assessment of treatment-associated changes in the temporomandibular joint and the mandibular symphysis. *Am J Orthod.* Vol.84, N°6, pp:443-65.

Behlfelt K, and al (1989) : Dentition in children with enlarged tonsils compared to control children. *Eur J Orthod,* Vol 11, N°4, pp:416-29.

Clifford FO. (1971) : Cross-bite correction in the deciduous dentition : principles and procedures. *Am J Ortthod.*Vol.59 :343-9

Cozza P and al. (2005) : Early orthodontic treatment of skeletal open-bite malocclusion: a systematic review.*Angle Orthod.*Vol.75, N°5, pp:707-13.

Dale JG. (2000) Serial extraction ... nobody does that anymore. *Am J Orthod Dentofacial Orthop.*Vol.117, N°5, pp:564-6.

Delaire J.(1971) Confection du masque ortopédique. *Rev Stomat Paris* Vol.72, pp: 579- 84

Demisch A.(1972).: Effects of activator therapy on the craniofacial skeleton in classe II, division 1 malocclusion. *Trans. Eur. Orthod. Soc.,*pp :295-310.

Droschl H.(1973) : The effect of heavy orthopedic forces on the maxilla in the growing Saimiri sciureus. *Am J Orthod Dentofacial Orthop.,* Vol.63, pp:449-61

Elder JR., Tuenge,RJ. (1974) : Cephalometric and histologic changes produced by extra-oral high pull traction of the maxilla of macaca Mulatta. *Am J Orthod Dentofacial Orthop.*Vol.66, pp:599-617.

Egermark-Eriksson I, and al.(1990) :A longitudinal study on malocclusion in relation to signs and symptoms of cranio-mandibular disorders in children and adolescents. *Eur J Orthod*Vol.12, N°4, pp:399-407.

Freunthaller P.(1967) : Cephalometric observation in Class II, Division I malocclusions treated with the activator. *Angle Orthod.*Vol.37, N°1, pp:18-25.

Gugino CF, Dus I. (1998) :Unlocking orthodontic malocclusions: an interplay between form and function.*Semin Orthod.* Vol.4, N°4, pp:246-55.

Ghafari J, and al. (1998) : Headgear versus function regulator in the early treatment of Class II, division 1 malocclusion: a randomized clinical trial. *Am J Orthod Dentofacial Orthop.*Vol.114, N°2, pp:162-5.

Gianelly AA, Arena SA, Bernstein L. (1984): A comparison of Class II treatment changes noted with the light wire, edgewise, and Fränkel appliances. *Am. J.Orthod.*Vol.86, N°4, pp:269-76.

Graber TM. (1971) : Serial Extraction. *AmJ Orthod* Vol.60, pp:541-575.

Graber TM., Profitt WR. (2007):Contemprary orthodontics. 4th St Louis,pp: 689- 707.

Guyer EC, Ellis EE 3rd, Mc Namara JA Jr (1986): Components of class III malocclusion in juveniles and adolescents. *Angle orthod.*Vol.56, N°1, pp:7-30.

Ingervall B, Thilander B. (1975) : Activity of temporal and masseter muscles in children with a lateral forced bite. *Angle Orthod* Vol.45, N°4, pp:249-58.

Janson M, Hasund A (1981). : Functional problems in orthodontic patients out of retention. *Eur J Orthod.* Vol.3, N°3, pp:173-9.

Kelly JE, Sanchez M, Van Kirk LE.(1973) : An assessment of the occlusion of teeth of children 6-11 Years. *Washington, DC : National center for health Satatistics*

Keski-Nisula K, and al. (2004) :Occurrence of malocclusion and need of orthodontic treatment in early mixed dentition.*Am J Orthod Dentofacial Orthop.* Vol 125, N°3, pp :20A

Hotz RP. (1947) : Active supervision of the eruption of the teeth by extraction. *Trans Eur Orthod Soc,* Vol.48, N°34,pp :47.

King EW. (1957) : Cervical anchorage in classe II, division 1 treatment : a cephalometric appraisal. *Angle Orthod.,*Vol.27, pp: 98-104

King EW. (1960) : Variation in profile change and their significance in timing treatment. *Angle Orthod.* Vol.30, pp :141-53

Kjellgren, Birger (1947): Serial extraction as a corrective procedure in dental orthopedic therapy,*Trans. Eur. Orthod. Sot.,* pp. 134-160.

Kreit LH, Burstone C, Delman L. (1968) : Patient cooperation in orthodontic treatment. *J Am Coll Dent.* Vol.35, N°4, pp:327-32.

Kurol J, Berglund L. (1992) Longitudinal study and cost-benefit analysis of the effect of early treatment of posterior cross-bites in the primary dentition. . *Eur J Orthod*Vol.14, N°3, pp:173-9.

Kutin G, Hawes RR.(1969) : Posterior cross-bites in the deciduous and mixed dentitions. *Am J Ortthod.* Vol.56, pp :491-504

Larsson E.(1986) : The effect of dummy-sucking on the occlusion: a review. *Eur J orthod*Vol.8, N°2, pp:127-30.

Linder-Aronson S. Adenoids. (1970) : Their effect on mode of breathing and nasal airflow and their relationship to characteristics of the facial skeleton and the dentition. A biometric, rhino-manometric and cephalometro-radiographic study on children with and without adenoids. *Acta Otolaryngol Suppl*N°265, pp:1-132.

Little RM, Riedel RA, Engst ED.(1990):Serial extraction of first premolars-Postretention evaluation of stability and relapse. *Angle Orthod*N°60, pp:255-262.

McNamara JA.(1973): Neuromuscular and skeletal adaptations to altered function in the orofacial region. *Am J Orthod.*Vol.64, N°6, pp:578-606

McNamara JA Jr, Bookstein FL, Shaughnessy T.(1985) :Skeletal and dental changes following functional regulator therapy on class II patients. *Am J Orthod.*Vol.88, N°2, pp:91-110.

McNamara JA Jr (1987) : An orthopedic approach to the treatment of Class III malocclusion in young patients. *J Clin Orthod.*Vol.21, N°9, pp:598-608.

McNamara JA Jr, Brudow WL.(1993): Orthdodontic and orthodpedic treatment in the mixed dentition. *Ann Arbor, Mich. : Needham Press.*

McNamara JA Jr. (2002) :Early intervention in the transverse dimension: is it worth the effort? *Am J Orthod Dentofacial Orthop*Vol.121, N°6, pp:572-4.

Nartallo-Turley PE, Turley PK.(1998): Cephalometric effects of combined palatal expansion and facemask therapy on Class III malocclusion. *Am J Orthod.* Vol.68, N°3, pp:217-24.

Ngan P, Fields HW(1997): Open bite: a review of etiology and management. *Pediatr Dent.* Vol.19, N°2, pp:91-8.

O'Mullane DM. (1973) : Some factors predisposing to injuries of permanent incisors in school children. *Br Dent J.*Vol.17, N°8, pp:328-32.

Persson M, Persson E, Skagies S. (1989) : Long-term spontaneous changes following removal of all first premolars in Class I cases with crowding. *EurJ Orthod* Vol.11, pp:271-282.

Poulton DR. (1967): The influence of extraoral traction. *Am J Orthod.* Vol.53, N°1, pp:8-18.

Proffit WR, Fields HW, Moray LJ (1988) : Prevalence of malocclusion and orthodontic need in the United State estimate from the H-HANES III survey. *Int J Adult Orthod Orthognath Surg.* Vol.13, pp:97-106

Proffit WR, Tulloch JF. (2002) : Preadolescent Class II problems: treat now or wait? *Am J Orthod Dentofacial Orthop*Vol.121, N°6, pp:560-2.

Richardson A. (1981): A classification of open bite. *Eur J Orthod.* Vol.3, pp: 289-96

Righellis EG.(1983) : Treatment effects of Fränkel, activator and extraoral traction appliances. *Angle Orthod.* Vol.53, N°2, pp:107-21.

Sakamoto T. (1981): Effective timing for the application of orthopedic force in the skeletal class III malocclusion. *Am J Orthod.* Vol.80, N°4, pp:411-6.

Sassouni V. (1969) :A classification of skeletal facial types. *Am J Orthod.*Vol.55, N°2, pp:109-23.

Stöckli PW, Willert HG.(1971): Tissue reactions in the temporomandibular joint resulting from anterior displacement of the mandible in the monkey. *Am J Orthod.*Vol.60, N°2, pp:142-55

Sugawara J, Asano T, Endo N, Mitani H. (1990) : Long-term effects of chincap therapy on skeletal profile in mandibular prognathism.*Am. J. Orthod.,*Vol.98, N°2, pp:127-33.

Tollaro I, and al. (1983): Contiributo cefalometrico alla di daignosi del morso aperto. Nota 1: morso aperto scheletrico. *Mondo Orthod.* 1983; Vol.8, N°3, pp: 47-59

Troelstrup B, Moller E. (1970) : Electromyography of the temporalis and masseter muscles in children with unilateral cross-bite. *Scand J Dent Res.*Vol.8, pp :425-30

Tulley WJ. (1969) : A critical appraisal of tongue-thrusting. *Am J Orthod.* Vol.55, N°6, pp:640-50.

Watson WG. (1972) : A computerized appraisal of the high-pull face-bow. *Am J Orthod.* Vol.62, N°6, pp:561-79

Wieslander L ., Tandlakare L. (1963) : The effect of treatment on the concurrent development of the craniofacial complex. *Am J Orthod.,*Vol.49, pp : 15-27

Wigdorowicz-Makowerowa N, and al.(1979): Epidemiologic studies on prevalence and etiology of functional disturbances of the masticatory system. *J.prosthet.Dent.*Vol.41, N°1, pp:76-82.

12

Maxillary Lateral Incisor Agenesis (MLIA)

Teresa Pinho

PhD in Orthodontics and Odontopediatrics in University of Porto; French Board of Orthodontics; Centro de Investigação Ciências da Saúde (CICS), Instituto Superior de Ciência da Saúde_Norte / CESPU Portugal

1. Introduction

In the permanent dentition, the type of congenital missing teeth varies from author to author and the demographic and geographic profiles. In Europeans, the mandibular second premolar is the most frequently absent tooth, followed by the maxillary lateral incisor and the maxillary second premolars (Bergstrom, 1977; Rolling, 1980; O'Dowling & McNamara, 1990; Aasheim & Øgaard, 1993; Nordgarden et al., 2002). In the Malaysian (Nick-Hussein & Majid, 1996), Israeli (Chosack et al., 1975) and American populations (Muller et al., 1970), the most frequently missing teeth are the maxillary lateral incisors. Focusing on MLIA the prevalence varies between 0.8 and 4.25% (Horowitz, 1966; Muller et al., 1970; Thilander & Myrberg, 1973; Magnusson, 1977; Rolling, 1980; Aasheim & Øgaard, 1993; Johannsdottir et al., 1997; Tavajohi-Kermani et al., 2002). In the Portuguese population a prevalence of 1.3 per cent was estimated, with a slightly higher frequency in females and also a unilateral occurrence more common than the bilateral occurrence (Pinho et al., 2005). Unilateral agenesis is often associated with dysmorphia or microdontia of the corresponding contralateral tooth (Pinho et al., 2009). This discovery led to the presumption that maxillary lateral incisors microdontia may represent a different expression of these molecular changes that lead to a defective development of the maxillary lateral incisors and it should therefore be considered with particular emphasis in the clinical diagnosis or in family history, allowing us to suspect of tooth agenesis (Pinho et al., 2010a). Hypodontia in the temporary dentition is a rare occurrence (0.4–0.9 per cent) and, when present, occurs more frequently in the incisor region, generally including an upper lateral incisor or a lower central or a lateral incisor (Ravn, 1971; Bennett & Ronk, 1980; Järvinen & Lehtinen, 1981; Johannsdottir et al., 1997; Pinho et al., 2005). When hypodontia occurs in the temporary dentition, most authors report 100 per cent absence of the permanent successor (Ravn, 1971; Bennett & Ronk, 1980; Järvinen & Lehtinen, 1981; Johannsdottir et al., 1997; Pinho et al., 2005) (Figure 1).

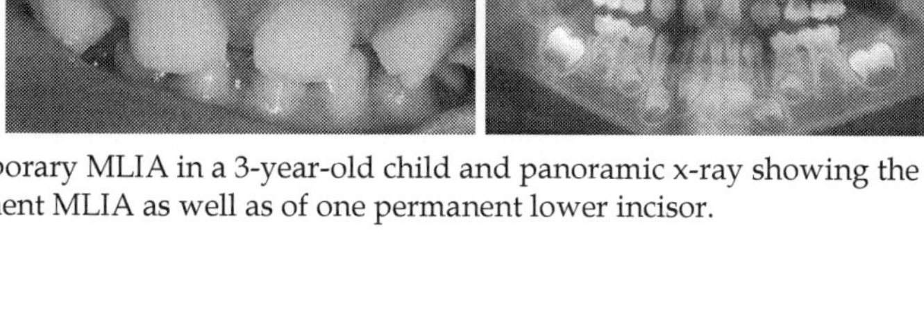

Fig. 1. Temporary MLIA in a 3-year-old child and panoramic x-ray showing the temporary and permanent MLIA as well as of one permanent lower incisor.

There is also a strong association between double teeth formation (fusion) in the temporary teeth and hypodontia in the permanent dentition (Ravn, 1971; Nick-Hussein & Majid, 1996). When a mandibular temporary lateral incisor and a canine are fused, agenesis of the permanent mandibular lateral incisor is a constant fact (Ravn, 1971; Johannsdottir et al., 1997). In cases where the fusion occurs only in incisors, they are rarely changed at the permanent dentition (Ravn, 1971). However, in Figure 2 we can see a case with temporary mandibular left central fusion and permanent lateral incisor agenesis on the same side. Cases of germinations at the temporary dentition are usually followed by normal permanent dentition (Ravn, 1971).

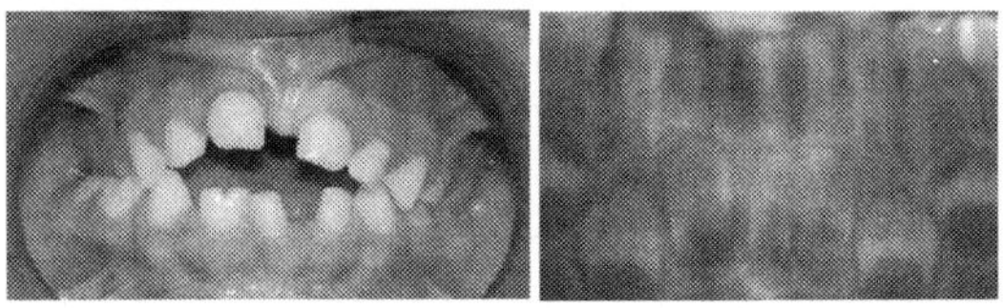

Fig. 2. Double tooth by fusion in temporary mandibular left central and lateral incisors in a 3-year-old child; Panoramic x-ray showing agenesis in a permanent incisor on the same side of the double teeth.

2. Etiology

Several etiological factors have been suggested for the development failure of the permanent tooth germ, thus leading to its absence, such as: physical obstruction, dental lamina rupture, limitation of space or functional anomalies. In spite of recent progress, the etiopathogenesis of hypodontia remains largely unknown (Kuchler et al., 2010; Vastardis, 2000; Kapadia et al., 2007). There is evidence that congenital tooth absence can be the result of environmental or hereditary causes, or even of their interaction (Schalk-van der Weide & Bosman, 1996; Swinnen et al., 2008).

The development of human dentition in terms of structure and organization is under genetic control and involves several factors, therefore it is logical to assume that mutations in some genes encoding these factors may affect the normal development of teeth and, eventually, may cause their absence.

Non-syndromic hypodontia is more common than the syndromic type. The evidence of a genetic cause for non-syndromic hypodontia came from the identification of significant family aggregation of MLIA and suggest microdontia of maxillary lateral incisors as part of the same phenotype, segregating as an autosomal dominant trait with incomplete penetrance (Pinho et al., 2010a); however, modes of transmission linked to X-chromosome and of polygenic or multifactorial type have also been proposed (Chosack et al., 1975).

Candidate genes in early steps of tooth development regulation (MSX1, PAX9, AXIN2, TGFa, Activin-b A, LEF1, RUNX2, BMP4, MMP1, MMP20), have been screened for putative mutations in affected families (Kuchler et al., 2010; Lin et al., 2008; Tummers &Thesleff, 2009).

Some mutations associated with tooth agenesis have been identified in humans at the MSX1 (Vastardis et al., 1996; Lidrali et al., 1998; Lidral & Reising, 2002; Mostowska et al., 2006) and PAX9 (Schuffenhauer et al., 1999; Stockton et al., 2000; Nieminen et al., 2001; Das et al., 2002; Pereira et al., 2006; Hansen et al., 2007; Tallon-Walton et al., 2007; Zhao et al., 2007; Guala et al., 2008) genes. Nevertheless, these genes might be fundamentally implicated in the

odontogenesis of posterior teeth (Pinho et al. 2010b). Lammi et al., (2004), reported that a nonsense mutation in the AXIN2, an essential component of the WNT/b-catenin pathway, caused familial oligodontia with a severe phenotype. In addition to oligodontia, those authors also found that a mutation in AXIN2 predispose the individual to colorectal cancer.
Considering the discrepancy between the high prevalence rate of tooth agenesis and the relatively small number of reported causative mutations in the PAX9, MSX1, and AXIN2 genes, the genetic contribution to hypodontia/oligodontia seems quite heterogeneous (Gerits et al., 2006). Environmental and epigenetic factors as well as genes regulating odontogenesis require further *in vivo* and *in vitro* investigation in order to better explain the phenotypic heterogeneity and to increase our knowledge about the odontogenic process (Swinnen et al., 2008).
In spite of recent developments, data regarding the genes responsible for the less severe forms of hypodontia are still scarce and controversial (Kuchler et al., 2010). A study of familiar aggregation in a Portuguese population of sixty-two probands with MLIA and 142 first-degree relatives showed that the relative risk (RR) for a first-degree relative of an individual with MLIA to have the same type of agenesis was 15 times higher when compared with a relative of an individual without that agenesis. Published results support a significant familial aggregation of MLIA and show that MLIA almost never segregates with other forms of agenesis, and suggest that microdontia of maxillary lateral incisors is part of the same phenotype (Pinho et al. 2010a). However previous search for mutations in the PAX9 and MSX1 genes, and their potential association with the MLIA phenotype in 12 Portuguese families, didn't show a clear association between those genes and the MLIA phenotype (Pinho et al., 2010b).

3. Craniofacial repercussions

There is no consensus on whether the changes that may occur during maxillary development are correlated or not with dental agenesis. However, some authors described a possible correlation (Wisth et al., 1974; Woodworth et al., 1985; Pinho et al., 2011a).
According to Pinho et al. (2011a) MLIA is associated with an upper maxilla shortening, and also a negatively conditioned anterio-superior facial height dimension. Woodworth et al. (1985) showed that the decrease in maxillary length in individuals with MLIA is more frequently associated with skeletal Class III. However, others concluded that dental agenesis of few teeth, have little or no effect on craniofacial structure, as there is a higher prevalence ratio of skeletal Class I in patients with agenesis (Dermaut et al., 1986; Yuksel & Ucem, 1997; Pinho et al., 2011a).
Patients with severe congenital teeth absence have unique dental and skeletal patterns (Ben-Bassat and Brin 2009) probably caused by reduced occlusal support (Nodal et al., 1994). Dentofacial development in individuals with severe hypodontia, may be due to skeletal and functional compensation rather than being motivated by a different growth pattern (Ogaard & Krogstad, 1995).

4. Clinical manifestations

Early diagnosis of dental anomalies are essential when evaluating the pediatric patient and for treatment planning (Pilo et al., 1987).
There are some direct and indirect clinical signs that can allow us to suspect of tooth agenesis. Among individuals with missing teeth, those who most frequently request

treatment are those with missing maxillary anterior teeth, namely the lateral incisors, probably for esthetic reasons. Hypodontia / oligodontia can be directly or indirectly supposed (Fig 3 and 4). The persistence of a temporary lateral incisor in the arch, beyond the expected date of eruption of its successor (Baccetti, 1998; Taylor, 1998), and / or asymmetric loss of temporary teeth (Millar & Taylor, 1995; Peck et al., 1996), dental midline shift in those who had unilateral agenesis on the same side of the agenesis and a molar Class II relation, which can be translated as a dental compensation towards the mesial sectors to camouflage the MLIA, are all indirect examples of this (Pinho et al., 2005, 2009, 2011b).

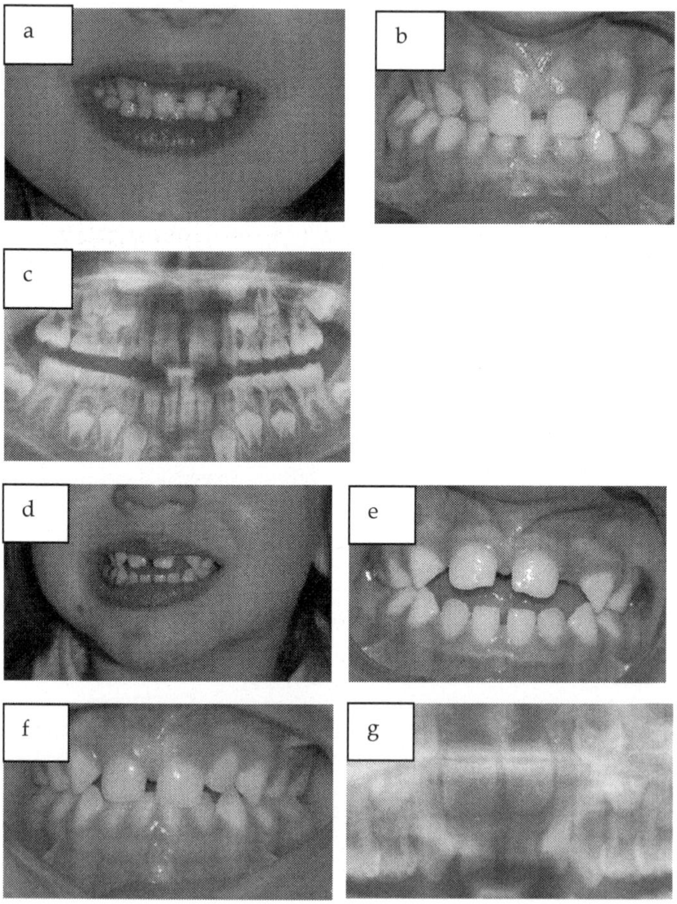

Fig 3. a, b) Temporary left MLIA in a 3-year-old child with a dental midline shift to the same side. (c) Panoramic x-ray showing bilateral permanent MLIA; d, e) Her sister with 2 years of age with no eruption of bilateral temporary lateral incisor; f) and only at 4 years of age the left one erupted; g) Panoramic x-ray showing bilateral permanent MLIA.

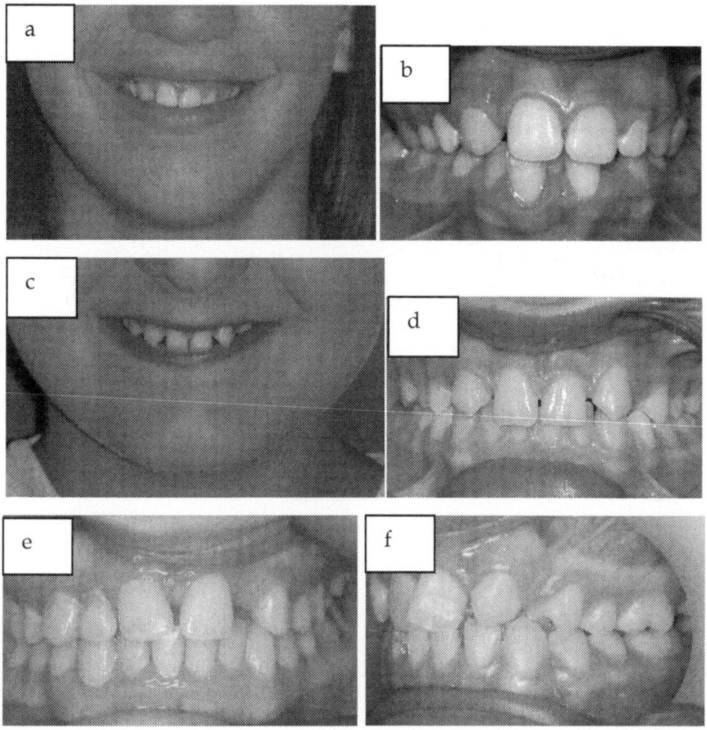

Fig. 4. a, b) Left MLIA in a 13-year-old girl with a dental midline shift to the same side; c, d) Bilateral MLIA in a 13-year-old male with centered dental midline; e) Persistence of a maxillary temporary lateral incisor in a 18 years old girl with bilateral MLIA; f) MLIA with a Class II molar and canine relation.

In multiple congenital absences, you can also find other signs: attrition of the correspondent temporary persistent tooth, atypical tooth migration, ankylosis, infra-occlusion of temporary molars, supra-eruption of the permanent teeth, contralateral microdontia and diastemas (Bergendal et al., 1996, Dhanrajani, 2002) (Figure 5).

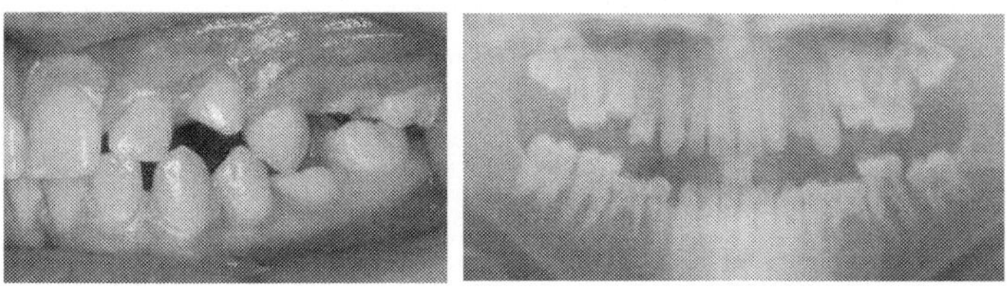

Fig. 5. a) Multiple congenital absences, with atypical tooth migration, ankylosis, infra-occlusion of temporary molars, and supra-eruption of the permanent teeth; b) Panoramic x-ray.

A radiographic examination should be used to complement the study of the patient, allowing confirmation of the number of absences and their location. Taking a panoramic radiography for routine was defended (Pilo et al., 1987) as a methodology to adopt for individuals who are less than 8 years old, whenever an incisor is missing in the arcade. This would facilitate an early diagnosis of tooth agenesis (Hobkirk et al., 1994; Bergendal et al., 1996).

According to Garn & Lewis (1970), crown size reduction associated with congenitally missing teeth is more significant in multiple agenesis than in cases of third molar agenesis, and occurs more frequently in women. Schalk-van der Weide et al. (1994) observed that patients with oligodontia (more than 6 teeth agenesis) had a reduction on both mesio-distal and labio-lingual dimensions of the tooth crowns (Figure 6). The reduction in size of some teeth in relatives may be an important factor for the determination of familiar occurrence of missing teeth (Schalk-van der Weide & Bosman, 1996). Yaqoob et al. (2011) stated that isolated bilateral absence of maxillary lateral incisors is associated with reduced mesiodistal tooth widths of both maxillary and mandibular anterior segments.

Some authors stated that permanent tooth agenesis, maxillary lateral incisor microdontia, palatally displaced canines, and distoangulation of mandibular second premolars are frequently associated with maxillary lateral incisor agenesis, providing additional evidence of genetic interrelationship as cause for these dental anomalies (Garib et al., 2010). For others, the factors involved in third molar agenesis and that of other teeth are probably the same (Baum & Cohen, 1971).

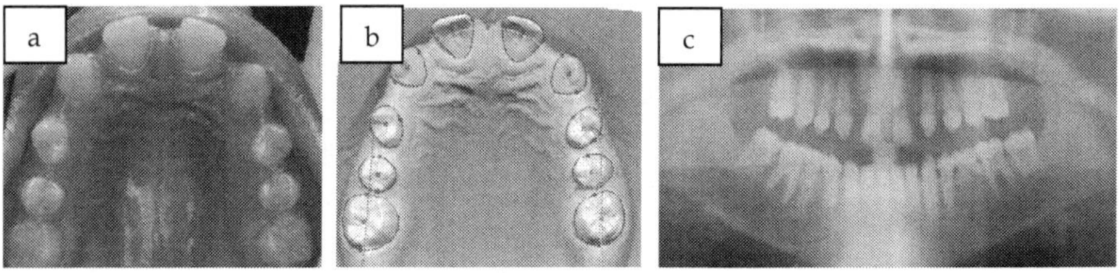

Fig. 6. a) Multiple diastemas associated with generalized microdontia and multiple dental agenesis in a 12 years old female; b) Generalized microdontia confirmed by models measurements c) Panoramic x-ray confirming the congenital absence of 18, 16, 12, 22, 26, 28, 38, 35 and 48 teeth.

In addition, some authors (Becker et al., 1981; Peck et al., 1996; Pirinen et al., 1996; Baccetti, 1998; Peck et al., 2002), referred that in early detection, we must take also into account the importance of the lateral incisor in the eruption of the canine tooth. The frequency of paradoxical bad positioning of the canine in cases of agenesis and / or lateral incisors microdontia demonstrates the importance of these teeth in guiding the way to canine eruption (Figure 7).

Other authors (Zirberman et al., 1990; Peck et al., 1996; Pirinen et al., 1996; Peck et al., 2002) suggested that these situations can be caused by the same genetic factor. Despite this strong evidence, there are also those who disagree (Brenchley & Oliver 1997; Pinho et al., 2005, 2009) and do not associate an ectopic canine with microdontia or with agenesis of maxillary lateral incisor but with malocclusions of Class II Div 2, due to the typical displacement of the labiopalatine adjacent lateral incisor (Millar & Taylor 1995).

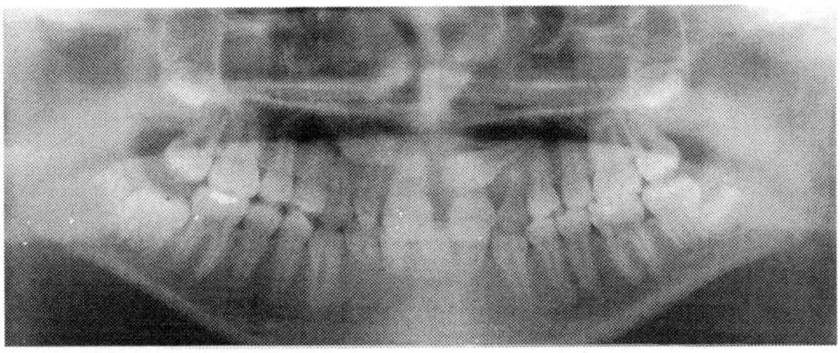

Fig. 7. Panoramic x-ray of a 14 years old female with maxillary canines included. Conical appearance of UR2 (12), agenesis of UL2 (22) and persistence of temporary UR3 (53) and UL3 (63).

The simultaneous occurrence of agenesis and supernumerary teeth is uncommon (Ranta & Tulensalo 1988; Zhu et al., 1996; Zhu et al., 1996; Pinho et al., 2005; Anthonappa et al., 2008) and it is more frequent in the permanent than in the primary dentition (Ranta & Tulensalo, 1988; Pinho et al., 2009) (Figure 8).

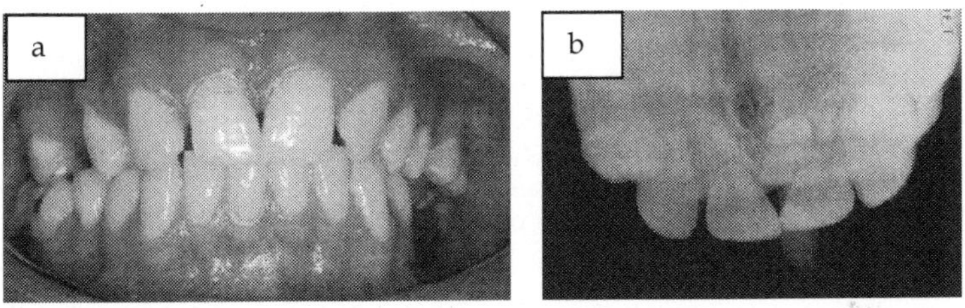

Fig. 8. a) Bilateral MLIA in a 25 years old male with spontaneous canine mesialization; b) Occlusal x-ray with a mesiodens placed between divergent roots of the central incisors.

In some syndromes there are typical patterns of hypodontia, while in others the congenital reduction in teeth number is described as sporadic. Anodontia (congenital absence of all teeth) is rare (Burzynski & Escobar, 1983) and is often associated with ectodermal dysplasia (Marques & Till, 1994).

Hypohidrotic ectodermic dysplasia is the most common form of ectodermic dysplasia in humans and is estimated to affect at least 1 in 17.000 people worldwide (ghr.nlm.nih.gov/hypohidrotic-ectodermal-dysplasia). Most people with hypohidrotic ectodermic dysplasia have hypohidrosis, hypotricosis and absent or malformed teeth (Marques & Till 1994; Itthagarun & King 1997; Kobielak et al., 2001) (Figure 9). There are other syndromes like Rieger's syndrome where hypodontia is also a main feature (Prabhu et al., 1997). For Schalk-Van Der Weide et al. (1994), patients with oligodontia/I (isolated) showed a low degree association of extra-oral signs with combinations of just one or two ectodermic anomalies. On the contrary, patients with oligodontia/S (Syndrome) show a strong tendency to present a combination of three or more ectodermic anomalies.

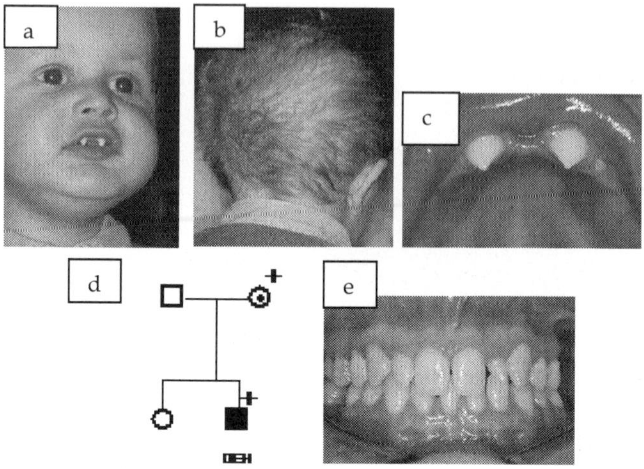

Fig. 9. a, b, c) 2 years old male with Hypohidrotic Ectodermal Dysplasia Syndrome (DEH); d, e) his mother with conical appearance of the lateral incisor.

5. Treatment

Of all missing teeth, those that most often motivate treatment request, probably for esthetic reasons, are the early absent maxillary teeth, namely the lateral incisors.
There are clinical situations in which the residual spaces are minimal and the patients feel fully satisfied with their esthetic appearance (Figure 10). Sometimes, though not completely satisfied, they are not motivated or economically capable for orthodontic treatment (Figure 11 and 12).

Clinical case 1 (Fig 10a-e)

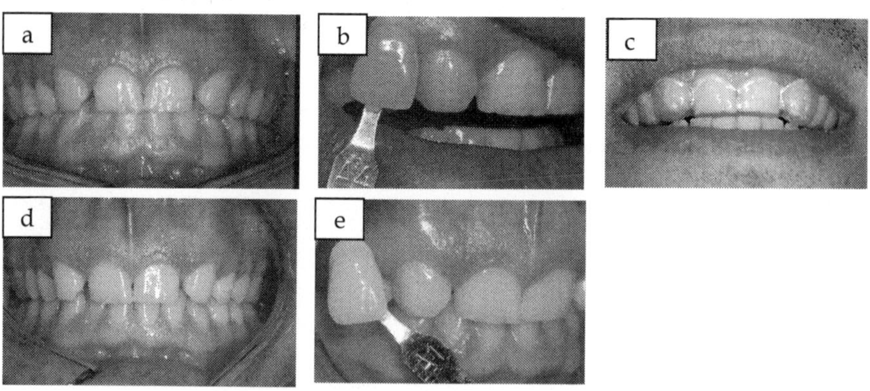

Fig. 10. a) Canine mesialized with unsightly color; b) Canine color corresponding to an A4 (range of Vita ®); c) canines bleaching ; d) Final aesthetic result after nighttime use of bleach; e) color change to an A1.

Clinical case 2 (Fig 11a-d and Fig 12a-d)

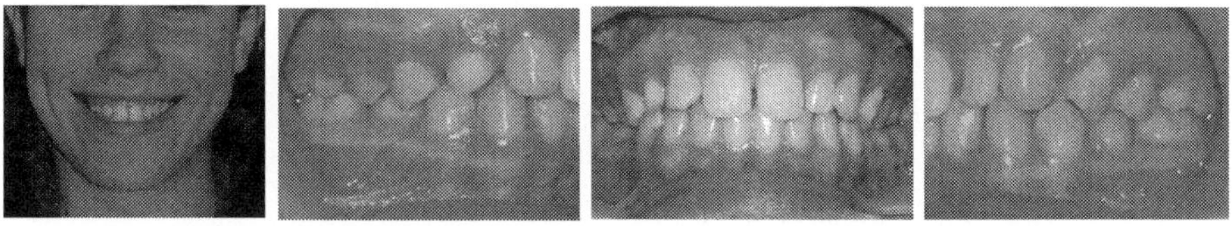

Fig. 11. Slight diastemas, unilateral agenesis of UR2 (12) with the UR3 (13) totally mesialized and the persistence of the temporary URC (53) distally positioned in relation to the corresponding permanent tooth. UL2(22) with conical appearance.

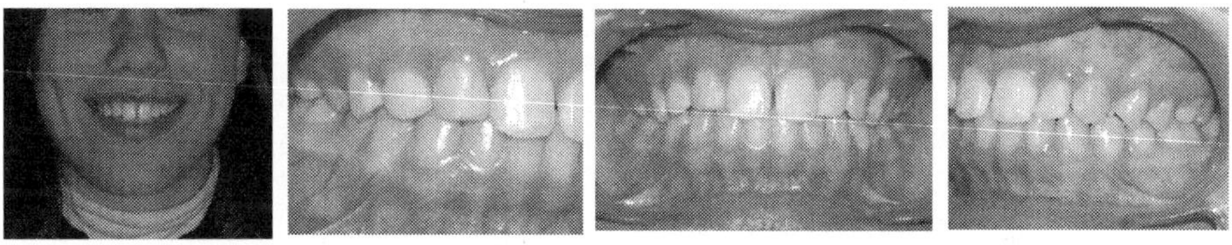

Fig. 12. Improvement of the UL2 (22), and the temporary UR3 (53) shape by an adhesive composite restoration in combination with cusp reshaping and adhesive composite restoration of the UR3 (13) mesial face.

If uni- or bilateral agenesis of the maxillary lateral incisors leads to situations that are esthetically unpleasant or unacceptable, therapeutic options should be orthodontic space closure or opening. The choice between these two types of treatment should not be made empirically. In most instances, the presence or absence of major occlusion problems serves as the primary criterion for either space closure or space opening.

There are several factors, and sometimes several interrelated factors, that limit different treatment options. Before starting any treatment the professional is obliged to inform patients of the various options, their clinical implications, advantages and disadvantages, and what should be the best plan for their particular case.

Several factors such as molar ratio, degree of incisors protrusion, facial patterns, skeletal arches interrelation, dental arch configuration, dental inclination, tooth shape, incisal contact, gingival margins contour, black triangles smile line, lip shape, and esthetic results should be considered in therapeutic options (Pinho & Neves 2001, 2003; Park et al., 2010). Also, we have to take in consideration the position of the lip attachment at the nasolabial junction that has a profound effect on the esthetics of the profile (Park et al., 2010).

5.1 Bilateral maxillary lateral incisors agenesis

5.1.1 Closure of the space

Closing the space means definitive treatment with orthodontic mesialization of the canine, replacing the missing lateral incisor, thus closing the anterior diastema. For many authors this is the treatment of choice since it is able to get a good esthetic (Millar & Taylor 1995; Pinho, 2003; Park et al., 2010). When the solution is space closure, to obtain an optimal esthetic and functional result it must be assumed that the canines will be modified, so to look and function as lateral incisors. The canine tooth requires, in cases associated with orthodontic mesialization, reduction of the mesial and distal face, as well as cutting of the cusp tip and palate face, and remodeling of the convexities in contact areas in order to create vertical interproximal areas, which are more agreeable with the contact points morphology of the lateral incisors and does not induce occlusal interferences (Bowden & Harrison, 1994; Millar & Taylor, 1995; Miller, 1995).

5.1.1.1 Indications

Some consideration factors, when closing the space, must be followed: Negative maxillary tooth disharmony (DDM), with crowding in the anterior area (Bowden and Harrison 1994); Class I with crowding, where extractions at the lower arch are indicated (Millar and Taylor 1995; Rosa & Zachrisson, 2001); Mesialized canine and easily modified with an acceptable color, compatible with the adjacent teeth (Millar & Taylor, 1995); the yellowish color of the canines can be improved using the technique of selective vital teeth bleaching (Pinho, 2003); Value of incisors relation with Class II division 1 (Bowden & Harrison 1994); Malocclusion that do not require extraction of mandibular teeth, with respect to Class II canine and molar (Pinho, 2003; Park et al., 2010).

5.1.1.2 Advantages

The benefits obtained by the closure of spaces corresponding to the missing lateral incisors are the following (Millar & Taylor, 1995): Solving of any previous crowding; avoiding artificial teeth; limiting treatment to orthodontics, decreasing costs by eliminating prosthetic treatment.

5.1.1.3 Disadvantages

The main disadvantage is the loss of the canine Class I.
Some authors (Rosa & Zachrisson, 2001) stated that no difference existed in adequacy of the occlusal function between canine-protected and group function (with remodeling procedures and occlusal adjustment, the group function is satisfactory). So, for these authors the elimination of the prosthetic solution makes this alternative the first option whenever possible.

Clinical case 3 (Figure 13 and 14)
Bilateral MLIA, with space closure in a 23 years old male.
Diagnosis: Bilateral agenesis of UR2 (12) and UL2 (22); canine and molar Class I relation on the right side, canine and molar Class II relation on the left side; bi-protrusion with pro-inclinated incisors in a hyperdivergent biotype with labial protrusion; overjet and overbite were 0 mm and -1 mm (open bite) respectively; the patient used a removable prosthesis with microdontic lateral incisors due to minimal space in the arcade. Due to esthetic factors, like bilabial protrusion and a closed naso-labial angle, space closure was the best option combined with extraction of the two mandibular first premolars (Figure 13).
After treatment, improvement of the incisors position and labial aesthetics can be observed. The harmony between the gingival margin of the central incisors, canines and first premolars was good, despite the mesio-distal canine dimension. Shorter canine gingival margin in relation to both central incisors, and first premolars more bucally positioned to bring them to a canine appearance (Figure 14).

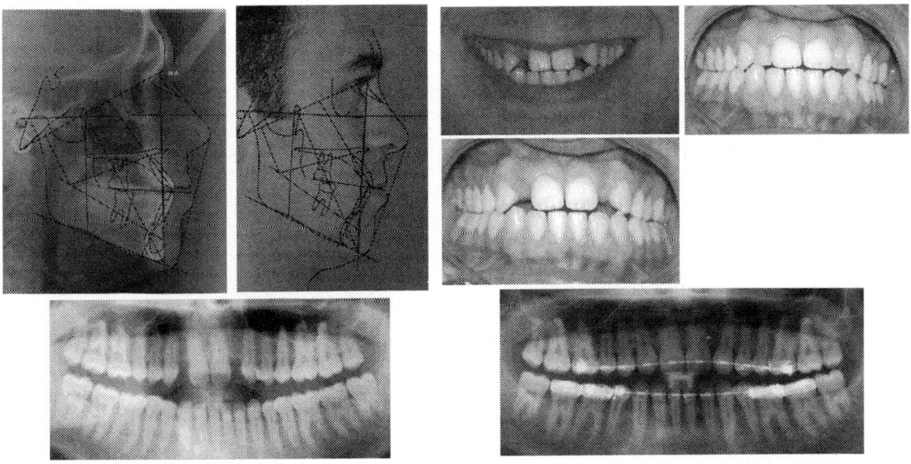

Fig. 13. Pre-treatment documentation, and panoramic x-ray at the middle of the treatment.

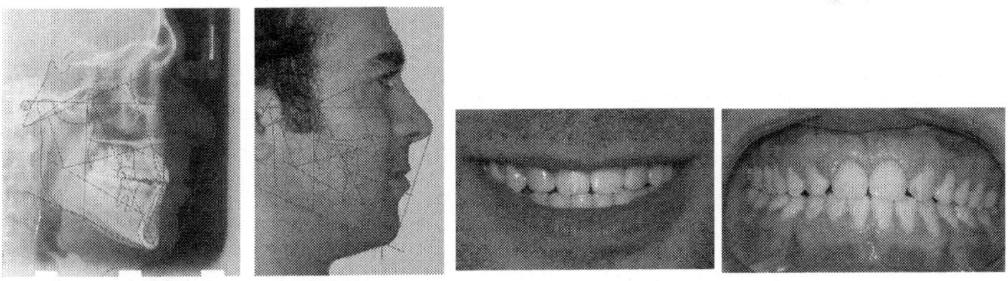

Fig. 14. Pos-orthodontic treatment documentation.

Clinical case 4 (Figure 15-17)

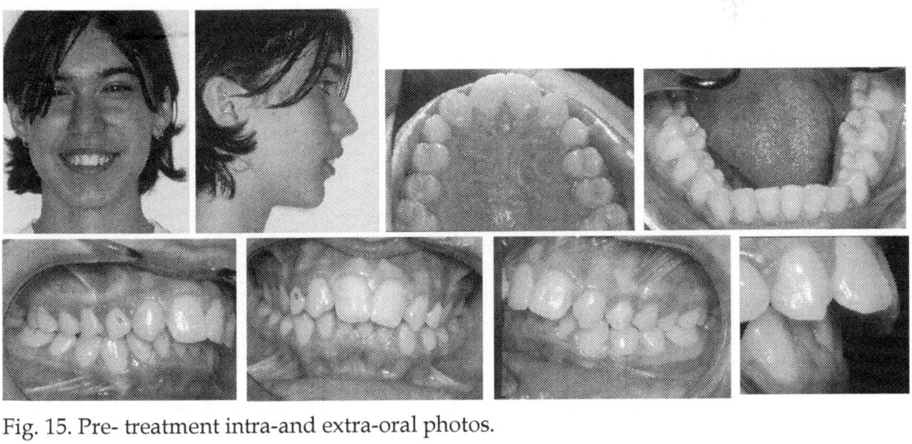

Fig. 15. Pre- treatment intra-and extra-oral photos.

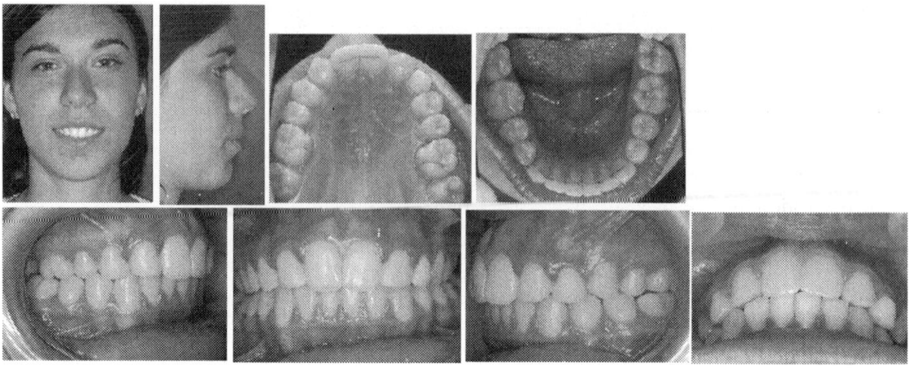

Fig. 16. Intra-and extra-oral photos after orthodontic treatment, bleaching and composite restorations.

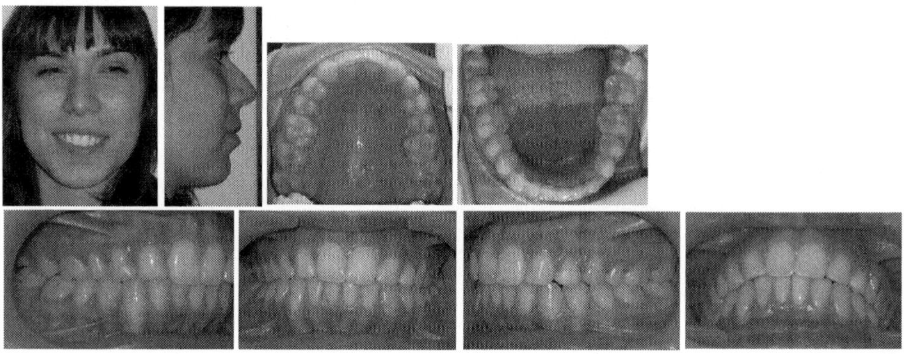

Fig. 17. Intra-and extra-oral photos, 8 years after orthodontic treatment.

Clinical case 4: Bilateral MLIA, with space closure in a 16 years old female.
Diagnosis: Bilateral agenesis of UR2 (12) and UL2 (22), convex facial profile with an increased lower facial third, lip incompetence and high smile line; mesialization of both canines, persistence of the deciduous canines, right-sided Class II molar relation and a left-sided Class I relation, with a 4.6-mm overbite and a 11.6-mm overjet, highly pronounced Spee curve, due to the extrusion of lower incisors; 4mm left deviation of the upper dental midline and right 1mm deviation of the lower dental midline ; despite these deviations, no facial asymmetry was detected (Figure 15).
The treatment aims were maintenance of the deciduous canine at the molar and canine Class I side and extraction the deciduous canine at the molar and canine Class II side. These steps aimed to allow the overjet and upper midline correction by retrusion of the anterior sector and deviation of the upper midline to the right. Improvement of the overbite and crowding, by intrusion and protrusion of the lower incisor group, and the maintenance of enough bone space at the level of the deciduous left upper canine in order to place an implant later.
After treatment we can observe improvement of the incisors position, as well as a more aesthetic labial position. Four months after orthodontic treatment ending, canines were

remodeled, by proximal aspects rectification and vestibular aspect modification and remodeling with a composite resin (final documentation, a-f). Eight years after, the results remained stable (Figure 17).

5.1.1.4 Interceptive treatment

Interceptive extractions of the deciduous upper lateral incisors and canine should be considered, while they are relatively high in the alveolus, in order to promote mesialized canine eruption and therefore spontaneous closure of the residual space caused by the absence of lateral incisors. Also, second deciduous molars interceptive extraction promote mesial migration of posterior teeth, causing an eruption of the permanent molars in a molar Class II relation, thus reducing the need for further treatment (Bowden & Harrison, 1994; Millar & Taylor, 1995). It is important to consider any coexisting malocclusion, a factor that may influence the decision to extract or not teeth. For example, in a nine years-old patient with a Class I (or Class III) relation, the extraction of the temporary maxillary canine and lateral incisor may allow an advance of the posterior teeth, whenever combined with the temporary loss of the second molars to help this advancement. However, in severe Class II, extractions should be done with additional caution because, they can curb the anterosuperior sector growth, or can facilitate the advancement of posterior sector making it impossible to fix Class II (bloking central incisor retrusion) (Millar & Taylor, 1995)

Clinical case 5 (Figure 18-23)

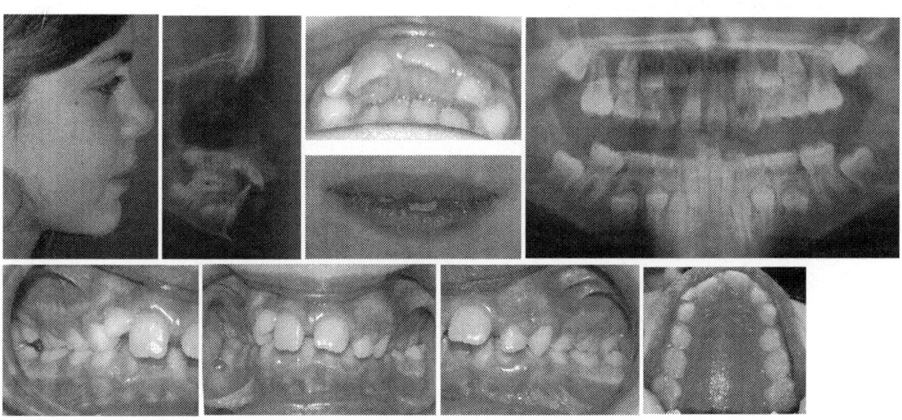

Fig. 18. Extra- and intra-oral photos; lateral telerradiography and panoramic x-ray, before interceptive treatment.

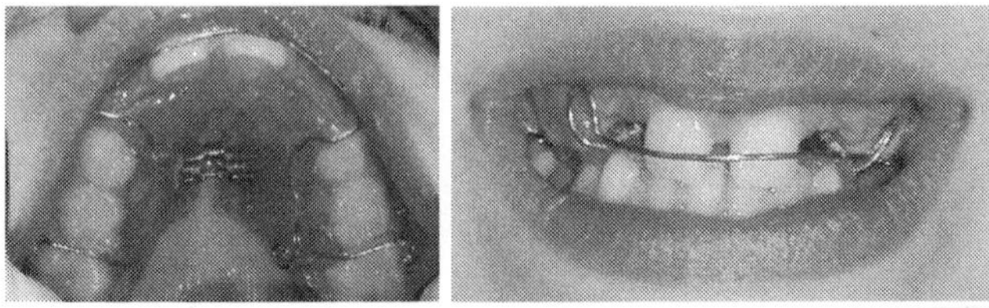

Fig. 19. Oclusal and smile photos during the use of removable appliance in interceptive treatment.

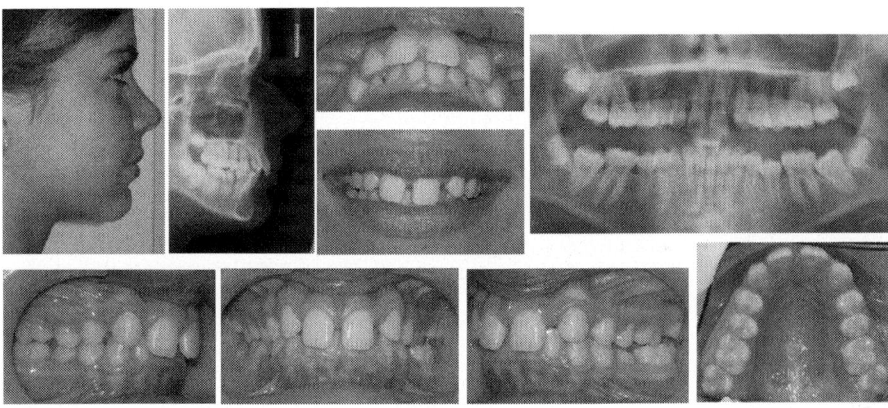

Fig. 20. Extra- and intra-oral photos; lateral telerradiography and panoramic x-ray, after interceptive treatment.

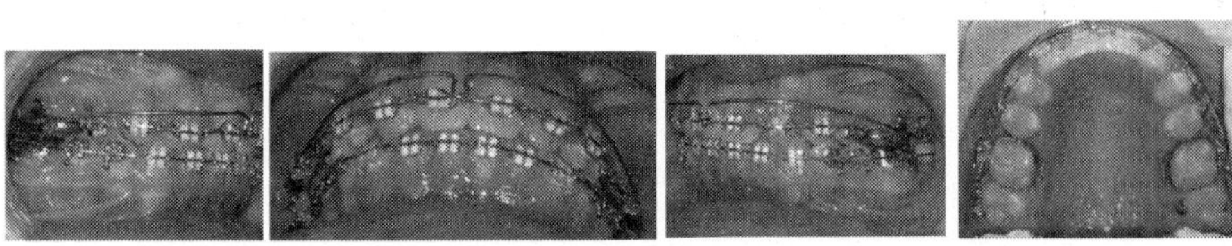

Fig. 21. Intra-oral photos, during straight wire technique treatment, with an overlay activated to improve the left posterior cross-bite.

Clinical case 5:
Unilateral MLIA, interceptive treatment, space closure with symmetry in a 7 years old female, at the beginning of the treatment.
Diagnosis: Unilateral agenesis of UR2 (12) with included microdontic UL2 (22) and retained temporary UL2 (62); bilateral Class II molar relationship, pro-maxilla, increased overjet, labial incompetence, protruded UL1 (21) with lower lip interposition; right 5 mm deviation of the upper dental midline and centered lower dental midline; crossbite of the UL6 (26) and LL6 (36) (Figure 18).

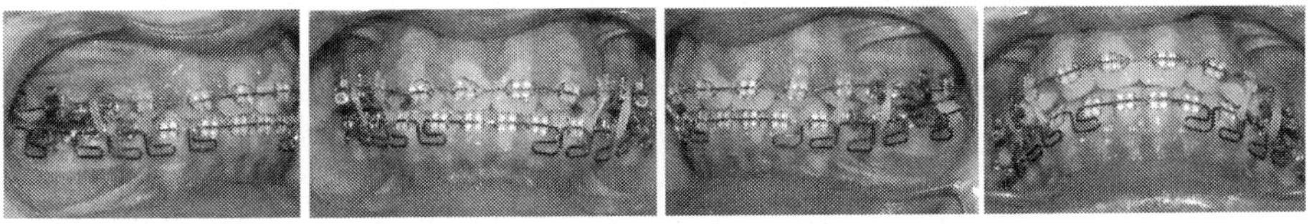

Fig. 22. Intra-oral photos, during Multiloop Edgewise Arch Wire (MEAW) in lower arch.

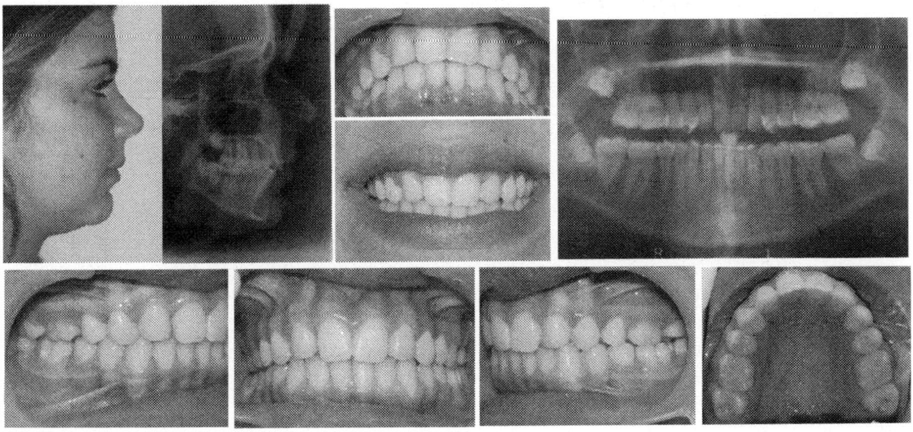

Fig. 23. Extra, intra oral photos; lateral telerradiography and panoramic x-ray, after orthodontic treatment.

Interceptive treatment: extraction of the included microdontic UL2 (22), the retained temporary UL2 (62), the temporary UR3 (53) and UL3 (63) when the patient was 8 years old. A removable appliance was placed for 1 year in order to improve the UL1 (21) position (Figure 19).

The extraction program led to a mesialized canine eruption and hence a spontaneous closure of residual space occurred and the upper dental midline was improved as well as the overjet (Figure 20).

Two years and six months after the use of the removable appliance ended, a bilateral fixed appliance allowed the improvement of the incisors position and of the dental intermaxillary relation; at the first stage a Straight-Wire technique (Figure 21) was used and, followed by a second stage with Multiloop Edgewise Arch-Wire (Figure 22) at the lower arch to finish the case with stable sagittal and vertical occlusion relationships between maxillary and mandibular arches.

The harmony between the gingival margin of the central incisors, canines and first premolars was good, despite the mesio-distal canine dimension. The facial profile improved and in spite of lateral incisor space closure, a stable dental articulation was accomplished with balanced occlusion with molar and canine bilateral Class II relation. Both midlines arches were aligned with the facial midline, and a correct overjet and overbite relationship were obtained (Figure 23).

5.1.2 Opening or maintaining space

The placement of an intraosseous implant in the edentulous area, followed by placement of a crown should be the first therapeutic option in cases of orthodontic space opening in post growth patients (Bowden & Harrison, 1994; Thilander et al., 1994; Small, 1996; Pinho & Neves, 2001; Zarone et al., 2006). Diagnosis and treatment of growing children with missing lateral incisors can be a problem because implants cannot be placed until facial growth is complete (Kokich, 2002, 2005). Females mature faster than males, and their adolescent growth spurt occurs sooner.

Space will be determined ultimately by the occlusion. Canines should be placed in a position that allows canine disclusion along the central incisors in a position that will provide optimal esthetics. Remaining space should be ideal for lateral incisor restoration, generally with 5 to 7 mm (Kokich, 2005). For Bergendal et al., (1996) minimum interdental space required for an implant is 6 mm mesio-distal and 5 mm in a buccolingual direction. However there are biologic limits of the bone dimension around implants that influence soft tissue esthetics. From the mesiodistal view, the distance between an implant and a tooth should not be less than 1.5mm, and if this minimum distance is not maintained, the attachment on the tooth side will undergo resorption, causing reduction or loss of the interproximal papilla (Esposito et al., 1993). From the buccolingual view, a 1.5mm-wide crater will also appear on the buccal side of the implant head (Spray et al., 2000).

In MLIA this ideal amount of bone is not available in the majority of cases, with the consequence of a high risk for soft tissue recession after an implant placement and prosthetic restoration. So, in these situations with a very esthetically demanding case, bone augmentation procedure will be needed (Grunder et al., 2005).

An x-ray examination, using periapical and panoramic techniques and, if necessary, computed tomography, gives us information that may be necessary for the proper assessment of the receptor site for the implant.

Autotransplantation is a viable option for treating missing teeth when a donor tooth is available (Bae et al., 2010).

5.1.2.1 Indications (Bowden & Harrison, 1994; Millar & Taylor, 1995, Pinho, 2001, 2004)

A canine that is difficult to remodel esthetically, as it presents a negative color to the bleaching technique or an unfavorable morphology; Concave profile; Widespread microdontia; Positive DDM, with multiple diastemas; Some cases of Class III malocclusion; Insignificant malocclusion, with Class I, without associated anomalies; Good intercuspidation; Some cases of cleft palate.

This option is recommended when a molar and canine Class I relation is the goal, with canine-protection as the basis of laterality.

Because some restorative options are possible, it is important to perform a clinical examination to decide which treatment plan best suit each patient. The solution with an implant is a viable option for replacing congenitally missing lateral incisors and should be seen as a definitive treatment plan, provided that all permanent teeth have erupted and skeletal growth is completed (Thilander et al., 1994; Small, 1996).

5.1.2.2 Advantages and disadvantages

The intercuspidation is maintained within the neutrality, preserving both canine and molar Class I relation. However, it is necessary to have different prosthetic solutions (Pinho & Neves, 2001).

5.1.2.3 Early treatment

Early diagnosis and the effective clinical management of hypodontia are important because the condition can lead to esthetic, physiologic, and functional problems (Tunc et al., 2011). In order to maintain various treatment options in the future, some authors defended that early orthodontic intervention may eliminate some of the periodontal and restorative problems that could arise in these patients as adults (Kokich 2005). For example, as a result of extracting the maxillary primary lateral incisor and guiding the eruption of the permanent canine into the lateral incisor space, an excellent implant site can be developed in the mixed dentition. In contrast, other authors stated that deciduous teeth should be retained if present, in order to preserve alveolar bone after tooth extraction, since alveolar bone resorbs rapidly after tooth extraction (Bowden & Harrison 1994).

Clinical case 6 (Figure 24-27)

Bilateral MLIA, with space opening in a 14 years old male.
Diagnosis): Bilateral agenesis of UR2 (12) and UL2 (22) and bilateral total mesialization of canines; concave soft-tissue profile, right molar Class I and left molar Class II relation (Figure 24).
Treatment goals involved regaining space for implant placement at the areas corresponding to UR2 (12) and UL2 (22). At the end of the treatment a bilateral molar Class I relationships was obtained. At the first treatment stage a Straight-Wire technique was used for twelve months, to allow alignment and levelling and, at the second stage, an occlusal plane modification and mandible repositioning was achieved with Multiloop Edgewise Arch-Wire (MEAW), used for six months. Different MEAW activation on both sides and short Class I vertical elastics in the anterior area on the right side and Class II on the left side were important to apply different orthodontic forces (Figure 25). This procedure made it possible to finish the case with stable sagittal and vertical occlusion relationships between maxillary and mandibular arches (Figure 26). A removable retainer has been used with a denture tooth to replace bilateral MLI until complete vertical and horizontal growth of the jaws (Figure 27).

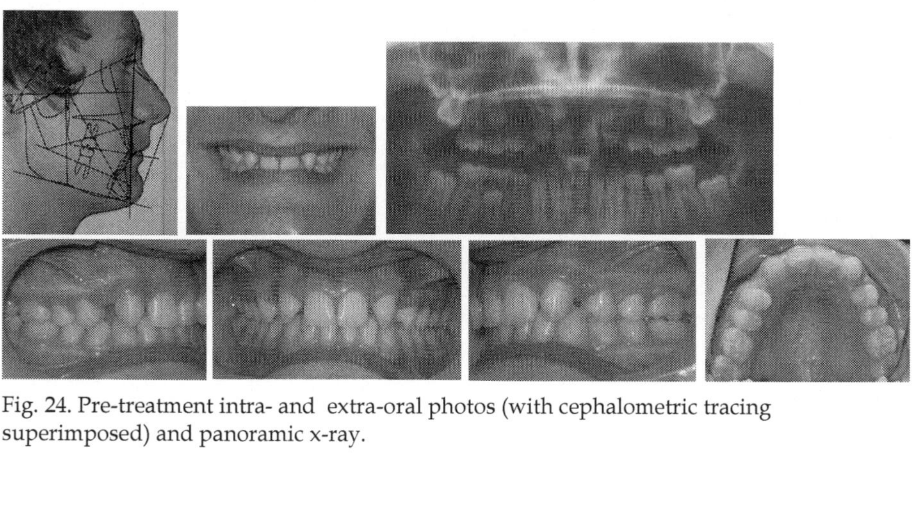

Fig. 24. Pre-treatment intra- and extra-oral photos (with cephalometric tracing superimposed) and panoramic x-ray.

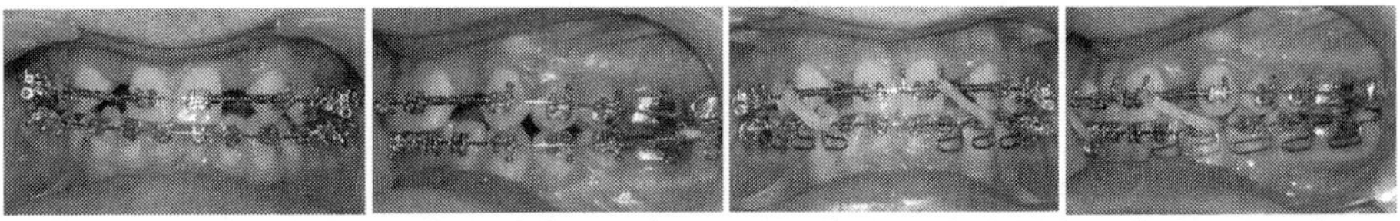

Fig. 25. Intra-oral photos with Multiloop Edgewise Arch Wire (MEAW) in the lower arch.

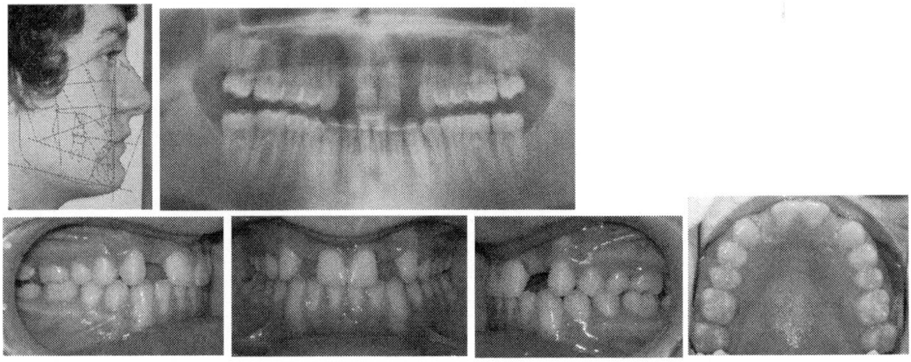

Fig. 26. Intra- and extra-oral photos (with cephalometric tracing superimposed) and panoramic x-ray after the orthodontic treatment.

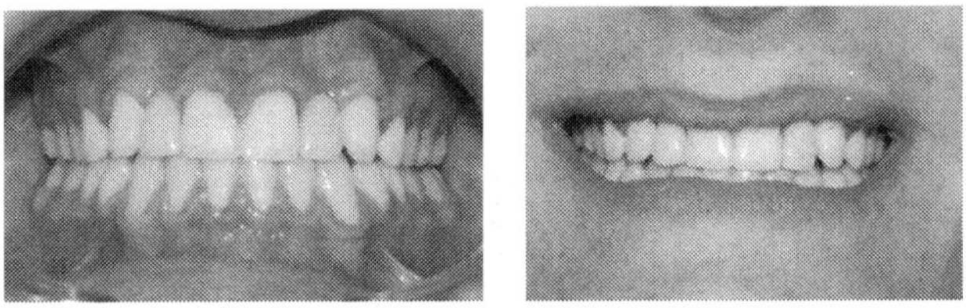

Fig. 27. Removable retainer with denture teeth to replace bilateral MLIA.

Clinical case 7 (Figure 28 and 29)

Bilateral MLIA, space opening in a 14 years old female with implants placement when the patient was 18 years old.

Diagnosis: Diastemas in the maxillary anterior region and partial bilateral mesialization of canines, due to bilateral agenesis of UR2 (12) and UL2 (22); concave soft-tissue profile with an open nasolabial angle, lip competence and a normal smile line, in relation to the facial midline, upper dental midline deviated to the left and centered mandibular dental midline; LL5 (35) agenesis with the persistence of the correspondent temporary; bilateral molar and canine Class II relationship (Figure 28).

Treatment involved space recovery for implant placement at the areas with congenital absences of UR2 (12) and UL2 (22), when the patient was 18 years old. Bilateral molar and canine Class I relationship obtained due to a lateral and posterior teeth distalization and mesial reposition of the mandible (Figure 29).

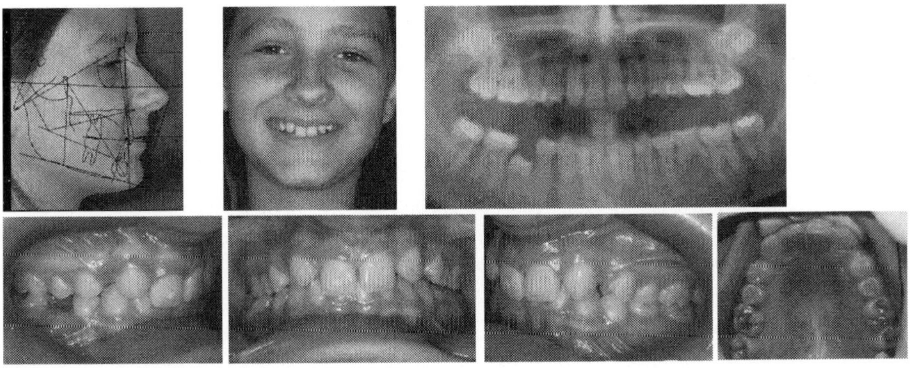

Fig. 28. Pre- treatment intra- and extra-oral photos (with cephalometric tracing superimposed) and panoramic x-ray.

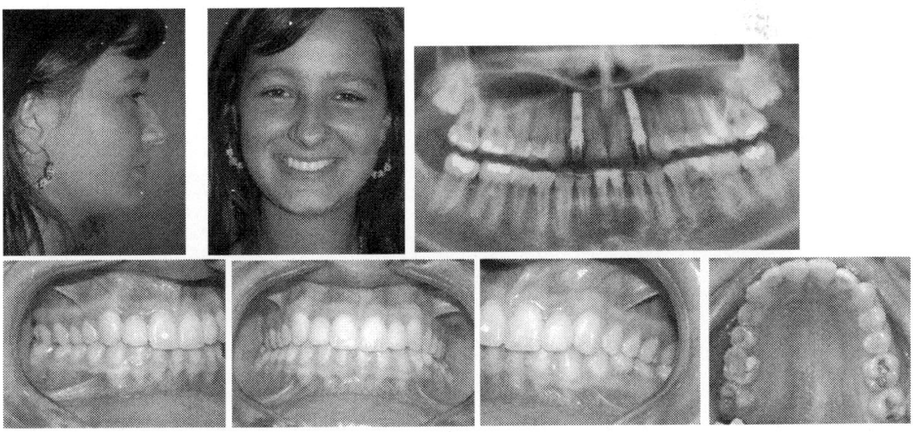

Fig. 29. Intra- and extra-oral photos and panoramic x-ray after orthodontic treatment.

5.2 Unilateral maxillary lateral incisors agenesis

When the lateral incisor microdontia is marked and / or root malformation is associated, it is preferable that the incisor extraction and the canine mesialization happens simultaneously, thus creating a symmetrical situation with preservation of the midline (Bowden & Harrison, 1994). If the option is to maintain the tooth, even if microdontic, we create mesial and distal spaces to the tooth to allow for later restoration by composite resin full ceramic crown, if at the root level no significant changes are seen.

If the lateral incisor is present in the arcade and is normal in size, the treatment option will depend on what has been mentioned, mainly the initial molar relations and the maxillary symmetry.

Not all solutions in unilateral agenesis should be based on predefined criteria, and an adequate clinical sense must always be present at the time of decision. When the occlusion is not appropriate to carry out the treatment plan with the opening or closure of spaces, some secondary criteria may help our choice. The position of the lip during smiling should be assessed, since the difference of color among teeth, lip contour, canine and adjacent teeth, as well as the difference in height between gingival margins will be less evident in patients with a low smile line. However, in patients with a high smile line, differences will be more detectable. These are the cases where there is always more difficulty, whether the option is the replacement with prosthesis or the space closure.

The harmony between the gingival margin of the front six maxillary teeth plays an important role in the aesthetic appearance (Kokich, 1996). The gingival contour depends on various factors like the periodontal biotype and the tooth shape. The gingival margin should follow the contour of the line-cementum junction, while the apex of the interproximal papilla must be situated midway between the incisal edge and the cervical margin of each anterior tooth, filling all the interproximal space. There are two acceptable standards for the height of the gingival margin of the six anterior-superior teeth: Standard Class 1, in which the gingival margins of the two central incisors (ICS) and upper canines (CS) must be within the same level and the lateral incisors (ILS) is positioned 1-2 mm more incisal; Standard Class II, in which the ICS, ILS and CS are at the same height (Chiche, 1994).

Clinical case 8 (Figure 30-32)

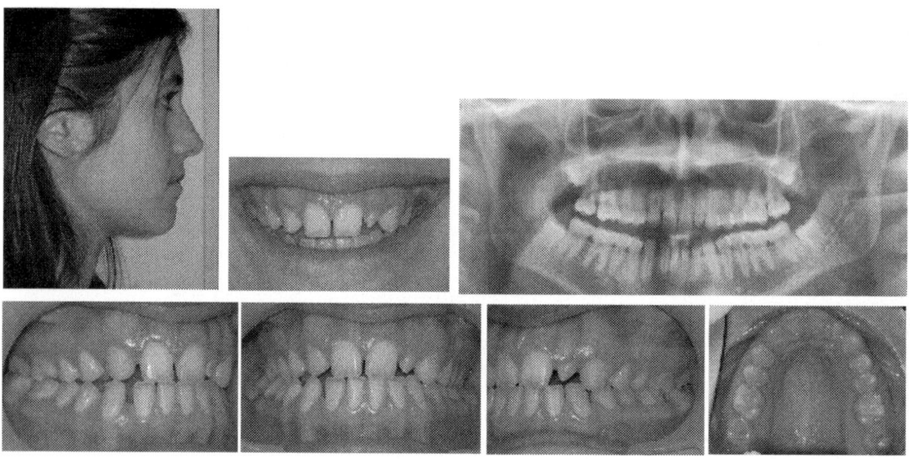

Fig. 30. Pre-treatment intra-and extra-oral photos and panoramic x-ray.

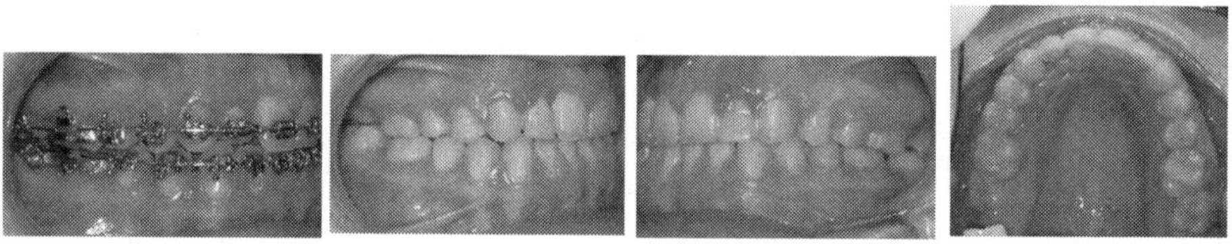

Fig. 31. Intra-oral photos during and at the end of the orthodontic treatment.

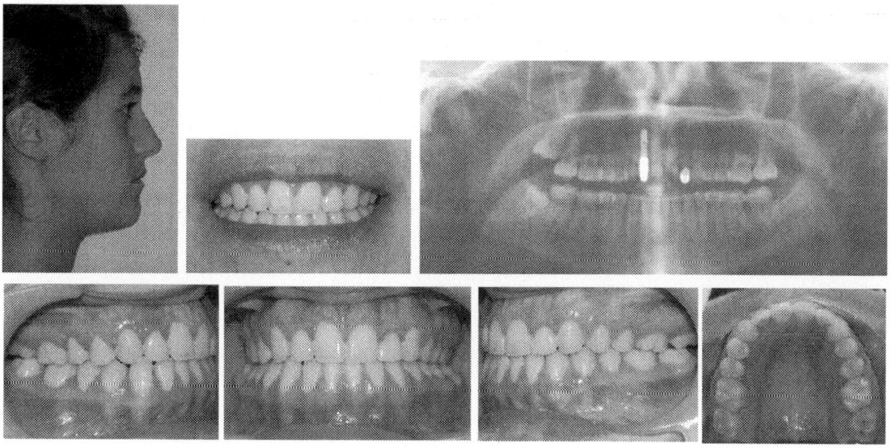

Fig. 32. Intra-and extra-oral photos 2 years after orthodontic treatment; panoramic x-ray. .

Clinical case 8: Symmetric space opening, in a 23 years old female.
Diagnosis: Unilateral agenesis of the UR2 (12) with a conical contralateral UL2 (22) and a mesialized UR3; molar and canine Class II relation on the right side and a molar and canine Class I on the left side; no dental crowding in the manbibular arch and some mesial and distal spaces related to the LR3 (43). Overjet and overbite were approximately 0mm. Panoramic x-ray revealed a mesialized root of the UR3 (13) (Figure 30).
The main factor that influenced the decision for the opening of space preserving symmetry was the high smile-line and thin lips that the patient presented.
The treatment was carried out in order to create symmetry, opening of space for placing an implant to replace tooth agenesis. The right molar Class I relation was obtained due to distalization of all 1st quadrant teeth and mesial movements of the posterior-inferior sector to close the existing mesial and distal diastema at the LR3 (43).
After opening the space a temporary prosthesis tooth was placed to improve the aesthetics. In order to improve the symmetry of the smile a gingival recontouring and a crown was performed on the UL2 (22) (Figure 31). Two years after the treatment the occlusion remained stable (Figure 32).

Clinical case 9: (Figure 33-35)

Symmetric space opening and lower incisor extraction, in a 12 years old female.
Diagnosis: Unilateral agenesis of the UR2 (12) with a microdontic contralateral UL2 (22); bilateral molar and canine Class I relation; severe dental crowding of the manbibular incisors; normal overjet and overbite, labial incompetence; crossed UL5 (25), UL6 (16), LL5 (35) and LL6 (36) . Panoramic x-ray confirmed mesial position of the UR3 (13) (Figure 33).
The main factor that influenced the decision to symmetrically open the space and extraction of LL1 (31) was the severe dental crowding of the manbibular incisors associated with a fine gingival biotype at the level of LL1 (31) and LR2 (42), labial incompetence and the existence of Bolton discrepancy due to the UL2 (22) microdontia (Figure 34).
The treatment was carried out in order to create enough space to allow the placement of an implant with the same dimension of the prosthetic tooth corresponding to the microdontic lateral incisor. At the end, left side bite was uncrossed (Figure 34). Six years after the treatment the occlusion remained stable (Figure 35).

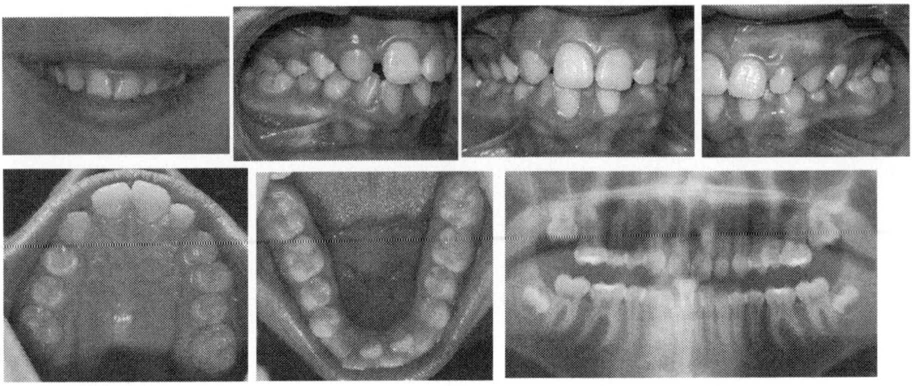

Fig. 33. Pre- treatment intra-and extra-oral photos and panoramic x-ray.

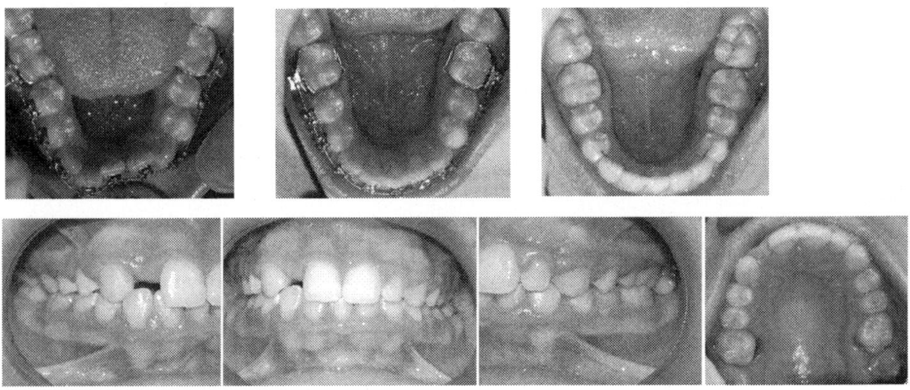

Fig. 34. Intra-oral photos during orthodontic treatment after the lower incisor extraction and at the end of the treatment.

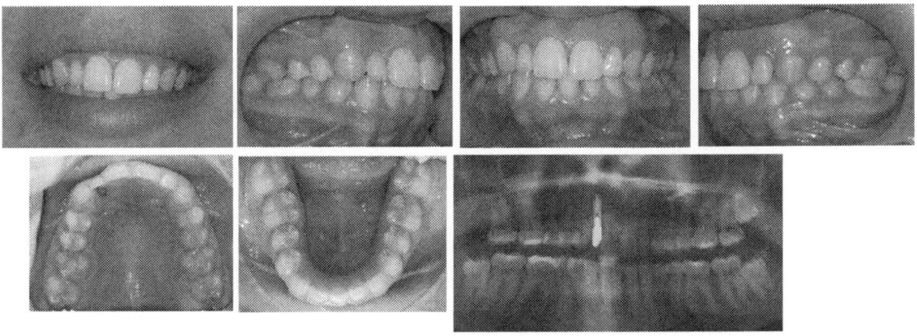

Fig. 35. Intra-and extra-oral photos, 6 years after orthodontic treatment; panoramic x-ray.

Clinical case 10 (Figure 36-39)

Symmetric space opening, in a 28 years old female.
Diagnosis: Unilateral agenesis of UR2 (12) with the UR3 (13) totally mesialized and persistence of the temporary URC (53) with distal positioned corresponding permanent tooth; contralateral UL2 (22) with conical appearance and a large periapical lesion; high vertical inclination of the incisors with an hypodivergent biotype; incomplete molar and canine Class II relation on both sides, except at the UR3 (13) where it is complete; overjet and overbite were 4.5mm and 8mm, respectively (Figure 36).
Due to esthetic factors originated by the smile line, as well as the periapical lesion of UL2 (22), the option was to extract UL2 (22) as well as the URC (53), to close the space with symmetry, aligning the permanent canines in order to replace the lateral incisors (Figure 37).
After treatment an improvement of the torque and the vertical position of upper incisors, was achieved. The option for leaving the upper canines slightly tilted towards a mesial position was to allow greater stability at the contact points with the central incisors, thereby preventing space reopening, taking into account the existing hypodivergent facial pattern (Figure 38). The improvement of the canines color and shape was possible though a bleaching of the canines and a combination of cupid reshaping and adhesive composite restoration of the mesial face (Figure 39).

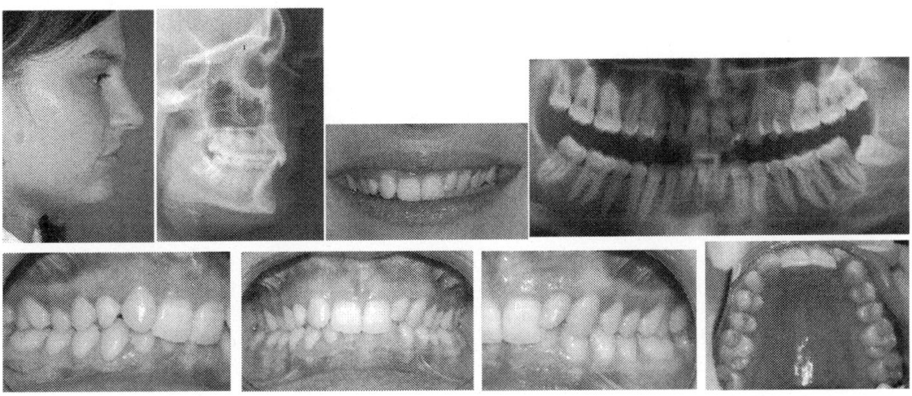

Fig. 36. Pre- treatment intra-and extra-oral photos; lateral telerradiography and panoramic x-ray.

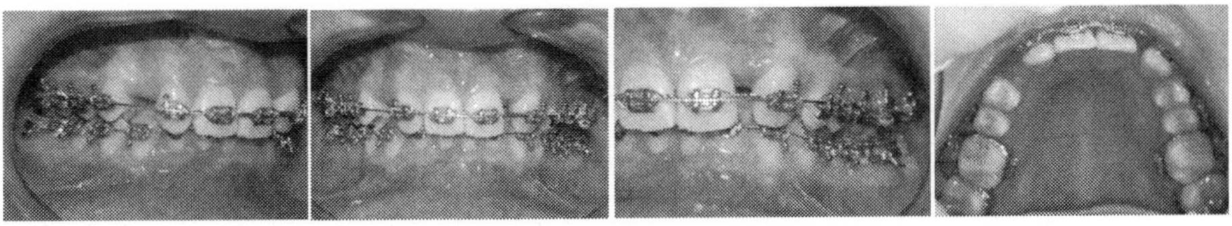

Fig. 37. Intra-oral photos, during orthodontic treatment

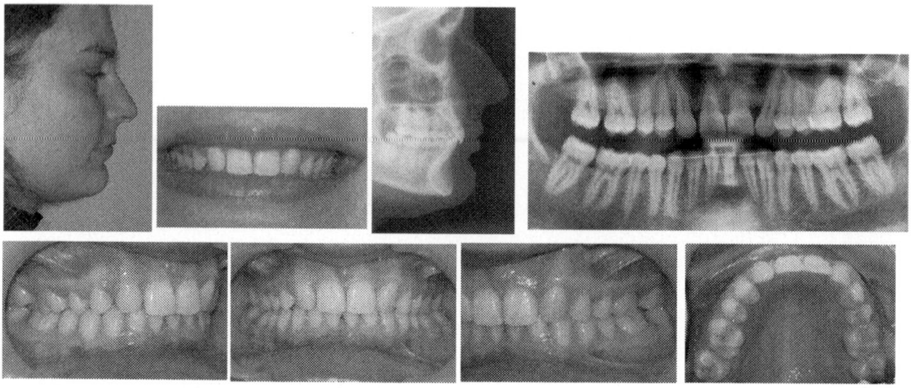

Fig. 38. Intra-and extra-oral photos after orthodontic treatment; lateral telerradiography and panoramic x-ray.

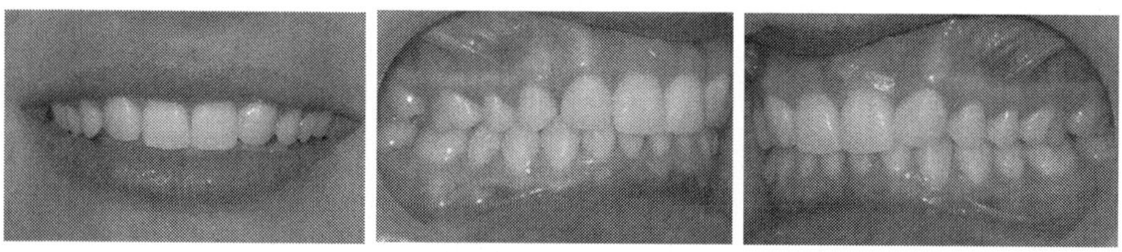

Fig. 39. Intra-and extra-oral photos 2 years after orthodontic treatment.

Clinical case 11 (Figure 40-44)

Asymmetric space closure, in a 12 years old female.

Diagnosis: Unilateral agenesis of the UR2 (12) with the UR3 (13) not totally mesialized; the contralateral UL2 (22) presented conical appearance; overjet increased due to high pro-inclination of the upper incisors; molar and canine Class II relation on the right side, being incomplete at the molar and full at the canine; on the left side a molar Class I and a canine Class II, due to a distal space at the UL3 (23); protruded upper lip with a closed nasolabial angle tendency. Panoramic x-ray revealed a considerable space between the root of UR1 (11) and the UR3 (13) (Figure 40).

The main factor that influenced the decision to close the space with asymmetry was the lower smile-line without visibility of the gingival margin during a forced smile.

The treatment was carried out in order to close space only on the right side with asymmetry, aligning the UR3 (13) with cupid reshaping to replace the UR2 (12). On the contralateral side the right molar Class I relation was maintained and the conical UL2 (22) was restored by adhesive resin composite that was done before the orthodontic treatment to facilitate the brackets bonding and then improved at the end of treatment. At the first stage a Straight-Wire technique was used (Figure 41) and then at the second stage a Multiloop Edgewise Arch-Wire technique was also used in order to improve occlusal relations between maxillary and mandibular arches (Figure 42).

After treatment, improvement of the incisors and anterior upper teeth gingival margin positions, as well as an esthetics labial position, instead of dental asymmetry can be observed (Figure 43).

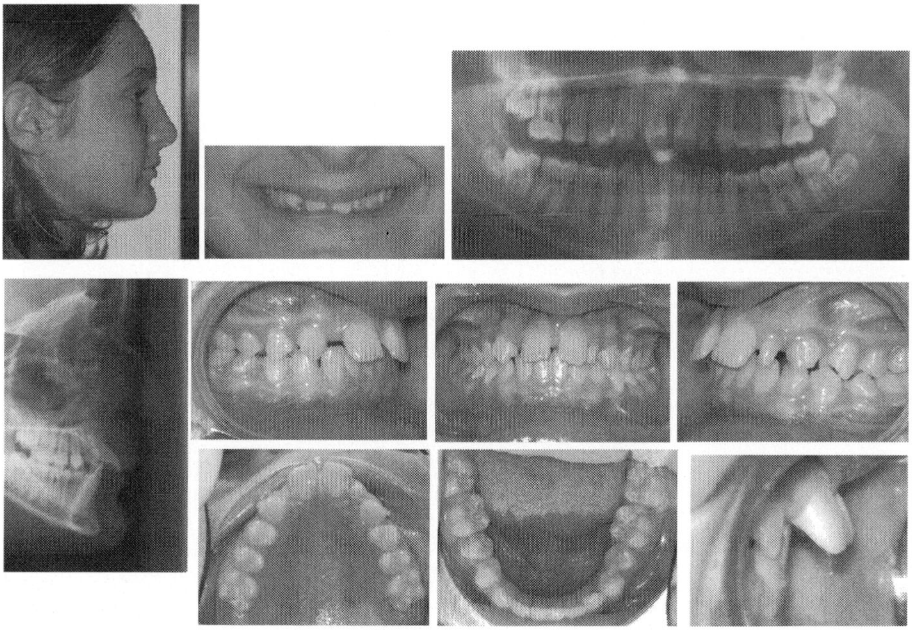

Fig. 40. Pre- treatment intra-and extra-oral photo; lateral telerradiography and panoramic x-ray.

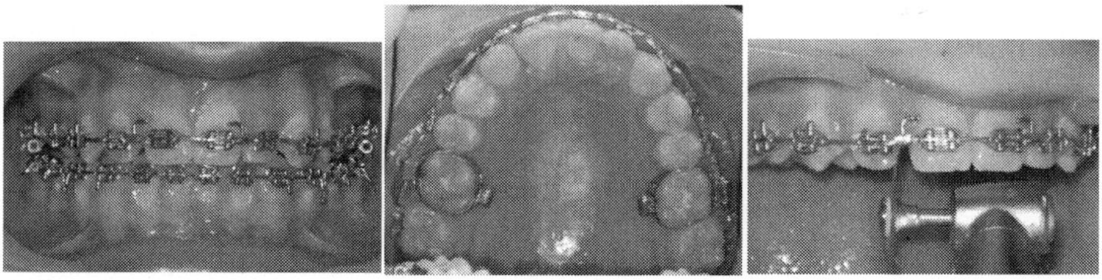

Fig. 41. Intra oral photos, during straight wire technique treatment.

In order to improve the symmetry of the smile a gingival recontouring was performed on the maxillar left lateral incisor, and resin composite reconstructions were done on the mesial face of UR3 (13) and UL2 (22). On the right side, lateral mandibular movements were guided by the first premolar, and in the left side by the canine. In the protusion movement there is a disocclusion of the posterior teeth (Figure 44).

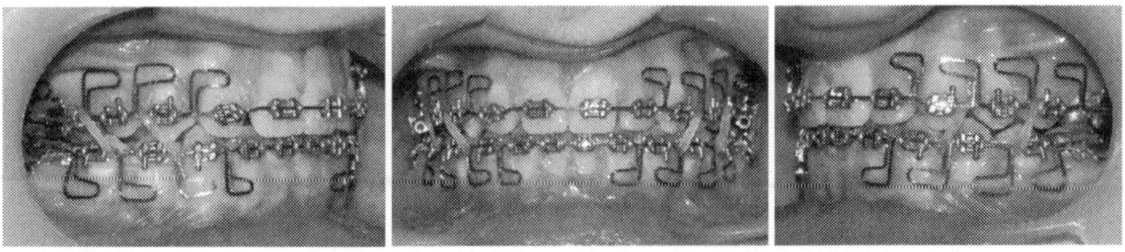

Fig. 42. Intra oral photos, during Multiloop Edgewise Arch Wire (MEAW).

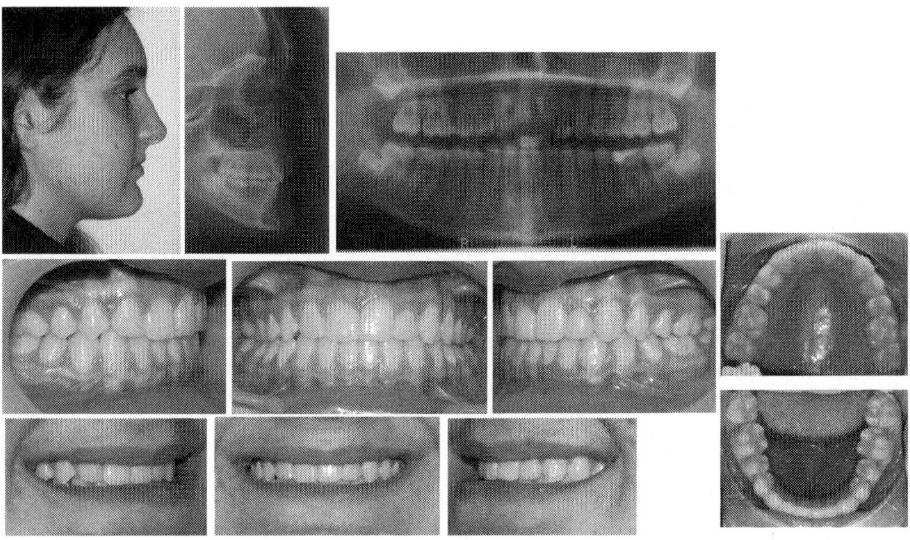

Fig. 43. Intra-and extra-oral photos after orthodontic treatment; and after UR3 (13) and UL2 (22) composite resin remodelation; lateral telerradiography and panoramic x-ray.

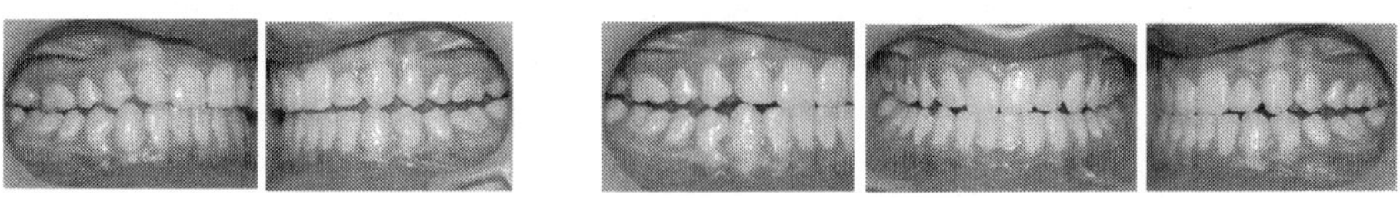

Fig. 44. Lateral and protrusive mandibular movements.

6. Final considerations

Orthodontists frequently face patients with maxillary lateral incisor agenesis (Pinho et al., 2005). Results obtained from Portuguese data showed that the risk for a first-degree relative of an individual with MLIA to have the same kind of agenesis is about 15 times higher than that of the general population (Pinho et al., 2010a). So, it is thus probable that different genes are involved in different phenotypes (Pinho et al., 2010a, 2010b).

In the diagnosis of agenesis of maxillary lateral incisors it is necessary to perform a good clinical examination and subsequent radiographic confirmation in order to observe not only the absence itself but also all the anomalies that may be associated (Pinho et al. 2005, 2009, 2011a, 2011b).

In the treatment plan for agenesis of the lateral incisors and the consequent choice for orthodontic therapy with closure or opening of the space we have to take into account esthetic, skeletal, dental, periodontal and functional factors (Pinho et al, 2001, 2003, 2004). Questionable situations should be based on predefined criteria, taking into account the clinical sense at the time of decision. In unilateral agenesis, the main factor that influences the decision to close the space with asymmetry is the position of the lip during forced smile.

7. References

Aasheim, B. & Øgaard B. (1993). Hypodontia in 9-year-old Norwegians related to need of orthodontic treatment. *Scandinavian Journal of Dental Research*, 101(5): 257-260.

Anthonappa, R. P.; Lee, C. K. et al. (2008). Hypohyperdontia: literature review and report of seven cases. *Oral Surgery, Oral Medicine, Oral Pathology, Oral Radiology & Endodontics*, 106(5): e24-30.

Baccetti, T. (1998). A controlled study of associated dental anomalies. *Angle Orthodontist* 68(3): 267-274.

Bae, J. H.; Choi, Y. H. et al. (2010). Autotransplantation of teeth with complete root formation: a case series. *Journal of Endodontics*, 36(8): 1422-1426.

Baum, B. J. & Cohen, M. M. (1971). Agenesis and tooth size in the permanent dentition. *Angle Orthodontist*, 41(2): 100-2.

Becker, A.; Smith, P. et al. (1981). The incidence of anomalous maxillary lateral incisors in relation to palatally-displaced cuspids. *Angle Orthodontist*, 51(1): 24-29.

Ben-Bassat, Y. & I. Brin (2009). Skeletal and dental patterns in patients with severe congenital absence of teeth. *American Journal of Orthodontics and Dentofacial Orthopedics*, 135(3): 349-356.

Bennett, C. G.; & Ronk S. L. (1980). Congenitally missing primary teeth: report of case. *ASDC Journal of Dentistry for Children*, 47(5): 346-348.

Bergendal, B., Bergendal, T. et al. (1996). A multidisciplinary approach to oral rehabilitation with osseointegrated implants in children and adolescents with multiple aplasia. *European Journal of Orthodontics*, 18(2): 119-129.

Bergstrom, K. (1977). An orthopantomographic study of hypodontia, supernumeraries and other anomalies in school children between the ages of 8-9 years. An epidemiological study. *Swedish Dental Journal*, 1(4): 145-157.

Bowden, D. E. & Harrison J. E. (1994). Missing anterior teeth: treatment options and their orthodontic implications. *Dental Update*, 21(10): 428-434.

Brenchley, Z. & Oliver R. G. (1997). Morphology of anterior teeth associated with displaced canines. *British journal of orthodontics*, 24(1): 41-5.

Burzynski, N. J. & Escobar V. H. (1983). Classification and genetics of numeric anomalies of dentition. *Birth Defects*, 19(1): 95-106.

Chiche, G. P., A. (1994). Esthetics of anterior fixed prosthodontics. Chicago: *Quintessence Books*, 13-32.

Chosack, A.; Eidelman E. et al. (1975). Hypodontia: a polygenic trait--a family study among Israeli Jews. *Journal of Dental Research*, 54(1): 16-19.

Das, P.; Stockton, D. W. et al. (2002). Haploinsufficiency of PAX9 is associated with autosomal dominant hypodontia. *Human Genetics*, 110(4): 371-376.

Dermaut, L. R.; Goeffers, K. R. et al. (1986). Prevalence of tooth agenesis correlated with jaw relationship and dental crowding. *American Journal of Orthodontics and Dentofacial Orthopedics*, 90(3): 204-210.

Dhanrajani, P. J. (2002). Hypodontia: etiology, clinical features, and management. *Quintessence International*, 33(4): 294-302.

Esposito, M.; Ekestubbe A., et al. (1993). Radiological evaluation of marginal bone loss at tooth surfaces facing single Branemark implants. *Clinical Oral Implants Research*, 4(3): 151-157.

Garib, D. G.; Alencar, B. M. et al. (2010). Agenesis of maxillary lateral incisors and associated dental anomalies. *American Journal of Orthodontics and Dentofacial Orthopedics*, 137(6): 732 e1-6; 732-733.

Garn, S. M. & Lewis, A. B. (1970). The gradient and the pattern of crown-size reduction in simple hypodontia. *Angle Orthodontist*, 40(1): 51-8.

Gerits, A.; Nieminen, P. et al. (2006). Exclusion of coding region mutations in MSX1, PAX9 and AXIN2 in eight patients with severe oligodontia phenotype. *Orthodontic Craniofacial Research*, 9(3): 129-136.

Grunder, U.; Gracis, S., et al. (2005). Influence of the 3-D bone-to-implant relationship on esthetics. *International Journal of Periodontics & Restorative Dentistry*, 25(2): 113-119.

Guala, A.; Falco, V., et al. (2008). Deletion of PAX9 and oligodontia: a third family and review of the literature. International Journal of Paediatric Dentistry.

Hansen, L.; Kreiborg, S. et al. (2007). A novel nonsense mutation in PAX9 is associated with marked variability in number of missing teeth. *European Journal of Oral Sciences*, 115(4): 330-333.

Hobkirk, J. A.; Goodman, J. R., et al. (1994). Presenting complaints and findings in a group of patients attending a hypodontia clinic. *British Dental Journal*, 177(9): 337-339.

Horowitz, J. M. (1966). Aplasia and malocclusion: a survey and appraisal. *American Journal of Orthodontics*, 52(6): 440-453.

Itthagarun, A. and N. M. King (1997). Ectodermal dysplasia: a review and case report. *Quintessence International*, 28(9): 595-602.

Järvinen, S. & Lehtinen L. (1981). Supernumerary and congenitally missing primary teeth in Finnish children. An epidemiologic study. *Acta Odontologic Scandnavian*, 39(2): 83-86.

Johannsdottir, B.; Wisth, P. J. et al. (1997). Prevalence of malocclusion in 6-year-old Icelandic children. *Acta Odontologic Scandnavian*, 55(6): 398-402.

Kapadia, H.; Mues, G. et al. (2007). Genes affecting tooth morphogenesis. *Orthodontic Craniofacial Research*, 10(4): 237-44.

Kobielak, K.; Kobielak, A. et al. (2001). Mutations in the EDA gene in three unrelated families reveal no apparent correlation between phenotype and genotype in the patients with an X-linked anhidrotic ectodermal dysplasia. *American Journal of Medical Genetics*, 100(3): 191-197.

Kokich, V. (2005). Early Management of Congenitally Missing Teeth. *Seminars in Orthodontics* 11: 146-151.

Kokich, V. G. (1996). Esthetics: the orthodontic-periodontic restorative connection. *Seminars in Orthodontics*, 2(1): 21-30.

Kokich, V. O. Jr. (2002). Congenitally missing teeth: orthodontic management in the adolescent patient. *American Journal of Orthodontics and Dentofacial Orthopedics*, 121(6): 594-5.

Kuchler, E. C.; Menezes, R. et al (2010). MMP1 and MMP20 contribute to tooth agenesis in humans. *Archives of Oral Biology*, [Epub ahead of print]

Lammi, L., S. Arte, et al. (2004). Mutations in AXIN2 cause familial tooth agenesis and predispose to colorectal cancer. *American Journal of Human Genetics*, 74(5): 1043-1050.

Lidral, A. C. & Reising, B. C. (2002). The role of MSX1 in human tooth agenesis. *Journal of Dental Research*, 81(4): 274-8.

Lidral, A. C.; Romitti, P. A. et al. (1998). Association of MSX1 and TGFB3 with nonsyndromic clefting in humans. *American Journal of Human Genetics*, 63(2): 557-568.

Lin, Y.; Cheng, Y. S. et al. (2008). FGFR2 in the dental epithelium is essential for development and maintenance of the maxillary cervical loop, a stem cell niche in mouse incisors. *Development Dynamics*, 238(2): 324-330.

Magnusson, T. E. (1977). Prevalence of hypodontia and malformations of permanent teeth in Iceland. *Community Dentistry and Oral Epidemiology*, 5(4): 173-178.

Marques, A. P. F. & Till, M. J. (1994). Ectodermal Dysplasia: treatment considerations and case reports. *Revista Portuguesa Cirurgia Maxilofacial*, 35(1/2): 17-22.

Millar, B. J. & Taylor, N. G. (1995). Lateral thinking: the management of missing upper lateral incisors. *British Dental Journal*, 179(3): 99-106.

Miller, T. E. (1995). Implications of congenitally missing teeth: orthodontic and restorative procedures in the adult patient. *Journal of Prosthetic Dentistry*, 73(2): 115-122.

Mostowska, A.; Biedziak, B. et al. (2006). A novel c.581C>T transition localized in a highly conserved homeobox sequence of MSX1: is it responsible for oligodontia? *Journal of Applied Genetics*, 47(2): 159-164.

Muller, T. P.; Hill, I. N. et al. (1970). A survey of congenitally missing permanent teeth. *Journal of the American Dental Association*, 81(1): 101-107.

Nick-Hussein, N. N. & Majid, Z. A. (1996). Dental anomalies in the primary dentition: Distribution and correlation with the permanent dentition. *Journal of Clinical Pediatric Dentistry*, 21(1): 15-19.

Nieminen, P.; Arte, S. et al. (2001). Identification of a nonsense mutation in the PAX9 gene in molar oligodontia. *European Journal of Human Genetics*, 9(10): 743-746.

Nodal, M.; Kjær, I. et al. (1994). Craniofacial morphology in patients with multiple congenitally missing permanent teeth. European Journal of Orthodontics, 16(2): 104-109.

Nordgarden, H.; Jensen, J. L. et al. (2002). Reported prevalence of congenitally missing teeth in two Norwegian counties. Community. *Dental Health*, 19(4): 258-261.

O'Dowling, I. B. & McNamara, T. G. (1990). Congenital absence of permanent teeth among Irish school-children. *Journal of the Irish Dental Association*, 36(4): 136-138.

Ogaard, B. & Krogstad O. (1995). Craniofacial structure and soft tissue profile in patients with severe hypodontia. *American Journal of Orthodontics and Dentofacial Orthopedics*, 108(5): 472-477.

Park, J. H.; Okadakage, S. et al. (2010). Orthodontic treatment of a congenitally missing maxillary lateral incisor. *Journal of Esthetic and Restorative Dentistry*, 22(5): 297-312.

Peck, S.; Peck, L. et al. (1996). Prevalence of tooth agenesis and peg-shaped maxillary lateral incisor associated with palatally displaced canine (PDC) anomaly. *American Journal of Orthodontics and Dentofacial Orthopedics*, 110(4): 441-443.

Peck, S.; Peck, L. et al. (2002). Concomitant occurrence of canine malposition and tooth agenesis: evidence of orofacial genetic fields. *American Journal of Orthodontics and Dentofacial Orthopedics*, 122(6): 657-660.

Pereira, T. V.; Salzano, F. M. et al. (2006). Natural selection and molecular evolution in primate PAX9 gene, a major determinant of tooth development. *Proceeding of the National Academy of Science of the USA*, 103(15): 5676-5681.

Pilo, R.; Kaffe, I. et al. (1987). Diagnosis of developmental dental anomalies using panoramic radiographs. *ASDC Journal Dentistry for Children* 54(4): 267-272.

Pinho, T. (2003). Agenesis of upper lateral incisors- case study: orthodontic and restaurative procedures. *Gnathos*, 2(2): 35-42.

Pinho, T. (2004). Skeletal Class III in a case with upper lateral incisors agenesis. *Gnathos*, 5: 33-41.

Pinho T. & Lemos C. Dental repercussions of maxillary lateral incisor agenesis. *European Journal of Orthodontics* 2011; doi: 10.1093/ejo/cjr084.

Pinho, T.; Maciel, P. et al. (2010a). Familial aggregation of maxillary lateral incisor agenesis. *Journal of Dental Research*, 89(6): 621-625.

Pinho, T.; Maciel, P. et al. (2009). Developmental disturbances associated with agenesis of the permanent maxillary lateral incisor. *British Dental Journal*, 207(12): E25.

Pinho, T. & Neves, M. (2001). Tratamento da ausência congénita de incisivos maxilares quando a opção é manter ou abrir o espaço. *Dental Sapiens*, 1(1): 7-16.

Pinho, T.; Pollmann, C. et al. (2011b). Craniofacial Repercussions in Maxillary Lateral Incisors Agenesis. *International Orthodontics*, 9:274-285.

Pinho, T.; Silva-Fernandes, A. et al. (2010a). Mutational analysis of MSX1 and PAX9 genes in Portuguese families with maxillary lateral incisor agenesis. *European Journal of Orthodontics*, 32(5): 582-588.

Pinho, T.; Tavares, P. et al. (2005). Developmental absence of maxillary upper lateral incisors in the Portuguese population. *European Journal of Orthodontics*, 27(5): 443-449.

Pirinen, S.; Arte, S. et al. (1996). Palatal displacement of canine is genetic and related to congenital absence of teeth. Journal of Dental Research, 75(10): 1742-1746.

Prabhu, N. T.; John, R. et al. (1997). Rieger's syndrome: a case report. *Quintessence International*, 28(11): 749-52.

Ranta, R. & Tulensalo, T. (1988). Symmetry and combinations of hypodontia in non-cleft and cleft palate children. *Scandinavian Journal of Dental Research*, 96(1): 1-8.

Ravn, J. J. (1971). Aplasia, supernumerary teeth and fused teeth in the primary dentition. An epidemiologic study. *Scandinavian Journal of Dental Research*, 79(1): 1-6.

Rolling, S. (1980). Hypodontia of permanent teeth in Danish schoolchildren. *Scandinavian Journal of Dental Research*, 88(5): 365-369.

Rosa, M. & Zachrisson B. U. (2001). Integrating esthetic dentistry and space closure in patients with missing maxillary lateral incisors. *Journal Clinic Orthodontic*, 35(4): 221-234.

Schalk-van der Weide, Y.; Beemer, F. A. et al. (1994). Symptomatology of patients with oligodontia. *Journal of Oral Rehabilitation*, 21(3): 247-261.

Schalk-Van Der Weide, Y.; Beemer, F. A. et al. (1994). Symptomatology of patients with oligodontia. *Journal of Oral Rehabilitation*, 21: 247-261.

Schalk-van der Weide, Y. & Bosman F. (1996). Tooth size in relatives of individuals with oligodontia. Archives of Oral Biology, 41(5): 469-472.

Schalk-van der Weide, Y.; Steen, W. H. et al. (1994). Reductions in size and left-right asymmetry of teeth in human oligodontia. *Archives of Oral Biology*, 39(11): 935-939.

Schalk-van der Weide, Y.; W. H. Steen, et al. (1992). Distribution of missing teeth and tooth morphology in patients with oligodontia. *ASDC Journal of Dentistry for Children*, 59(2): 133-140.

Schuffenhauer, S.; Leifheit, H. J. et al. (1999). De novo deletion (14)(q11.2q13) including PAX9: clinical and molecular findings. *Journal of Medical Genetics*, 36(3): 233-236.

Small, B. (1996). Esthetic management of congenitally missing lateral incisors with single-tooth implants: A case report. *Quintessence International*, 27(9): 585-590.

Spray, J. R.; Black, C. G. et al. (2000). The influence of bone thickness on facial marginal bone response: stage 1 placement through stage 2 uncovering. *Annals of Periodontology*, 5(1): 119-228.

Stockton, D. W.; Das, P. et al. (2000). Mutation of PAX9 is associated with oligodontia. Nature Genetics, 24(1): 18-19.

Swinnen, S.; Bailleul-Forestier, I. et al. (2008). Investigating the etiology of multiple tooth agenesis in three sisters with severe oligodontia. *Orthodontic Craniofacial Research*, 11(1): 24-31.

Tallon-Walton, V.; Manzanares-Cespedes, M. C. et al. (2007). Identification of a novel mutation in the PAX9 gene in a family affected by oligodontia and other dental anomalies. *European Journal of Oral Sciences*, 115(6): 427-432.

Tavajohi-Kermani, H.; Kapur, R. et al. (2002). Tooth agenesis and craniofacial morphology in an orthodontic population. *American Journal of Orthodontics and Dentofacial Orthopedics*, 122(1): 39-47.

Taylor, R. W. (1998). Eruptive abnormalities in orthodontic treatment. *Seminars in Orthodontics*, 4(2): 79-86.

Thilander, B. & Myrberg N. (1973). The prevalence of malocclusion in Swedish schoolchildren. *Scandinavian Journal of Dental Research*, 81(1): 12-21.

Thilander, B.; Odman, J. et al. (1994). Osseointegrated implants in adolescents. An alternative in replacing missing teeth? *European Journal of Orthodontics*, 16(2): 84-95.

Tummers, M. & Thesleff I. (2009). The importance of signal pathway modulation in all aspects of tooth development. *Journal of Experimental Zoology* Part B: Molecular and Developmental Evolution.

Tunc, E. S.; Bayrak, S. et al. (2011). Dental development in children with mild-to-moderate hypodontia. *American Journal of Orthodontics and Dentofacial Orthopedics*, 139(3): 334-338.

Vastardis, H. (2000). The genetics of human tooth agenesis: new discoveries for understanding dental anomalies. *American Journal of Orthodontics and Dentofacial Orthopedics*, 117(6): 650-656.

Vastardis, H.; Karimbux, N. et al. (1996). A human MSX1 homeodomain missense mutation causes selective tooth agenesis. *Nature Genetics*, 13(4): 417-421.

Wisth, P. J.; Thunold, K. et al. (1974). The craniofacial morphology of individuals with hypodontia. *Acta Odontologic Scandnavian*, 32(4): 281-290.

Woodworth, D. A.; Sinclair, P. M. et al. (1985). Bilateral congenital absence of maxillary lateral incisors: a craniofacial and dental cast analysis. *American Journal of Orthodontics*, 87(4): 280-293.

Yaqoob, O.; Dibiase, A. T. et al. (2011) Relationship between bilateral congenital absence of maxillary lateral incisors and anterior tooth width. *American Journal of Orthodontics and Dentofacial Orthopedics*, 139(3): e229-233.

Yuksel, S. & Ucem T. (1997). The effect of tooth agenesis on dentofacial structures. *European Journal of Orthodontics*, 19(1): 71-78.

Zarone, F.; Sorrentino, R. et al. (2006). Prosthetic treatment of maxillary lateral incisor agenesis with osseointegrated implants: a 24-39-month prospective clinical study. *Clinical Oral Implants Research*, 17(1): 94-101.

Zhao, J.; Hu, Q. et al. (2007). A novel missense mutation in the paired domain of human PAX9 causes oligodontia. *American Journal of Medical Genetics*, 143A(21): 2592-2597.

Zhu, J. F.; Crevoisier, R. et al. (1996). Congenitally missing permanent lateral incisors in conjunction with a supernumerary tooth: case report. *Pediatric Dentistry*, 18(1): 64-66.

Zhu, J. F.; Marcushamer, M. et al. (1996). Supernumerary and congenitally absent teeth: a literature review. *Journal of Clinical Pediatric Dentistry*, 20(2):87-95.

Zirberman, Y.; Cohen, B. et al. (1990). Familial trends in palatal canines, anomalous lateral incisors, and related phenomena. *European Journal of Orthodontics*, 12: 135-139.

13

Orthodontics and Caries

Farid Bourzgui, Mourad Sebbar and Mouna Hamza
Department of Orthodontics, Faculty of Dentistry, University of Hassan II Ain Chok, Casablanca, Morocco

1. Introduction

The purpose of orthodontics is to achieve correct dental occlusion, while at the same time improving aesthetic appearance. However, we know today that orthodontic treatment increases the risk of carious lesions, which harm patients and jeopardize the successful outcome of the treatment. The formation of carious lesions as a result of orthodontic treatment can be ascribed to inadequate elimination of dental plaque due to hindrance by intrabuccal appliances.

To forestall these particularly harmful collateral effects, thorough knowledge of how caries form and the associated risk factors is necessary. The risk factors specific to each patient should therefore be accurately evaluated before any orthodontic treatment is undertaken, and then monitored throughout the treatment so that health-damaging carious lesions do not become established.

The aim of this chapter is to define caries and its aetiological factors, pinpoint its various risk factors in orthodontics, describe a preventive, prophylactic approach to be taken before, during and after orthodontic treatment, and make recommendations.

2. Caries

Dental caries is the result of bacteria-induced breakdown of the hard tissues of the tooth by progressive local demineralization (Muller et al,1998; Rillard et al, 2000).

2.1 Etiological factors

The aetiology of caries is multifactorial. Caries are formed under the simultaneous action of several factors (Fig.1): cariogenic bacteria in dental plaque, food, terrain and a time scale sufficient for the carious lesion to grow (Charland et al, 2001).

2.1.1 Cariogenic bacteria

The inside of the mouth and dental plaque contain a broad variety of bacteria. *Streptococcus mutans* is the main micro-organism responsible for human caries. This bacterium uses carbohydrates as a nutrient and energy source, metabolizing them to form lactic acid, which lowers pH and thereby causes the demineralization of tooth enamel (Rillard et al, 2000). This infectious disorder develops with a prevalence that is related to the degree of oral sepsis present.

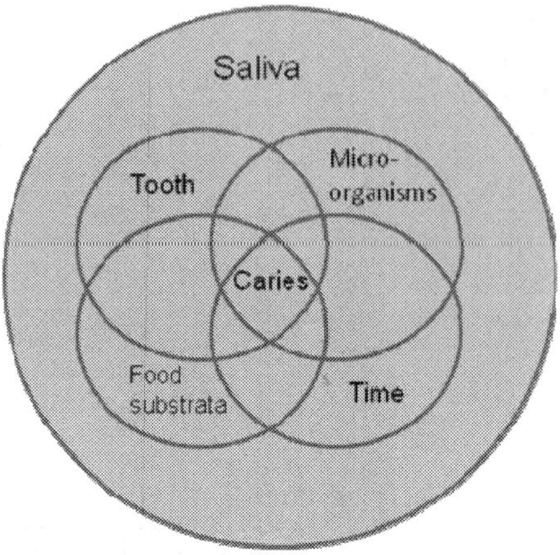

Fig. 1. Aetiological factors in dental caries

2.1.2 Food

Food plays an essential part in the formation and spread of caries (Haikel & Hemmerle, 1993, 2001). Cariogenic bacteria can survive in the mouth and act there only if they find fermentable food sugars to meet their metabolic requirements *in situ* (Haikel, 2001). Sucrose is the commonest food carbohydrate. It is naturally present in most fruits and vegetables, but is also deliberately added to many food products (Miller et al, 2000).

Essential aetiological food-related factors include the duration of the cariogenic conditions, oral retentiveness and the physical form of the food, the types and concentrations of carbohydrates present, and the patient's eating habits (Droz & Blique, 1999).

2.1.3 Terrain

Dental anatomy can constitute a host-related risk factor. Deficient dental contact points favour the development of dental plaque and caries. Caries can also start in the pits and crevices of the back teeth, which form anfractuous areas that even the finest bristles of a toothbrush cannot easily penetrate.

Saliva also plays an important part in the cariogenic process. Its action is essentially carioprotective, through its mechanical "wash-out" action, responsible for eliminating food waste, and through some of its constituents that act on the remineralization of the enamel. Thus any modification of saliva flow will favour the development of caries (Haikel & Hemmerle, 1993).

Like any disease, caries evolves according to the unstable equilibrium between the intensity of the pathological factors cited above and the biological defence response (Haikel, 1993). Caries appear when the balance between demineralization and remineralization at the tooth surface is disturbed. Dental caries is a dynamic process with periods of progression alternating with stationary phases. This cariogenic process is generally reversible in its initial stages in favourable conditions, but it is irreversible once it has reached an advanced stage (Charland & Salvail, 2003).

2.2 Orthodontic treatment and increased risk of caries

Alongside the usual risk factors for dental caries, orthodontic treatments are also a non-negligible risk factor (Gorton & Featherstone, 2003; Travess et al, 2004; Derks et al, 2007). Introducing a fixed appliance in the mouth favours the build-up of dental plaque, makes oral hygiene very difficult, restricts salivary self-cleaning and so creates an environment that favours the onset of caries (Ahn & Kho, 2003; Derks et al, 2007; Lovrov et al, 2007).

The fitting of orthodontic appliances causes a modification of the oral ecosystem, with an increase in the numbers of cariogenic bacteria (Batoni et al, 2001; Sukontapatipark et al, 2001). This change upsets the balance between the processes of demineralization and remineralization, thereby increasing the patient's individual risk of caries (Fig. 2).

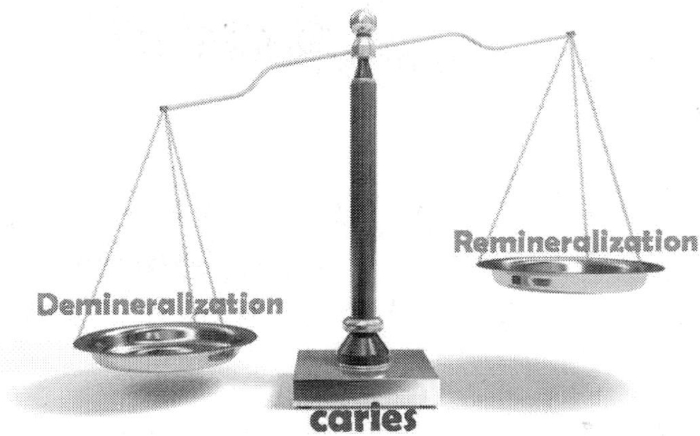

Fig. 2. Increased individual risk of caries in a patient due to imbalance between the processes of demineralization and remineralization.

In addition, orthodontic treatment is most often applied during adolescence, when the permanent teeth have recently erupted and so are more vulnerable to caries because of their young enamel. This greatly compounds the risk of caries, and so orthodontic treatment at this age will favour the formation of carious lesions. These can be caries in pits and grooves, which make up more than 60% of lesions diagnosed according to Chaussain (Chaussain et al, 2009). However, the carious lesions can also be localized on smooth surfaces, giving the amelar demineralization lesions known as "white spots" (Zimmer & Rottwinkely, 2004; Sudjalim et al, 2006). According to Kamp, these "white spots", or initial lesions of the enamel, are present in 25-30% of patients who are following an orthodontic treatment (Jordan, 1998).

The teeth most vulnerable to demineralization are the maxillary incisors and the first permanent molars. The three locations most at risk of demineralization are: the cervical areas, the areas located under the bands and the enamel adjacent to cemented brackets (O'Reilly & Featherstone, 1987; Jordan & LeBlanc, 2002).

This initial lesion that occurs during orthodontic treatment appears clinically as an opaque whitish or greyish halo at the junction between the cement and the enamel, and generally at the gum level at the base of the half moon bracket. If the mineral loss continues, then an irreversible cavity formation ensues (Fig. 3.4.5).

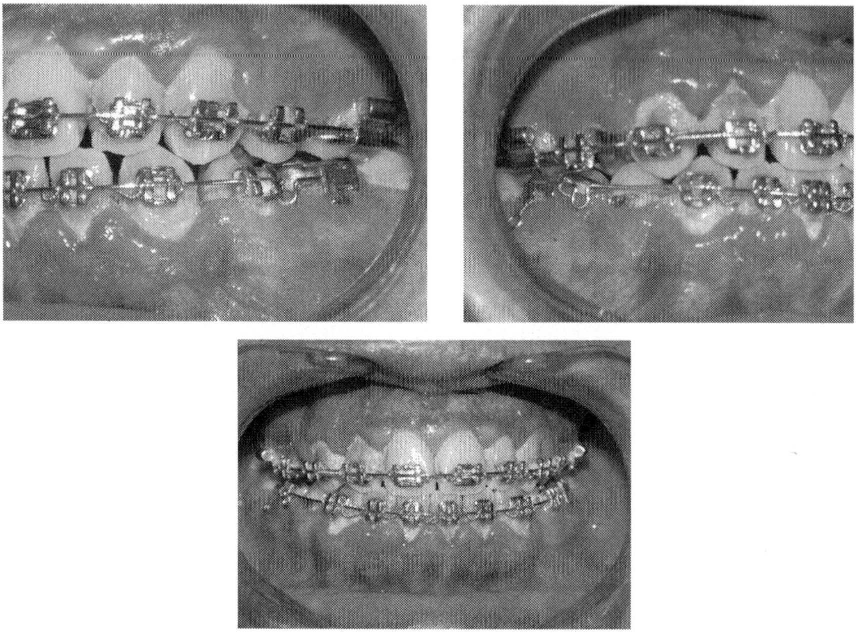

Fig. 3. 4. 5 Patient who had been wearing a brace for 7 years presented for consultation with this buccodental state.

3. Study conducted at the faculty of Dentistry, Casablanca

The department of dentofacial orthopaedics of the faculty of dentistry at Casablanca conducted an internal survey to evaluate the prevalence of dental caries and associated risk factors in orthodontics (Bourzgui et al, 2010). A total of 155 patients were followed up for 3 months and 19 days. Their average age was 21.13 ± 8.22 years. The survey included patients wearing fixed orthodontic appliances with vestibular cemented brackets. Patients fitted with lingual appliances, plates or prosthetic devices, and those displaying tooth tissue abnormalities were excluded. Of the included patients, 27.1% had worn their orthodontic appliances for less than 6 months, 36.8% for between 6 and 18 months and 36.1% for more than 18 months.

All the patients used a toothbrush and toothpaste: 52.3% brushed their teeth three times a day, 63.8% for less than 3 minutes, and 63.9% using the up-and-down method. A mechanical toothbrush was used by 94.2% and an electric toothbrush by 5.8%; 43.9% used no dental floss, inderdental brushes or toothpicks; 88.4% used fluoride toothpaste and 3.9% used fluoride mouthwash, but none used fluoride gels or fluoride varnishes.

Plaque index was between 0.5 and 1 in 33.6% of the patients and between 1 and 1.5 in 36.1%. Overall it was between 0.08 and 2.4 with an average of 1.12 ± 0.48 (Fig. 3).
Gingival index was less 0.5 in 34.9% of the patients and between 0.5 and 1 in 41.2%. Overall it was between 0 and 2 with an average of 0.67 ± 0.43 (Fig. 4).
Excessive consumption of carbohydrates in soft drinks was reported in 31.6% of the patients, and 45.8% were in the habit of snacking essentially on sweetened foods. No preventive sealing of pits and grooves of permanent molars had been carried out on 87.1% of the patients.
Before the orthodontic treatment, 72.2% of the subjects presented caries, and 27.8% of these lesions had appeared during the orthodontic treatment; 89.7% of the caries occurred on the back teeth and 56.7% were occlusal; 7.7% had developed white spots on their teeth during the treatment, on front teeth in 25%, back teeth in 25% and both front and back teeth in 50% of cases.

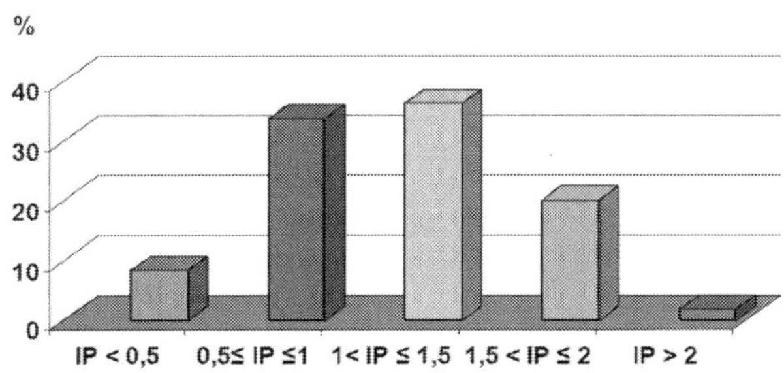

Fig. 6. Distribution of subjects by plaque index

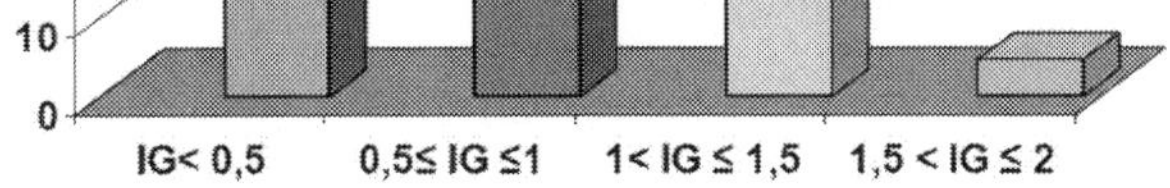

Fig. 7. Distribution of subjects by gingival index

4. Prevention of caries risk in orthodontics

Patients wearing orthodontic appliances should be considered as patients at risk, for whom a preventive, prophylactic approach should be implemented before, during and after the orthodontic treatment (Terrie et al, 2004).

4.1 Before orthodontic treatment

4.1.1 Clinical interview

First of all a clinical interview of the patient should be conducted to determine his or her patterns of behaviour, eating habits, dental hygiene and, if possible, the history of any fluoride treatments undergone (Fortier et al, 1997; Kuhn & Besnault, 2000; Zimmer & Rottwinkel, 2004).

In the case of children, this interview can also assess the degree to which their families are ready, willing and able to help the treatment succeed, an essential factor in ensuring a good quality follow-up of the different treatments proposed (Terk, 1993; Fortier et al, 1997). This interview is followed by a full clinical and radiological dental examination.

4.1.2 Clinical examination

Right at the start the buccodental state should meet certain criteria to facilitate orthodontic treatment and not be likely to cause any local complications that could be wrongly interpreted as being directly due to the orthodontic treatment itself, and so be blamed on it (Fortier et al, 1997).

The role of the practitioner, whether a paedodontist or a general practitioner, is to undertake a systematic search for disorders and abnormalities, both visible and invisible, and make a complete assessment of them.

The dental report: should:

- state the number of teeth present, absent, and treated;
- record all the clinically visible carious lesions and their complications;
- identify any structural abnormalities liable to produce areas of special fragility.

4.1.3 Radiological examination

In addition to the dental examination, an accurate, systematic radiological examination should be performed (Fortier et al, 1997).

Its aim should be:

- to determine the extent of any carious lesions and their possible complications;
- to visualize any relapsed carious lesions under fillings;
- to monitor the progress of apexogenesis or apexification treatment.

4.1.4 Dental care treatment

After this examination, an appropriate treatment plan should be drawn up to carry out the different dental care treatments needed before the orthodontic treatment can in turn be initiated. This pre-orthodontic buccodental preparation is an essential step (Fortier et al, 1997).

The orthodontist should be personally involved at this stage and ensure that all preventive precautions are taken and all necessary treatment is carried out, jointly with the paedodontist or general practitioner.

The following should be performed:

- treatment of all caries;
- treatment of all pulp disorders due to caries;
- restoration of anatomic and functional integrity of teeth used as supports for orthodontic treatment;
- Preventive sealing of grooves, pits and crevices in all permanent teeth (Haikel, 2001; Gontijo et al, 2007).

4.1.5 Education and motivation

Before undertaking curative and preventive treatment, prime importance should be given to dietary recommendations: the patients should be informed and made aware of the cariogenic potential of foods and bad eating habits such as snacking, and be taught to eat sensibly (Blique & Droz, 1999; Miller & Blique, 2000).

In addition, motivation and awareness of buccodental hygiene should be emphasized in the treatment plan. The patient should display a satisfactory level of oral hygiene before the orthodontic treatment is started, and be expected to maintain this level of hygiene throughout the treatment (Burkland, 1999; Sukontapatipark et al, 2001). The rules of hygiene should become a routine habit, which should even so be reinforced at intervals.

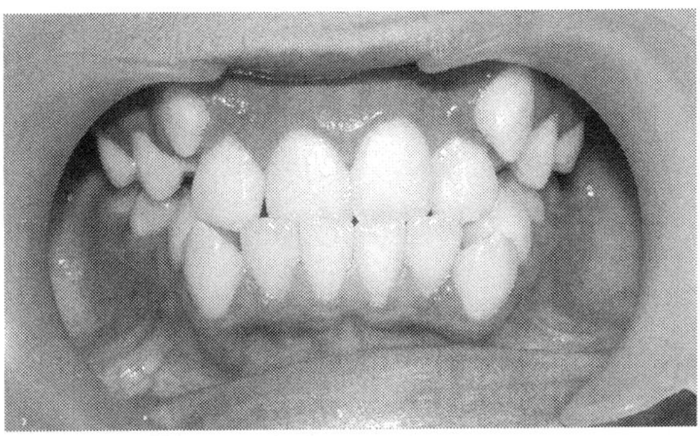

Fig. 8. Patient with dental crowding; preparation before orthodontic treatment

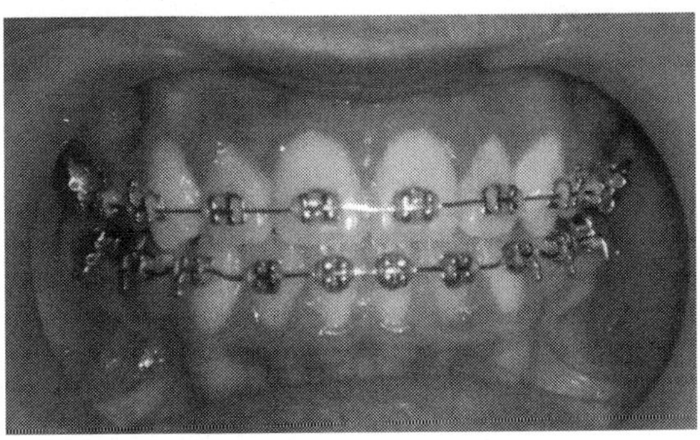

Fig. 9. Maintenance of buccodental hygiene during treatment

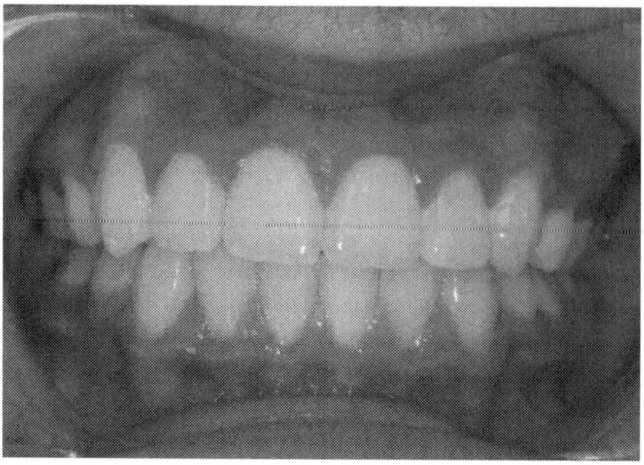

Fig. 10. End of orthodontic treatment with a satisfactory aesthetic outcome and healthy enamel.

4.2 During orthodontic treatment

Special attention should be paid to the choice of bonding material and to fluoride-based prevention.

4.2.1 Fitting of the orthodontic appliance

The close fitting of bands on teeth is recommended, but this is sometimes insufficient to maintain the protection of the cement if pressure and chewing impact are high (Terk, 1993).
Glass ionomer cement has been used for some years and offers a good solution to this problem. It is less friable than oxyphosphate, bonds equally to metal and enamel, and releases fluoride, thus helping to protect the teeth. Its use marks an important advance that greatly reduces the occurrence of demineralization under bands (Evrenol et al, 1999).
Successful outcome of orthodontic treatment also depends on the quality of bracket bonding. Cementing of brackets should always be preceded by treatment of amelar surfaces with prophylactic brushing to remove plaque and other debris. Satisfactory bonding is obtained using phosphoric acid combined with composite resin. The choice of cementing material should take into account both bonding strength and cariostatic power. Composite resins are generally most often used, but studies have shown that bacterial plaque builds up more readily on these resins than on enamel, which can cause demineralization around the brackets.
Glass ionomer cements can also be used to cement brackets: the teeth need no prior acid etching and there is no change in amelar surfaces after removal. Results show a significant reduction in carious lesions when a glass ionomer cement is used to cement orthodontic brackets. The use of this material also significantly reduces the number of white spots observed after removal of the appliance (Dubroc et al, 1994; Donly et al, 1995; Foley et al, 2002; Pascotto et al, 2004; Benson et al, 2005; Cacciafesta et al, 2007; Sudjalim et al, 2007; Lin et al, 2008). Fluoridated bonding resins have anticariogenic power, reducing the occurrence of demineralization adjacent to orthodontic devices by releasing fluoride at

specific sites (Evrenol et al, 1999; Wilson & Donly, 2001). The use of this material should thus be encouraged during orthodontic treatment, especially in patients with high levels of *Streptococcus mutans*.

When braces are removed, excess composite remaining on the teeth must be eliminated: if left in place it will retain bacterial plaque and favour caries formation. Likewise, the peripheral joint should be well chamfered to facilitate saliva flow and tooth brushing.

4.2.2 Buccodental hygiene

Clinical maintenance is essential throughout any orthodontic treatment. Elimination of plaque and food debris is a foremost requirement for buccodental hygiene (Fortier et al, 1997; Haikel , 2001). Concern for oral hygiene should be constant, not only among all practitioners, but also among patients: throughout the treatment period the patient should successfully maintain a satisfactory level of oral hygiene despite the hindrance of the appliance.

Teaching the patient to achieve good oral hygiene, plus follow-up by the orthodontist, is certainly the easiest preventive therapy that can be set in place (Alexander & Ripa, 2000; Kuhn & Besnault, 2000). A method of brushing teeth should be taught that takes into account the patient's age (young child or adult), socio-cultural level, dexterity and any disabilities (Kuhn & Besnault, 2000; Adel Lees, 2003; Zuhal, 2006; Ay et al, 2007). Electrically operated brushes may be preferred if the patient is unable to ensure correct oral hygiene by simple mechanical brushing (Petersson, 2000; Costa et al, 2007); an electric toothbrush reduces dental plaque more completely than a mechanical toothbrush (Kaklamanos & Kafkas, 2008).

Tooth brushing should be done with a fluoridated toothpaste, as it is currently acknowledged that fluoridated toothpastes exert a cariostatic effect (Sommermater & Bigeard, 1993; Arnold et al, 2006; Farhadian et al, 2008). The use of a fluoridated toothpaste appreciably reduces dental plaque, and increases fluoride levels in the biofilm, where it acts as a powerful inhibitor of several bacterial enzymes. The need for at least two daily brushings should be emphasized in order to favour a continuous exchange of fluoride ions between the salivary medium and the enamel surface (Sommermater & Bigeard, 1993; Farhadian et al, 2008). The use of fluoridated toothpastes can reduce the frequency of caries by 15–30%, the best results being obtained with high-fluoride toothpastes (Modesto et al, 2000; Derks et al, 2004).

The follow-up of oral hygiene also allows an appraisal of the patient's motivation. In some particularly unfavourable cases, where the quality of hygiene is inadequate or even severely lacking, the orthodontic treatment should de discontinued with no hesitation, temporarily or definitively, based on an assessment of the likelihood of achieving a healthy buccodental state, adequate motivation and improved oral hygiene and eating habits (Fortier et al, 1997). This approach will forestall the occurrence of not only caries but also parodontal lesions that can take various forms (hyperplasic gingivitis, receding gums, etc.).

For the interproximal areas, which are difficult to get at, there are other ways to eliminate plaque (Petersson, 2000; Haikel, 2001). The use of orthodontic dental floss and interdental brushes is necessary in addition to brushing. Water jets have shown undeniable efficacy for eliminating food debris and form an excellent adjunct to mechanical brushing, being particularly recommended for wearers of appliances.

orthodontiques (Haikel , 2001).

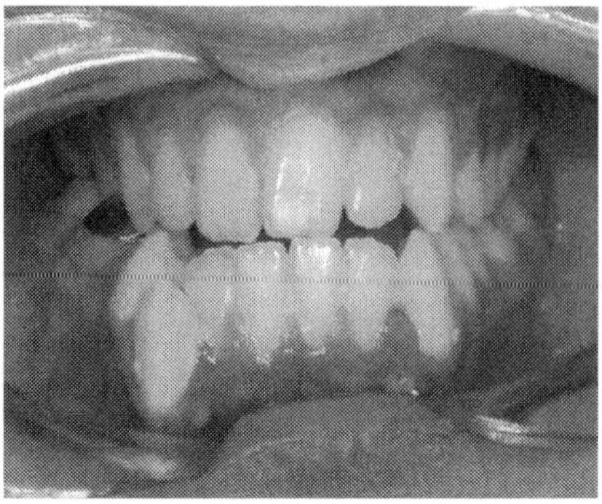

Fig. 11. Photograph at the start of treatment; presence of bacterial plaque due to poor hygiene

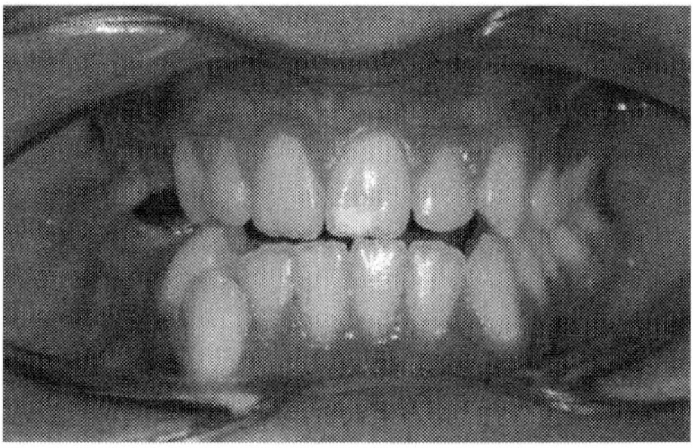

Fig. 12. Good oral hygiene before fitting of brackets

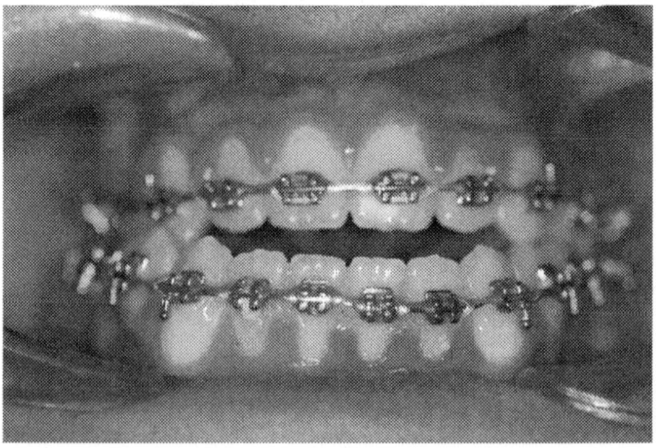

Fig. 13. Regular maintenance of oral hygiene throughout the orthodontic treatment.

4.2.3 Control of dental plaque by professional prophylactic cleaning

Besides oral hygiene at home, professional prophylactic cleaning is designed to reduce bacterial load, enhance the efficacy of brushing and facilitate cleaning by the patient (Kuhn & Besnault, 2000; Arnold et al, 2006). Professional tooth cleaning two or three times a year maintains a healthy mouth and reduces the number of caries (Petersson, 2000). It allows proper cleaning of the areas that are hard for the patient to brush.

The coronal surfaces can be polished using fluoridated pastes of progressively finer particle size, and elastomer polishing cups or brushes, to impede the mechanical retention of bacteria (Arrow, 1998).

4.2.4 Screening for caries

Whatever type of appliance is used, the attack of hard tissue, when it occurs, starts by demineralization of the enamel. With multibracket appliances this attack can begin close to cemented brackets or under bands when the cement breaks down and mouth fluids get between the metal and the enamel, where proper cleaning is impossible. (Terk, 1993). Thus the joints between back teeth and bands should be regularly inspected to prevent salivary percolation. If there is any doubt about the quality of the seal the bands should be removed and refitted (Fortier et al, 1997).

4.2.5 Sealing of pits and crevices

Pits and crevices are especially vulnerable to dental caries. These anfractuous areas cannot be readily brushed out and topical fluoride application provides only weak protection (Sommermater & Bigeard, 1993). Caries can always be prevented by sealing grooves, pits and crevices in all growing permanent teeth: premolars and especially the second permanent molars that erupt during orthodontic treatment (Fortier et al, 1997).

The purpose of sealing grooves and crevices on the occlusal faces of teeth is to reduce the bacterial load by smoothing highly anfractuous occlusal shapes that favour food and bacteria retention, and thereby making cleaning easier (Kuhn & Besnault, 2000).

4.2.6 Topical fluorotherapy

The favourable action of fluorides is now well established. The fluoride ion has a preventive effect against caries (Haikel & Hemmerle, 2001; Featherstone, 1999; Modesto et al, 2000; Kuhn et Besnault, 2000; Miller et al, 2004(a), 2004(b); Farhadian et al, 2008). It:

- modifies bacterial metabolism in dental plaque, by inhibiting some enzyme processes;
- inhibits the production of acids, by acting on the composition of the bacterial flora and (or) on the metabolic activity of micro-organisms;
- reduces demineralization and favours the remineralization of early carious lesions, by exerting a remineralization effect, especially at low concentrations. During recurrent episodes of lowered pH, the incorporation of fluoride in the surface layers of the enamel is facilitated (Benson et al, 2004, 2005; Sudjalim et al, 2007).

The main cariostatic effect of topical fluoride preparations is due to the formation of calcium fluoride, which precipitates onto healthy surfaces or in the micropores of active lesions that are not yet at the cavity stage. When the amelar surface is exposed to fluoride, fluoride ions adhere to the surface and form crystals of calcium fluoride. These then act as potential reservoirs from which fluoride can be released (Evrenol et al, 1999; Farhadian et al, 2008).

The more fluoride that is supplied in the first days of treatment, the better will be the structure of the calcium fluoride crystals formed. This is why it is most important to treat the enamel with fluoride just after acid etching (Evrenol et al, 1999).
The prophylactic action of fluoride depends on its concentration, but even more so on the frequency with which it is supplied to the mouth. The topical effects of fluorides are cumulative: the more a tooth is exposed to fluorides, the more resistant to caries it becomes (Sommermater & Bigeard, 1993; Farhadian et al, 2008). Even a small increase in fluoride concentration in the saliva and the plaque can provide a high protection against caries by favouring remineralization. Fluoride can be retained in the saliva at concentrations in the range 0.03–0.1 ppm for 2–6 hours (Featherstone, 1999). Thus in addition to the use of fluoride toothpaste, certain newly-formed shallow surface lesions can be treated early in the course of orthodontic treatment by topical application of painted varnishes, gels or fluoridated solutions to stimulate the remineralization of the enamel surface.

4.2.6.1 Mouthwashes

The use of fluoridated mouthwashes is the commonest method to help prevent caries (Benson, 2005). Fluoridated mouthwashes reduce demineralization and increase remineralization of the enamel near orthodontic bands and brackets (Adair, 1998). There are several different ways to use fluoridated mouthwashes. They can be administered (Sommermater & Bigeard, 1993; Petersson, 2000; Farhadian et al, 2008):

- in low doses (0.05% NaF) at frequent intervals, once or twice a day;
- in high doses (0.2% NaF), once a week or twice a month.

The reduction of caries is 25–30% (Haikel, 2001; Modesto et al, 2000).
For Zero et al. (Featherstone, 1999), NaF mouthwashes (0.05%–225 ppmF) used for 1 minute increase fluoride levels in saliva for 2–4 hours.

4.2.6.2 Fluoride gels

In fluoridated gels the concentration of fluoride can range from 10,000 to 20,000 ppm. These gels are most often acidified preparations of NaF, which favour ion exchange (Wilson & Donly, 2001). Their efficacy depends on how readily accessible the areas to be treated are: the vestibular and lingual areas are obviously best protected (Kuhn & Besnault, 2000).
High-fluoride gels (up to 20,000 ppm such as Fluocaril bi-fluoré 2000*) are applied using trays fitted by the practitioner and used in the dental surgery (Sommermater & Bigeard, 1993; Farhadian et al, 2008). It is recommended to leave the trays in place for 4 minutes; the patient must not mouth-rinse, drink or eat for an hour or an hour and a half after application of the fluoride gel. Two applications a year are recommended (Haikel, 2001).

4.2.6.3 Fluoride varnishes

Fluoride varnishes are used preventively around cemented brackets to reduce the cariogenic effects of bacterial plaque at the most vulnerable sites such as proximal edges and cervical surfaces (Fortier et al, 1997; Vivaldi-Rodrigues et al, 2006; Gontijo et al, 2007; Farhadian et al, 2008; Shafi, 2008; Martinez-Mier, 2009). They do not elicit the patient's cooperation.
These varnishes were developed to adhere to the enamel surface for long periods (up to 12 hours or more) and release their fluoride slowly on the enamel surfaces, so reducing the time spent by the patient in the dentist's chair (Sommermater & Bigeard, 1993; Haikel, 2001; Schmitt et al, 2002; Demito et al, 2004; Stecksen-Blicks et al, 2007).
Fluoride varnishes are usually applied twice a year on specific areas with incipient lesions on smooth surfaces.

Three types of varnish are currently on the market:

- Fluor Protector* with 0.1% fluoride,
- Duraphat* with 2.2% fluoride,
- Bifluoride* with 5% fluoride.

Fluoride varnishes should be used in weakly motivated patients in an intensive treatment schedule (three days running), repeated every three or four months, or twice or three times a year. The varnishes are thus used as a preventive measure to reduce demineralization of the enamel around the brackets, promote the remineralization of the carious lesions and avert further lesions (Petersson, 2000; Gontijo et al, 2007; Farhadian et al, 2008).

4.2.6.4 Combined fluoride varnishes and chlorhexidine

Control by antimicrobial agents has also given excellent results in combination with fluoride in high-risk patients (Petersson, 2000; Haikel, 2001; Alves et al, 2008). Fluoride and chlorhexidine form a powerful combination: the fluoride acts to protect the hard tissues, while the chlorhexidine reduces buccal pathogens present in the saliva and dental plaque (Petersson, 2000; Ogaard et al, 2001; Beyth et al, 2003; Attin et al, 2006; Derks et al; 2008)

Antibacterial varnishes (1% such as Cervitec*) are applied locally on at-risk sites, e.g. incipient lesions that have to be cleaned up to allow remineralization (Haikel, 2001; Kuhn & Besnault, 2000). They lower the numbers of *Streptococcus mutans* in the plaque close to fixed appliances (Madlena et al, 2000; Alves et al, 2008; Derks et al, 2008).

Applying a chlorhexidine-based varnish is straightforward. It is painted on with a brush and dried on the tooth surface with a gentle air stream. The patient then has to wait at least one hour after application of the varnish before eating or drinking (Petersson, 2000).

Like gels, chlorhexidine varnishes have to be applied repeatedly, two or three times in the space of a few days, and every three or four months to be effective.

The combined use of an antibacterial varnish and a fluoride varnish is more efficacious in averting new carious lesions (Ogaard et al, 2001).

4.2.7 Maintenance and follow-up during orthodontic treatment

The odontologist should remain fully involved throughout the orthodontic treatment, and draw up a follow-up schedule jointly with the orthodontist and the patient to keep the risk of caries at a low level. Thus regular maintenance consultations with the odontologist must be planned. This follow-up schedule should be adapted to each patient's individual risk of caries. For children at very low risk, two or three annual visits are recommended. For children at higher risk, a visit every 2 months will be necessary.

4.3 After orthodontic treatment

The treatment ends when the planned result has been achieved (Fortier et al, 1997). After the brackets have been removed, residues of cement remain on the teeth, requiring a thorough polishing of the dental surfaces (Osorio et al, 1998).

The paedodontist or general practitioner should then carry out a careful examination of the entire mouth to diagnose and treat:

- any proximal caries;
- any caries that have formed under the molar bands and in areas where brushing between the brackets and the gingival festoon has been deficient.

Traces of demineralization, which cannot be foreseen, are often discovered at the end of treatment, requiring continued preventive fluoride treatment (Terk, 1993). In this case it is important to make topical applications of fluorides in a solution, gel or varnish to facilitate surface remineralization of incipient carious lesions. If there are no lesions, in the most favourable cases these applications are the only precautions that need to be taken at the end of the orthodontic treatment (Fortier et al, 1997; Willmott, 2004). O'Reilly and Featherstone (Featherstone, 1999) have shown that demineralization around the brackets can be completely eliminated by a combination of fluoride toothpaste and daily rinsing with 0.05% NaF solution.

Another study (Kleber et al, 1999) concerning remineralization with fluoride after removal of orthodontic devices has shown that:

- the use of a fluoride toothpaste twice a day leads to remineralization after 2 months;
- combining fluoride toothpaste and fluoride gels speeds up remineralization (1 month).

5. Conclusion and recommendations

Patients wearing orthodontic appliances should be considered as being at high risk of dental caries. Thus before starting an orthodontic treatment, it is essential to treat all existing tooth decay. Pits and crevices in first and second permanent molars should be filled with a sealant in all patients younger than 20 years old who are at high cariogenic risk.

A screening and consultation schedule should be presented to the patient and parents. Clinical and radiological examinations (retroalveolar and retrocoronal views) should be performed to look for white spots and caries.

The orthodontist should teach the patient to use a suitable brushing method. The use of interdental brushes and dental floss should be encouraged, besides brushing teeth after every meal. Emphasis should be placed on the importance of diet, and patients should be encouraged to reduce their sugar consumption.

Prophylaxis with topical fluoride application should be implemented: high-fluoride toothpastes, fluoride mouthwashes, gels and varnishes during and after the orthodontic treatment, especially for patients at high cariogenic risk.

Finally, close collaboration throughout with paediatric odontologists and conservative dentists is indispensable.

6. References

Adair, S.M. The role of fluoride mouthrinses in the control of dental caries: a brief review. *Pediatr Dent 1998* Mar-Apr; Vol 20, n°2: 101-104.

Adel Lees, M. A comparison between written, verbal and videotape oral hygiene instruction for patients with fixed appliances. *J. Orthod.* 2003; 27: 323-327.

Ahn, S.J. & Kho, H.S. Adhesion of oral streptococci to experimental bracket pellicules from glandular saliva. *Am. J. Orthod. Dentofacial. Orthop.* 2003; Vol 124, n°2: 198-203.

Lovrov, S.; Hertrich, K. & HIRSCHFELDER U. Enamel demineralization during fixed orthodontic treatment-incidence and correlation to various oral-hygiene parameters. *J. Orofac. Orthop.* 2007; Vol 68, n°5: 353-363.

Alexander, S.A. & Ripa, L.W. Effects of self-applied topical fluoride preparations in orthodontic patients. *Angle Orthod.* 2000; Vol 70, n°6: 424-430.

Alves, P.V.M.; Alviano, W.B., Bolognese, A.M. & Nojima, L.I. Treatment protocol to control streptococcus mutans level in an orthodontic patient with high caries risk. *Am. J. Orthod. Dentofacial Orthop.* 2008; 133: 91-4.

Arnold, W.H; Dorow, A.; Langenhorst, S.; Ginter, Z.; Banoczy, J. & Gaengler, P. Effect of fluoride toothpastes on enamel demineralization. *BMC Oral Health* 2006;Vol 6, n°8: 1-6.

Arrow, P. Oral hygiene in the control of occlusal caries. *Com. Dent. Oral Epidemiol.* 1998; 26: 324-330.

Attin, R.; Ilse, A.; Werner, C.; Wiegand, A. & Attin, T. Antimicrobial effectiveness of a highly concentrated chlorhexidine varnish treatment in teenagers with fixed orthodontic appliances. *Angle Orthod.* 2006; Vol 76, n°6: 1022-1027.

Ay, Z.Y.; Sayin, M.O.; Ozat, Y.; Goster, T.; Atilla, A.O.& Bozkurt, F.Y. Appropriate ral hygiene motivation method for patients with fixed appliances. *Angle Orthod.* 2007; Vol 77, n°6: 1085-1089.

Batoni, G.; Pardini, M.; Ota, F. & Guica, M.R. Effect of removable orthodontic appliances on oral colonisation by mutans streptococci in children. *Eur. J. Oral Sci.* 2001; 109: 388-392.

Benson, P.E.; Parkin, N.; Millet, D.T.; Dyer, F.E., Vine S., & Shah A. Fluorides for the prevention of white spots on teeth during fixed brace treatment. *Cochrane Database Syst Rev.* 2004; (3): CD003809.

Benson, P.E.; Shah, A.A.; Millet, D.T; Dyer, F.; Parkin, N. & Vine, P.S. Fluorides, orthodontics and demineralization: a systematic review. *J. Orthod.* 2005; Vol 32, n°2: 102-114.

Beyth, N.; Redlich, M.; Friedman, M. & Steinberg, D. Effect of sustained-release chlorhexidine varnish on streptococcus mutans and actinomyces viscosus in orthodontic patients. *Am. J. Orthod. Dentofacial Orthop. 2003; Vol 123, n°3: 345-348.*

Blique, M & Droz, D. Contrôle du risque alimentaire et prophylaxie dentaire individuelle en omnipratique, 2éme partie: technique d'analyse et de conseil. *Inf. Dent.* 1999; Vol 81, n°23: 1673-1681.

Bourzgui, F.; Sebbar, M. & Hamza M. Le risque carieux en orthodontie: étude descriptive d'un échantillon de 155 patients. *Rev. Stomatol. Chir. Maxillofac.* 2010; 111: 276-279.

Burkland, G. Hygiene and the orthodontic patient. *J. Clin. Orthod.* 1999; Vol 33, n°8: 443-446.

Cacciafesta, V.; Sfandrini, M.F.; Tagliani, P. & Kiersy, C. In vitro fluoride release rates from 9 orthodontic bonding adhesives. Am. J. Orthod. Dentofacial Orthop. 2007; 132: 656-62.

Charland, R.; Voyer, R.; Cudzinowski, L.; Salavail, P. & Abelardo, L. La carie dentaire: étiopathogénie, diagnostic et traitement: encore beaucoup à découvrir. *J. Dent. Québec* Novembre 2001; Vol 38, pp. 409-416.

Charland, R.& Salvail P. Les fluorures: quoi de neuf ? *J. Dent. Québec* Vol 20, Janvier 2003, pp. 11-16.

Chaussain, C.; Opsahl Vital, S.; Viaillon, V.; Vermelin, L.; Haignere, C. & SIXOU, M. Interest in a new test for caries risk in adolescents undergoing orthodontic treatment . *Clin. Oral Investig.*; 2009.

Costa, M.R.; Silva, V.C.; Miqui, M.N.; Sakima, T.; Spolidorio, D.M.& Cirelli, J.A. Efficacy of ultrasonic, electric and manual toothbrushes in patients with fixed orthodontic appliances. *Angle Orthod* 2007; Vol 77, n°2: 361-366.

Demito, C.F; Vivaldi-Rodrigues, G; Ramos, A.L & Bowman, S.J. The efficacy of a fluoride varnish in reducing enamel demineralization adjacent to orthodontic brackets: an in vitro study. *Orthod. Craniofac. Res. 2004*; Vol 7, n°4: 205-210.

Derks, A.; Katsaros, C.; Frencken, M.A. & Kuijpers-Jagtman, A.M. Caries-inhibiting effect of preventive measures during orthodontic treatment with fixed appliances; a systematic review. *Caries Res.* 2004; Vol 38, n°5: 413-420.

DerkS, A.; Kuijpers Jagtman, A.M., Frencken, J.E., Van't Hof, M.A. & KATSARAS, C. Caries preventive measures used in orthodontic practices: an evidence-based decision?. *Am. J. Orthod. Dentofacial Orthop. 2007; 132: 165-170.*

Derks, A.; Frencken, J.; Bronkhorst, E., Kuijpers-Jagtman, A.M. & Katsaros, C. Effect of chlorhexidine varnish application on mutans streptococci counts in orthodontic patients. *Am J Orthod Dentofacial Orthop 2008;* Vol 133, n°3: 435-439.

Donly, K.J.; Istre, S. & Istre, T. In vitro remineralization at orthodontic band margins cemented with glass ionomer cement. *Am J Orthod Dentofacial Orthop* 1995 May; Vol 107, n°5: 461-464.

Dubroc, G.C.; Mayo, J.A. & Rankine, C.A. Reduction of caries and demineralization around orthodontic brackets: effect of a fluoride-releasing resin in the rat model. *Am J Orthod Dentofacial Orthop.* 1994 Dec; Vol 106, n°6: 583-587.

Droz, D. & Blique, M. Contrôle du risque alimentaire et prophylaxie dentaire individuele en omnipratique, 1ère partie: Connaître les facteurs de risque essentiels pour mieux les identifier. Poser le problème de l'alimentation cariogène. *Inf Dent.* 1999; Vol 81, n°20: 1405-1411.

Evrenol, B.I.; Kucukkeles, N.; Arun, T. & Yarat, A. Fluoride release capacities of four different orthodontic adhesives. *J. Clin Pediatr Dent* 1999, *Vol* 23, n°4: 315-320.

Farhadian, N.; Miresmaeili, A.; Eslami, B. & Merhabi, S. Effect of fluoride varnish on enamel demineralization around brackets: an in-vivo study. *Am. J. Orthod. Dentofacial Orthop.* 2008; 133: S95-98.

Featherstone, J.D.B. Prevention and reversal of dental caries: role of low level fluoride. *Community Dent Oral. Epidemiol.* 1999; 27: 31-40.

Foley, T.; Aggarwal, M. & Hatibovic-Kofma, N. A comparison of in vitro enamel demineralization potential of 3 orthodontic cements. *Am J Orthod Dentofacial Orthop* 2002; Vol 121, n°5: 526-530.

Fortier, J.P; Villette, F.; Aldin, P. & Brasseur, B. L'odontologie pédiatrique et le traitement orthodontique. *Réalités Cliniques* Vol.8 n°3, 1997: 225-241.

Gontijo, L.; Cruz, A. & Brandao, P. Dental enamel around fixed orthodontic appliances after fluoride varnish application. *Braz. Dent. J.* 2007; Vol 18, n°1: 49-53.

Gorton, J. & Featherstone, J.D.B. In vivo inhibition of demineralization around orthodontic brackets . *Am. J. Orthod. Dentofacial Orthop.* 2003; Vol 123, n°1: 10-14.

HaïkeL, Y. & Hemmerle, J. Thérapeutique étiopathogénique de la carie. *Encycl. Méd. Chir., Stomatologie et Odontologie,* 23-010-F-10, 1993, 11p.

Haïkel, Y. Thérapeutique étiopathogénique de la carie. *Encycl. Méd. Chir., Stomatologie et Odontologie,* 23-010-F-10, 2001, 21p.

Jordan, C.N. Prevention of white spot enamel formation during orthodontic treatment. *Gen. Dent.* Sep-Oct 1998:498-502.

Jordan, C. & LeBlanc, D.J. Influences of orthodontic appliances on oral populations of mutans streptococci. *Oral Microb. Immun.* 2002; 17(2): 369-447.

Kaklamanos, E.G. & Kalfas, S. Meta-analysis on the effectiveness of powdered toothbrushes for orthodontic patients. *Am. J. Orthod. Dentofacial Orthop.* 2008; 133: 187.e1-187.e5.

Kleber, C.J.; Milleman, J.L.; Davidson, K.R.; Putt, M.S.; Triol, C.W. & Winston, A.E. Treatment of orthodonyic white spot lesions with a remineralizing dentifrice applied by toothbrushing or mouth trays. *J Clin Dent 1999;* Vol 10, 1 Spec No: 44-49.

Kuhn, G. & Besnault, C. Prophylaxie, prévention et dentisterie non invasive. *Revue d'Odontostomatologie* 2000, Tome 29, n°4: 179-187.

Lin, Y.C; Lai, Y.L; Chen, W.T & Lee, S.Y. Kinetics of fluoride release from reuptake by orthodontic cements. Am. J. Orthod. Dentofacial Orthop. 2008; 133: 427-434.

Madlena, M.; Vitalyos, G.; Marton, S. & Nagy, G. Effect of chlorhexidine varnish on bacterial levels in plaque and saliva during orthodontic treatment. *J Clin Dent 2000;* Vol 11, n°2: 42-46.

Martinez-Mier, E.A. Fluoride varnish applications may reduce the formation of white spot lesions (WSL) adjacent to orthodontic fixed appliances. *J. Evid. Based Dent. Pract.* 2009; Vol 9, n°1: 16-17.

Miller, C.; Blique, M. & Lasfargues J.J. Les conseils diététiques en dentisterie préventive. *Réalités cliniques*, Vol 11, n° 1, 2000, pp. 33-49.

Miller, C.; Ten Cate, J.M. & Lasfargues, J.J. La reminéralisation des lésions carieuses (1): le rôle essentiel des fluorures. *Réal. Clin.* 2004(a); Vol 15, n°3: 249-260.

Miller, C.; Ten Cate, J.M. & Lasfargues, J.J. La reminéralisation des lésions carieuses (2): synergies thérapeutiques. *Réal. Clin.* 2004(b); Vol 15, n°3: 261-275.

Modesto, A.; Lima, K.C &, Uzeda, M. Effects of solutions used in infants' oral hygiene on biofilms and oral microorganisms. *Journal of Dentistry for children* , September-October 2000: 338-344.

Muller, M., Lupi, L., Jasmin, J.R. & Bolla, M. Etiologie de la carie . *Encycl Méd Chir, Odontologie*, 23-010-A30, 1998, 6p.

Ogaard, B.; Larsson, E.; Henriksson, T.; Birkhed, D. & Bishara, S.E. Effects of combined application of antimicrobial and fluoride varnishes in orthodontic patients. *Am J Orthod Dentofacial Orthop* 2001 Jul; Vol 120, n°1: 28-35.

O'Reilly, M.M. & Featherstone, J.D. Demineralization and remineralisation around orthodontic appliances: an in vivo study. *Am. J. Orthod. Dentofacial Orthop.* 1987; Vol 92, n°1: 33-40.

Osorio, R.; Toledano, M.& Garcia Godoy, F. Enamel surface morphology after bracket debonding. *Journal of Dentistry for children* , September-October 1998: 313-317.

Pascotto, R.; Navarro, M.F.; Filho, L.C. & Cury, J.A. In vivo effect of resin- modified glass ionomer cement on enamel demineralization around orthodontic brackets. *Am J Orthod Dentofacial Orthop 2004;* Vol 125, n°1:36-41.

Petersson, L.G. Prévention: santé buccale, une vision et un défi pour le praticien. *Réalités Cliniques* 2000; Vol 11, n°4: 375-390.

Rillard, F.; Khelifa, N. & Colon P. Données actuelles sur la pathogénie de la maladie carieuse. *Rev odontosomatol*, Tome 29, n°4, pp 189-196.

Shafi, I. Fluoride varnish reduces white spot lesions during orthodontic treatment. *Evid. Based Dent* 2008; Vol 9, n°3; p. 81.

Schmitt, J.L.; Staley, R.N.; Wefel, J.S.; Kanellis, M.; Jakobsen, J.R. & Keenan, P. Effect of fluoride varnish on demineralization adjacent to brackets bonded with RMGI cement. *Am. J. Orthod. Dentofacial Orthop.* 2002; Vol 122, n°2: 125-134.

Sommermater, J.I. & Bigeard, L. Méthodes de prévention au cabinet dentaire chez l'enfant et le jeune. *Réalités Cliniques* Vol.4 n°3, 1993: 283-304.

Stecksen-Blicks, C.; Renfors, G.; Oscarson, N.D.; Bergstrand, F. & Twetman, S. Carie-preventive effectiveness of a fluoride varnish: a randomized controlled trial in adolescents with fixed orthodontic appliances. *Caries Res.* 2007; 41: 455-459.

Sudjalim, T.R.; Woods, M.G. & Manton, D.J. Prevention of white spot lesions in orthodontic practice: a contemporary review. *Aust. Dent. J.* 2006; Vol 51, n°4: 284-289.

Sudjalim, T.R.; Woods, M.G.; Manton, D.J. & Reynolds, E.C. Prevention of demineralization around orthodontic brackets in vitro. *Am. J. Orthod. Dentofacial Orthop.* 2007; 131(6): 705e1-9.

Sukontapatipark, W.; El Agroudi, M.A. & Sellisetth, N.J. Bacterial colonisation with fixed appliances; a scanning electron microscopy study. *Eur. J. Orthod.* 2001; Vol 23, n°5: 475-484.

Terk, B. Motivation à l'hygiène chez les enfants traités en orthodontie. *Réalités Cliniques* Vol.4 n°3, 1993: 375-385.

Terrie, B.; Bounoure, G. & Vaysse, F. Prévention des lésions carieuses lors des traitements orthodontiques: rôle du pédodontiste et de l'orthodontiste. *Rev. Orthop. Dento Faciale* 2004; 38: 253-270.

Travess, H., Roberts-Harry, D. & Sandy J. Orthodontics. Part 6: Risks in orthodontic treatment. *Br. Dent. J.* 2004; Jan 24; Vol 196, n°2: 71-77.

Vivaldi-Rodrigues, G.; Demito, C.F.; Bowman, S.J. & Ramos, A.L. The effectiveness of fluoride varnish in preventing the development of white spot lesions. *World J. Orthod.* 2006; Vol 7, n°2: 138-144.

Willmott, D.R. White lesions after orthodontic treatment: does low fluoride make a difference? *J. of Orthodontics* 2004; Vol. 31: 235-242.

Wilson, R.M. & Donly, K.J. Demineralization around orthodontic brackets bonded with resin-modified glass ionomer cement and fluoride-releasing resin composite. Pediatr Dent 2001 May-Jun; Vol 23, n°3: 255-259.

Zimmer, B.W. & Rottwinkel, Y. Assessing patient-specific decalcification risk in fixed orthodontic treatment and its impact on prophylactic procedures; *Am. J. Orthod. Dentofacial Orthop.* 2004; Vol 126, n°3: 318-324.

ZuhaL, Y.A. Appropriate Oral Hygiene Motivation Method for Patients with fixed appliances. *Ang. Orthod.* 2006; Vol 77, n°6:1085–1089.

14

New Strategies for Class II Fixed Functional Orthodontics, Including MRI Diagnostics, Manual Functional Analysis and Physiotherapy

Douglas Edward Toll, Nenad Popović and Nicole Drinkuth
Orthodontic Group Practice
Germany

1. Introduction

Frequently, Angle Class IIs display a retrognathic mandible rather than a prognathic maxilla [McNamara, Connelly & McBride, 1975[1]]. Since the mandible appears to be the primary cause, it is logical to focus on it when treatment options are discussed. Consequently, all major fixed and removable Class II correction appliances attempt to improve mandibular growth and position. Several types are available on the market: Fixed Functionals like the MARA (Mandibular Anterior Repositioning Appliance), the Herbst appliance and William Clark's Twin Block are, however, by far, more effective than removable appliances in more difficult cases and in cases with lacking or insufficient patient compliance. [O'Brien, Wright, Conboy et al., 2003[2]]

The primary difference between Class II/1 and Class II/2 is the angle of upper incisor inclination: In Class II/1s, the upper anteriors are proclined, creating a large sagittal step with the lingual, gingival part of the upper incisors holding the mandible posteriorly. This often causes enormous pressure on the TMJs and thus damage to the structures of the TMJ. In Class II/2s, the bite is usually very deep, and the upper incisors are retroclined, also producing a force vector that is directed distally, toward the TMJs. The bite in Class II/2s is not seldomly extremely deep, and the vertical height of the lower face is often reduced (brachycephalic growth).

A great help for optimal diagnostics and treatment planning in orthodontic patients, esp. in patients with TMD (Temporomandibular Disorder) symptoms, has been MRI (Magnetic Resonance Imaging). MFA (Manual Functional Analysis) has recently evolved in the Netherlands and Germany as an important complement to MRI scanning. It covers very well the functional aspects of TMD, because it is a thorough orthopaedic type of musculoskeletal examination. Although dynamic imaging has been developed to diagnose mandibular mobility and disc behaviour, the MFA is also still a valuable adjunct as a diagnostic tool. Combining the very important MRI with MFA, the clinician gains very important knowledge of the condition of the TMJs and if the condyles can be advanced or not. MRI scanning and MFA also are the decisive factors as to the type of manual therapy / physiotherapy that is indicated as complement to mechanical anterior mandibular advancement. The latter is crucial, because - without proper manual therapy -, it is much more difficult or even impossible to obtain satisfactory and stable treatment results.

V4

Douglas E. Toll, D.D.S, M.S., B.S., F.I.D.C.
Zahnarzt für Kieferorthopädie/Doctor of Dental Surgery
Northwestern University Chicago, Illinois / USA
Kronberger Str. 10 · 65812 Bad Soden/Ts. · Frankfurt · Germany

Telefon: +49 (0) 61 96 24 007
Fax: +49 (0) 61 96 61 865
E-Mail: TollOrtho@t-online.de
Website: http://www.Praxis-Toll.de

Dear colleague, Bad Soden, den__________________

Please take MRIs of both temporo-mandibular joints of our patient ____
for important diagnostic purposes.

Initial diagnosis with suspected:

right side...	**left side...**
☐ **partial anterior disc/dorsal condyle displacement**	☐ **partial anterior disc/dorsal condyle displacement**
☐ **total anterior disc/dorsal condyle displacement**	☐ **total anterior disc/dorsal condyle displacement**
☐ **condylar hypermobility**	☐ **condylar hypermobility**
☐ **condylar head degeneration**	☐ **condylar head degeneration**
☐ **joint surface alterations with/without arthrosis**	☐ **joint surface alterations with/without arthrosis**
☐ **disc adhesion**	☐ **disc adhesion**
☐ **verify disc position**	☐ **verify disc position**
☐ **reason for tinnitus/ acute hearing loss/ vertigo migraine/ trigeminus neuralgia**	☐ **reason for tinnitus/ acute hearing loss/ vertigo migraine/ trigeminus neuralgia**

☐ **cervical vertebra degeneration**

☐______________________________ ☐______________________________

☒ **Surface coil** ☐ **Proton density-weighted** ☐ **Fat suppressed** ☐ **T2-weighted** ☒ **Contrast agent**

Seq. 1: ☐ **Bite 0:** parasagittal (CO=Where patients normally chew), with mouth closed and maximal contact on the posterior teeth. During the sequence patient should bite together as tightly as possible without jiggling.

Seq. 2: ☐ **Bite A:** parasagittal (CR=Lower jaw forced as far back as possible) with mouth closed posterior teeth **must absolutely** be in contact! **Bite registration A has a 1mm x 4cm plastic strip, e.g. Copyplast.** During this sequence, the patient should bite together as tightly as possible and without jiggling. Additionally the lower jaw should be placed as far back as possible. If there is no detectable CO-CR difference, this sequence is not necessary.

Seq. 3: ☐ **Bite B:** The patient should bite into **Bite B** as follows: open mouth widely, push lower jaw forward as far as possible (if possible with clicking) and then move the mandible backwards into Bite B. In this position the bite is opened approx. 3mm and forward approx. 3mm. This is a slightly exaggerated, estimated desired jaw position, i.e. near the muscular physiological position.

Seq. 4: ☐ **Paracoronal** sequence - with **Bite registration B only!**

Seq. 5: ☐ **Bite C:** Bring lower jaw forward as much as possible and open mouth ca. 10mm. Midlines need not be straight and as always without jiggling.

Seq. 6: ☐ **Bite registration with cork:** parasagittal, mouth maximally opened and maximally forward with cork. This sequence is only necessary, if the lower jaw's anterior mobility is very limited and then replaces Bite C. Sometimes the cork bite is additionally desired for research purposes.

Seq. 7: ☐ The **pilot view lines to measure the condylar angle** should only be visible on the side being examined (not on the opposite side).

Seq. 8: ☐ **In case of possible sinus/nasal septum problems (e.g. deviation)** please take the necessary vertical slices to see the sinus or nasal septum adaquately (can be a paper hardcopy).

Seq. 9: ☒ **Dynamic imaging of the jaw joint movements**, if possible animated and real-time sequences.

Please show molars in all parasagittal slices. If necessary, please readjust the display caudally. In some cases, if the condylar angle diverges too far from the position of the molars, please make a new, separate display. Exception: if there are brackets and bands in the mouth.

We ask you to give the patient your original images, even if you have not yet written the report.
☒ **CD-ROM** ☐ **3D-CT** ☐ **with stereolithografic model** ☐ **Dental-CT regio ____**
☐ **Volume-CT** **Enclosed:** ☐ **OPG** ☐ **lateral headplate** ☐ **previous MRIs**

☐ **Please call us back regarding muscular examinations or lymph node problems.**

Thank you very much!

Fig. 1. Detailed MRI prescription form containing suspected diagnoses, (if applicable) T1, T2, PD weighting, etc. and instructions for each static sequence. Dynamic sequences are also included: animated sequences and video sequences.

In Class II patients, we often find severe TMJ degeneration in MRI scans and MFA [Toll, Popović & Drinkuth, 2010[3]]. This degree of condylar and disc degeneration and displacement is frequently not accompanied by the expected associated symptoms (craniofacial pain, muscular tenseness, dizziness, tinnitus, etc.). [45 years of empirical data from own practice[4]]

Fixed Functional orthodontic treatment in combination with flat build-ups on the last molars in the mandible can be used to unlock the bite, advance the condyles and give physiological TMJ decompression. Sometimes, sagittal (mesio-distal) stabilisation of the achieved results is necessary for a lifetime.

2. Magnetic Resonance Imaging (MRI) diagnostics and Manual Functional Analysis (MFA)

In our practice, magnetic resonance imaging has been in use for over 14 years. Gradually, this method has evolved into the most significant method for the clinical diagnostics of temporomandibular pathologies. Our MRI scans comprise 7 to 9 different sequences, oriented parasagittally, paracoronally and transversally. The static sequences include 4 different bite positions - for which silicon bites are individually made. These bites dictate where the radiologists are to make the imaging position. In our practice, these silicone bites are made as follows: bite 0 (habitual occlusion, equals CO), bite A (CR, the most dorsally forced mandibular position), bite B (slightly overcorrected desired anterior mandibular position), and bite C (the most anterior mandibular position possible, with mouth opened approximately 10 mms). Bite B is the clinically most significant one: It tells us, if the patient's discs can be reduced, as the lower jaw is advanced to a slightly overcorrected, physiological position. A detailed MRI prescription is shown in fig. 1.

The MFA examination is a very thorough way to assess the condition of the upper craniofacial system. It begins with a good medical anamnesis, including especially a report on pain sensations, limited mobility, altered visual facial aspect (asymmetry), neurological problems (paraesthesias, paralyses, dystonias) and pre-existing conditions like rheumatism.

The MFA is actually an orthopaedic examination, designed to test the components of the craniomandibular system in terms of condition, tightness and degree of mobility. This includes muscles, cartilage, bone and ligaments. The presence or absence of pain and its severity during specific manipulations (movement, palpation, and auscultation) is recorded. One advantage of the MFA is that conditions like disc adhesion, muscular problems (tightness, myogeloses) or tightness of the joint capsule can be diagnosed directly and without great difficulty.

3. Physiotherapy

We feel, the professional field "physiotherapy" comprises a number of different techniques and disciplines, some of which are used interchangeably and synonymously with the term "physiotherapy". Some disciplines that come under physiotherapy are:

- Manual Therapy
- Osteopathy
- Cranio-Sacral Therapy
- Chiropractic

Sometimes, the above (Osteopathy, Cranio-Sacral Therapy, Chiropractic) are lare listed as specialised discipline of manual therapy and manual therapy as a field in medicine (manual medicine) - as opposed to physiotherapy, which is often a trained profession.

- Physiotherapy/ professional training
  - Manual Therapy/ medicine
  - Osteopathy
  - Cranio-Sacral Therapy
  - Chiropractic

Manual therapy or physiotherapy should be used in gnathology to treat muscular imbalances and other functional disorders of the musculoskeletal system (including the ligaments). One is able to treat, e.g., undesirably hypertonic retractor muscles with intramuscular Botulinum A injections, mostly in severe cases. In less severe cases, primarily physiotherapy can be used to strengthen selected hypotonic muscles or muscle groups and loosen tight muscles, ligaments and/ or joint capsules.

Again, usually, physiotherapy is the main treatment to strengthen the mandibular protractors and to detonise the retractors, to give them normal strength. The TMJ capsules and ligaments sometimes are also too tight and should be treated with physiotherapy. Build-ups are necessary to permanently unlock the bite, so the desired mandibular positional changed can be carried out. Physiotherapy, it has become obvious, is very helpful in assisting to unlock the bite.

4. Orthognathic-orthodontic treatment for class IIs and class IIIs

Previously, we have surgerised many of our more severe Class II patients with and without TMJ problems. The maxillo-mandibular relation and the sagittal/ transverse/ vertical dimensions were corrected into Class I and neutral occlusion. Our task as orthodontists was, then, to correct the patient's occlusion into a Class I dental occlusion and to stabilise the obtained results. Sometimes, Class II correction involved the use of some type of Class II elastics and/or headgears to maintain the Class I dental occlusion.

Today, however, the number of Class II patients in our practice undergoing surgery has decreased greatly, thanks to the success of Class II Fixed Functional correction. Orthognathic surgery, in turn, is playing an increasingly important role for surgical Class I and Class III correction.

5. Our recommended fixed functional treatment of Class II malocclusions

Functional orthodontics is not a new discovery. In Germany, this kind of orthodontics has been in use for centuries. There are many functional orthodontic appliances available on the market. However, the fact remains, that they are removable and therefore depend upon the patient's compliance.

In easy patients with healthy TMJs and good patient compliance, however, removable appliances usually work well. If cases are difficult and require long hours of functional correction, it is easier, quicker, and more stable to give them a fixed functional appliance.

What makes a "difficult" case?

1. More than 3 mm sagittal correction
2. TMJ pathologies, such as disc and/or condylar degeneration and displacement
3. Positive findings in an MFA examination in dorsally, cranially or laterally forced condylar positions

4. Decreased mobility of the mandible in one or more directions

An effective way of tackling the problem is to combine European functional orthodontics with fixed appliances as were primarily developed in the United States. This achievement was actually done by Emil Herbst, in the beginning of the 20th century in Germany: the Herbst appliance. Several appliances have followed in its wake since its important rediscovery in the 1970s by Professors Pancherz and Ruf (Gießen/Germany). One of them is the MARA. In 1991, Dr. Toll introduced Dr. James Eckhart to the MARA. Dr. Eckhart had been using the Herbst appliance. First, two different concepts for the MARA were developed: a bite-jumper with an almost 90° elbow used mostly in the USA, and an angled German/ European version that incorporates the patient's condylar path and is sometimes also used in the USA.

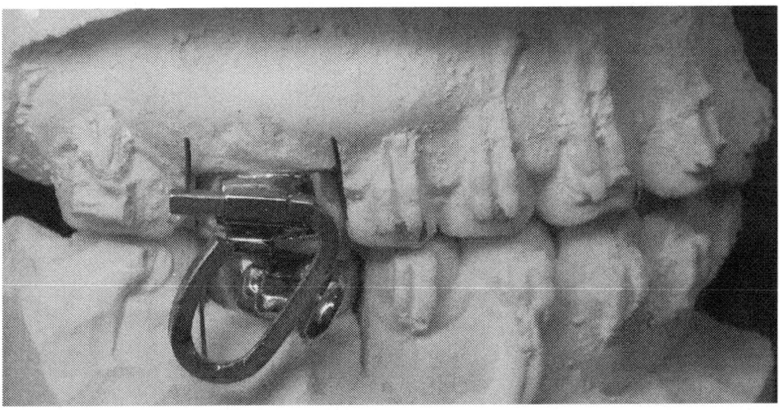

Fig. 2. Right lateral view of the Mandibular Anterior Repositioning Appliance, mounted on a plaster model.

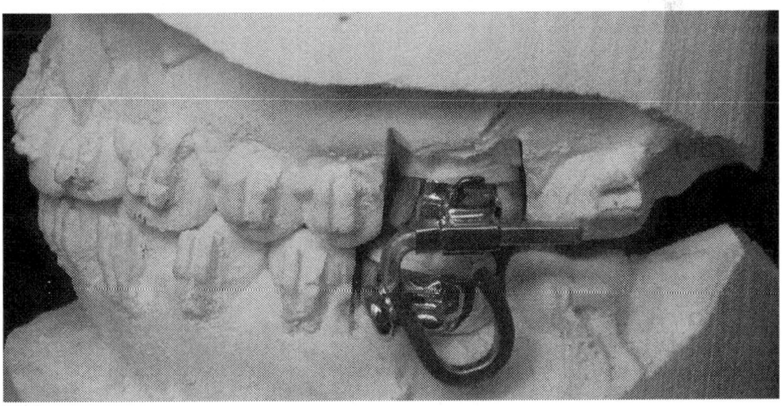

Fig. 3. Left lateral view of the Mandibular anterior Repositioning Appliance, mounted on a plaster model.

The MARA is usually cemented on the upper and lower 6s. The part designed for the lower jaw consists, among other, of special crowns or "beefy" bands, i.e. thicker bands, because the normal bands sometimes may break, unless soldered or welded correctly on the band without any band-weakening potential. Together, in cooperation with AOA (Allesee Orthodontic Appliances), Dr. Toll and Dr. Eckhart developed the first serial versions of that appliance in 1995. Fig. 2 and 3 show a lateral view of the MARA, mounted on a plaster model. It was decided by AOA that the version by Dr. Eckhart was preferable, so there is no danger of bringing the lower dental arch too far forward. For some time, however, important improvements have been made to the MARA, including the redesign that was mentioned and variations with different attachments and differently shaped elbows. The new design of the MARA usually incorporates a buccal shield on the lower part of the MARA, so the lower arm, fixed to the buccal, does not bother the cheek. This happens rarely, but it is a possibility in patients with strong buccal muscles [Allan-Noble, 2002[5]]. Actually, this effect is beneficial, because most patients with narrow jaws, i.e. transverse compression, need to have the muscular tone normalised. Hypertonic buccal muscles prevent stable transverse expansion. In our practice, maxillary lip-bumpers are a very good first phase treatment modality to normalise muscular tone, so the cheeks do not become irritated. In addition, a lip-bumper as a modified Fränkel appliance helps expand the maxilla, which is almost always desirable in a Class II case. With the MARA, as other Fixed Functionals, the usual expansion of the maxilla is necessary. In younger patients, this can be done first, followed by Class II correction with the MARA. When orthodontic treatment achieves transverse and sagittal overcorrection of the maxilla of almost one millimetre, the case will remain stable.

In the MARA, it is easy to take out the upper removable leg while leaving the rest of the appliance in, in order to check that the patients do not have an unstable anterior overcorrection. Another method is to make the upper removable leg much smaller to make sure the case stays stable before removing the appliance totally.

The MARA is used to advance the mandible, to encourage condylar growth enhancement in children and adolescents, and to stabilise the desired anterior repositioning. Even in adults, condyles and fossae usually show remodelling, bringing further functional improvement. It appears that there are no MARA cases as of today that have shown any occurrence of TMJ problems under MARA treatment and its condylar advancement. The opposite is the case: The MARA usually decreases or eliminates the problem (such as tinnitus, clicking, etc.). A study on 58 patients conducted in our practice shows that the TMD symptoms tend to improve greatly under MARA therapy [Toll, Popović & Drinkuth, 2010[3]]. A successful disc recapture achieved by anterior repositioning of the mandible is shown in fig. 4.

In conjunction with the MARA, other orthodontic appliances can be worn like brackets, Class II elastics, lip bumpers, surgical or non-surgical suture splits for the maxilla (rapid palatal expander), etc. The MARA, if used alone, is usually worn with a standard lower lingual arch and an upper palatal bar or expander.

It is definitely better to use the vertical leg in the upper jaw in cases where it is undesirable to advance the lower anterior teeth. The reason for this is: With the vertical version, the patients do not have a propulsion effect on the lower teeth, as with all other Functionals. The Class II correction is done by neuromuscular reprogramming, to advance the mandible and, thus maintaining the condyles in an advanced position. Another advantage of the MARA is that it does not create a permanent connection between maxilla and mandible, but allows the mandible to "float" freely. Also, it prevents the patients from biting in Class II:

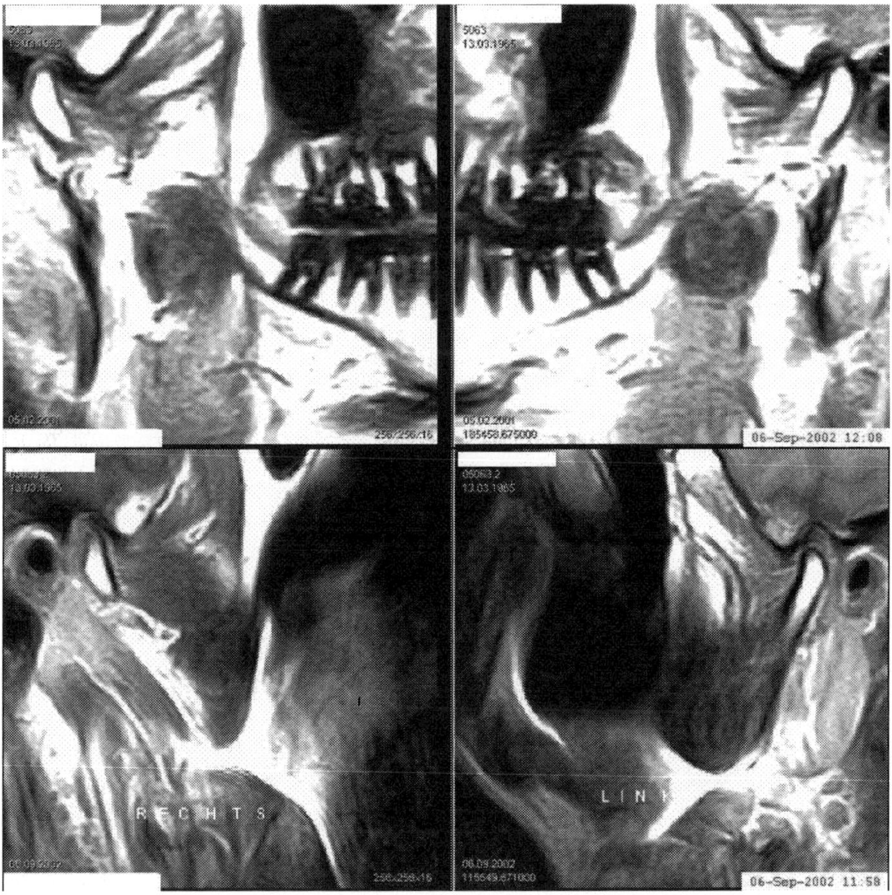

Fig. 4. Pre (top)- and post-treatment (bottom) TMJ MRI showing an anteriorly prolapsed disc pre-, and a recaptured disc post treatment.

When the patients try to bite retrally, the lower arm collides with the upper elbow. This prevents the jaw from closing, forcing the patients to bite anteriorly, in Class I, in order to be able to close the jaw. Thus, the mandibular advancement is solely a neuromuscular one, not one enforced by propulsion mechanics. There is a proprioceptive feedback loop between masticatory muscular activity and mandibular/ occlusal position. When the mandible stays anteriorly, muscular activity and reflexive pathways adapt. The time it takes the muscles and ligaments to adapt to the new functional position is not easy to predict. Sometimes, the patients adapt within 2 -3 months, esp. if they start with a dorso-cranial condylar position. In contrast, the adaption sometimes may take over a year, particularly in patients with unhealthy TMJs, which can be demonstrated well in MRIs. With any type of appliance, it is important to retain the patients in this advanced position and to test them constantly with a so-called speech-centric test, with the upper arms removed and in which the clinician watches the patients speak as they sit in the chair. To have the patients reclined a little bit is even a more thorough test to see if, despite what gravity does to the position of the mandible, it stays in the anterior position. Because the MARA has no fixed connection from the maxilla to the mandible, it does not ever interfere with speech and with chewing and therefore is a very comfortable appliance.

6. Our treatment concept

The "entrapped mandible syndrome" is a combination of deep bite, retruded mandible and undesirably steep upper incisor angulation. This combination of factors is most often found in Class II/2 patients. To treat this "entrapped mandible syndrome" effectively and to stop present TMJ degeneration from growing worse, it is important to 1) eliminate the deep bite. This gives the mandible the "freedom" to advance on its own. This ability strongly depends upon how tight the joint capsules and the ligaments are. We call this "unlocking the bite". 2) Once "unlocked", it is crucial to allow the mandible to advance to its physiological position by correcting incisor angulation and by using a Fixed Functional, like the MARA.

This unlocking of the bite is done with temporary crowns on the 6s or sometimes even the 7s. Additionally, flat composite build-ups can be cemented on the other molars to totally eliminate any bucco-lingual or antero-posterior interdigitation, freeing the mandible.

Not only do we need to unlock the bite with build-ups, as described above. It is also very important that, in deep bites, simultaneous intrusion of the upper and lower anteriors is done, so the "entrapped mandible" is totally "free". It appears that, at no time during the entire treatment, should the incisors and cuspids have any contact. The mandible must be totally free to grow and advance optimally. An important recommendation is that, during the night, light up-and-down elastics should be worn from the upper to the lower 6s, so the mandible cannot open wide and propulsion is lost. The MARA also works well on Class II open bites. It is important, here, that the patients learn to be able to close their lips. If any complications exist in the upper respiratory passage they need to be eliminated (enlarged tonsils, conchae, or adenoids, etc.). This means, of course, that mouth breathing should be treated in all orthodontic patients simultaneously during orthodontic correction, i.e. open bite patients should also be treated with the MARA, but one must be sure to eliminate the cause of the open bite simultaneously during treatment. Mouth breathing increases the amount of necessary correction and decreases stability. At the end of treatment, in our view, it is important to have delayed front tooth disclusion and cuspid guidance, so that the mandible can settle and stabilise in its new position.

When orthodontic treatment is finished, including very slight overcorrection, it is better to continue treating with the MARA for a slightly longer period of time than to try to prevent a relapse in a Class II direction with Class II elastics. During this time, the build-ups should remain in the mouth, so there is no cuspal interference. Class II elastics cause undesirable anterior tipping. Holding the Class II correction with the MARA, which is not visible, is the preferable way of making sure that the case remains stable. Mini-screws in the maxillary cuspid area to miniscrews in the mandibular molar area are another way of holding the Class II correction without undesirable tooth tipping, such as the lower arch slipping anteriorly.

A hypomochlion, i.e. a pivot in the 7s region, produces a TMJ decompression. Pivots on the 6s on teenagers do not cause TMJ decompression. In younger children, when the 7s have not erupted yet, the pivots can be inserted on the 6s, which does give some decompression. As soon as the 7s erupt, however, they should be removed from the 6s and put on the 7s.

7. Summary

Fixed Functionals are always indicated in difficult Class II cases. It is important to do the previously mentioned tests or examinations to see if the case is in any way difficult or easy. If the first is the case, it is strongly recommendable to use a Fixed Functional. The bite must be jumped and under no condition allowed to relapse distally during treatment. The cases should be monitored in the retention phase, so that the problem does not return. It is our opinion that, in Fixed Functionals, this is the only way to be assured that the Class II correction can be stably maintained.

Any of the removable functional appliances work well in patients with mild to moderate forms of the Class II malocclusion and/ or excellent patient compliance. Here, it is perhaps not necessary to use Fixed Functionals, as soon as the TMJs are proven (with MRI and MFA) to be healthy. In such a case, we usually use a positioner activator in our practice, because it is the only functional appliance that provides 4-dimensional control of the teeth.

8. References

[1] McNamara JA, Connelly TG & McBride, MC (1975) Histological Studies of Temporomandibular Joint Adaptations. In: Determinants of Mandibular Form and Growth. J.A. McNamara, Monography No. 4. Craniofacial growth Series, Ed. Ann Arbor Center for Human Growth and Development: 209-227

[2] O'Brien K, Wright J, Conboy F (2003) Effectiveness of treatment for class II malocclusion with the herbst or twin-block appliances: a randomized, controlled trial. AJO-DO (124)2: 128-137

[3] Toll DE, Popović N & Drinkuth N (2010) The Use of MRI Diagnostics in Orthognathic Surgery - Prevalence of TMJ Pathologies in Angle Class I, II, III Patients. J Orof Orthop (71)1: 68-80

[4] 45 years of empirical data from own practice

[5] Allan-Noble PS (2002) Clinical Management of the MARA – A Manual for Orthodontists and Staff. PDF-file by Allesee Orthodontic Appliances, version 02/2002 (URL http://www.aoalab.com/index/cms-filesystem-action? file=AOALab-Education-PDF/clinicalmanagementmara2002-manuals.pdf)

Treatment and Long Term Follow-Up of a Patient with an Impacted Transmigrant Canine

Neslihan Üçüncü[1], Belma Işık Aslan[1] and H. Tuğçe Oğuz Türel[2]
[1]*Gazi University/Faculty of Dentistry/ Department of Orthodontics*
[2]*Bayındır Hospital / Ankara*
Turkey

1. Introduction

Impacted teeth are those with a delayed eruption time or those which are not expected to erupt completely based on clinical and radiographic assessment (Richardson & Russell, 2000). All teeth can be impacted. However, third molars, maxillary canines, maxillary and mandibular premolars, and maxillary central incisors are the teeth most frequently involved (Rajic et al., 1996).

Impactions are twice as common in females (1.17 %) as in males (0.51 %). The prevalence of impacted maxillary canines is 0.9–2.2%, but mandibular canine impaction occurs 20 times less frequently than maxillary canines (Alaejos-Algarra et al., 1998; Aydin et al., 2004; D'Amico et al., 2003). It is an even more rare phenomenon when such an impacted mandibular canine migrates to the other side of the mandible, crossing the mandibular midline (Joshi, 2001). Shah et al. (1978) found 8 unerupted mandibular canines in 7886 individuals. Grover and Lorton (1985) found 11 impacted mandibular canines in 5000 individuals. Ericson and Kural (1986) estimated the incidance of mandibular canine impaction to be 0.35 %.

The etiology of impacted teeth is unknown, though several mechanisms have been proposed. Tumors, cysts, and odontomes may cause malposition of teeth if they lie in the path of eruption of teeth. Other possible etiologic factors suggested by some authors are premature loss of deciduous teeth, prolonged retention or early loss of the deciduous canine, crowding, spacing, supernumerary teeth, abnormal position of the tooth bud, excessive length of the crown of the mandibular canines, dilaceration of the root, iatrogenic origin and idiopathic condition with no apparent cause cystic lesions, an abnormally strong eruption force and heredity (Bishara, 1992; Javid, 1985; Joshi & Shetye, 1994).

The treatment options for impacted canines are no treatment, surgical intervention, removal, transplantation, prosthetic or restorative treatment or surgical exposure with or without orthodontic traction to align the malpositioned tooth. The preferred option is surgical exposure and alignment (Blair et al.,1998). Successful treatment of impacted canines is dependent on the position of the tooth in both the sagittal and transversal planes, ankylosis and dilaceration of the tooth. It has generally been accepted that the more a canine is horizontally impacted, the less successfull the tooth will be brought into its correct position (Odegaard, 1997). Since prevention of impacted canines provides the best long-term results, intervention with surgical attachment of an orthodontic button or bracket should be implemented only as a second alternative (Crawford, 2000).

Transmigration was defined as a phenomenon of an unerupted mandibular canine crossing the mandibular midline (Tarsitino et al., 1971). Later Javid (1985) stated that the midline was required to be crossed by one-half or more of the length of the tooth. However in 2006, Auluck et al., suggested that the tendency of a canine to cross the barrier of the mandibular midline suture is a more important consideration than the distance of migration after crossing the midline.

Until recently most studies have reported that the mandibular canine is the only tooth in the dental arch that migrated across the midline. Yet recently, Kara et al. (2011) have encountered two transmigrant laterals and three transmigrant premolars in 90 transmigrant teeth. In other studies, transmigration of a lateral incisor (Camilleri, 2007), a premolar (Alves et al., 2008) and maxillary canines (Aydin & Yilmaz, 2003; Shapira & Kuftinec, 2005) have been detected.

Different incidences have been reported in the rate of transmigrant teeth. Zvolanek (1986) failed to find any cases in a sample of 4,000 patient series. Javid (1985) reported that a radiographic survey of 1000 students revealed only 1 transmigrated impacted mandibular canine. In the studies considering the Turkish population, Aydın et al. (2004) observed 0.31%; Aktan et al. (2010) found 0.34%; Büyükkurt et al. reported (2007) 0.33 ratio of transmigration and recently Kara et al. (2011) found 0.075 percentages of transmigrant teeth.

Joshi (2001) stated that 89 % of the transmigratory mandibular canines were impacted and 91 % were unilateral. The left canine is more involved than the right canine, and women tend to have this condition more frequently than do men (Joshi, 2001; Kara et al., 2011). Although unilateral migration is more common, bilateral transmigration of mandibular canines has also been reported (Kuftinec et al., 1995). Transmigrant teeth may erupt ectopically at the midline or on the opposite side of the arch (Camilleri & Scerri, 2003). The transmigrated teeth maintain their nerve supply from the original side (Fiedler & Alling, 1968).

Stafne (1963) reported that a transmigrated mandibular canine always moves in the direction of the cusp tip and deviates mesially. The transmigrant canine usually travels along the labial side of the incisor roots and migrates as far as the roots of the first molar on the opposite side (Camilleri & Scerri, 2003; Javid, 1985). Ando et al. (1964) and Stafne (1963) stated that movement of transmigratory canine is more rapid before the formation of its root, yet Dhooria et al. (1986) observed a fairly rapid movement even after completion of the root formation.

The exact mechanism of transmigration is not yet known although numerous theories exist in the literature to explain their occurrence. One of the theory is that the transmigrant teeth could be the result of a malpositioning of the dental lamina during the embryonic stage of tooth development (Joshi, 2001). Heredity has been hinted as a causative factor. Most of the time, the canine just migrates without any pathological entity, but rarely a cyst or odontoma accompanies such a tooth (Kara et al., 2011).

Clinical and radiographic examination is usually required to diagnose transmigrant teeth for they are usually detected within the symphysis of the mandible. In the existence of overretention of the primary canine, a radiographic examination should have be done to check the permanent mandibular canines. (Joshi & Bhatt, 1971).

When a transmigrant mandibular canine reaches a horizontal position where there is no obstruction by the roots of the incisors, it may travel forward toward the midline, cross the symphysis and assume a position where the entire tooth may be situated on the opposite

side of the mandible (Stafne, 1963). Thoma (1963) states that horizontally impacted transmigrated canine "almost always have to be removed".
The aim of this case report is to demonstrate that a horizontally transmigrated mandibular canine can be treated by using surgical exposure and orthodontic treatment mechanics and to show the long-term results.

2. Case report

The patient was a 10 year 1 month-old white female when she first applied for an orthodontic consultation. The medical history revealed no medical problems. There was no history of trauma to the craniofacial complex. She was in the early mixed dentition and complete orthodontic records were obtained. In clinical investigation, a crossbite in upper left region and Angle Class III malocclusion were observed. Panoramic and cephalometric radiograph analysis revealed a horizontally impacted mandibular right canine with its crown located slightly distal to the right central incisor root apex (Figure 1,2,3,4).

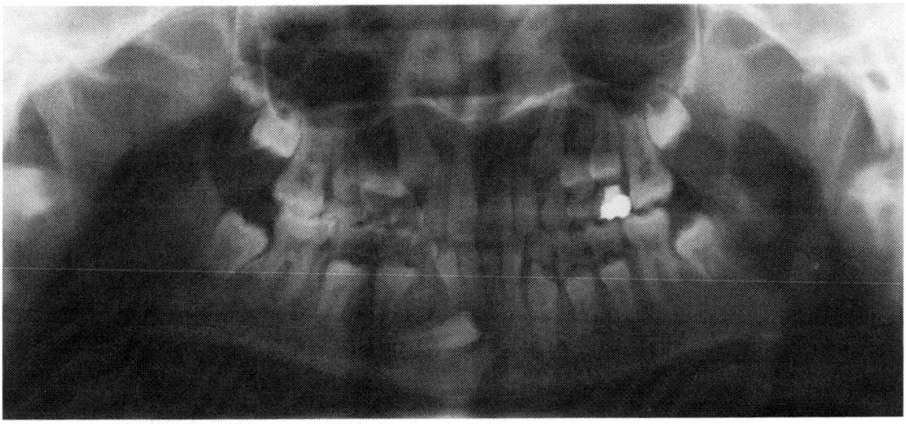

Fig. 1. Panaromic radiograph of patient at age 10 years, 1 month.

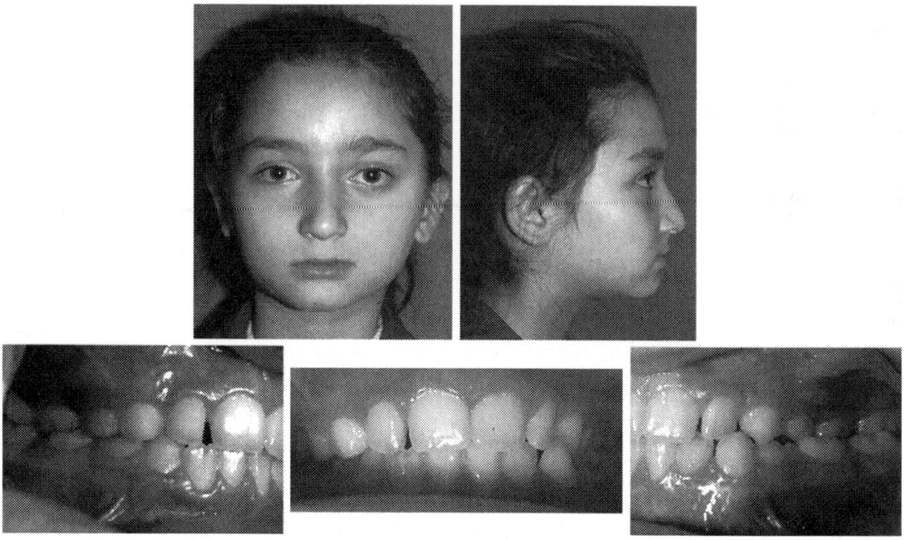

Fig. 2. Intraoral and extraoral photographs of patient at age 10 years,1 month.

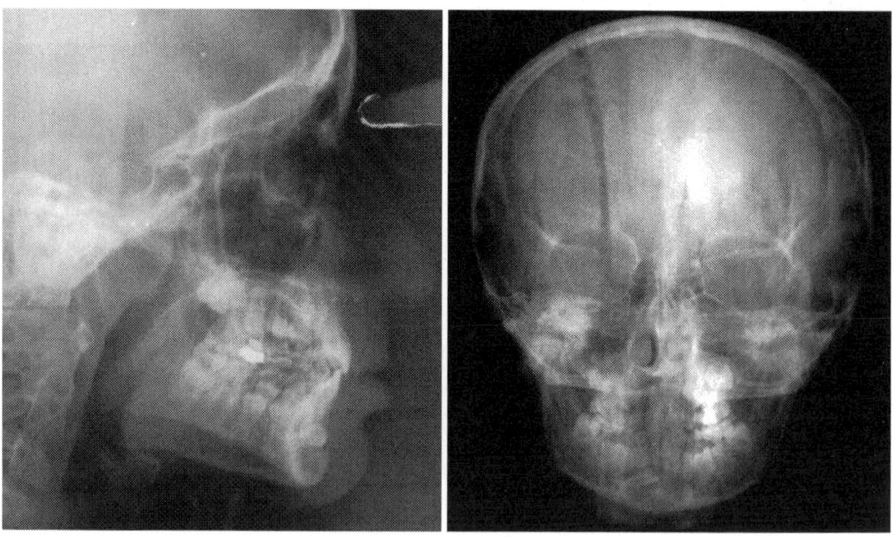

Figs. 3.4. Lateral cephalometric and anteroposterior radiographs of patient at age 10 years 1 month.

A maxillary Schwarz appliance was used to correct the posterior crossbite. In the retention period of the Schwarz appliance, a panaromic radiograph of the patient was taken. According to the panaromic radiograph, it was observed that the horizontally right impacted canine migrated mesially, crossed the midline and became a transmigrant tooth (Figure 5).

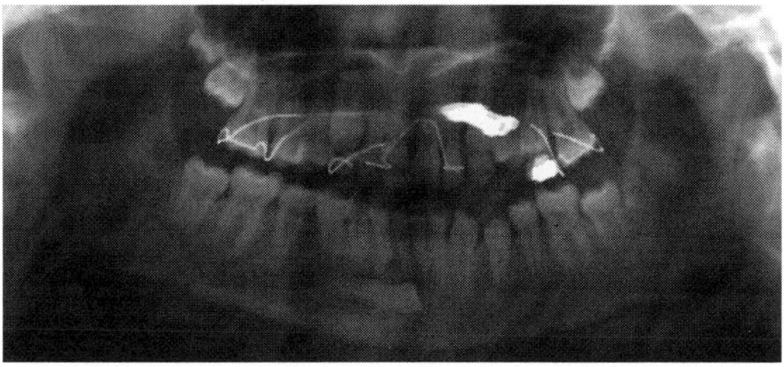

Fig. 5. Panaromic radiograph of patient at the retention period of Schwarz appliance.

2.1 Treatment plan

Treatment options were surgical removal, surgical exposure and orthodontic traction or autotransplantation of the impacted tooth. We didn't prefer the autotransplantation option since the root of the tooth was already completed. All of the treatment alternatives were explained to the patient and her parents. They accepted the surgical exposure and orthodontic traction option. If orthodontic traction had not been successful, the impacted tooth would have been extracted and implant or prothetic approaches could have been performed.

2.2 Treatment progress and results

First, the patient was referred to an oral surgeon for the elimination of follicule epithelium. Three weeks later, an open approach was performed and a window was opened on the mucosa through cauterization, then an orthodontic bracket with 0.30 mm. ligature wire extending into the oral cavity was surgically attached to the canine (Figure 6).

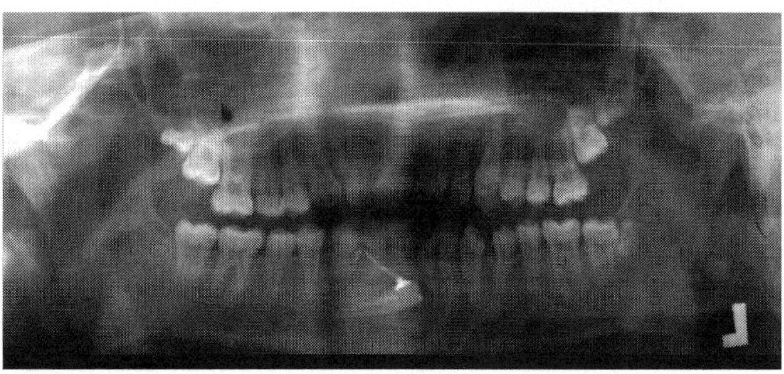

Fig. 6. Panaromic radiograph of patient showing surgically attached of an orthodontic attachment to the canine.

Two weeks later, 50 gr orthodontic force was applied to transmigrated canine through elastics hanged between Schwartz appliance and the canine (Figure 7).

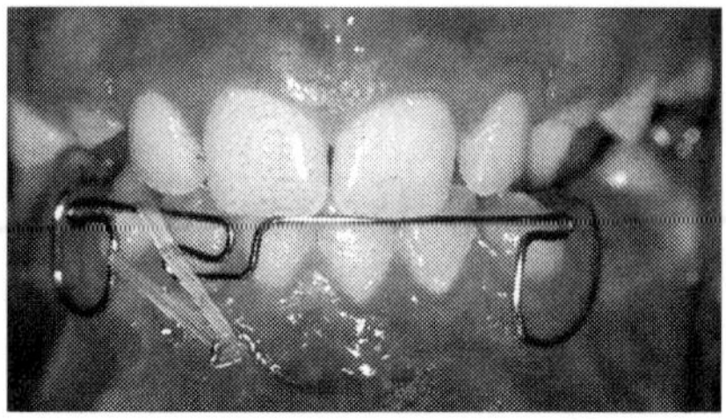

Fig. 7. 50 gr orthodontic force applied to transmigrated canine with elastics towards the Schwartz appliance.

This application continued for 9 months. At the end of 9 months, a new appliance was done and the traction force was increased to 90 grams. After one year, the crown of the transmigrant canine was seen intraorally (Figure 8,9,10).

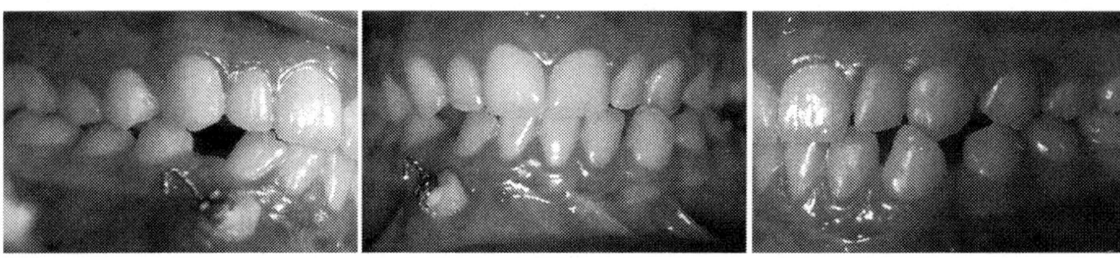

Fig. 8. Intraoral photographs of patient when the transmigrant canine seen intraorally.

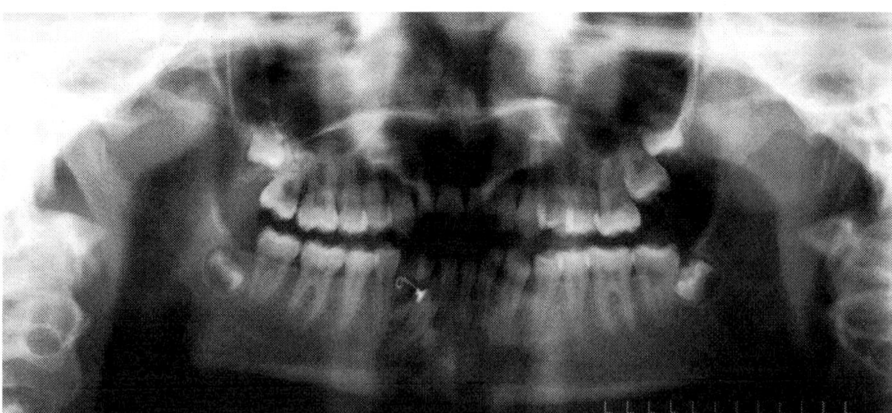

Fig. 9. Panaromic radiograph of patient when the transmigrant canine seen intraorally.

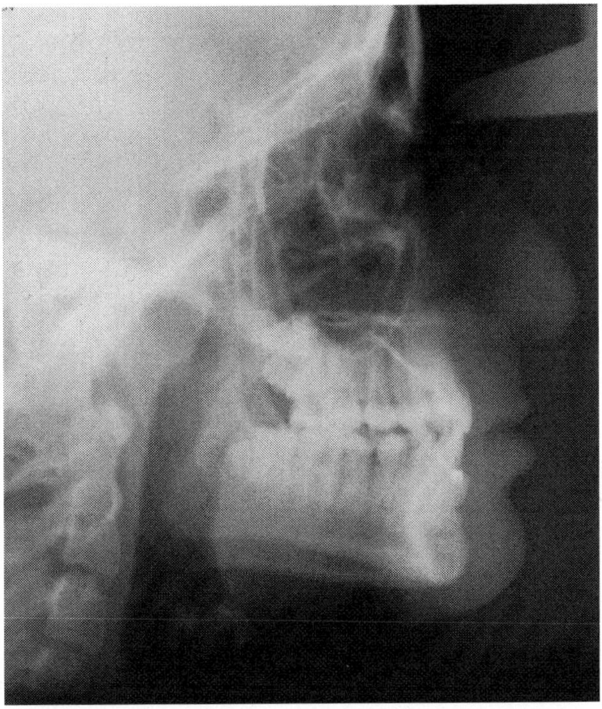

Fig. 10. Lateral cephalometric radiograph of patient when the transmigrant canine seen intraorally.

Comprehensive orthodontic records were secured, and it was decided to attempt a non-extraction mode of treatment, with 0.018″ x 0.022″ slot Roth appliances. In the aligning period of the mandibular arch, 0.014″ and 0.016″ NiTi was used with an open coil spring which was placed between 42 and 44 to create space for the transmigratory tooth. After providing adequate space, 0.016″ SS arch wire with stopper bends was applied to the mandibular arch. An intra-mandibular elastic applying 90 grams force was hanged between 43 and 46 for the distalization of 43. Then 44, 45, 46 and 41, 42, 31, 32, 33 were figurated to strengthen their anchorage. An extrusive force was applied to 43 by a chain elastic hanged between 44 and 42. Meanwhile 0.014″ and 0.016″ NiTi arch wires were applied for the alignment of the maxillary arch. Then 0.016″ x 0.022″ NiTi, 0.017″x 0.022″ Ni-Ti and SS arch wires were applied respectively to maxillary and mandibulary arches to maintain torque. The fixed orthodontic treatment elapsed 2 years. Class I molar and canine relationship bilaterally were achieved. The arches were successfully aligned and leveled, and ideal overbite and overjet were established. Comprehensive orthodontic records were obtained and Hawley appliances were prepared for retention (Figure 11,12,13). Superimposition and cephalometric analysis of the patient before and after orthodontic treatment are shown in Figure 14 and Table 1. The Hawley appliances were used for 8 months all day and the following 8 months only at night.

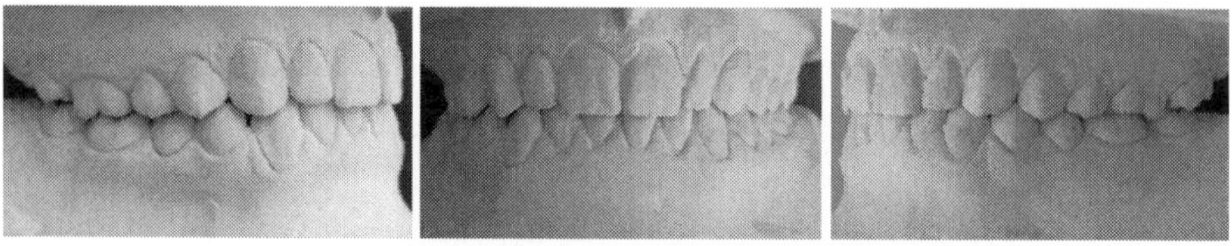

Fig. 11. Intraoral photographs of patient after fixed orthodontic treatment

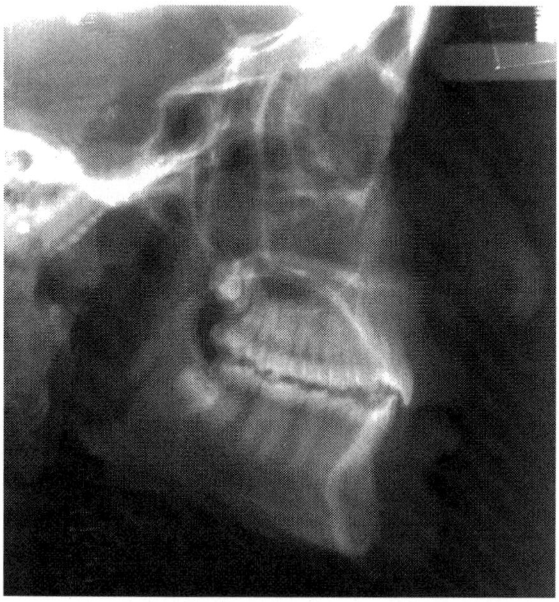

Fig. 12. Lateral cephalometric radiograph of patient after fixed orthodontic treatment

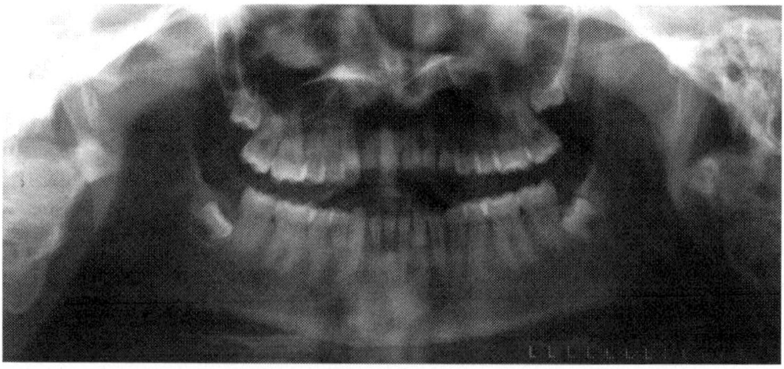

Fig. 13. Panaromic radiograph of patient after fixed orthodontic treatment.

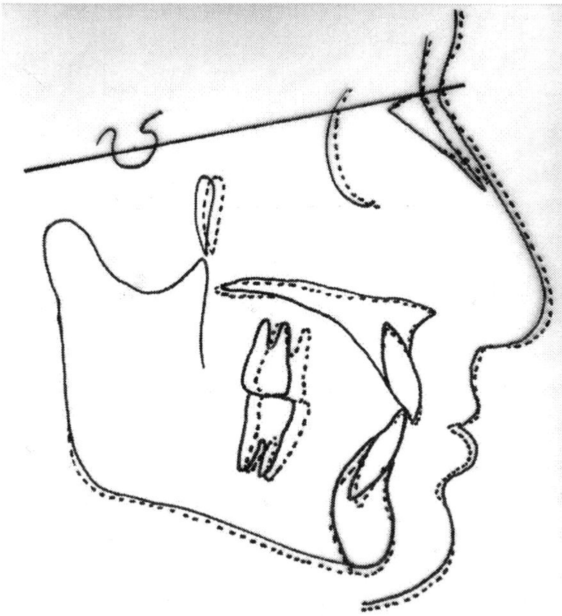

Fig. 14. Cephalometric superimpositions of patient before and after full fixed orthodontic treatment

	T1	T2
SNA	76°	76°
SNB	73.5°	73°
ANB	2.5°	3°
SNGoGn	27.5°	27.5°
N-ANS	49 mm	50 mm
N-Me	109 mm	111 mm
S-Go	75 mm	76.5mm
U1-NA	1 mm/16.5°	2.5mm/20°
L1-NB	2.5 mm/25°	3.5 mm/21°
U1/L1	136°	137.5°
Overjet	1.5mm	2mm
Overbite	3mm	3mm

Table 1. Cephalometric measurements at the beginning (T1) and the end (T2) of full fixed therapy

Three years later from retention which is in fact four and a half years later from fixed orthodontic treatment, the patient was recalled to check the stability of the treatment and the position of third molars. Full orthodontic records were obtained (Figure 15,16). The patient was referred to oral surgeon for the removal of 18, 28 and 48 to provide the occlusion stability. The retention records demonstrated good results.

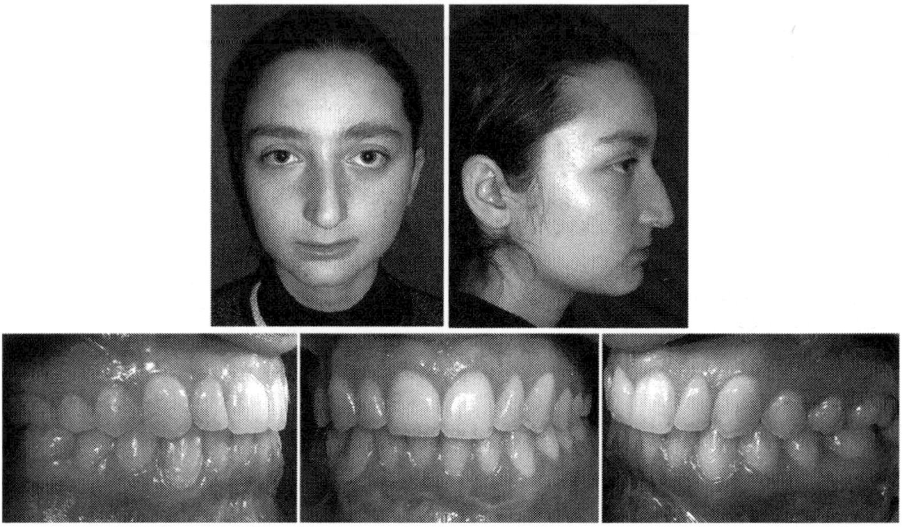

Fig. 15. Intraoral and extraoral photographs of patient 4.5 years after fixed orthodontic treatment.

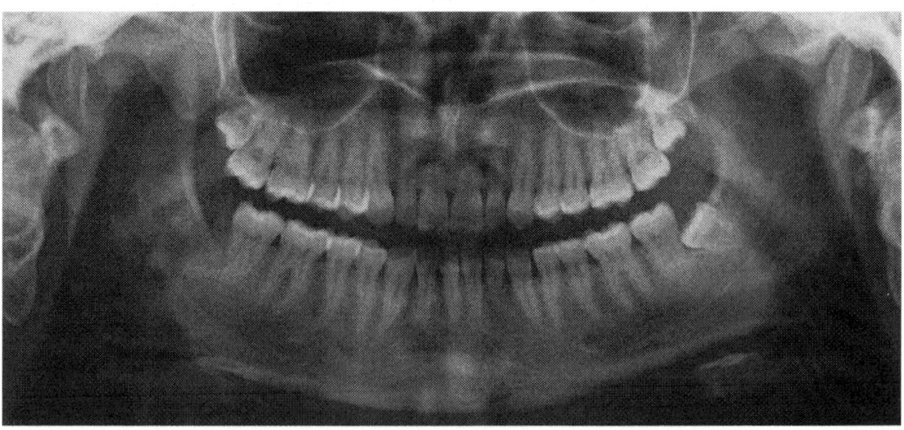

Fig. 16. Panaromic radiograph of patient 4.5 years after fixed orthodontic treatment.

3. Discussion

Transmigration of the mandibular canine across the mandibular midline is a rare and elusive phenomenon. Mupparapu (2002) described five patterns of canine transmigration: Type 1 for a canine impacted mesio-angularly across the midline, labial or lingual to the anterior teeth; Type 2 for a canine horizontally impacted near the inferior border of the mandible inferior to the apices of the incisors; Type 3 for a canine erupting on the opposite side of the jaw; Type 4 for a canine horizontally impacted near the inferior border of the contralateral side and Type 5 regardless of eruption status, canine positioned vertically in the midline with the long axis of the tooth crossing the midline. Type 2 corresponds to our case. According to Mupparapu (2002), the most frequently encountered type of transmigrant teeth was type 1, followed by type 2 and then type 4. Type 5 was the least frequently seen.

Impacted and transmigrated mandibular canines are often symptomless. Patients in deciduous dentition demonstrating the absence of the permanent canine from the mandibular arch, may be suspected to have an impacted or transmigrated canine (McDonald & Yap,1986).

Treatment considerations for transmigratory teeth depend on the stage of development, distance of migration and the symptoms. When the root apices are closed, extraction often is the only choice. Clinical clues can help to diagnose this problem at an early stage to avoid extraction. Axial inclination of the canines can help to predict the likelihood of canine impaction and transmigration (Joshi, 2001). Canines lying within 25 ° to 30 ° of the midsagittal plane have a tendency for impaction, but they do not migrate to the midline. If canines are within an angle of 30 ° to 50 °, they tend to cross the midline yet those that are found at an angle greater than 50 °, transmigration is almost always the rule (Pratt, 1969). Stafne (1963) found that the greatest amount of tooth migration occurred before the root is completely formed. If these malpositioned teeth can be detected early, they may be surgically exposed and moved using orthodontic forces.

The other treatment options proposed for impacted mandibular canines include observation, surgical removal and transplantation (McDonald & Yap, 1986).

If the impacted teeth is asymptomatic, it can be left in its place, but a series of radiographs should be taken periodically (Plumpton, 1966). Surgical extraction could be planned in the following situations (Camilleri & Scerri, 2003):

1. Progressive deterioration of the position of the mandibular canine during a one year follow-up period.
2. If the patient has any associated abnormalities, such as a developing apical cyst, neuralgia, displacement of teeth or resorption of an adjacent tooth root.
3. Severe mandibular crowding which requires therapeutic extractions to correct the incisor crowding. This would reduce the orthodontic treatment time and also the hazardous orthodontic tooth movement.

Wertz (1994) advocated that, if a nonextraction method of orthodontic treatment is indicated, a surgical repositioning should probably be attempted just before extracting the transmigrated canine. However, if the diagnosis indicates an extraction mode of treatment in the lower arch, then the transmigrated canine should be extracted instead of the usual premolar, eliminating excessive treatment time. Howard (1976) expressed a similar viewpoint.

If adequate space for alignment of an impacted mandibular canine exists and it is mechanically possible to reposition an impacted mandibular canine into proper position, then surgical exposure and orthodontic treatment is indicated (Ferguson, 1990; McDonald & Yap, 1986).

In published reports, tranmigrant canines were treated mostly by surgical extraction (Gonzalez-Sanchez, 2007). Only Wertz (1994) reported three transmigrant canines corrected successfully by surgical exposure and orthodontic treatment.

Wertz (1994) reported that, if the tip of the crown has migrated past the opposite incisor area or if the apex has migrated past the apex of the adjacent lateral incisor root apex, it might be mechanically impossible to bring the aberrant canine into its normal place.

Autotransplantation is another approach to correct this problem. Camilleri and Scerri (2003) stated that when the mandibular incisors are in a normal position and space for transmigrated canine is sufficient, autotransplantation may be undertaken. However, an immature tooth is required for success, and the difficulty in removing the tooth in one piece complicates the procedure (Rebellato & Schabel, 2003).

In this case, the root development of the transmigrated mandibular canine was already completed. Therefore, surgical exposure and orthodontic traction was preffered instead of autotransplantation.

Some authors believe that the age of patient is an important factor in the success of proposed tooth movement (Machen, 1989). In patients under 14 years old, before extracting the tooth, other options should be considered and the case should be carefully assessed. In patients over 14 years old, significant changes are not expected and extraction should only be considered (Ando et al., 1964). In a recent retrospective study, Aras et al. (2011) reported that forced eruption in four teeth out of twenty mandibular impacted canine teeth applying a traction force resulted in failure. They claimed that high mean age could be the reason of failure. Orton et al. (1995) states that treatments starting after the end of a pubertal growth spurt are likely to be protracted. In this case, successful forced eruption of the transmigrated canine may also be due to the orthodontic treatment of the case at an early age.

Experimental studies have shown that the loss of periodontal attachment does not occur during orthodontic tooth movement providing the periodontium is maintained in a healthy state (Ericsson & Thilander, 1978). However, in clinical studies, the variable loss of periodontal support is observed which may reflect the hygiene challenge associated with fixed orthodontic appliances (Alstad & Zachrisson, 1979; Zachrisson & Alnaes, 1973). Except this condition, various periodontal problems can occur due to the surgical approach. Either an open or a closed surgical approach can be used to uncover the crown of impacted tooth and to place an orthodontic attachment. Open approach may lead to gingival recession, bone loss, decreased width of keratinized gingiva, delayed periodontal healing and gingival inflammation. With close approach method, less complications and more esthetically pleasing results are obtained (Frank & Long, 2002).

In this case, open approach was performed to uncover the crown of the impacted tooth because of the localization of the tooth and the direction of the orthodontic forces that would be applied. In the long term, no periodontal complications except mild gingival recession was detected. No root resorption or pulpal damage was observed in both the transmigrated canine and the adjacent teeth. An ideal Class I occlusion was maintained at the end of the treatment. The results were satisfying and stable 4.5 years after from the fixed orthodontic treatment.

4. Conclusion

This case demonstrated that a horizontally impacted transmigrant mandibular canine can be succesfully treated without the risk of root resorption, periodontal and pulpal damage by maintaining adequate plaque control, applying small and constant forces and preferring the appropriate surgical approach.

5. References

Aktan, A.M.; Kara, S.; Akgünlü, F. & Malkoç, S. (2010). The Incidence of Canine Transmigration and Tooth Impaction in a Turkish Subpopulation. *European Journal of Orthodontics*, Vol.32, No.5, (Epub March 2010), pp. 575-581, ISSN 1460-2210.

Alaejos-Algarra, C.; Berini-Aytes, L. & Gay-Escoda, C. (1998). Transmigration of Mandibular Canines: Report of Six Cases and Review of the Literature. *Quintessence International*, Vol.29, No.6, (June 1998), pp. 395-398, ISSN 0033-6572.

Alstad, S. & Zachrisson, B.U. (1979). Longitudinal Study of Periodontal Condition Associated with Orthodontic Treatment in Adolescents. *American Journal of Orthodontics*, Vol.76, No.3, (September 1979), pp. 277-286, ISSN 0889-5406.

Alves, D.B.; Pedrosa, E.F.; Andreo, J.C.; de Carvalho, I.M. & Rodrigues Ade, C. (2008). Transmigration of Mandibular Second Premolar in a Patient with Cleft Lip and Palate- Case Report. *Journal of Applied Oral Science*, Vol.16, No.5, (September-October 2008), pp. 360-363, ISSN 1678-7765.

Ando, S.; Aizawa, K.; Nakashima, T.; Sanka, Y.; Shimbo K, Kiyokawa K. (1964). Transmigration Process of the Impacted Mandibular Cuspid. *Journal of Nihon University School of Dentistry*, Vol.6, pp. 66–71, ISSN 0029-0432.

Aras, M.H.; Halicioğlu, K; Yavuz, M.S. & 3, Çağlaroğlu M. (2011). Evaluation of surgical-orthodontic treatments on impacted mandibular canines. *Medicina Oral Patologia Oral y Cirugia Bucal*, (January 2011), Available from: >PMID:21196853>.

Auluck, A.; Nagpal, A.; Setty, S., Pai, K. & Sunny, J. (2006). Transmigration of Impacted Mandibular Canines: Report of Four Cases. *Journal of the Canadian Dental Association*, Vol.72, No.3, (April 2006), pp. 249-252, ISSN 0709-8936.

Aydin, U. & Yilmaz, H.H. (2003). Transmigration of Impacted Canines. *Dentomaxillofacial Radiology*, Vol.32, No.3, (May 2003), pp. 198-200, ISSN 0007-1285.

Aydin, U.; Yilmaz, H.H. & Yildirim, D. (2004). Incidence of Canine Impaction and Transmigration in a Patient Population. *Dentomaxillofacial Radiology*, Vol.33, No.3, (May 2004), pp. 164-169, ISSN 0007-1285.

Bishara, S.E. (1992). Impacted Maxillary Canines: A Review. *American Journal of Orthodontics and Dentofacial Orthopedics*, Vol.101, No.2, (February 1992), pp. 159-71, ISSN 0889-5406.

Blair, G.S.; Hobson, R.S. & Leggat, T.G. (1998). Posttreatment Assesment of Surgically Exposed and Orthodontically Aligned Impacted Maxillary Canines. *American Journal of Orthodontics and Dentofacial Orthopedics*, Vol.113, No.3, (March 1998), pp. 329-332, ISSN 0889-5406.

Büyükkurt, M.C.; Aras, M.H.; Caglaroglu, M. & Gungormus, M. (2007). Transmigrant Mandibular Canines. *Journal of Oral and Maxillofacial Surgery*, Vol.65, No.10, (October 2007), pp. 2025-2029, ISSN 0278-2391.

Camilleri, S. & Scerri, E. (2003). Transmigration of Mandibular Canines. A Review of the Literature and a Report of Five Cases. *Angle Orthodontist,* Vol.73, No.6, (December 2003), pp. 753-762, ISSN 0003-3219.

Camilleri, S. (2007) Double Transmigration and Hyperdontia. *Angle Orthodontist,* Vol.77, No.4, (July 2007), pp. 742-744, ISSN 0003-3219.

Crawford, L.B. (2000). Four Impacted Permanent Canines: An Unusual Case. *Angle Orthodontist.* Vol.70, No.6, (December 2000), pp. 484-489, ISSN 0003-3219.

D'Amico, R.M.; Bjerklin, K.; Kurol, J. & Falahat, B. (2003). Long-term Results of Orthodontic Treatment of Impacted Maxillary Canines. *Angle Orthodontist,* Vol.73, No.3, (June 2003), pp. 231-238, ISSN 3219.

Dhooria, H.S.; Sathawane, R.S.; Mody, R.N. & Sakharde, S.B. (1986). Transmigration of Mandibular Canines. *Journal of the Indian Dental Association,* Vol.58, No.9, (September 1986), pp. 348-351, ISSN 0019-4611.

Ericson, S.; Kurol, J. (1986). Radiographic Assessment of Maxillary Canine Eruption in Children with Clinical Signs of Eruption Disturbances. *European Journal of Orthodontics.* Vol.8, pp. 133-140, ISSN 0141-5387.

Ericsson, I. & Thilander, B. (1978). Orthodontic Forces and Recurrence of Periodontal Disease. An Experimental Study in the Dog. *American Journal of Orthodontics,* Vol.74, No.1, (July 1978), pp. 41-50, ISSN 0889-5406.

Ferguson, J.W. (1990). Management of the Unerupted Maxillary Canine. *British Dental Journal,* Vol.169, No.1, (July 1990), pp. 11-17, ISSN 0007-0610.

Fiedler, L.D. & Alling, C.C. (1968). Malpositioned Mandibular Canine: Report of a Case. *Journal of Oral Surgery,* Vol.26, No.6, (June 1968), pp. 405-407.

Frank, C.A. & Long, M. (2002). Periodontal Concerns Associated with the Orthodontic Treatment of Impacted Teeth. *American Journal of Orthodontics and Dentofacial Orthopedics,* Vol.121, No.6, (June 2002), pp. 639-649, ISSN 0889-5406.

Gonzalez-Sanchez, M.A.; Berini-Aytés, L. & Gay-Escoda, C. (2007). Transmigrant Impacted Mandibular Canines: A Retrospective Study of 15 Cases. *The Journal of The American Dental Association,* Vol.138, No.11, (November 2007), pp. 1450-1455, ISSN 0002-8177.

Grover, P.S. & Lorton, L. (1985). The Incidence of Unerupted Permanent Teeth and Related Clinical Cases. *Oral Surgery Oral Medicine Oral Pathology,* Vol.59, No.4, (April 1985), pp. 420-425, ISSN 1079-2104.

Howard, R.D. (1976). The Anomalous Mandibular Canine. *British Journal of Orthodontics,* Vol.3, No.2, (April, 1976), pp. 117-119, ISSN 0007-0610.

Javid, B. (1985). Transmigration of Impacted Mandibular Cuspids. *International Journal of Oral Surgery,* Vol.14, No.6, (December 1985), pp. 547-549, ISSN 0300-9785.

Joshi, M.R. & Bhatt, N.A. (1971). Canine Transposition. *Oral Surgery Oral Medicine Oral Pathology,* Vol.31, No.1, (January 1971), pp. 49-53, ISSN 1079-2104.

Joshi, M.R.; Shetye, S.B. (1994). Transmigration of Mandibular Canines: A Review of the Literature and Report of Two Cases. *Quintessence Internnational,* Vol.25, No.4, (April 1994), pp. 291-294, ISSN 0033-6572.

Joshi, M.R. (2001). Transmigrant Mandibular Canines: A Record of 28 Cases and a Retrospective Review of the Literature. *Angle Orthodontist,* Vol. 71, No.1, (February 2001), pp. 12-22, ISSN 0003-3219.

Kara, M.I.; Ay, S.; Aktan, A.M.; Şener, I.; Bereket, C.; Ezirganlı, Ş. & Demirkol, M. (2011). Analysis of Different Type of Transmigrant Mandibular Teeth. *Medicina Oral Patologia Oral y Cirugia Bucal,* (January 2011), Available from: > PMID:21196850>.

Kuftinec, M.M.; Shapira, Y. & Nahlieli, O. (1995). Bilateral Transmigration of Impacted Mandibular Canines. *The Journal of the American Dental Association,* Vol.126, pp. 1022–1024, ISSN 0002-8177.

Machen, D.E. (1989). Legal Aspects of Orthodontic Practice: Risk Management Concepts. The Impacted Canine. *American Journal of Orthodontics and Dentofacial Orthopedics,* Vol.96, pp. 270-271, ISSN 0889-5406.

McDonald, F. & Yap, W.L. (1986). The Surgical Exposure and Application of Direct Traction of Unerupted Teeth. *American Journal of Orthodontics and Dentofacial Orthopedics,* Vol.89, pp. 331-340, ISSN 0889-5406.

Mupparapu, M. (2002). Patterns of Intra-osseous Transmigration and Ectopic Eruption of Mandibular Canines: Review of Literature and Report of Nine Additional Cases. *Dentomaxillofacial Radiology,* Vol.31, pp. 355-60, ISSN 0007-1285.

Odegaard, J. (1997). The Treatment of a Class I Malocclusion with Two Horizontally Impacted Maxillary Canines. *American Journal of Orthodontics and Dentofacial Orthopedics,* Vol.111, pp. 357-65, ISSN 0889-5406.

Orton, H.S.; Garvey, M.T. & Pearson, M.H. (1995). Extrusion of the Ectopic Maxillary Canine Using a Lower Removable Appliance. *American Journal of Orthodontics and Dentofacial Orthopedics,* Vol.107, pp. 349-59, ISSN 0889-5406.

Plumpton, S. (1966). The Extraction of Mandibular Teeth via an Extra-oral Approach. *British Journal of Oral Surgery,* Vol.4, pp. 127-131.

Pratt, R.J. (1969). Migration of Canine Across the Mandibular Mid-line. *British Dental Journal,* Vol.126, pp. 463–464, ISSN 0007-0610.

Rajic, S.; Muretic, Z. & Percac, S. (1996). Impacted Canine in a Prehistoric Skull. *Angle Orthodontist,* Vol.66, pp. 477-80, ISSN 0003-3219.

Rebellato, J. & Schabel, B. (2003). Treatment of a Patient with an Impacted Transmigrant Mandibular Canine and a Palatally Impacted Maxillary Canine. *Angle Orthodontist,* Vol.73, pp. 328-336, ISSN 0003-3219.

Richardson, G. & Russell, K.A. (2000). A Review of Impacted Permanent Maxillary Cuspids: Diagnosis and Prevention. *Journal of the Canadian Dental Association,* Vol.66, pp. 497-501, ISSN 0709-8936.

Shah, R.M.; Boyd, M.A. & Vakil, T.F. (1978). Studies of Permanent Tooth Anomalies in 7886 Canadian Individuals II: Congenital Missing, Supernumerary and Peg Teeth. *Dental Journal,* Vol.44, pp. 265-268, ISSN 0007-0610.

Shapira, Y. & Kuftinec, M.M. (2005). Unusual Intraosseous Transmigration of a Palatally Impacted Canine. *American Journal of Orthodontics and Dentofacial Orthopedics,* Vol.127, pp. 360-3, ISSN 0889-5406.

Stafne, E.C. (1963). Malposed Mandibular Canine. *Oral Surgery Oral Medicine Oral Pathology,* Vol.16, pp. 1330, ISSN 1079-2104.

Tarsitano, J.; Wooten, J. & Burditt, J. (1971). Transmigration of Nonerupted Mandibular Canines: Report of Cases. *The Journal of the American Dental Association,* Vol.82, No.6, pp. 1395-7, ISSN 0002-8177.

Thoma, K.H. (1963). Oral Surgery 4 th ed., CV Mosby, St Louis, pp. 273 (as quoted) Wertz, R.A. (1994) Treatment of Transmigrated Mandibular Canines. *American Journal of Orthodontics and Dentofacial Orthopedics*, Vol.106, pp. 419-427, ISSN 0889-5406.

Wertz, R.A. (1994). Transmigrated Mandibular Canines. *American Journal of Orthodontics and Dentofacial Orthopedics*, Vol.106, pp. 419-27, ISSN 0889-5406.

Zachrisson, B.U. & Alnaes, L. (1973). Periodontal Condition in Orthodontically Treated and Untreated Individuals I. Loss of Attachment, Gingival Packet Depth and Clinical Crown Height. *Angle Orthodontist*, Vol.43, pp. 402-11, ISSN 0003-3219.

Zvolanek, J.W. (1986). Transmigration of an Impacted Mandibular Canine. *Illinois Dental Journal*, Vol.55, pp. 86-7, ISSN 0019-1973.

Part 4

Orthognathic Surgery

16

Orthodontic Contribution to Orthognathic Surgery Cases

Nikolaos Topouzelis
Aristotle University of Thessaloniki, Dental School
Greece

1. Introduction

Skeletal malocclusion (dysgnathia) is defined as the congenital or acquired abnormal position or morphology of one or both jaws. There might be symmetry or asymmetry with disruption of the maxillomandibular relationship or the relationship of the jaws to the skull base combined with malocclusion or joint disruption. The main treatment objectives for serious skeletal malocclusions are aesthetic, functional and psychological rehabilitation. For this kind of cases these goals may be achieved. The orthodontist can move teeth and alveoli but this has no substantial impact on the adult basal jaw bone. The main orthodontist's task is teeth alignment. The oral & maxilofacial surgeon is responsible for the surgical correction of jaws and their associated structures. Generally speaking, the diagnosis and treatment plan of orthognathic cases require a systematic team approach. Although team member composition may differ depending on conditions at any given time, an ideal team should include an orthodontist, a maxillofacial surgeon, a phychiatrist or a clinical phychologist, a prosthetologist and a specialised dental technician. Orthognathic surgery involves risks and this is why we need to proceed with it only after careful planning. It is particularly important to understand the patient's view; this establishes trust and communication and helps achieve high quality results.

The management protocol for dentofacial abnormalities, treated through the cooperation of orthodontics and orthognathic surgery involves taking detailed medical and dental history of the patient, clinical examination, casts analysis, photographs, radiographs analysis (leading to diagnosis and treatment plan), presurgical orthodontics, actual surgery and post-surgical orthodontics.

2. Medical history

Taking a comprehensive medical history is of the utmost importance. Most orthognathic patients are young individuals and their health normally allows then to undergo general anaesthesia and extensive surgery. However, there are specific disorders, such as blood diseases (coagulation disorders), hormonal disorders, heart diseases, allergies, rheumatic diseases, respiratory diseases (sleep apneoa), which require special treatment (Harris & Hunt, 2008).

Very serious facial disproportions might be associated with systemic diseases, such as acromegaly (Class III cases) or chronic juvenile arthrities and muscular dystrophy (Class II cases with open bite). Such medical problems complicate orthognathic treatment and may lead to a generally unstable result if not sufficiently controlled. Furthermore, patients' psychological assessment is essential so as to ensure that their expectations are realistic. Besides, the case of dysmorphobia should be examined, because such patients are totally unsuitable for orthognathic treatment, as they are bound to be disappointed by the result (Winchester & Young, 2007).

3. Dental history

When taking the patient's dental history, existing teeth should be recorded and any caries or periodontal problems identified and treated before orthodontic treatment and orthognathic surgery, in coooperation with specialised dentists. However, there might be problems such as missing teeth which would be better treated after orthognathic surgery. Orthodontic intra-oral examination must include: a) assessment of static and functional occlusion and dental base relationships in the three spatial dimensions. It is important to check and record if there are extreme lateral or protrusive mandibular movements along the mandible elevation path, in cases of anterior or posterior cross-bite and in cases of disruption of the relationship between the upper and lower midline or the relationship between the upper and lower midlline the midline of the face; b) the presence of tooth spacing or crowding in relation to possible tooth size or morphology disorders; c) the presence of tooth displacement or rotation; d) the presence of anterior teeth inclination, since upper incisors become apparent when they are labially inclined, while lower incisors become apparent in patients with Class III skeletal dyscrepancy when these teeth are lingually inclined; e) checking incisal overbite and overjet. In cases of open bite, it should be checked whether there is a step at the occlusal plane in the upper arch and the anterior teeth are positioned higher than the lower ones; f) occlusal plane disorders, which are checked in the anteroposterior and vertical dimensions using the curve of Spee and in the transverse dimension using the curve of Wilson, which assesses the buccal-lingual position of the occlusal surface of posterior upper and lower teeth; g) the morphology of the dental arches and the palate. In cleft cases, a careful analysis of their type and extension is necessary as well as an examination of bone deficits that require grafts (Harris & Hunt, 2008); h) tongue assessment. A sizeable tongue (macroglossia) may lead to dental and skeletal problems and undermine the stability of the outcome of the orthodontic and orthognathic treatment; it may also cause problems with mastication, speech and breathing; i) examination of tonsil size, since their excessive size may cause respiratory problems; j) recording problems related to masticatory muscles and the temporomandibular joint, so that if related problems appear after treatment, there will be no confusion as to whether they preexisted or not; if possible, such problems should be dealt with before treatment starts. It is important to advise patients to ensure they fully comprehend that orthognathic surgery takes place so as to correct dento-mandibular disorders and its impact on a preexisting temporomandibular dysfunction is unpredictable; in fact the problem may be exacerbated postoperatively (Onizawa et al., 1995).

4. Clinical examination of the face

Clinical examination in regard to facial aesthetics and symmetry is more successful when the patient is sitting comfortably, with the horizontal Frankfurt plane parallel to the ground or in a normal position, with the dental arches in central occlusion and the lips totally relaxed. The aim of the clinical examination, in combination with cephalometric radiography and photographs is to recognise whether the maxilla, the mandible or both jaws are pathological and to note other important facial features.

4.1 Frontal clinical examination

The frontal facial view is what the patient sees in the mirror and it is also what is usually seen by other people in personal interaction. This is why this view is of particular significance. Numerous major facial parameters can be assessed in frontal view in regard to both the vertical and the transverse dimension. Maximum facial width should be assessed through the inter-zygomatic width. The ratio of facial height to width should be 1.3:1 for women and 1.35:1 for men (Fig. 1). Another quite significant measurement is the bigonial width, which should be around 30% shorter than the bizygomatic width (Fig. 1). However, according to current beauty standards, faces where the bigonial width is longer than normal are preferred (Winchester & Young, 2007). The conventional way to assess the vertical dimension of the face is to ensure that there are three equal vertical parts (Fig. 1). The upper part is between the hairline and the eyebrows, the middle part between the eyebrows and the base of the nose and the lower part from the base of the nose to the gnathion. It is important to examine if the vertical height of the three parts is excessive or deficient, in particular regarding the middle third that entails the maxilla and the lower third that entails the mandible (Sarver et al., 2003). In the lower facial third, the ratio of the upper lip height to the lower lip and chin height should be 1:2 (Fig. 1). A pronounced labiomental fold may indicate a reduced anterior facial height, while a shallow fold an increased height.

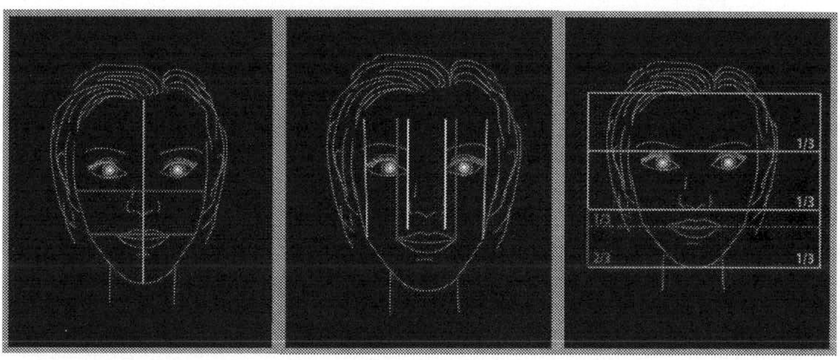

Fig. 1. Facial proportions

When assessing the transverse dimension of the face, it is important to initially note any asymmetry of the middle or lower third of the face. When the upper or lower dental midlines of a patient do not coincide or do not agree with the skeletal midlines (Fig. 9) differential diagnosis is essential in order to follow the right treatment.

The nose is a central structure of the face and plays a particularly important role during clinical examination. Traditionally, among Caucasians, it was acceptable that the alar base width as measured from the lateral aspects of the alar cartilages of the nose, should be more or less equal to the inter-canthal distance, as measured between the medial canthi of the eyes (Fig. 1). This assessment is important when maxillary impaction is planned (Harris & Hunt, 2008). The width of the mouth should be more or less equal to the distance between the medial borders of the iris (Fig. 1). Similarly, the width of the mandible at the level of the gonion should be more or less equal to the distance between the lateral canthi of the eyes (Sarver et al., 2003).

Dentolabial relationships play an important role in facial aesthetics and they should be assessed at a resting position as well as in function while the patient is smiling. The visible part of the teeth and gingivae under the upper lip is important when making a decision concerning maxillary depression or lower maxillary repositioning. At rest, 2-3 mm of the incisors should be visible. Higher figures, up to 5 mm, have also been proposed (Arnett & Bermann, 1993a, 1993b) following the rationale that more exposure of the teeth is acceptable among women than among men. When laughing, the whole of the central incisor up to the level of marginal gingivae should be visible or even including 1-2 mm of the attached gingivae. More extensive exposure of the attached gums is more acceptable among women than among men. (Guariglia & Ronchi, 2005).

4.2 Profile clinical examination

When examining the face from its side view, what is first reviewed are, again, the previously referred vertical proportions (Fig. 2) and any balance and harmony problems in the sagittal dimension.

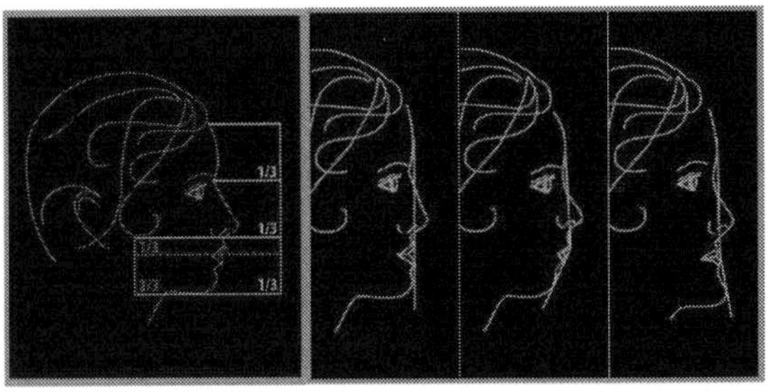

Fig. 2. Vertical proportions and reference lines for facial profile assessment

The nose and its features are also examined because nasal appearance may often undergo related and anatomical alterations in many osteotomies. So, in a Le Fort I osteotomy, maxillary impaction will tend to elevate the tip of the nose and restrict the nasal hump. What should also be assessed is the nasolabial angle; higher values tend to be more acceptable among women, while lower values among men. An acute nasolabial angle may be associated with maxillary hypoplasia and, therefore, may be improved with surgical maxillary protrusion. Controlling maxillary and mandibular protrusion or retrusion is assessed with two vertical lines. The first line goes through the most prominent part of the forehead (Fig. 2) and the second line goes through the soft tissue nasion. In a harmonious face, the end of the lips should touch the first line while maxillary soft tissues should be about 2-3 mm anterior to the second line and the chin should be 2 mm posterior to the second line (Winchester & Young, 2007).

In cases of sagittal disorder of the maxillomandibular relation, differential clinical aetiology diagnosis may become apparent in Class III cases, by filling the upper lip with soft wax or cotton (Fig. 3) until the relationship between the lips and the facial profile approximates what is considered normal. Similarly, surgical correction of a retruded mandible may be represented by asking the patient to slide the mandible forward.

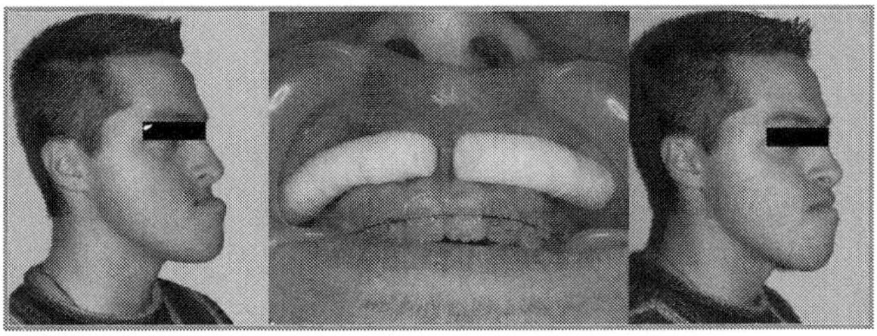

Fig. 3. Change in the facial profile after filling the upper lip with cotton

The submental region should be examined to check for the presence of excessive fat or a double-chin appearance, which is often associated with a short neck. Sometimes, mandibular set back may enhance this subcutaneous tissue deposit. This may be a contra-indication for mandibular set back or may make liposuction or plastic surgery necessary. However, among young patients, the submental region is usually spontaneously contoured after the operation.

5. Laboratory examinations

5.1 Casts

Casts should represent all the teeth that are present, the alveolar processes, the frenulums and the grooves (gingivolabial, gingivo-buccal, gingivolingual). The bases of the casts are trimmed in the intercuspal or central occlusion position, with the help of the corresponding bite records. The casts provide the best data for the assessment of dental problems and static occlusion. Initially they are examined separately in regard to arch shape (parabolic, triangular, square), rotations, deviations and ectopic and infraoccluded teeth. Crowding or spacing is evaluated through the correlation of dental width and the alveolar bone available. The symmetry between the left and right half in the upper and lower dental arches in all three dimensions is assessed, since there might be asymmetries at the vertical level that concern teeth, groups of teeth or the whole of the dental arch, causing an inclination to the transverse occlusal plane. The orientation of the occlusal plane is assessed on the basis of the curve of Spee in regard to the anteroposterior dimension, and on the basis of the curve of Wilson frontally (Fig. 4). In cases of posterior cross-bite with an increased curve of Wilson, it is very difficult or impossible to achieve proper occlusion with orthodontic, orthopaedic or even surgical maxillary expansion. The solution for such cases is maxillary expansion with multiple section osteotomies. Buccal inclination of posterior lower teeth is often associated with macroglossia or tongue protrusion (Wolford et al., 2004).

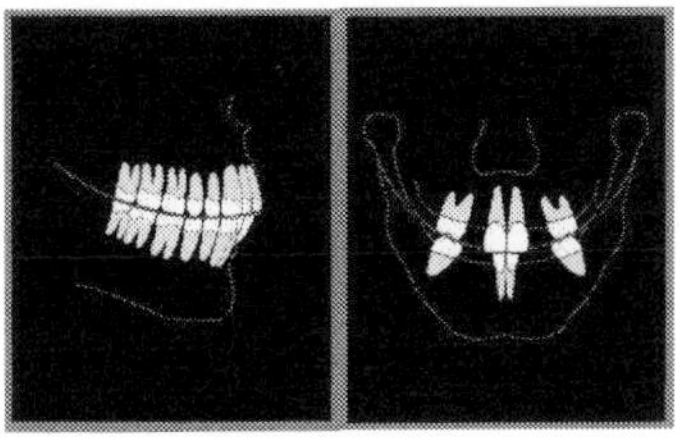

Fig. 4. The curve of Spee and of Wilson

Assessment of the width of the upper and lower dental arches is performed by measuring the inter-canine, inter-premolar and inter-molar distances and comparing them with the recommended normal values, which, however, is purely indicative in nature and changes depending on race and an individual's size. Disorders in the transverse plane affect preoperative orthodontics and determine the surgical treatment necessary. A practical way to reveal width discrepancies, as well as upper and lower arch discrepancies in general, is to mount the casts manually, so that the first molars are in Class I malocclusion.

Casts help us perform Bolton analysis, which is a method that compares the magnitude of the mesio-distal dimension of the upper and lower teeth. It may concern the anterior teeth or the whole set of teeth of the two arches. If there are discrepancies in tooth width, alignment and intercuspation are obstructed. Such disorders are usually caused by small upper lateral incisors or wide lower ones. Along with Bolton analysis, one should take into account the incisors' labiolingual width and their axial inclination. Assessing tooth size discrepancies is very important because this is also a factor determining the goals of presurgical orthodontics and surgical treatment. An even more accurate assessment is possible with a diagnostic wax set up on the casts.

A pair of casts is mounted on an anatomical articulator with facebow record, although a hinge articulator might be suitable for cases that require only mandibular surgery. The need to mount casts during the initial stages of treatment planning is a controversial issue, but may be necessary if maxillary impaction is being planned, so as to define the effect of mandibular autorotation. In cases of significant displacement, it might also be useful to mount casts in central occlusion so as to help treatment planning. In most cases, however, it is sufficient to use manual mounting of casts so as to determine arch intercuspation, avoiding the need of a facebow record (Winchester & Young, 2007).

5.2 Photographs

Photographs are an auxiliary tool for the clinical examination and cephalometry when investigating the aesthetic and functional restoration of the dentition and the face. Initially, two frontal photographs should be taken, one with the lips at rest position and one with the person laughing; then a ¾ photograph of the face and a profile photograph should taken. In cases of asymmetries, it would be useful to take photographs of both profiles. In order to make better use of extra-oral photographs, hair, beard and moustache should be removed from the face. Intra-oral photographs should include anterior teeth and the left and right buccal segments parts in occlusion as well as photographs of the occlusal surfaces of the upper and lower arch using a mirror. Photographs sometimes provide a more objective view than clinical examination, particularly in cases of asymmetry. Photographs should be taken before and after surgery to help the intervention or to serve teaching purposes; rarely, they might also be used for medico-legal purposes.

5.3 Radiographs

In order to plan an orthognathic case, it is necessary to have a panoramic and a lateral cephalometric radiograph. The overview of the panoramic radiograph indicates the presence of pathological conditions, such as impacted teeth that have not erupted, congenitally missing teeth or supernumerary teeth, caries, periodontal disease, apical lesions or cysts as well as the inclination or course of dental roots. The panoramic radiograph provides images of various forms of the mandibular open or closed angle as well as the relative position, morphology and integrity of the condyles (Fig. 5). In cases of condyledamage, the radiograph should be complemented by axial tomography or even three dimensional scans of the temporomandibular joint (3 - dimensional CT scan) (Kapila et al., 2011). Periapical radiographs are useful for a more accurate evaluation of inter-root spaces, when inter-dental osteotomies are to be performed. An occlusal radiography is often useful to clarify regions with a particular pathology, e.g. in order to locate the position of impacted teeth and to determine bone deficits in cleft cases.

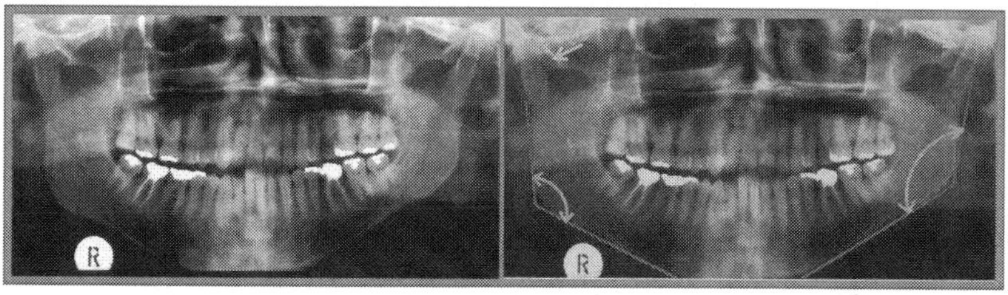

Fig. 5. Panoramic radiograph of a patient with asymmetry

5.3.1 Lateral cephalometric radiograph

Cephalometric analysis performed on the lateral cephalometric radiograph provides details about skeletal structure relationships as well as relationships between skeletal structures and the teeth and facial soft tissues, which cannot be observed in any other way. The catalytic role of such imaging on the complexity of the stomatognathic system and the knowledge of the functional impact of various facial patterns has been included not only in orthodontics but in other fields as well, such as orthognathic surgery.

Although cephalometric analysis is extremely useful to provide information concerning the diagnosis and treatment plan, this is not an absolutely exact scientific method (Baumrind & Frantz, 1971). Furthermore, it should not be considered as a primary diagnostic tool; it should be considered that the treatment aims are a proportional and harmonious facial structure, without necessarily aspiring at ideal cephalometric measurements. When there are significant discrepancies between clinical evaluation and cephalometric analysis data, the clinical assessment is much more significant in preparing the treatment plan (Chaconas & Fragiskos, 1991). Today there is a wide range of cephalometric radiograph analysis methods, which are either linear-descriptive or structural ones (Muller, 1962). Cephalometric radiograph analysis methods are usually based on measurements, which are compared to corresponding ones within normal range; this, however, presents inherent difficulties (Ricketts, 1975; Sassouni 1971), due to racial or ethnic differences, age and gender differences, possible differences in radiographic techniques (orientation in regard to the horizontal Frankfurt plane or in accordance to the natural head position) or differences that concern the criteria for selecting the 'normal' sample, such as occlusal features and skeletal background, at any given time (Miethke, 1995). In essence, though, what is important is whether there is harmony or discrepancy between the functional structures of the craniofacial complex in the same individual rather than the agreement of cephalometric data of the individual under study when compared to the normal sample range, as this was defined by the researcher at any given time (McNamara & Brudon 1993; Sassouni, 1971). Linear and descriptive analysis in lateral cephalometric radiographs is based on the study of jaw relationships with the cranial base and each other, the relationships of teeth with each other and their corresponding bone bases and the relationships of soft tissues in the profile view of the face. Measurements performed concern the maxilla, the mandible, the teeth and soft tissues.

5.3.1.1 Maxillary measurements (Fig. 6)

1. The S-N-A Angle: this provides an indication about the anteroposterior position of the maxillary base in relation to the anterior cranial base. Its normal value is 82°±2 for men and 81°±2 for women. A high value indicates a protruding maxilla, while a low one a retrusive maxilla. 2. The angle formed by the Frankfurt plane and the line defined by the nasion and point A. This is called maxillary depth and its mean value is 90°±3. This angle indicates the anteroposterior position of the maxilla in relation to the horizontal plane. Skeletal Class II type caused by the maxilla presents values over 90°, while, Class III types present lower values. This angle also presents lower values in cases of palatal clefts. 3. The distance of point A from the McNamara line (drawn through point N perpendicularly to the horizontal Frankfurt plane): this indicates the position of the maxilla in relation to the anterior part of the skull and, normally, point A lies near this line. Values above +3 mm indicate maxillary protrusion, while values under -3 mm indicate maxillary retrusion. Anteroposterior maxillary assessment should also take into account that the position of point A is affected by potential alveolar protrusion and by any pronounced inclination of the upper incisors. 4. The N-CF-A Angle (CF is the intersection point of the Frankfurt plane with the PTV plane). This is called maxillary height and its mean value is 56°±3. It indicates the vertical position of the maxilla in the face. In cases of skeletal open bite caused by the maxilla, the values of this angle are low, which indicates a short upper face.

5.3.1.2 Measurements concerning the mandible (Fig. 6)

1. The S-N-B Angle. This indicates the anteroposterior position of the mandible in relation to the anterior base of the skull. Its normal value is 80°±2 for men and 78°±2 for women. A high value indicates a protruding mandible, while a low value a retrusive one. It should be taken into account that the values of the S-N-A and S-N-B angles are influenced by the inclination and lenght of the anterior cranial base S-N. 2. The facial angle, formed by the Frankfurt plane and the facial plane N-Pg. Its mean value is 90°±3. This angle assesses the anteroposterior position of the mandible and determines whether a skeletal Class II or III is caused by the mandible. 3. The distance of point Pg from the vertical line going through point N. This indicates the anteroposterior position of the mandible in relation to the base of the skull. Normally, its values range from -4 mm to 0 mm for individuals of medium facial size (McNamara, 1984). Among adults, point Pg usually lies 2 mm behind this line. Values under -5 mm indicate a retrusive mandible, while values above +3 mm indicate a protrusive maxilla (Stroud, 1997). 4. The angle formed by the mandibular plane (Go-Me) and the Frankfurt plane. This is the FMA Angle of Tweed. Its mean value is 25°±4. This angle provides an indication as to the vertical height of the mandibular ramus and the posterior facial height. This measurement indicates the vertical type of the face. An open angle indicates a long face and, in cases of skeletal anterior open bite, that it is caused by the mandible. On the contrary, a closed angle indicates a short type of face and in cases of skeletal deep bite this is caused by the mandible. A high value indicates a long and narrow face with narrow dental arches. On the contrary, patients with a small angle tend to have a relatively high posterior facial height and increased activity of the masticatory muscles. Furthermore, they have a tendency for an overbite and muscular spasm particularly of the

temporalis and the medial pterygoid muscle, predisposing for TMJ problems (Chaconas & Gonidis, 1986).

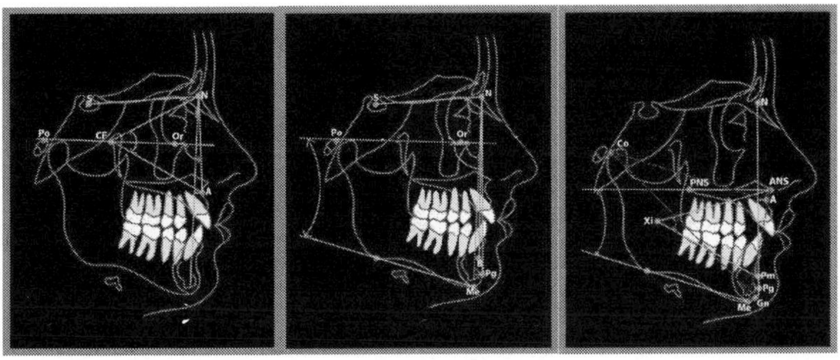

Fig. 6. Cephalometric measurements concerning maxilla, mandible and their relationship

5.3.1.3 Measurements concerning the relationship between maxilla and mandible (Fig.6)

1. The convexity of the face, which is the distance of point A from the facial plane N-Pg. Its mean value among adults is 1.7 mm±2. If point A lies in front of the N-Pg line, then the profile is convex and it is a skeletal Class II case, either because the chin is retrusive or because the maxilla is protruding or because there is a combination of the two. On the contrary, if point A lies behind the N-Pg line, then the profile is concave and the case is one of skeletal Class III, either because the chin is protruding or because the maxilla is retrusive or because the two conditions co-exist. The highest acceptable convexity among adults is 4 mm (Langlande, 1981). 2. The ANS-Xi-Pm angle indicates the lower facial height. Its mean value among adults is 47°±4. If this angle value is higher, it indicates the presence of open bite, while a lower value indicates the presence of deep bite. 3. The angle formed by the maxillary plane (ANS-PNS) and the mandibular plane (Go-Me). Its mean value is 27°±4. This angle is important because it indicates the posterior facial height and reflects the surgically significant pterygo-masticatory muscle and ligament height. For example, a patient with a high value for this angle, e.g. exceeding 35°, tends to have a relatively short posterior facial height and, therefore, an equally short posterior height of the muscles and ligaments involved. Any attempts to stretch this posterior connective tissue by rotating the anterior mandibular body upwards, in an anti-clockwise direction, around a fulcrum formed by the posterior molar occlusion is condemned to fail and lead to early surgical relapse (Hunt, 2008a). It should be noted here that the position of the mandible is not only affected by its size and its position due to the inclination of the cranial base, but also by the vertical dimension. For example, if the vertical dimension is excessive, the mandible might appear to be insufficient in relation to the maxilla. Therefore, it would be relatively retrusive, but only due to the vertical dimenstion. The opposite would be true in vertical deficits. If the vertical dimension is not normal, additional measurements often help clarify the analysis (Stroud LP. (1997), such as those recommended in McNamara's method. McNamara's method (McNamara, 1984) attempts to individualise patients, given that there is indeed a stable linear relationship between the relative length of the maxilla (distance between Condyle Co, i.e. the most superior lateral point of the mandibular condyle, and point A) and the relative length of the mandible (distance between the Condylium Co from the anatomical Gn). For

every relative length of the maxilla of a specific individual, there is one relative length of the mandible within a given width. This relationship also takes into account the vertical dimension, as this is defined by the anterior lower facial height (ANS-Me) (Fig. 6). In other words, what is characteristic about the McNamara method is the presence of the triangle formed by the maxilla, the mandible and the anterior lower facial height and their interrelationship as shown in the tables of composite values resulting from the combination of the three cephalometric samples (Table 1). So, the "originality" of this method lies in the fact that it directly correlates maxillary and mandibular lengths with lower facial height, regardless of the gender or the age of an individual. This leads to a useful combination of measurements with the substantial advantage of using it for diagnostic and therapeutic purposes in cases of skeletal problems, particularly when a combination of orthodontic treatment and orthognathic surgery is required (Sinclair & Proffit, 1991).

5.3.1.4 Measurements concerning dental relations (Fig. 7)

1. The angle formed by the lognitudinal axis of the upper incisor and the palatal plane (1/ANS-PNS). Its mean value is 109°±5. In cases of Class III dentoalveolar disorder, this angle often presents increased values, since the incisors have an increased labial inclination in order to compensate for or alleviate the malocclusion present. 2. The angle formed by the lognitudinal axis of the upper incisor and the anterior cranial base (1/S-N). Its mean value is 103°±2. This angle becomes particularly significant in cases when the palatal plane is to surgically change inclination, as in some open bite cases. In these cases, its coassessment with Angle 1/ANS-PNS indicates to the orthodontist the necessary preoperative movement of upper incisors. 3. The distance of the labial surface of the upper incisor from a vertical line going through point A and drawn so as to be parallel to the vertical line going through the nasion. This measurement determines the anteroposterior position of the upper incisor in relation to the mandible. Its mean value is 4-6 mm. Upper incisor positions more posterior than 1 mm to this line are considered to be lingual positions, while upper incisors situated more than 7 mm anterior to this line are prominent incisors. 4. The angle formed by the lognitudinal axis of the lower incisor and the mandibular base plane (ī /Go-Me). Its mean value is 90°±5. This angle indicates the anatomical position of the lower incisor in relation to the base of the mandible. A reduced value of this angle is almost always encountered in Class III malocclusion cases, as a compensatory factor. However, in cases of Class II malocclusion, this angle is increased (Guariglia & Ronchi, 2005). 5. The angle formed by the lognitudinal axis of the lower incisor and the dentoalveolar plane A-Pg (ī /A-Pg). Its mean value is 22°±4. This angle indicates the inclination of the lower incisor in relation to the

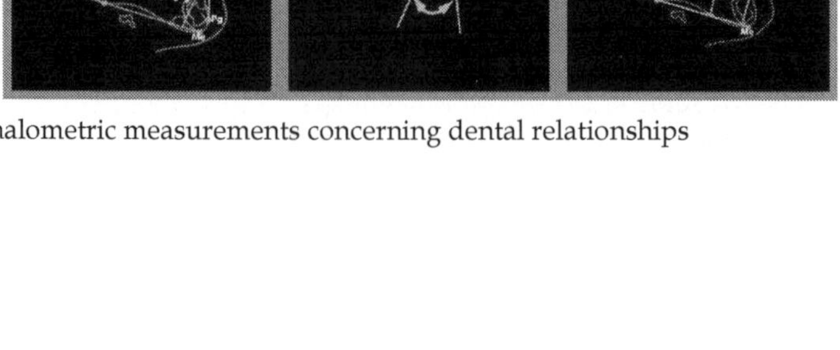

Fig. 7. Cephalometric measurements concerning dental relationships

dentoalveolar plane A-Pg and it adapts to the facial skeletal type; it is increased in short facial types and decreased in long types. 6. The distance of the lower incisal edge from the dentoalveolar plane A-Pg ($\bar{1} \rightarrow$A-Pg). Its mean value is 2.4 mm±2 and it indicates the projection of the lower incisor. Incisors lying more than 5 mm in front of the line are protruding, while incisors behind the line are retrusive. 7. The distance of the lower incisal edge from the occlusal plane. Its mean value is 1.25 mm±2 and it indicates overeruption of the lower incisor; it shows whether the abnormal deep bite is due to theintrusion orextrusion of the lower or upper incisor (Ricketts, 1982). 8. The distance of the upper incisal edge from the palatal plane ($\underline{1} \rightarrow$ANS-PNS). Its mean value is 33 mm±3 and it indicates the anterior dentoalveolar height. 9. The distance of the lower incisal edge from the mandibular plane ($\bar{1} \rightarrow$Go-Me). Its mean value is 44 mm±2 for men and 40 mm±2 for women. It indicates the lower anterior dentoalveolar height. It should be noted that these measurements of the anterior upper and lower dentoalveolar height reflect aspects of the lower height of the face. In other words, if the anterior lower height of the face is increased, then the upper and lower anterior dentoalveolar height will also be increased, with the exception of some open bite cases. (Hunt, 2008a). 10. The distance of the tip of the medial cusp of the lower first molar from the mandibular plane ($\bar{6} \rightarrow$Go-Me). Its mean value is 38 mm±3 and it indicates the posterior lower dentoalveolar height. 11. The distance of the tip of the medial cusp of the upper first molar from the palatal plane ($\underline{6} \rightarrow$ANS-PNS). Its mean value is 28 mm±3 and it indicates the posterior upper dentoalveolar height. Low values of the upper and lower posterior dentoalveolar height might indicate ankylosis or eruption failure. On the contrary, high values indicate supraeruption and are blamed for skeletal anterior open bite (Langlande, 1986). 12. The angle formed by the occlusal plane and the horizontal Frankfurt plane. The occlusal plane is defined by points corresponding to the middle of the overlapping of the cusps of premolars and molars. Mean angle value is 8°±4 and it indicates the inclination of the occlusal plane. This plane is very important from a functional point of view, in relation to mandibular movement. Along with the anterior and posterior decisive factors for occlusion, it determines how teeth get disengaged (Stroud, 1997). The occlusal plane has a significant impact on function and aesthetics, particularly in cases of bimaxillary osteotomy (Wolford, 2007).

5.3.1.5 Measurements concerning facial soft tissues (Fig. 8)

1. The ratio of the middle third to the lower third of facial soft tissues is 1:1. The middle third is the distance determined by points Gs (the most anterior part of the forehead corresponding to the glabella) and Sn (the most posterior point of the nasal base, where it joins the upper lip). The lower third is the distance defined by points Sn and Mes (the lowest point of chin soft tissues). In most orthognathic surgery patients, abnormalities are located in the lower third of the face, which is increased in relation to the middle third, either due to vertical excess of the posterior maxillary region or due to increased anterior vertical height of the mandible. In cases of reduced lower third of the face, the cause expected is either vertical maxillary hypoplasia or reduction of the anterior vertical height of the mandible or forward rotation of the mandible (Reyneke, 2003). 2. The length and eminence of the nose is the projection of the Sn - Pn distance on a straight line parallel to the horizontal Frankfurt plane and going through point Sn. Its mean value is 18±2 mm. Aesthetically it is more acceptable for women to have less eminent noses than men (Lines et al., 1978). When planning maxillary osteotomy, the impact it might have on the nose should be taken into account. 3. The distance of the subnasal point Sn from point Sts (the lowest point of the

upper lip) is the upper lip height. Its normal value is 22±2 mm in men and 20±2 mm in women. If measurements indicate values below normal ones, then the upper lip is short. The upper lip height is a decisive factor for the vertical dimensions of the lower third of the face, because it represents one third of this distance and because it is not easy for the upper lip height to change. This measurement is the basis that can determine the vertical height of the lower two thirds of the lower third of the face.

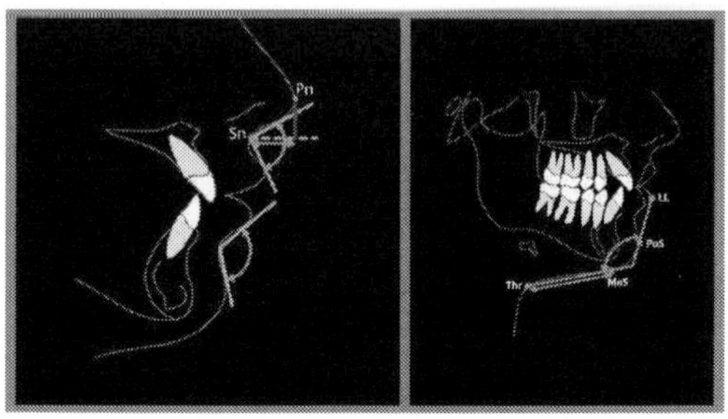

Fig. 8. Measurements concerning facial soft tissues

4. The distance of point Sts from the upper incisal edge, when the lips are at rest. Its normal value is 2.5 ± 1.5 mm (Arnett & Bergman, 1993; Fish & Epker, 1980; Miethke, 1995; Proffit, 1993). This measurement is affected by the upper lip height, the height of the maxilla, the height of the upper incisal crown, the thickness of the lips and the inclination and anteroposterior position of the upper incisors. This assessement is particularly important when determining the vertical dimensions of the face, particularly when there are vertical maxillary dysplasia (Wolford, 2007). Lack of upper incisor exposure might indicate vertical maxillary hypoplasia, while exposure exceeding 4 mm may indicate vertical maxillary excess, if the the upper lip height is normal (Reyneke, 2003). 5. The nasolabial angle, formed by a tangent on the columella which goes through the subnasal point Sn and a straight line connecting point Sn with the most anterior point of the upper lip (UL). An angle of 85°-105° is considered normal and this value varies depending on race (Burstone, 1967; Lines et al., 1978). The angle is usually acute in Class III cases, while Class II patients present a more obtuse nasolabial angle. A straight line going through point Sn and parallel to the horizontal plane separates the nasolabial angle into a superior and an inferior part. The upper/lower nasolabial angle ratio is of particular importance and should be one to four (Fig. 8). Ratios above 25% indicate an eminent upper lip or an upward tipping nose. On the contrary, lower ratios may indicate a retrusive upper lip or reduced eminence of the nose tip (Stella & Epker, 1990). It should be taken into account that when the maxilla is surgically shifted upward and backward, this causes loss of upper lip support, an increased nasolabial angle and flattening of the nose, which results in bad aesthetics due to a premature aging effect. 6. The mentolabial angle, formed by the straight line that goes through the most posterior point of the mentolabial sulcus (Sm) and it is tangent to the lower lip and the chin tangent that also goes through point Sm. Its mean value is 130°±10, with lower values preferable for men than for women. This angle is usually acute in Class II cases with anteroposterior mandibular hypoplasia, due to the pressure exercised by the upper incisors on the lower lip or in cases of macrogenia. The angle is flattened in microgenia cases or due to lower lip tension in Class III malocclusion cases. When planning genioplastic osteotomy, what should

be considered is not only the anteroposterior position of the chin but also the menton shape and the mentolabial sulcus. 7. The mentocervical angle, formed by the straight line going through the most posterior point of the menton (PoS) and the most anterior point of the lower lip (LL) and a straight line going through the lowest point of the menton (MeS) and the neck-throat joint point (Thr). The mean value of this angle is 110°±8. It is more acute in skeletal Class III cases and less acute in skeletal Class II cases, in which mandibular disorders are involved. 8. The throat length is the distance between the neck-throat joint point (Thr) and the lowest point of the menton (MeS). Its mean value is 40±5 mm. The throat length is increased in cases of mandibular macrognathia and it is shorter in cases of mandibular micrognathia. This measurement is useful to ensure differential diagnosis between anteroposterior mandibular excess and maxillary hypoplasia. The menton-throat angle and the throat length are of particular importance when planning surgical anteroposterior shift of the mandible, genioplastic osteotomy (protrusive or reductive) or submental liposuction. Thus, in individuals with a short throat length and mandibular protrusion, backward surgical shift of the mandible would be particularly unaesthetic (Proffit, 1991). To ensure proper assessment of these measurements, radiographs should be taken in the natural head position. 9. The eminence of the upper and lower lips and the chin are assessed on the basis of distances of points UL, LL and PoS from a straight line that goes through point Sn and is perpendicular to the Frankfurt plane. Mean values of these distances are as follows: 2±2 mm for the upper lip, 0±2 mm for the lower lip and -3.5±2 mm for the chin (Bass, 1991: Fish & Epker, 1980; Wolford, 1990). The eminence of the lips, according to Ricketts are the distances of points UL and LL from the aesthetic plane PoS-Pn. Normally, the lips lie behind the aesthetic plane: the upper lip at 4 mm and the lower lip at 2 mm. These measurements indicate the balance or lack of balance of the soft tissue between the lips and the nose - chin profile (Ricketts et al., 1982).

5.3.1.6 Cephalometric prediction of surgical orthodontic treatment

Cephalometric prediction of the surgical orthodontic treatment outcome allows the direct visualization of both dental and skeletal movement and projects the probable post-surgical patient profile. It can be of assistance to both orthodontists and maxillofacial surgeon in planning the treatment and to patients in comprehending postoperative changes and, mainly, the change in the appearance of their faces. Various manual cephalometric methods have been proposed (Fish & Epker 1980; McNeil et al., 1972; Proffit, 1991; Wolford et al., 1985; Worms, 1976). Manual cephalometric techniques are implemented either using the overlay method or templates. The overlay method by Proffit (Proffit, 1991) is the simplest prediction method for mandibular osteotomies; it is restricted to surgeries that do not affect the vertical position of the maxilla and is not time consuming. These are its stages, in brief (Fig. 9) : a) drawing the initial cephalometric tracing (CT) and the surgical reference line; b) a second acetate paper is placed over the initial tracing, so called the overlay tracing; Drawing on the overlay tracing the skeletal structures that are not going to change during surgery, including the surgical reference line; c) Movement of the CT mandible backward, on the overlay so as to achieve the desirable overjet and overbite and the proper intercuspation of posterior teeth. Drawing on the overlay the lower teeth and the part of the mandible in front of the surgical line; d) Superimposition on the cranial base and measurement of the backward movement of the lower incisor and skeletal chin movement; calculation of the predicted position of the lower lip and soft chin, using data regarding ratios of soft tissue changes relative to respective skeletal movements (the response of the lower lip represents 60% of skeletal changes, while the chin response is absolute, i.e. 1:1)

(Jensen et al., 1992). Measurement of the distance between the surgical reference lines to determine the surgical movement in millimetres; e) Superimposition at the mandible and drawing the lower lip outline and the chin; f) Superimposition at the cranial base; drawing the predicted soft tissue profile. The template method is implemented in all types of osteotomy and it is very useful in repositioning of the chin and almost necessary when the maxilla is plan to be moved on the vertical plane. However, the implementation of this method is time-consuming. In cases of one or two pieces osteotomies, the entire maxilla outline is drawn while in three-piece osteotomies an outline of the anterior and posterior maxillary pieces and the mandibular outline are drawn. The mandible rotates around the condyle (Proffit & Sarver, 2003).

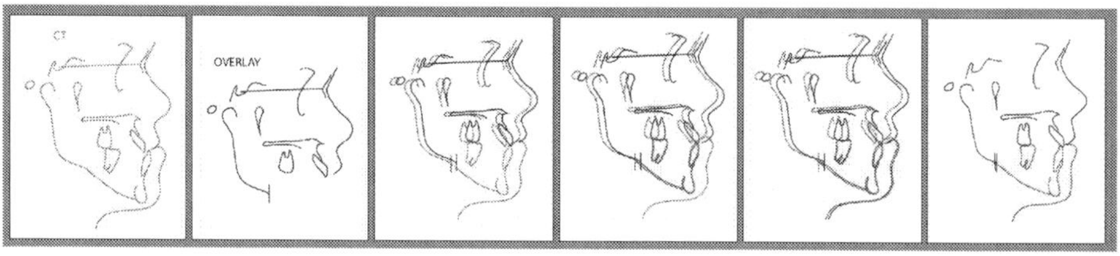

Fig. 9. The stages of Proffit's overlay method

Cephalometric prediction using a computer presupposes digital tracing of the cephalometric radiograph; it can be performed either by using software programmes alone or a combination of software and video images (Athanasiou & Kragskov, 1995). The operator shifts the cursor to various points, depending on the type of surgery, until the desirable aesthetic outcome is achieved. Then the predicted postoperative profile is printed and surgical movements can be calculated on it. This way, it is possible to save and analyse graphic data, to diagnose and plan the orthognathic cases as well as to predict the patient's postoperative profile. Computerized cephalometric prediction combined with video images is performed through automatic superimposition of the cephalogram on the patient's profile by the software programme, which is visible on the video monitor. All movements are of actual size. Today three-dimensional prediction methods are available. Computer prediction facilitates physician-patient communication, but there are certain inaccuracies involving mainly the lip area and the chin region (Eales et al., 1994; Kaipatur & Flores-Mir, 2009; Kolokitha et al., 1996; Kolokitha, 2007).

5.3.2 Anteroposterior cephalometric radiography

Anteroposterior analysis based on cephalometric radiographs is mainly useful for studying transverse asymmetries of the craniofacial complex. This analysis provides information about the width and inclination of the dental arches in relation to their osseous bases at the transverse plane. The analysis also provides an opportunity to assess the width of transverse maxillomandiubular relations and the vertical dimensions of corresponding skeletal parts or points of the dentition of the two facial halves and the nasal cavity, while analysing any asymmertries at the transverse or vertical planes. The study of facial symmetry is not always a mathematical measurement, according to certain authors. The symmetry can also be 'roughly' assessed, i.e. just by looking at the face. Vion considers it easier to assess asymmetry by placing the tracing on millimetre graph paper (Vion, 1976). Ricketts recommends the use of measurements, the most important of which for orthognathic surgery candidates are the following (Ricketts, 1982) (Fig. 10): 1. The distance between the maxilla (zygomatic process) and the frontal facial plane (JR →ZR) and (JL →ZL). Its mean value for adults is 15±1.5 mm and it indicates the left and right width of the maxilla and the mandible. It determines whether posterior cross-bite is skeletal. High values indicate skeletal lingual cross-bite, while low values indicate skeletal buccal cross-bite. 2. The angle formed by the maxillary midline (ANS - middle of ZR - ZL) and the mandibular midline (ANS - Me). Its mean value is 0°±2. In cases of asymmetry, this angle determines whether it is caused by dental or skeletal causes or by functional shift of the mandible. When the two midlines coincide there is symmetry and they both go through the incisal contact points. 3. The difference between the height of the occlusal plane at the left and right molars, measured in relation to the ZR - ZL line. Its mean value is 0±2 mm. Deviation from the mean value indicates asymmetry accompanied by structural abnormality of the maxilla or the mandible or both jaws. True skeletal asymmetry accompanied by an inclined occlusal plane is usually a warning sign for TMJ dysfunction. 4. The difference between the right and left angles, formed by points ZR-GA-AZ on the right and ZL-AG-ZA on the left. Its mean value is 0°±2. It indicates the position of the mandible and helps explain the nature of the asymmetry. Where the difference exceeds 4° it should be examined whether the asymmetry is of a structural or functional aetiology. These angles are significantly affected by a head turn on the headrest. Langlande also recommends the use of the distance between point DC (top of the condyle head) and the corresponding anti-gonion point AG, as well as the distance between point Me and the corresponding anti-gonion point so as to assess asymmetry (Fig. 10). These measurements make it possible to judge whether the asymmetry is due to the ramus or the body of the mandible (Langlande, 1981).

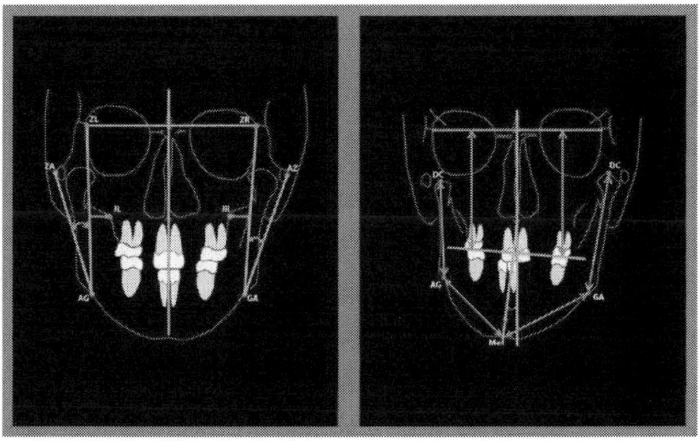

Fig. 10. Measurements concerning anteroposterior cephalometric radiographs

6. Preoperative orthodontics

The goals of preoperative orthodontic treatment are to allow for maximum surgical correction of the abnormality, to facilitate potential sectional surgical procedures and to provide the possibility for creating an ideal, stable occlusion (Tompach et al., 1995). The major part of orthodontic treatment takes place before surgery and might last one and a half to two years (Slavnic & Marcusson, 2010; Diaz et al., 2010). However, there are those who prefer to leave the major part of orthodontic treatment for after the surgery. Extensive preoperative treatment and limited postoperative treatment is usually better tolerated by the patient and provides smoother cooperation (Lee, 1994). The goals of preoperative orthodontic treatment are achieved with the alignment and flattening of the arches, the exacerbation of dental relations by removing all dentoalveolar compensation for the skeletal abnormality and with arch coordination.

6.1 Arch alignment

The first goal of preoperative orthodontics is to align the dental arches or their parts so that they might be compatible with each other. Correcting crowding and rotations, management of impacted teeth and arch length discrepancies is mainly a concern of preoperative orthodontics, because it facilitates arch intercuspation; otherwise, the surgical result would be restricted. If arch length is to be reduced, and the incisors need to be shifted backwards, then extractions are performed, as, for example, in Class III cases, when the upper incisors need to be moved backward or in Class II cases, when the lower incisors have to be moved backward to achieve exacerbation (Proffit & White, 1991) (Fig. 11). When sectional surgery is being planned, the deviation of dental roots close to the osteotomies starts with the initial wire and it is monitored through periapical radiographs. The modern preconstructed brackets of fixed devices and straight Ni-Ti wires have significantly simplified modern orthodontics. Selecting the slot size is a matter of personal preference, although the 0.022 inch system can better immobilise intraoperatively with rigid 19 X 25 wires. Ceramic brackets are pleasant, because they provide aesthetic solutions; however, their disadvantage is that they break easily during surgical manipulations. Most preconstructed bracket systems have been designed to tip the roots of canines distally and, thus, create sufficient space between them and the roots of lateral incisors.

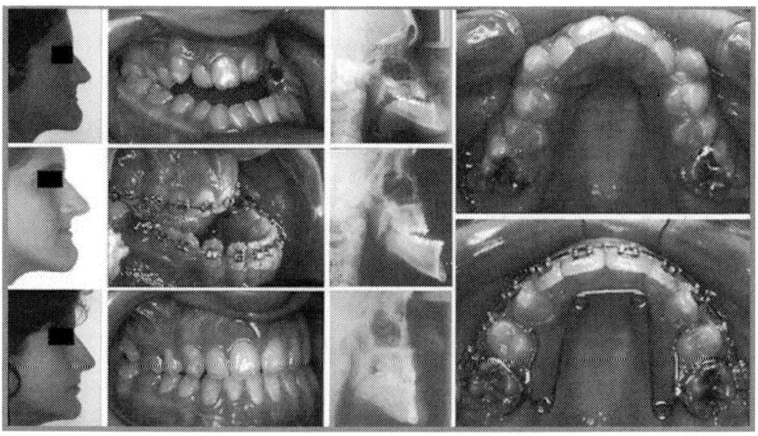

Fig. 11. A Class III case, with preoperative extractions of the first upper premolars to manage crowding and to move the upper incisors in order to achieve exacerbation of the negative overjet, which was completed with labial tipping of the lower incisors

This space is useful in cases where interdental osteotomies are to take place in the maxilla. When osteotomy incisions are performed distally to the canines, the use of brackets on the contralateral canines warrants that the integrated distal tipping of the brackets keeps the apices anteriorly and outside surgical incisions (Hunt, 2008b).

6.2 Arch flattening

The planning of dental arch flattening is particularly important. The general principle is that extrusion is easier postoperatively, while intrusion needs to be completed preoperatively or intra-operatively. Dental flattening and alignment are ususally a common one-step process in conventional orthodontics. This is not the case for all surgical cases. When the mandible is surgically moved forward or backward, the position of the lower incisor is what determines the lower facial height. In surgical correction of Class II, when the lower facial height is reduced, it is preferable not to correct the curve of Spee in the lower dental arch, either through orthodontics or surgically. Surgical protrusion of the mandible creates lateral open bite and a tripod-like occlusal relation; only the last molars and incisors are in an occlusal relationship. Besides, the lower facial height increases as the chin moves downward. Before the operation, the teeth are aligned and the anteroposterior relationship of the incisors has been determined. However, the curve of Spee remains in all wire arches, including the final stabilising wire (Proffit & Fields, 2007). The lateral open bite is treated with extrusion of the teeth involved, using vertical elastic forces during postoperative orthodontics. Numerous clinicians think that 2mm of extrusion in every arch is the maximum that may be achieved and remain stable without relapse (Hunt, 2008b). If the intentional lateral open bite that remains after surgery is deemed to be too much, then the curve of Spee will have to be reduced preoperatively, with the inevitable limitation that the increment of the lower anterior facial height will be limited postoperatively.

If the incisors are intruded preoperatively in a patient with deep bite, the operation tends to move the mandible upwards at the chin and downwards in the menton region, due to pivot effect. This increase of the posterior facial height will stretch the masticatory muscles (muscular stretching) and this is why it is unstable. However, when the incisors are not intruded preoperatively, the operation will move the chin downwards and the mandibular angle upwards, thus causing clockwise rotation of the mandible, which, generally speaking, is more stable in relation to the anti-clockwise mandibular rotation (Lake et al., 1981). (Fig. 12). On the contrary, when the lower facial height is increased, the pronounced curve of Spee has to be flattened preoperatively by intrution of the anterior part or surgically flattened with base osteotomy following sectional orthodontic flattening. Often a combined operation involving the maxilla is necessary to avoid the downward movement of the menton angle and further increase of the facial height, which is undesirable. If intrusion is necessary, the technique of sectional arches is indicated for preoperative orthodontics using mild forces in the order of 10 - 20 g per tooth, so that root resorption may be avoided, particularly if the teeth are fine. If this approach leads to lack of dental position control, it is preferable to have a continuous arch from molar to molar, with an anterior step for the incisors and canines. Continuous straight arches may achieve flattening, but probably with undesirable incisor tipping, which can be managed with extractions that allow the posterior movement of incisors. Surgical flattening is rarely indicated for the lower dental arch (Hunt, 2008b; Levander & Malmgren, 1988). When surgically correcting open bite, in cases of increased lower facial height, it is preferable not to correct the curve of Spee preoperatively in the upper dental arch, since multiple section osteotomies are indicated in such cases. During preoperative orthodontics, the aim is to exacerbate open bite with extrusion of posterior teeth and intrusion of anterior ones. During the operation, the final flattening of sections takes place, which allows the forward rotation of the mandible. If a one piece Le Fort I osteotomy is decided, with greater intrusion of the posterior part of the maxilla, preoperative orthodontic flattening is required, but anterior teeth extrusion should be avoided before the operation, because even mild orthodontic relapse may cause postoperative opening of the bite (Proffit & Fields, 2007). The importance of orthodontic movements of sectional flattening, which are usually unstable, is that it allows an attempt to minimise postoperative relapse. Following the removal of fixed orthodontic devices, the intruded incisors tend to infraocclude again and the extruded molars and premolars tend to intrude once again, thus compensating for the trend of the open bite to recur as a result of surgical relapse or undesirable growth rotation. (Houston, 1988; Lake et al., 1981). Sectional flattening is achieved if a step is made preoperatively to the upper wire arch at the occlusal plane or two lateral and one labial sectional arches are inserted. Other orthodontic devices that may be used are upper wire arches with increased curve of Spee, lower wire arches with inversed curve of Spee, inter-arch elastics to extrude posterior teeth, neck-traction headgear on the upper molars, J-pull headgear on the upper incisors or mini screws in order to intrude them (Winchester & Young, 2007).

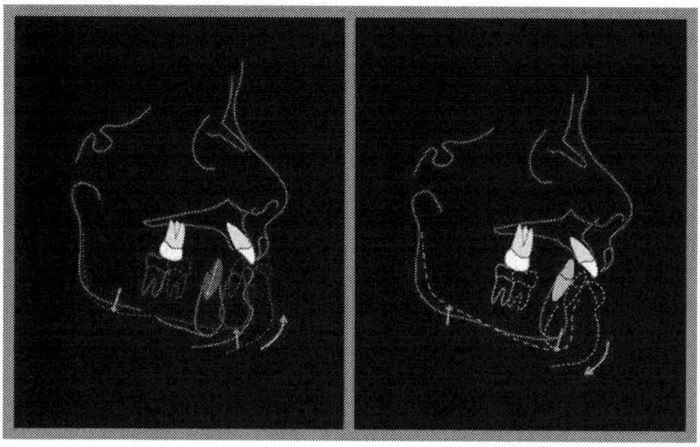

Fig. 12. Schematic representation of a Class II case surgical correction, where there is reduced lower facial height and the curve of Spee is pronounced. The red colour indicates chin and menton movements if the incisors are intruded (A) preoperatively and the green colour indicates what happens if they are not (B).

6.3 Exacerbation

In serious skeletal discrepancies, the teeth try to maintain some contact, under the effect of external and internal forces, so as to compensate for the skeletal problem. Although this compensation improves occlusal relationships and the patient's appearance, it restricts the extent of surgical correction. In skeletal Class III cases, the upper incisors are often labially inclined, while the lower ones are lingually inclined. On the contrary, in cases of skeletal Class II the upper incisors are often upright and the lower labially inclined. A consequence of these compensatory changes is that the overjet is virtual in regard to the actual magnitude of the skeletal discrepancy. Preoperative orthodontics aims at exacerbating dental relationships, by removing the camouflage effect and placing the incisors in normal inclination for the skeletal bases, if this is feasible (Jacobs & Sinclair, 1983). (Fig. 20, 21) Removing compensation exacerbates the malocclusion preoperatively, but reveals the true magnitude of the skeletal problem, thus allowing optimal surgical correction without limitations or occlusal interference. So, if dental compensation from the incisors in Class II, type 1 cases is removed, twice as much forward movement of the mandible is possible, as opposed to what would have achieved if the compensation had not been removed. Similarly, in Class III cases, the mandibular backward movement allowed is five times as much when compensation is removed. (Fig. 13) (Worms et al., 1976). In Class II, type 1 cases, extractions of the first lower premolars may be performed to achieve exacerbation (Fig. 13) and Class III inter-gnathic elastic forces may be used. In Class III cases, there is often a small maxilla with crowding and the upper first premolars might have to be extracted along with the expansion, so as to achieve exacerbation. Furthermore, in Class III cases, when the goal is anteroposterior exacerbation, Class II inter-gnathic elastic forces may be used (Jacobs & Sinclair, 1983). The use of Roth's brackets on incisors with increased crown torque might be an advantage in Class II cases, but undesirable in surgical Class III cases (Winchester & Young, 2007). The exacerbation extent of the incisors is affected by postoperative skeletal stability; this means that full and extensive exacerbation might not always be the goal for a sound surgical outcome. In a Class III case, the exacerbation of the incisors might lead to such great discrepancy, that two-jaw osteotomy might be required for correction and a stable postoperative outcome; on the contrary, limited compensation might only need mandibular surgery. Furthermore, the extent of the exacerbation is restricted in cases of insufficient alveolar bone, when the roots of the incisors are fine or partly resorbed or if there are teeth with poor prognosis. When there is a very narrow attached gum zone or thin periodontium in the lower anterior region, it might be advisable to place a free gum graft before labial dental movement, so as to avoid resorption of the labial alveolar process and denuding of the roots (Boyd, 1978). In the case of maxillary depression at different levels, full exacerbation of the upper incisors is not necessary. The posterior region of the maxilla is depressed more than its anterior part. The consequence of such surgery is that the incisors are palatally inclined. So, when orthodontics is performed in this case, preoperative preparation migth intentionally leave the upper incisors with a slight labial inclination (Hunt N, 2008b).

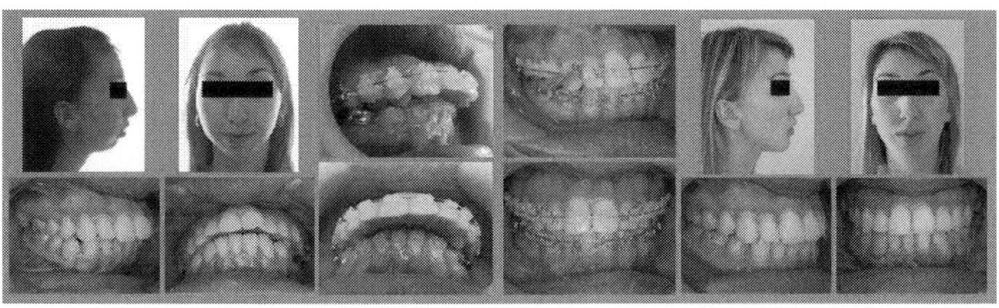

Fig. 13. A Class II case, where the lower anterior teeth, after extractions of the first lower premolars, were moved backwards to achieve exacerbation and allow forward surgical movement of the mandible. During postoperative treatment, Class II elastic forces were used to support sagittal correction.

6.4 Intercuspation of the two arches

One of the goals of preoperative orthodontics is to achieve harmonisation of dental arches at all levels during surgery. Controlling dental arch harmonisation is initially achieved by the use of snap models (mounting the casts manually in occlusion) before surgery. Anteroposterior changes in skeletal relationships sometimes require modification in the transverse width of the arches, and expansion of the upper dental arch, in particular, so as to achieve harmonisation of intermolar and intercanine width. The way to achieve expansion depends on its magnitude and the initial bucco-lingual inclination of upper posterior teeth. Usually, this occurs spontaneously with the use of coordinated upper and lower continuous wire arches and the quad-helix device, which are useful for progressive expansion (Proffit & White, 2003). The quad helix device might result in a deviating movement, but it has the advantage of allowing differential expansion in the right and left buccal sections. Rapid maxillary expansion is not recommended for adults, dut to potential risk for the roots and the periodontium, although surgically assisted rapid maxillary expansion may be performed (Barber & Sims, 1981).

Transverse problems are often overlooked because posterior dental compensation is less apparent than sagittal skeletal discrepancies of the incisors. However, these become apparent during simulated cast surgery. In surgery simulation of a serious skeletal Class II case, by moving the initial casts manually, a bilateral cross-bite occlusion appears, which was not apparent before, because the lower arch has moved to a narrower region of the upper arch. On the contrary, a posterior cross-bite in Class III may not need preoperative management, because it might well be resolved automatically with the posterior surgical mandibular movement, as the lower arch moves to a wider part of the upper arch or as the upper arch moves to a narrower part of the lower arch in cases of surgical maxillary protrusion. Furthermore, in Class III cases with narrow upper arches, the palatal cusps of the molars often interfere with the postoperative position planned, due to insufficient control of the torque. The use of Roth's molar rings with increased torque helps prevent this problem. Thick, rigid, rectangular wire arches are necessary to control torque and maintain the expansion achieved (Winchester & Young, 2007). The transverse problem needs to be diagnosed from the start. It is also essential to note if it is of dental or skeletal aetiology and if correction is to be achieved through orthodontics, sectional surgery or surgically assisted palatal expansion. Orthodontic expansion should not be attempted preoperatively in patients who are going to undergo surgical expansion. Finally, the only way to check if arch compatibility has been achieved in surgical patients is to mount the study casts on the articulator (Sabri, 2006).

Before the end of the preoperative phase, upper and lower rigid rectangular wires need to be passively in position for eight weeks before surgery. Some type of hooks or brackets with thick attachments should be placed on the wires Kobayashi so as to facilitate immobilisation during surgery. Preoperative orthodontics should have been completed in twelve months and the case needs to be planned in such a way for postoperative treatment, that the final correction may be achieved within six months.

7. Postoperative orthodontics

The aim of postoperative orthodontics is to bring the teeth to their final positions and secure balanced occlusion; finally retention planning should be achieved. This phase of the treatment starts two to four weeks later, after a satisfactory range of mandibular movement has been achieved and there is good bone healing. At first the occlusal splint is removed as well as the rigid stabilising wires, which are replaced by continuous working wires. This replacement is quite significant, particularly when there are occlusal surfaces only in two or three teeth after the splint is removed, which means that proprioceptive stimuli make the patient try to find a new position with more contact points. This, however, is not desirable because it might complicate the completion of treatment and the healing of recent osteotomies. This problem is avoided if teeth are allowed to freely come to full contact immediately after splint removal. This is better achieved with light, round wires combined with light, box elastics (Sabri, 2006). Postoperative correction of tripod occlusion with a pronounced curve of Spee and lateral open bite usually includes a combination of elastic wire arches with vertical intergnathic elastics and may last slightly longer than usual. When the upper dental arch is flat, a stable upper rectangular arch is maintained, while an elastic arch, for example a braided steel wire, may be placed on the lower arch. When both arches need extrusion, the rectangular arches may be cut and elastics can be applied between the upper and lower sections (Hunt, 2008b). The elastics are not necessarily vertical, but can have an anterior or posterior contributing force to support sagittal correction. For mandibular protrusion Class II elastics should be used (Fig. 13), whereas mandibular retrusion needs Class III elastics. The orthodontist needs to see the patient every two to three weeks at this stage, to continue the controlled guidance towards final occlusion relationships through the elastics and to avoid displacement or deviations of the mandible. Usually patients wear the elastics continously, even when eating, for the first four weeks, continuously but not at meal times for the next four weeks and only at night for another four weeks (Proffit & Fields, 2007). In cases with a predisposition for open bite, postoperative use of elastics in the buccal sections needs to last the shortest possible time, so as to avoid opening the bite. The use of elastics is terminated after stable occlusion has been achieved. In cases when multiple section osteotomies have been performed and the canine brackets had been preoperatively reversed, it is necessary for them to be reattached, by placing them in the proper position so as to create the right deviation of their longitudinal axes. If palatal expansion was performed intraoperatively, postoperative flexible wires cannot prevent transverse relapse; In order for transverse control to be achieved, a palatal bar can be used (Winchester & Young, 2007).

The postoperative phase of the treatment needs to be completed within 4-5 months (Slavnic & Marcusson, 2010) after the operation, because mobilisation and cooperation on the part of patients dwindle after this period (Kiyak et al., 1984).

8. Retention

Retention is not different from that of usual orthodontic treatment for adult patients. So, dental movements achieved through preoperative and postoperative orthodontics, need a retention period that follows the removal of fixed appliances. This allows the alveolar bone and periodontal tissues to be reinforced. Where incisors' rotation has been corrected or large spaces closed, a fixed, stable, attached lingual or buccal retention mechanism is used. In other cases, a movable retention appliance may be used (Hunt, 2008b). When surgical or orthodontic expansion has been achieved, it should be maintained with retention for at least 1 year, because it is usually unstable (Phillips et al., 1992).

9. References

Arnett GW, Bergman RT. (1993a). Facial keys to orthodontic diagnosis and treatment planning. Part I. *American journal of orthodontics and dentofacial orthopedics*, Vol. 103, No. 4, pp. 299-312, ISSN 0889-5406.

Arnett GW, Bergman RT. (1993b). Facial keys to orthodontic diagnosis and treatment planning. Part II. *American journal of orthodontics and dentofacial orthopedics*, Vol. 103, No. 5, pp. 395-4ll, ISSN 0889-5406.

Athanasiou AE, Kragskov J. (1995). Computerized Cephalometric Systems. In: *Orthodontic Cephalometry*, Athanasiou AE, pp. 231-239, Mosby-Wolfe, ISBN 0 7234 2045 9, London.

Barber AF, Sims MR. (1981). Rapid maxillary expansion and external root resorption in man: a scanning electron microscope study. *American Journal of Orthodontics*. Vol. 79, No. 6, pp. 630-652, ISSN 0002-9416.

Bass NM. (1991). The aesthetic analysis of the face. *European Journal of Orthodontics*, Vol. 13, No. 5, pp. 343-50, ISSN 0141-5387.

Baumrind S, Frantz RC. (1971). The reliability of head film measurements. 1. Landmark identification. *American journal of orthodontics*, Vol. 60, No. 2, pp. 111-127, ISSN 0002-9416.

Boyd RL. (1978). Mucogingival considerations and their relationship to orthodontics. *Journaj of Periodontology*, Vol. 49, No 2, pp. 67-76, ISSN 0022-3492.

Burstone CJ. (1967). Lip posture and its significance in treatment planning. *American journal of orthodontics*, Vol. 53, No. 4, pp. 262-284, ISSN 0002-9416.

Chaconas SJ, Fragiskos FD. (1991). Orthognathic diagnosis and treatment planning: a cephalometric approach. *Journal of oral rehabilitation*, Vol. 18, No. 6, pp. 531-545, ISSN 0305-182X.

Chaconas SJ, Gonidis D (1986). A cephalometric technique for prosthodontic diagnosis and treatment planning. *The* Journal of Prosthetic Dentistry, Vol. 56, No. 5, pp. 567-74, ISSN 0022-3913.

Diaz PM, Garcia RG, Gias LN, Aguirre-Jaime A, Pérez JS, de la Plata MM, Navarro EV, Gonzalez FJ.(2010). Journal of Oral and Maxillofacial Surgery. Vol. 68, No. 1, pp. 88-92, ISSN 0278-2391.

Eales EA, Newton C, Jones ML, Sugar A. (1994). The accuracy of computerized prediction of the soft tissue profile: a study of 25 patients treated by means of the Le Fort I osteotomy. The *International Journal of Adult Orthodontics and Orthognathic Surgery*, Vol. 9, No. 2, 141-152, ISSN 0742-1931.

Fish LC, Epker BN. (1980). Surgical-orthodontic cephalometric prediction tracing. *Journal of clinical orthodontics*, Vol. 14, No. 1, pp. 36-52, ISSN 1079-5154.

Guariglia A, Ronchi P. (2005). Cephalometry in Dentofacial Anomalies, In: *Orthodontic-Surgical Treatment of Dentofacial Anomalies*, Ronchi P, pp. 35-45, Quintessenza, ISBN 88-7492-101-2, Milan Italy.

Harris M, Hunt N. (2008). General Assessment, In: *Fundamentals of Orthognathic Surgery*, Harris M, Hunt N, pp. 1-22, Imperial College Press, ISBN-13 978-1-86094-993-7, London UK.

Houston WJB. (1988). Mandibular growth rotations - their mechanisms and importance. European Journal of Orthodontics, Vol. 10, No. 4, pp. 369–373, ISSN 0141-5387.

Hunt N. (2008a). Radiographic Analysis and Imaging, In: *Fundamentals of Orthognathic Surgery*, Harris M, Hunt N, pp. 23-39, Imperial College Press, ISBN-13 978-1-86094-993-7, London UK.

Hunt N. (2008b). Orthodontic Preparation, In: *Fundamentals of Orthognathic Surgery*, Harris M, Hunt N, pp. 51-70, Imperial College Press, ISBN-13 978-1-86094-993-7, London UK.

Jacobs JD, Sinclair PM. (1983). Principles of orthodontic mechanics in orthognathic surgery cases. American journal of orthodontics. Vol. 84, No 5, pp. 399-407, ISSN 0002-9416.

Jensen AC, Sinclair PM, Wolford LM. (1992). Soft tissue changes associated with double jaw surgery. *American Journal of Orthodontist and Dentofacial Orthopedics*, Vol. 101, No. 3, pp. 266-275. ISSN 0889-5406.

Kaipatur NR, Flores-Mir C. (2009). Accuracy of computer programs in predicting orthognathic surgery soft tissue response. *Journal of Oral and Maxillofacial Surgery*. Vol. 67, No. 4, pp. 751-759. ISSN 0278-2391.

Kapila S, Conley RS, Harrell WE Jr. (2011). The current status of cone beam computed tomography imaging in orthodontics. *Dentomaxillofac Radiology*, Vol. 40, No. 1, pp. 24-34, . ISSN 0250-832X.

Kiyak HA, Hohl T, West RA, McNeil RW. (1984). Psychologic changes in orthognathic surgery patients: a 24 - month follow up. *Journal of Oral and Maxillofacial Surgery*, Vol. 42, No. 8, pp. 506-512, ISSN 0278-2391.

Kolokitha OE, Athanasiou AE, Tuncay O. (1996). Validity of computerized predictions of dentoskeletal and soft tissue profile changes after mandibular setback and maxillary impaction osteotomies. The *International Journal of Adult Orthodontics and Orthognathic Surgery*, Vol. 11, No. 2, pp. 137-154, ISSN 0742-1931.

Kolokitha OE. (2007). Validity of a manual soft tissue profile prediction method following mandibular setback osteotomy. *European Journal of Dental*, Vol. 1, No. 4, pp. 202-211. ISSN 0141-5387.

Lake SM, McNeill RW, Little RM, West RA. (1981). Surgical mandibular advancement: A cephalometric analysis of treatment response. *American journal of orthodontics*, Vol. 80, No. 4, pp. 376-394, ISSN 0002-9416.

Langlade M. (1981). *Diagnostic orthodontique*. Maloine S.A., ISBN 2-224-00738-8, Paris.

Langlade M. (1986). *Therapeutique orthodontique*. Maloine S.A., ISBN 2-224-00465-6, Paris.

Lee RT. (1994). The benefits of post-surgical orthodontic treatment. *British journal of orthodontics*. Vol. 21, No 3, pp. 265-74, ISSN:0301-228X.

Levander E, Malmgren O. (1988). Evaluation of the risk of root resorption during orthodontic treatment: a study of upper incisors. *European Journal of Orthodontics*, Vol. 10, No. 1, pp. 30-38, ISSN 0141-5387.

Lines PA, Lines RR, Lines C. (1978). Profilemetrics and facial esthetics. *American journal of orthodontics*, Vol. 73, No. 6, pp. 648-657, ISSN 0002-9416.

Liou EJ, Chen PH, Wang YC, Yu CC, Huang CS, Chen YR. (2011). Surgery-first accelerated orthognathic surgery: postoperative rapid orthodontic tooth movement. Journal of Oral and Maxillofacial Surgery. Vol.69, No.3, pp. 781-785, ISSN 0278-2391.

Luther F, Morris DO, Karnezi K. (2007). Orthodontic treatment following orthognathic surgery: how long does it take and why? A retrospective study. *Journal of Oral and Maxillofacial Surgery*. Vol.65, No.10, pp.1969-1976, ISSN 0278-2391.

McNamara JA. (1984). A method of cephalometric evaluation. *American journal of orthodontics,* Vol. 86, No. 6, pp. 449-469, ISSN 0002-9416.

McNamara JA, Brudon WL. (1993). Orthodontic and Orthopedic Treatment in the Mixed Dentition, pp. 13-54, Needham Press, ISBN 0-9635022-1-2, Ann Arbor USA.

McNamara JA, Ellis E. (1988). Cephalometric analysis of untreated adults with ideal facial and occlusal relationships. *The International journal of adult orthodontics and orthognathic surgery,* Vol. 3, No. 4, pp. 221-231, ISSN 0742-1931.

McNeill RW, Proffit WR, White RP. (1972). Cephalometric prediction for orthodontic surgery. The Angle orthodontist, Vol. 42, No. 2, pp. 154-164, ISSN 0003-3219.

Miethke R. (1995). Possibilities and Limitations of Various Cephalometric Variables and Analyses. In: *Orthodontic Cephalometry,* Athanasiou AE, pp. 63-103, Mosby-Wolfe, ISBN 0 7234 2045 9, London.

Muller L. (1962). *Cephalometrie et orthodontie,* SNPMD, ISBN 2-903482-06-3, Paris.

Onizawa K, Schmelzeisen R, Vogt S. (1995). Alteration of tem¬poromandibular joint symptoms after orthognathic sur¬gery: a comparison with healthy volunteers. Journal of oral and maxillofacial surgery, Vol. 53, No. 2, pp. 117-121, ISSN 0278-2391.

Phillips C, Medland WH, Fields HW, Profitt WR, White RP Jr. (1992). Stability of surgical maxillary expansion. The *International Journal of Adult Orthodontics and Orthognathic Surgery,* Vol. 7, No. 3, pp. 139-146, ISSN 0742-1931.

Proffit WR. (1991). Treatment planning: The search for wisdom. In: *Surgical Orthodontic Treatment.* Proffit WR, White RP Jr, pp. 142-191. Mosby, ISBN 0-8016-5291-X, St Louis USA.

Proffit WR, White RP Jr. (1991). Combined Surgical – Orthodontic Treatment: Who Does What, When?. In: *Surgical Orthodontic Treatment,* Proffit WR, White RP,Jr, pp. 192-224, Mosby, ISBN 0-8016-5291-X, St Louis USA.

Proffit WR, Fields HW. (1993). *Contemporary Orthodontics Second edition.* pp. 607-645, Mosby-Year Book, ISBN 0-8016-6393-8, St.Louis USA.

Proffit WR, Sarver DM. (2003). Treatment planning: Optimizing benefit to the patient. In: *Contemporary Treatment of Dentofacial Deformity.* Proffit WR, White RP,Jr, Sarver DM, pp. 172-244, Mosby, ISBN 0-323-01697-9, St.Louis USA.

Proffit WR, White RP, Jr. (2003). Combining Surgery and Orthodontics: Who Does What, When?. In: Contemporary Treatment of Dentofacial Deformity. Proffit WR, White RP,Jr, Sarver DM, pp. 245-267, Mosby, ISBN 0-323-01697-9, St.Louis USA.

Proffit WR, Fields HW. (2007). *Contemporary Orthodontics Fourth edition.* pp. 686-718, Mosby, ISBN 13: 978-0-323-04046-4, St.Louis USA.

Reyneke JP. (2003). *Essentials of Orthognathic Surgery,* Quintessence Publishing Co, ISBN 0-86715-410-1, China.

Ricketts RM, Roth RH, Chaconas SJ, Schulhof RJ, Engel GA. (1982). *Orthodontic diagnosis and planning Vol 1,* pp. 127-147, Rocky Mountain /Orthodontics, LCCN 82-62145, Denver, Colo. U.S.A.

Ricketts RM. (1975). A four-step method to distinguish orthodontic changes from natural growth. Journal of clinical orthodontics, Vol. 9, No. 4, pp. 208-28, ISSN 1079-5154.

Ricketts RM (1981). Perspectives in the clinical application of cephalometrics. The first fifty years. The Angle orthodontist, Vol. 51, No. 2, pp. 115-50, ISSN 0003-3219.

Sabri R. (2006). Orthodontic Objectives in Orthognathic surgery: state of the art today. *World Journal of Orthodontics,* Vol. 7, No. 2, pp. 177-191, ISSN 1530-5678.

Sassouni V (1958). Diagnosis and treatment planning via roentgenographic cephalometry. *American Journal of Orthodontist,* Vol. 44, No. 6, pp. 433-463, ISSN 0002-9416.

Sassouni V. (1971). *Orthodontics in dental practise,* Mosby, ISBN 8016-4300-7, St Louis USA.

Sinclair PM, Proffit WR. (1991). Class III Problems: Mandibular Excess - Maxillary Deficiency. In: *Surgical Orthodontic Treatment,* Proffit WR, White RP, pp. 428-482. Mosby, ISBN 0-8016-5291-X, St Louis USA.

Slavnic S, Marcusson A. (2010). Duration of orthodontic treatment in conjunction with orthognathic surgery. *Swedish Dental Journal,* Vol. 34, No. 3, pp. 159-166, ISSN 0347-9994.

Stroud LP. (1997). Mounted Study Casts and Cephalometric Analysis. In: *Science and Practice of Occlusion,* McNeill C, pp. 331-348, Quintessence Publishing Co, ISBN 9780867153040. Chicago USA.

Tompach PC, Wheeler JJ, Fridrich KL. (1995).Orthodontic considerations in orthognathic surgery. The *International Journal of Adult Orthodontics and Orthognathic Surgery.*Vol.10, No2, pp.97-107, ISSN 0742-1931.

Vion P. (1976). Anatomie teleradiographique en norma lateralis. *Revue d'Orthopédie Dento-Faciale,* Vol. 10, No. 4, pp. 449-537, ISSN 0337-9736.

Winchester LJ, Young DR. (2007). Orthodontic Role in Planning: Clinical Aspects, In: *Maxillofacial Surgery,* Booth PW, Schendel SA, Hausamen J-E, pp. 1211-1223, Churchill Livingstone Elsevier, ISBN-13 978-0-443-10053-6, St. Louis USA.

Wolford LM, Hilliard FW, Dugan DJ. (1985). *Surgical Treatment Objective. A Systematic Approach to the Prediction Tracing,* Mosby Year Book, ISBN 9780801656095, St Louis USA.

Wolford LM, Stevao ELL, Alexander CM, Goncalves JR. (2004). Orthodontics for Orthognathic Surgery, In: Peterson's Principals of Oral and Maxillofacial Surgery, Miloro M, Ghali GE, Larsen PE, Waite P, pp. 1111-1134, BC Decker Inc, ISBN 1-55009-234-0, Canada.

Wolford LM. (2007). Surgical Planning in Orthognathic Surgery, In: *Maxillofacial Surgery,* Booth PW, Schendel SA, Hausamen J-E, pp. 1155-1210, Churchill Livingstone Elsevier, ISBN-13 978-0-443-10053-6, St. Louis USA.

Worms FW, Isaacson RJ, Speidel TM. (1976). Surgical orthodontic treatment planning: prolile analysis and mandibular surgery. *The Angle orthodontist*, Vol. 46, No. 1, pp. 1-25, ISSN 0003-3219.

17

Long-Term Outcome of Orthognathic Surgery

Lisen Espeland and Arild Stenvik
University of Oslo
Norway

1. Introduction

Orthognathic surgery is treatment which often leads to great improvement in function and appearance, but is demanding to the patient, considerable resources are being spent, and risks for unwanted side effects are involved. Because of the elective nature of the treatment it is particularly important that the patient is well informed about all aspects of the provision and outcome of treatment before the decision to initiate treatment is reached. This information should be evidence-based. In this area it is, however, difficult to establish research materials that are both homogenous and of adequate size. The present chapter represents an attempt to summarize research findings from long-term follow-up of more than 1000 patients treated according to an established protocol over a period of 15 years.

2. Background

Since 1970 an orthognathic team of orthodontists and maxillofacial surgeons at the University of Oslo has monitored patients referred for advice and treatment planning, surgery, and a 3-year follow-up at regular intervals after the operation. The patient files comprise clinical recordings, photos, radiographs, and patient questionnaires. Cephalograms have been obtained 1 week before and 1 week, 2 and 6 months, and 1 and 3 years after surgery. The results presented here are based on observations from patients in whom the bony segments have been stabilized with rigid fixation only.

About 150 patients have been referred each year of whom 50 to 60% have undergone surgery. Pre-surgical orthodontic treatment lasts on average 18 months and post-surgical orthodontics 6 months (Dowling et al., 1999). The osteotomies that will be discussed in this chapter comprise one-piece LeFort I, bilateral sagittal split (BSSO) and extraoral vertical ramus osteotomies (EVRO), and genioplasty. Standardized protocols which have been followed over time have made it possible to establish homogenous subsamples of sufficient size for analyses of various aspects of treatment such as skeletal stability, sensory function, effect on airways and soft tissue profile, and patient satisfaction.

3. Stability

Skeletal relapse after orthognathic surgery may be due to biological factors like lack of neuromuscular adaptation and condylar resorption, as well as factors related to the surgical procedures. The extent of the relapse may be associated with the magnitude and direction of skeletal movements, the method of fixation, and the use of bone grafts. A hierarchy of stability based on initial anatomy and various surgical procedures has been proposed (Proffit et al., 1996). Relapse may be presented as the mean post-surgical change, or as the rate of subjects with a clinically significant relapse, usually defined as change of 2 mm or more. Another issue of importance is when the relapse occurs, and hence short- and long-term stability should be examined. Skeletal relapse may also to a varying extent impact on occlusal stability.

3.1 Skeletal stability

The results presented below is a compilation of findings from studies performed at the University of Oslo. The cephalometric variables have been recorded as x- and y-coordinates (Fig. 1). The x-axis was constructed 7° to the nasion-sella line. The most common osteotomies for management of Class II and III skeletal malocclusions will be addressed.

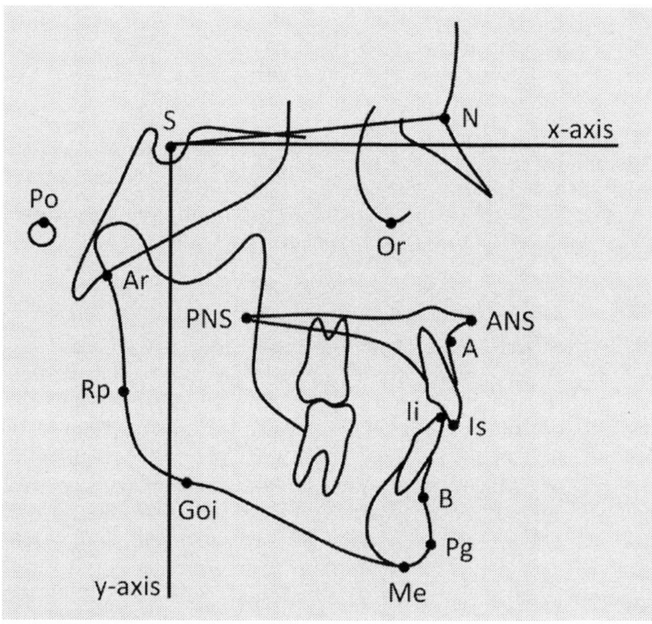

Fig. 1. Cephalometric landmarks used in analyses of stability

3.1.1 Class III: mandibular setback

The bilateral sagittal split osteotomy (BSSO) is a versatile and widely used approach for correction of mandibular prognathism. In a study of 80 (46 males, 34 females) consecutively operated patients (Mobarak et al., 2000a) this procedure appeared to be fairly stable. Three years post-surgery the mean relapse was 1.6 mm and represented 26% of the surgical setback at Pogonion (Pg) (6.3 mm). In 36% of the patients relapse was clinically significant (≥ 2 mm). Most of the relapse took place during the first 6 months after surgery (72%) (Fig. 2). The magnitude of the setback was to some extent associated with the amount of horizontal relapse ($r = 0.39$, $P < 0.01$). Gender differences in relapse were small.

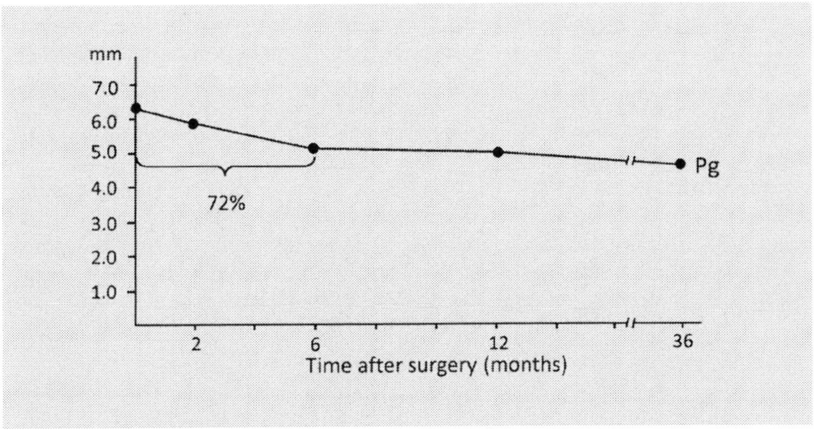

Fig. 2. Mean postsurgical horizontal change at Pg as a function of time in 80 mandibular setback (BSSO) patients.

An alternative approach to BSSO is the vertical ramus osteotomy (VRO). Traditionally the VRO has required intermaxillary fixation for 6-8 weeks. Since 1995, stable plate fixation has routinely been used with an extraoral incision by our team (Hoegevold et al., 2001) (Fig. 3). The main morphologic indication for applying the extraoral VRO (EVRO) has been a moderate setback without rotation. Another indication is related to reduced risk for sensory disturbances. In a 1-year follow-up study post-operative changes were mainly in the form of a small anterior relapse tendency of about 10% of the surgical setback. Mean relapse was 0.6 mm (SD 1.2 mm). A relapse ≥ 2 mm was observed in 14% of the subjects (Mobarak et al., 2000b).

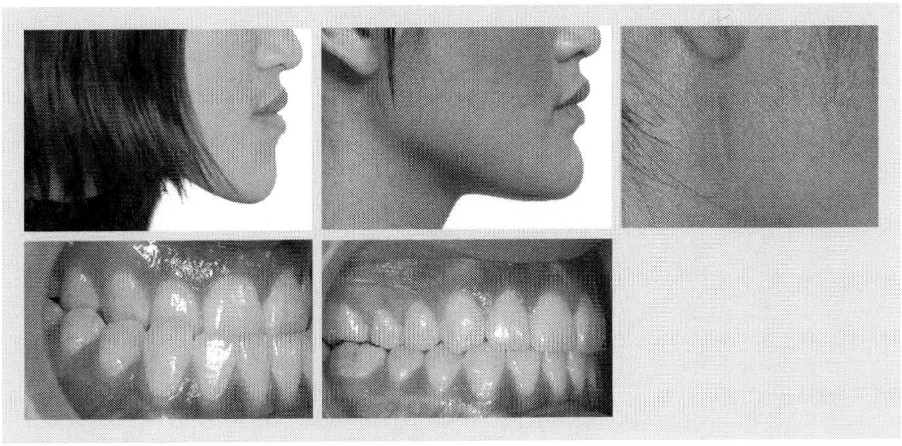

Fig. 3. Patient with mandibular prognathism before treatment and 3 years after EVRO. Facial scar after extraoral incision to the right.

3.1.2 Class III: maxillary advancement

After the LeFort I osteotomy became common in the 1970-ies, this is an increasingly used alternative to correct Class III malocclusion. This approach allows treatment based on the diagnosis in cases where the discrepancy is caused by a retrognathic maxilla (Fig. 4). In addition to be associated with few unwanted side-effects like nerve injuries, a negative impact on the airways which may occur after mandibular setback, is avoided.

In a sample of 43 individuals having had maxillary advancement of ≥ 2 mm (mean advancement 5 mm), the mean relapse was 0.9 mm (18%), and the relapse was clinically significant in 14% of the patients (Dowling et al., 2005). Almost all (89%) of the relapse took place during the first 6 months. Regression analysis identified large advancements and downward movement of the anterior maxilla as risk factors for horizontal relapse.

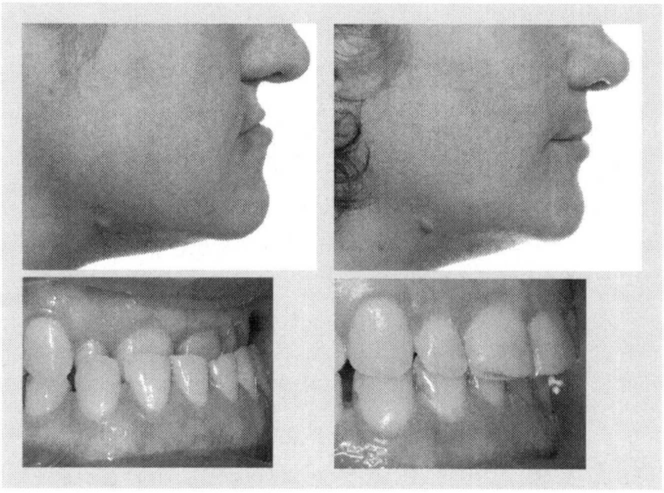

Fig. 4. Patient with retrognathic maxilla before and after maxillary advancement (one-piece LeFort I).

3.1.3 Class III: bimaxillary surgery

In patients with severe skeletal discrepancies single jaw surgery may not be possible or may have an unwanted effect on the patient's facial appearance. In later years, there has been a trend for increased use of a combination of mandibular setback and maxillary advancement. Severe skeletal Class III malocclusions are frequently associated with anterior open bite, which is more readily corrected with bimaxillary surgery and may also ensure optimal facial harmony (Fig. 5).

A study of stability comprised 81 patients (Jakobsone et al., 2011a) who pre-surgery had a mean negative overjet of -7 mm (range -18.9 to 3.2 mm) and a negative overbite of -1.8 (range -9.7 to 6.4 mm). Skeletal stability assessed 3 years after surgery varied depending on the direction and amount of the surgical repositioning. Maxillary advancement was stable, whereas a significant mean relapse was observed after mandibular setback (Fig. 6). About half of the 62 subjects with a setback of 2 mm or more, had a clinically significant relapse. Most of the skeletal relapse occurred during the first 6 months after surgery. Regression analysis showed that stability was increased when the setback was small and the posterior maxilla was impacted.

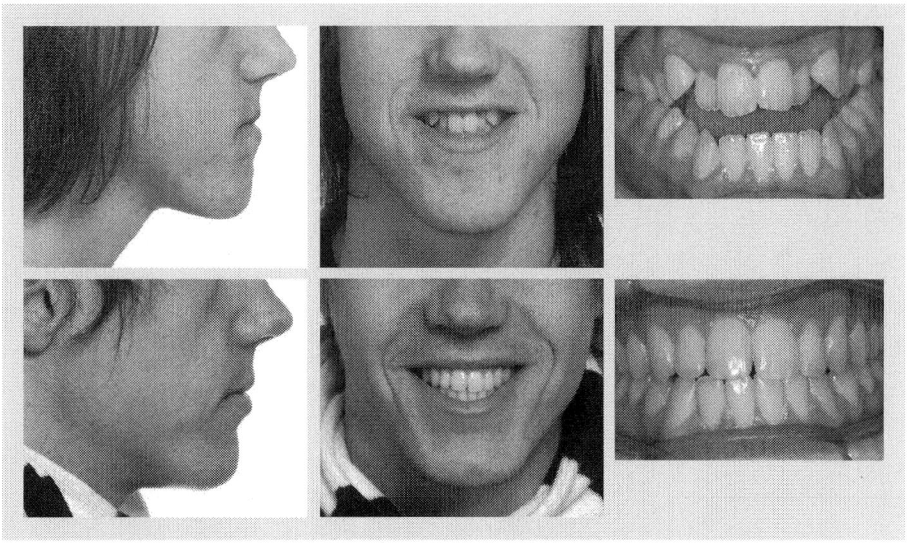

Fig. 5. Patient with severe Class III malocclusion and open bite corrected with one-piece LeFort I and BSSO (before treatment and 3 years after surgery).

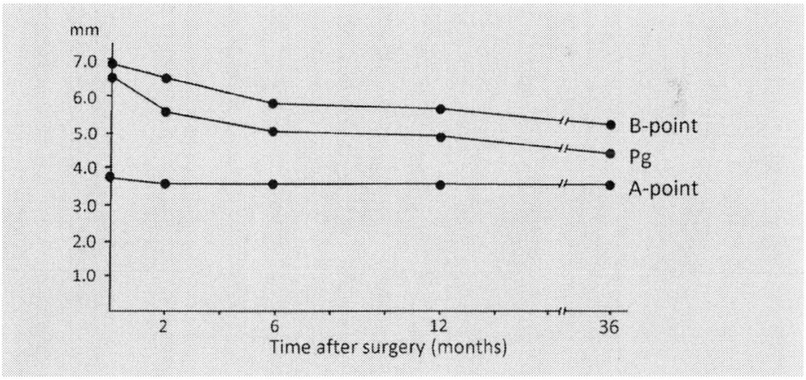

Fig. 6. Mean horizontal changes at various cephalometric landmarks as a function of time in 81 Class III patients having bimaxillary surgery (BSSO and one-piece LeFort I).

3.1.4 Class II: mandibular advancement

The BSSO is the most frequently used osteotomy for management of mandibular retrognatism. High-angle and low-angle Class II cases represent two distinct entities, with different facial patterns, treatment goals, and clinical challenges.

A study of stability analysed these two categories separately in 61 consecutive cases (Mobarak et al., 2001a). High- (n = 20) and low-angle (n = 20) patients had different patterns of surgical and post-operative skeletal changes. High-angle cases were associated with greater horizontal relapse. Relapse in the low-angle cases occurred early in the post-operative period, whereas in the high-angle cases, relapse was a more continuous process with a significant proportion occurring later in the follow-up period (Fig. 7). Increasing the anterior facial height (low-angle) was a relatively stable procedure, with on average 70% of the improvement remaining after 3 years.

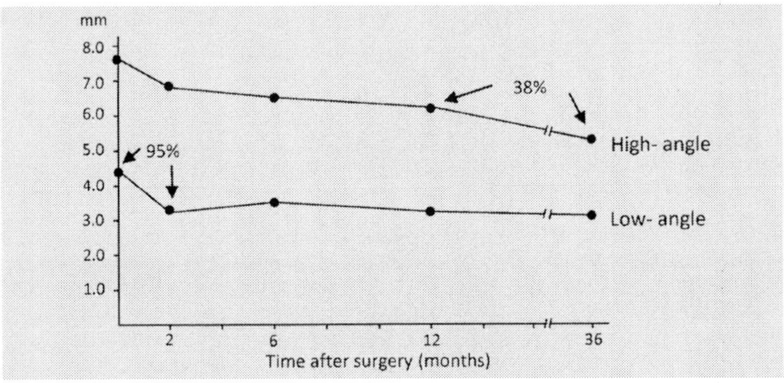

Fig. 7. Mean horizontal changes at Pg in low- and high-angle cases as a function of time. Mean surgical advancement appears from the vertical axis.

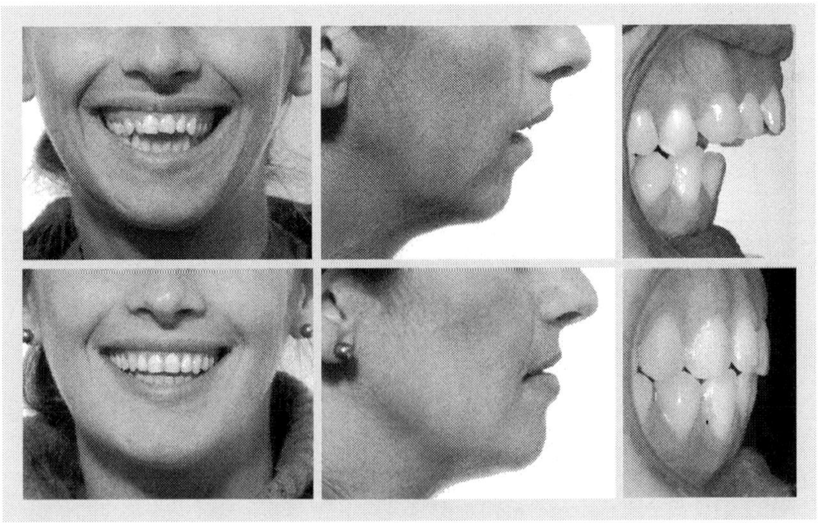

Fig. 8. Patient with severe Class II with open bite and high-angle facial pattern before treatment and 3 years after surgery with BSSO and one-piece LeFort I.

3.1.5 Class II: bimaxillary surgery

Our studies of stability after bimaxillary surgery to correct skeletal Class II malocclusion have focused on subjects with a high-angle facial pattern as this group represents the greatest challenge. In a study of 31 patients (ML/NSL > 38°) the stability of maxillary impaction and mandibular advancement varied considerably (Winter et al., 2010). Stable results (relapse < 2 mm) after maxillary impaction were observed in 77% of the subjects, whereas mandibular advancements were stable in only 42%. Despite the risk for relapse, some patients showed excellent results after 3 years (Fig. 8).

3.1.6 Class II: advancement genioplasty

Genioplasty allows 3-dimensional control of chin position, resulting in significant improvement of facial aesthetics whether performed separately or combined with other osteotomies. Of the actual corrections of the chin, advancement genioplasty to improve a receding chin is probably the most common.

Our study of stability after advancement genioplasty included 21 subjects who had no additional osteotomies (Shaughnessy et al., 2006) (Fig. 9). Mean advancement was 8.4 mm. The results 3 years after surgery showed that this was a stable procedure with a mean relapse of only 8% of the advancement. Some of the post-surgical change could be ascribed to remodelling in the area rather than instability of the segment.

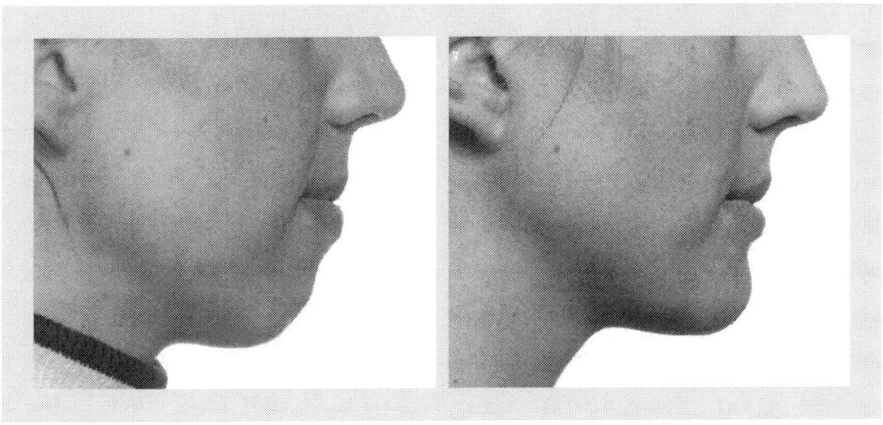

Fig. 9. Advancement genioplasty patient pre-treatment (left) and 3 years after surgery (right).

3.1.7 Open bite correction by isolated maxillary surgery

Open bite occurs both in Class I, II, and III malocclusions. When the sagittal discrepancy is moderate, the occlusion can usually be corrected by LeFort I impaction as the only procedure (Fig. 10). In a study of 40 consecutively operated patients (Espeland et al., 2008a) it was observed that impaction of posterior maxilla (≥ 2 mm) relapsed by one third. Inferior movement of the anterior maxilla relapsed about two thirds. Most of the relapse occurred during the first 6 months after surgery.

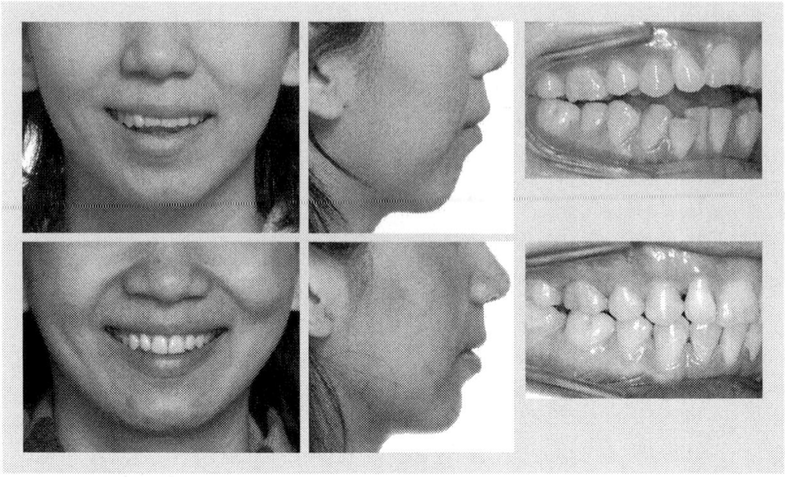

Fig. 10. Patient with open bite before treatment and after one-piece LeFort I with impaction of posterior maxilla.

3.1.8 Summary – skeletal stability

Fig. 11 summarizes frequencies of stable results (relapse < 2 mm) after various one-jaw osteotomies. The most stable results were observed after advancement of the maxilla, setback of the mandible (EVRO), and advancement of the chin. The least stable procedures were advancement of the mandible in patients with high-angle facial pattern and downward movement of the maxilla. In the literature a number of factors have been proposed which may explain skeletal relapse. For Class III anomalies early relapse has been associated with clockwise rotation of the proximal segment during BSSO-surgery (Proffit et al., 1996). In our study (Mobarak et al., 2000a), however, this did not seem to be responsible for marked relapse. Late relapse has often been ascribed to late mandibular growth which our findings also indicated. For Class II corrections by BSSO advancement, early relapse has been suggested to be due to suboptimal positioning of the condyle, whereas condylar resorption might be responsible for relapse occurring later. Risk factors for condylar resorption have been addressed in the literature, for example condylar morphology and bone quality (Hoppenreijs et al., 1999).

3.2 Occlusal stability

Despite some skeletal relapse after most surgical corrections, the anterior occlusion is generally stable. In the studies addressing stability referred to above, the incisor relationship was also examined. Below is a short summary of the main findings.

After Class III correction by one-jaw surgery, both with setback of the mandible (Mobarak et al., 2000a) and advancement of the maxilla (Dowling et al., 2005), all patients examined had a positive overjet 3 years after the operation. Bimaxillary surgery resulted in positive overjet in 79 of 81 patients (Jakobsone et al., 2011a). Relapse of open bite was observed in 8 subjects, and in 5 of these, the negative overbite was less than 1 mm.

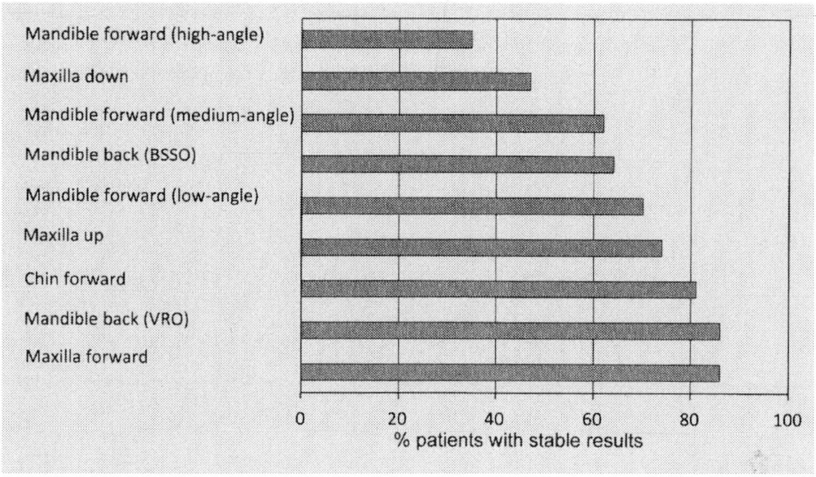

Fig. 11. Diagrammatic representation of stability after various one-jaw surgical procedures. Bars represent frequency of patients with relapse less than 2 mm 3 years after surgery.

After Class II correction with mandibular advancement, the difference in skeletal stability between patients with low- and high-angle facial pattern was reflected in the stability of the occlusion. After 3 years 85% of the low-angle patients had overjet less than 4 mm, whereas the corresponding figure for the high-angle subjects was 60%. In the group of 41 high-angle patients treated with bimaxillary surgery, one third of those having overjet > 6 mm before surgery, still had an overjet > 6 mm after 3 years.

Of 40 open-bite patients treated by isolated LeFort I impaction, 88% had positive overbite 3 years post-surgery (Espeland et al., 2008a). In all the remaining patients, the negative overbite was less than 1 mm. The skeletal relapse was counteracted by dentoalveolar compensation, which contributed to approximately 50% of the correction of the overbite.

For all categories of malocclusion, the skeletal relapse generally took place during the first 6 months. A negative effect on the occlusion was avoided for most patients by dentoalveolar compensation, which underlines the importance of post-surgical monitoring and orthodontic management if signs of relapse become apparent.

4. Soft tissue response

Software for prediction of the soft tissue response has become an integral part of treatment planning aiming to provide a realistic estimate of the outcome of surgery. Ratios (or percentages) for soft to hard tissue changes have focused in particular on nose, lips, mentolabial fold, and chin. It is important that the data which serve to generate software prediction programs are valid. Changes in sagittal and vertical dimensions as well as lip thickness have been addressed in studies at our department.

4.1 Class III: mandibular setback

The soft tissue response for the lower lip, mentolabial fold and soft tissue chin to the underlying hard tissues was about 1:1. Some effect was also seen for the upper lip (Fig. 12).

The main effect of mandibular setback on the soft tissue profile included an increase in facial convexity, straightening and lengthening of the upper lip with a concomitant increase in nasolabial angle, and deepening of the mentolabial fold (Mobarak et al., 2001b).

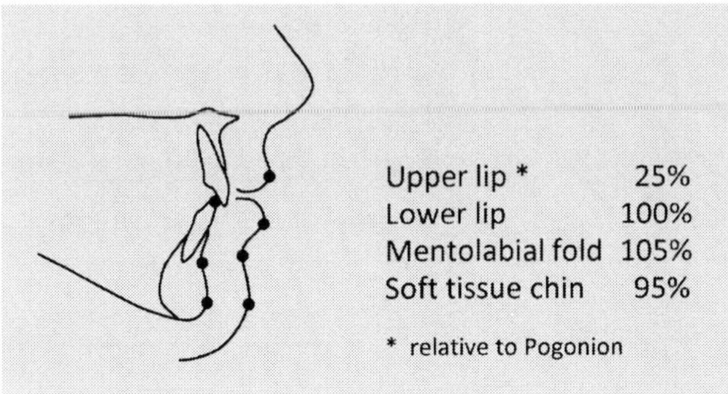

Fig. 12. Relationship between soft and hard tissue horizontal changes after mandibular setback in 80 patients (BSSO).

4.2 Class III: bimaxillar surgery

To quantify the relative soft tissue response to the skeletal changes, a sample of 80 patients were divided in 3 subgroups according to pre-operative characteristics: 1) open bite, 2) positive overbite and the upper lip resting on upper incisors, and 3) positive overbite and the upper lip resting on lower incisors (lip block) (Jakobsone et al., 2011b).

In the first two groups, there were strong correlations between the horizontal movement of upper incisors and upper lip (r = 0.77 and 0.85, respectively). The upper lip followed the maxilla with a ratio of 0.5:1. When the upper lip rested on lower incisors before surgery, the association between maxillary repositioning and upper lip changes were weak. In all groups a strong association between horizontal soft and hard tissue changes of lower lip and chin was observed. The vertical position of the tip of the nose was affected by both the vertical and horizontal repositioning of the maxilla. Several factors influencing the soft tissue response were identified. Software prediction programs should preferably take into account different pre-surgical characteristics.

4.3 Class II: mandibular advancement

The ratio for the soft to hard tissue response after mandibular advancement was about 1:1 for the chin and 0.6:1 for the lower lip. For the mentolabial fold, the ratio was on average 0.9:1, but varied somewhat according to vertical facial pattern (Mobarak et al., 2001c). Following mandibular advancement the facial profile became straighter. The mentolabial fold became more shallow, especially in low-angle subjects who also had an increase in anterior facial height.

4.4 Class II: advancement genioplasty

In our study of soft tissue response to advancement of the chin as the only surgical procedure, the results showed that the ratio for soft to hard tissue movement was 0.9:1 (Shaughnessy et al., 2006). The mentolabial depth increased as a result of treatment (Fig. 9).

5. Effect on upper airways

In addition to the changes in masticatory function and facial harmony, repositioning of the jaws may also impact on airway morphology. Mandibular advancement and setback osteotomies have been reported to influence the position of the hyoid bone, and consequently tongue position, pharyngeal airway morphology, and head flexion (Achilleos et al., 2000a,b). Studies have also shown that in adults, there is on average a reduction in the sagittal dimension of the minimal pharyngeal airway space with increasing age (Kollias & Krogstad, 1999). Over the last two decades the capacity of maxillo-mandibular osteotomies to induce or resolve obstructive sleep apnoea (OSA) has received increased attention. A challenge in the planning of orthognathic surgery is to balance concerns related to facial aesthetics and airway changes.

A recent study of bimaxillary correction of Class III malocclusion examined whether maxillary advancement and/or impaction had the potential to compensate for the negative effect of mandibular setback on airways (Jakobsone et al., 2011c).

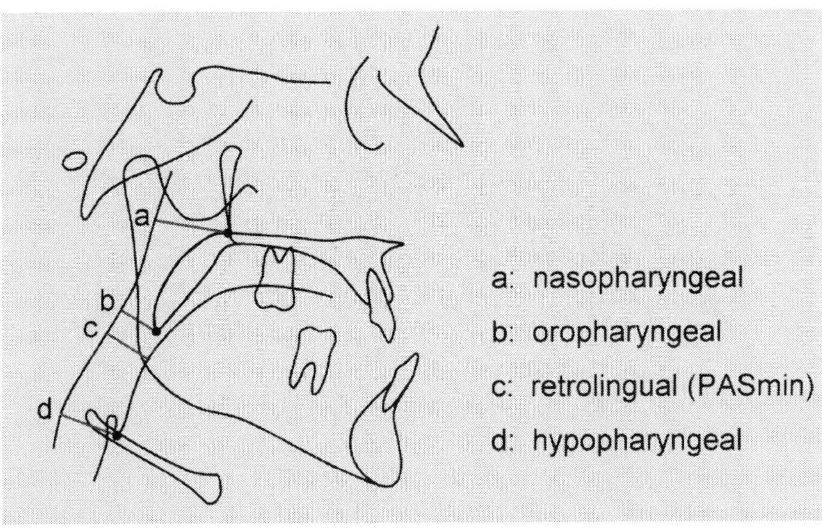

Fig. 13. The 4 levels in the upper airways which were cephalometrically examined.

Sagittal dimensions of the pharynx were measured on 4 different levels (Fig. 13) in 4 subgroups. The long-term change (3 years) at the various levels related to whether the maxilla was advanced and/or impacted or not, appears from Fig. 14. Advancement of the maxilla resulted in an increase of 15-20% at the nasopharyngeal level. At the hypopharyngeal level, advancement of the maxilla did to some extent compensate for the negative effect of mandibular setback. A decrease of 5-10% was observed at the oropharyngeal and retrolingual (PASmin) levels.

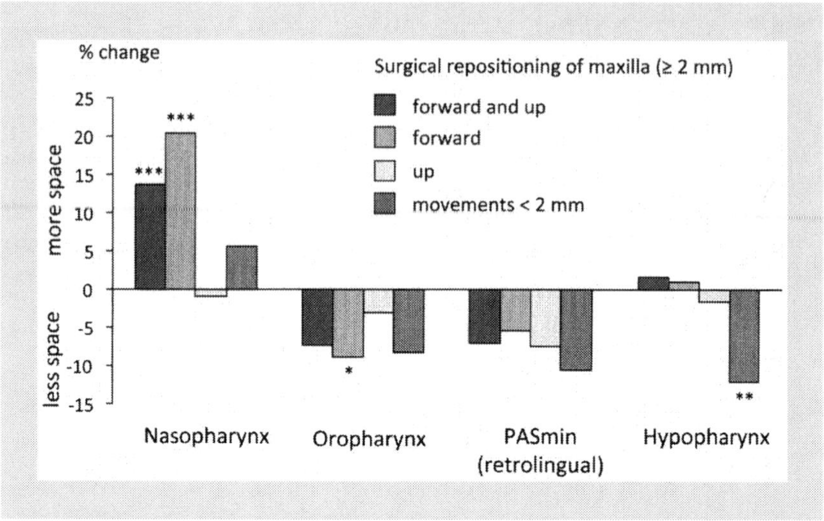

Fig. 14. Change (%) in sagittal dimension of the upper airways related to varying maxillary repositionings in subjects undergoing bimaxillary surgery for correction of Class III malocclusion.

6. Sensory function

Impairment of sensory function is the most common long-term side effect after orthognathic surgery, especially following sagittal split osteotomies (Westermark et al., 1999). In our sample of 381 patients operated with bilateral sagittal split osteotomy (BSSO), 47.8% reported altered sensory function 3 years after the operation (Table 1).

Patient's report	% patients
Normal / almost normal	52.2
Reduced	40.4
Increased	6.3
Complete loss	1.0

Table 1. Patients' reports of sensation in the lower lip and chin 3 years after bilateral sagittal split osteotomy.

Among patients with impaired sensation (n=181), 40.9% indicated that the impairment was of concern to them because it affected their daily life. A mild distress was reported by 28.2%, 8.3% reported a moderate distress, and 4.4% said the situation caused severe distress. The age at the time of surgery was significantly associated with self-reported alterations in sensory function ($P < 0.001$). Distress due to impaired sensation also increased with age ($P = 0.024$) (Fig. 15).

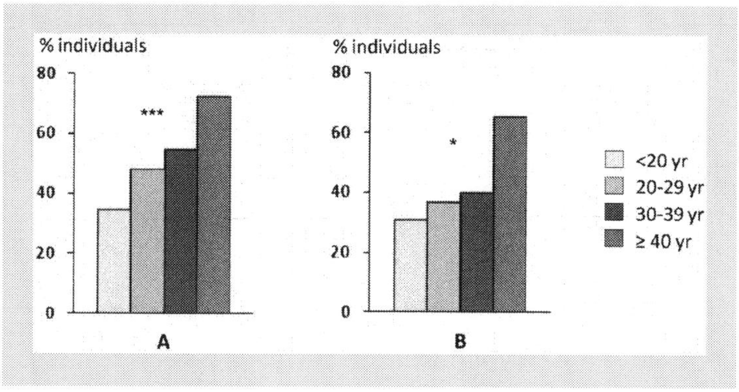

Fig. 15. **A:** Relative frequency of individuals reporting altered sensory function according to age among 381 subjects operated with BSSO. **B:** Relative frequency of individuals reporting varying levels of distress (mild, moderate, and severe combined) according to age among 181 who reported altered sensation. * $P < 0.05$, *** $P < 0.001$.

7. Patients' satisfaction with treatment results

Orthognathic surgery may have an impact on quality of life (Cunningham et al., 2002). At a clinical review 3 years after surgery, patients monitored by our team fill in a questionnaire addressing their opinions of the treatment result in terms of improvement in dental and facial appearance, chewing ability, speech, impact on social life, satisfaction with overall result, and whether they would re-elect surgery with their present experience (Espeland et al., 2008b). Findings among 705 consecutively operated patients appear from Tables 2-4. Totally 90.6% reported that they were satisfied with the overall treatment result, and 88.5% indicated that they would have re-elected surgery based on their present experiences. Of those expressing dissatisfaction, 47.0% stated that they would have made the same decision.

	Very satisfied	Satisfied	Somewhat dissatisfied	Very dissatisfied
Females (n=399)	56.6	31.1	10.5	1.8
Males (n=306)	64,4	30.1	4.9	0.7
Total (n=705)	60.0	30.6	8.1	1.3

Table 2. Patients' answers to a question about satisfaction with the treatment result (%). Significant difference between genders ($P = 0.017$).

	Satisfied (%)	Dissatisfied (%)
Skeletal Class I (n=97)	93.8	6.2
Skeletal Class II (n=214)	82.2	17.8
Skeletal Class III (n=394)	94.4	5.6

Table 3. Patients' reports on satisfaction/dissatisfaction related to skeletal malocclusion. Significant difference between categories ($P < 0.001$).

	Satisfied (%)	Dissatisfied (%)
Mandibular setback (n=226)	96.0	4.0
Mandibular setback and LeFort I (n=119)	94.1	5.9
Mandibular advancement (n=130)	83.1	16.9
Mandibular advancement and LeFort I (n=30)	76.7	23.3
Maxillary surgery (LeFort I) (n=124)	88.7	11.3
Other procedures (n=76)	90.8	9.2

Table 3. Patients' reports on satisfaction/dissatisfaction related to surgical approach. Significant difference between approaches ($P < 0.001$).

Relatively more males than females were satisfied, and correction of Class III malocclusion was associated with increased frequency of satisfied patients. The patients' stated reasons for dissatisfaction were allocated to the following categories: impaired nerve function (n=16), relapse (n=18), appearance (n=17), TMJ problems (n=8), occlusal function (6), and other reasons (n=11).

8. Concluding remarks

Orthognatic surgery may on the basis of systematic monitoring of outcomes according to our established protocols be regarded as a treatment modality that predictably leads to the correction of severe occlusal anomalies. Skeletal corrections are also generally stable and even if some relapse may occur, the occlusion is usually not affected due to orthodontic compensation during the first post-surgical months. Most patients are also satisfied with the result. Improvement in facial soft-tissue profile and the effect on upper airways are less predictable. Class II malocclusions represents a greater challenge compared to other anomalies, especially in patients with high-angle facial pattern.

9. Acknowledgment

The authors are greatly indebted to Håkon Størmer for excellent support in preparation of the illustrations.

10. References

Achilleos, S., Krogstad, O. & Lyberg T. (1979). Surgical mandibular advancement and changes in uvuloglossopharyngeal morphology and head posture : a short- and long-term cephalometric study in males. *European Journal of Orthodontics*, Vol.22, No.4, (August 2000a), pp. 367-381, ISSN 0141-5387

Achilleos, S., Krogstad, O. & Lyberg T. (1979). Surgical mandibular setback and changes in uvuloglossopharyngeal morphology and head posture : a short- and long-term cephalometric study in males. *European Journal of Orthodontics*, Vol.22, No.4, (August 2000b), pp. 383-394, ISSN 0141-5387

Cunningham S.J., Garratt, A.M. & Hunt, M.P. (1973). Development of a condition-specific quality of life measure for patients with dentofacial deformity: II. Validity and responsiveness testing. *Community Dentistry and Oral Epidemiology*, Vol.30, No.2, (April 2002), pp. 81-90, ISSN 0301-5661

Dowling, P.A., Espeland, L., Krogstad, O., Stenvik, A. & Kelly, A. (1986). Duration of orthodontic treatment involving orthognathic surgery. *The International Journal of Adult Orthodontics and Orthognathic Surgery,* Vol. 14, No.2, (Summer 1999), pp. 146-152, ISSN 0742-1931

Dowling, P.A., Espeland, L., Mobarak, K.A. & Hogevold, H.E. (1986). LeFort I maxillary advancement: 3-year stability and risk factors for relapse. *American Journal of Orthodontics and Dentofacial Orthopedics,* Vol.128, No.5 (November 2005), pp. 560-567, ISSN 0889-5406

Espeland, L., Dowling, P.A., Mobarak, K.A. & Stenvik, A. (1986). Three-year stability of open-bite correction by 1-piece maxillary osteotomy. *American Journal of Orthodontics and Dentofacial Orthopedics,* Vol.134, No.1, (July 2008a), pp. 60-66, ISSN 0889-5406

Espeland, L., Høgevold H.E. & Stenvik, A. (1979). A 3-year patient-centred follow-up of 516 consecutively treated orthognathic surgery patients. *European Journal of Orthodontics,* Vol.30, No.1, (February 2008b), pp. 24-30, ISSN 0141-5387

Hoppenreijs, T.J.M., Stoelinga, P.J.W., Grace, K.L. & Robben, C.M.G. (1986). Long-term evaluation of patients with progressive condylar resorption following orthognathic surgery. *International Journal of Oral and Maxillofacial Surgery,* Vol.28, No.6, (December 1999), pp. 411-418, ISSN 0901-5027

Høgevold, H.E., Mobarak, K.A., Espeland, L., Krogstad, O. & Skjelbred, P. (1987). Plate fixation of extra-oral subcondylar ramus osteotomy for correction of mandibular prognathism: clinical aspects and short term stability. *Journal of Cranio-maxillo-facial Surgery,* Vol.29, No.4, (August 2001), pp. 205-211, ISSN 1010-5182

Jakobsone, G., Stenvik A., Sandvik, L. & Espeland, L. (1986). Three-year follow-up of bimaxillary surgery to correct skeletal Class III malocclusion: stability and risk factors for relapse. *American Journal of Orthodontics and Dentofacial Orthopedics,* Vol.139, No.1, (January 2011a), pp. 80-89, ISSN 0889-5406

Jakobsone, G., Stenvik, A. & Espeland, L. Predicting the soft tissue profile changes after bimaxillary operations for Class III correction, *Proceedings of* EOS 2011 *87th Congress of the European Orthodontic Society,* Istanbul, Turkey, June 19-23, 2011b

Jakobsone, G., Stenvik, A. & Espeland, L. (1986). The effect of maxillary advancement and impaction on the upper airway after bimaxillary surgery to correct Class III malocclusion. *American Journal of Orthodontics and Dentofacial Orthopedics,* (April 2011c) (in press)

Kollias, I. & Krogstad, O. (1979). Adult craniocervical and pharyngeal changes - a longitudinal cephalometric study between 22 and 42 years of age. Part II: morphological uvulo-glossopharyngeal changes. *European Journal of Orthodontics,* Vol.21, No.4, (August 1999), pp. 345-355, ISSN 0141-5387

Mobarak, K.A., Krogstad, O., Espeland, L. & Lyberg, T. (1986). Long-term stability of mandibular setback surgery: a follow-up of 80 bilateral sagittal split osteotomy patients. *The International Journal of Adult Orthodontics and Orthognathic Surgery,* Vol 15, No.2, (Summer 2000a), pp. 83-95, ISSN 0742-1931

Mobarak, K.A., Krogstad, O., Espeland, L. & Lyberg, T. (1986). Stability of extraoral vertical ramus osteotomy: plate fixation versus maxillomandibular/skeletal suspension wire fixation. *The International Journal of Adult Orthodontics and Orthognathic Surgery,* Vol.15, No.2, (Summer 2000b), pp. 97-113, ISSN 0742-1931

Mobarak, K.A., Espeland, L., Krogstad, O. & Lyberg, T. (1986). Mandibular advancement surgery in high-angle and low-angle Class II patients: different long-term skeletal responses. *American Journal of Orthodontics and Dentofacial Orthopedics*, Vol.119, No.4, (April 2001a), pp. 368-381, ISSN 0889-5406

Mobarak, K.A., Krogstad, O., Espeland, L. & Lyberg, T. (1931). Factors influencing the predictability of soft tissue profile changes following mandibular setback surgery. *The Angle Orthodontist*, Vol.71, No.3, (June 2001b), pp. 216-227, ISSN 0003-3219

Mobarak, K.A., Espeland, L., Krogstad, O. & Lyberg, T. (1986). Soft tissue profile changes following mandibular advancement surgery: predictability and long-term outcome. *American Journal of Orthodontics and Dentofacial Orthopedics*, Vol.119, No.4, (April 2001c), pp. 353-367, ISSN 0889-5406

Proffit, W.R., Turvey, T.A. & Phillips, C. (1986). Orthognathic surgery: A hierarchy of stability. *The International Journal of Adult Orthodontics and Orthognathic Surgery*, Vol.11, No.3 (1996), pp. 191-204, ISSN 0742-1931

Shaughnessy, S., Mobarak, K.A., Høgevold, H.E. & Espeland L. (1986). Long-term skeletal and soft-tissue responses after advancement genioplasty. *American Journal of Orthodontics and Dentofacial Orthopedics*, Vol.130, No.1. (July 2006), pp. 8-17, ISSN 0889-5406

Westermark, A., Bystedt, H. & von Konow, L. (1986). Patients' evaluation of the final result of sagittal split osteotomy: is it influenced by impaired sensitivity of the lower lip and chin? *The International Journal of Adult Orthodontics and Orthognathic Surgery*, Vol.14, No.2, (Summer 1999), pp. 135-139, ISSN 0742-1931

Winter, B.U., Stenvik, A. & Espeland, L. Bimaxillary orthognathic surgery of high-angle skeletal Class II malocclusions - stability after 3 years, *Proceedings of WFO 2010 7th International Orthodontic Congress*, Sydney, Australia, Abstract 1505, February 6-9, 2010

18

Orthodontic-Surgical Treatment: Electromyographic and Electrognatographic Evaluation with Three Electromyographic Instruments

Giampietro Farronato, Cinzia Maspero, Lucia Giannini and Guido Galbiati
Fondazione IRCCS Ca' Granda, Ospedale Maggiore Policlinico, Milan, Italy

1. Introduction

The introduction of electromyography in orthodontics determined the beginning of some studies about neuromuscolar system's response to physiological and pathological oral alterations and the effect of masticatory muscles on facial morphology.[1,2]
Experimental studies demonstrated that a real change in muscolar function causes morphology alterations.[1]
Several studies in literature, from Watt e Williams, who studied in 1951 the effect of masticatory bolus on mouse maxillary and mandibular development, to Avis who in 1961 showed how muscolar function was important for gonial region development, connect morpholgy and function.[3,4]
In the last years masticatory muscles response to dento-skeletal discrepancies, alterations of breathing, swelling, speech and posture, to functional therapies, implant supported therapy and prosthetic rehabilitation has been studied.[5]
The definition of occlusion changed in time and it is now not based on mechanics theory but it includes functional aspects.[6-10]
In literature different positions about the compensatory muscolar aequilibrium in skeletal discrepancies can be found.
A correct diagnosis is based not only on clinical and radiographic examination, but it is also important to analyze informations obtaining from neuromuscolar system.[2]
Knowing muscular action allows to obtain a correct diagnosis, prognosis and treatment planning and helps in avoiding failures.[2]
Electromyography allows to evaluate neuromuscolar system and equilibrium, mandibular movements alterations and the effects of orthodontic therapy on stomathognatic system.[7]
Nowadays, different kind of electromyographic instruments are available, each of them constructed following specific protocols and with different aims.
It is well known that facial growth is influenced by both genetic and extrinsic factors and that muscle function exercises an important influence both on growth and on craniofacial morphology.[11]
Orthodontic-surgical treatment was born in order to reposition the skeletal bone basis in a normal position in subjects where their position was not correct.

Modifications of the facial skeleton have consequences on all masticatory muscles, even if the majority of studies in literature is referred to masseter and temporal muscle because this muscles are easy to study with surface analysis.[12,13]
Many studies in literature have tried to highlight the effect of orthognathic surgery on neuromuscular system.
Most authors explained that a first modification of the neuromuscular system can be seen during presurgical orthodontic phase besides Precious and Skulsky showed that maximum bite force is reduced after the beginning of the fixed orthodontic therapy.[14]
Also Dean, Throckmorton and Sinn showed that patients in orthodontic-surgical treatment were able to express a minor bite force in presurgical phase if compared to the one they could express before starting therapy.[15] Thomas et al affirmed that there was a reduction of the maximum mandibular opening movement and of its movement in vertical sense before and after the orthodontic phase, connected to the same protective mechanism which explains the maximum bite force reduction.[16] Morever, during mandibular movements, there was a painful action of brackets on teeth and of orthodontics thread in soft tissues of cheek and lips, which limited the patient in executing normal movements.
Furthermore the presurgical orthodontic treatment contributed to reduce the possibility of mandibular movements and the consequent reduction of occlusal contacts, increasing interferences between dental elements with reduction of mandibular excursion.[17-21]
Many studies analyzed the modifications consequent to a surgical reposition of bone basis.
Finn, Throckmorton, Bell and Legan did not show an increase of the maximum muscular force post surgical of muscular advancement and maxillary retroposition.[22]
Also Van den Braber et al affirmed that oral function is not influenced by mandibular advancement surgery.[23] On the contrary round Athanasiou had discovered that surgical correction of maxillary prognathism increased the intensity of occlusal contacts and hypothesized that such harmonization of the dentofacial skeleton would influence the neuromuscular system.[24] Kobayashi et al affirmed that the steadiness of the masticatory rhythm is improved by orthognathic surgery in subjects with mandibular prognathism. [25]
A Tatsumi et al study has proved that, after the surgical orthodontic treatment, an aesthetic improvement, a reduction of the duration of the masticatory cycle and an improvement of the activity of masticatory muscles are obtained.[26] These advantages suggest that patients who undergo this operation gain a functional readjustment in post-surgical phase Proffit reported a maximum bite force increase in some patients in post-surgical phase. Unfortunately, this increase was not an improvement compared to the beginning of the therapy, but a return to initial conditions before starting orthodontic therapy.
These changes underwent a huge variability, due to the different sensibility of patients on dental, muscular and articulation level. Besides, to explain the obtained results, the patient's will and emotional stress were probably more important than muscular advantages and biomechanics.
The majority of studies have analyzed only a single phase of the treatment.
The aim of this work consists in the evaluation of the neuromuscular functionality and mandibular kinesiology in 100 patients undergoing orthodontic surgical treatment.
Values obtained analyzing masticatory muscles in patients with important skeletal discrepancies using three different kind of electromyographic instruments were compared.

2. Material and methods

Study group

All patients during the orthognathic surgery treatment at the Orthodontic Section of the department of Surgical, Reconstructive and Diagnostic Sciences have been submitted to classical instrumental exams, clinical and radiographic, and also periodically to an electromyographic and electrokinesiographic evaluation.

The analyzed sample is composed of 100 patients [44 men and 56 women] at the end of growth.

Criteria followed in selecting patients were:

- adult age
- the presence of a dento-skeletal discrepancy
- the necessity of a combined orthodontic-surgical treatment

The three criteria had to coexist at the same time.

The electromiographic and the kinesiographic examination have been performed on orthodontic-surgical patients:

- during the first visit
- before the start of the orthodontic therapy
- during the presurgical phase of orthodontic bimonthly
- every month from three months before the surgical operation to three months after
- the day before the surgical operation
- during the intermaxillary fixation
- at the removal of the fixation
- during post-surgical orthodontic phase with the same terms (times) of pre-surgical orthodontic phase.
- at the removal of surgical bite
- at the end of the treatment
- during follow up

In every phase, patients executed two electromyographic examinations through two different electromyograms.

Before every tests clinicans asked patients if they had dental or muscolar pain in order to avoid errors.

The electromyographic instruments used in the work were the electromiography Freely [De Gotzen - Legnano - Italia], the electromiography and electrognatography K6-I EMG [Myotronics - Tukwila WA - USA] and the electromiography and electrognatography Biopak [Bioresearch Associate -USA].

The muscles considered have been the anterior temporal muscle and the masseter muscle.

In order to compare the data versus the healthy population, a control group has been settled. This group consists of patients in adult age, skeletal class I, with absence of temporal-mandibular problems and absence of a previous orthodontic or a combined orthodontic-surgical treatment.

Finally a statistic test evaluation has been performed with t test and ANOVA test.

Methods

The muscles considered in the electromyographic evaluation have been:

- the anterior temporal muscle
- the masseter muscle in its superficial component

- The patient was in a special totally undisturbed and noiseless room. He sat on a rigid stool with an adjustable height, so to have the angle between thigh and leg of 90° (degrees).

The legs were parallel to the floor, the back upright and the gaze beyond the horizon.
Head was in natural head position.
After skin cleaning with a wad soaked in Neoxinal (clorexidina 0,5% in hydroalcoholic solution with no less than 70% of alcohol) to reduce forehead impedance and facilitate adhesiveness, electrodes were positioned.
The electrodes position was the same for both the equipments and unmodified with the use of either equipment.
The electrodes were disposable and bipolar, Duo Trade Silver/ Silver Chloride previously gelled. The interpolar distance was of 21±1 mm, each pole was circular, 10 mm in diameter.
The bipolar electrodes were positioned according to the following procedure:

- for the masseter muscle: the operator, behind a seated subject, palpates the belly of the muscle while the patient clenches his teeth. To position the bipolar electrode parallel to the muscle fibres, the line connecting the commissura labiorum oris with the tragum is ideally drawn as well as the line connecting the the lateral part of eye and gonion.

The position of the electrode makes the superior pole in the intersection point between the two lines and its major axis is along the esocanto-goniac line.

- for the temporal muscle: the muscle is palpated while clenching thus localizing the major axis of the zygomatic process of the frontal bone.

The bipolar electrode is positioned along the line parallel to this process passing about a transverse finger posteriorly and superiorly to it; this way the electrode will be parallel to the muscle fibres and positioned more or less superficially in comparison with the frontoparietal suture.
A grounding electrode (monopolar) is positioned on a silent muscular area of the forehead. Such electrode may be positioned on the volar surface of the forearm, considered a possible silent area. The electromyographic instrument utilises such electrode as a reference eliminating part of all background noises. So, it can be considered a first filter to abolish interferences.
The tests with the two instruments are executed consecutively without taking off electrodes. An average of data collected by each patient was then done at every therapeutic phase.

3. Results

At the beginning of the treatment the patients present a compensatory equilibrium to malocclusion. During presurgical orthodontic phase electromyographic and electrognatographic values become worse and they continue worsening after surgical intervention. They improve in post surgical orthodontic phase.
After the removal of the orthodontic appliance, electromyographic values improve until they reach optimal values. Mandibular movement rehabilitation is satisfactory and constant also if it needs more time than muscular rehabilitation. At the end of the treatment maximum mandibular opening is still less than the preoperatory one. (fig. 1-14)
The three instruments have been planned through different principles, they are based on different ideas and they have different aims.
The different types does not avoid the possibility to obtain complementary data, not even in numeric values, but in their meaning. (fig. 15-21)

Data obtained from all instruments gives to the clinicians the same information, also if they are expressed in different ways.

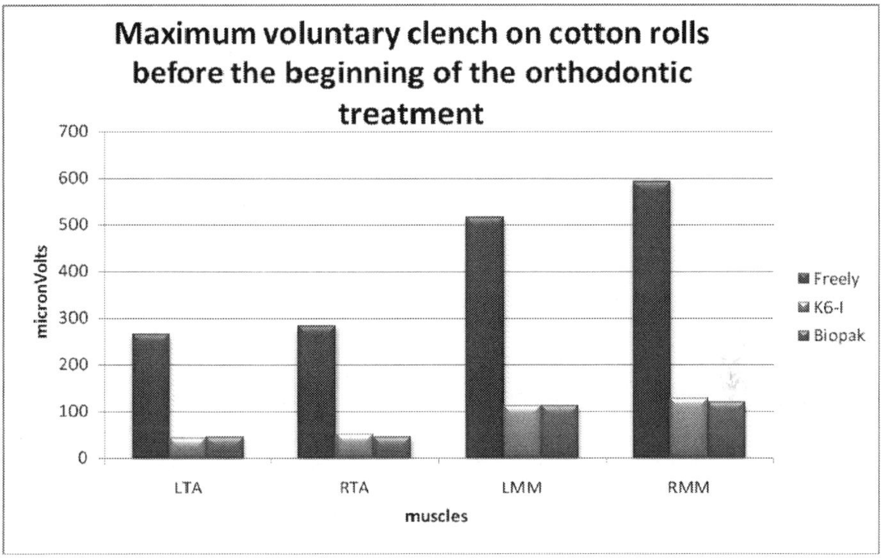

Fig. 1.

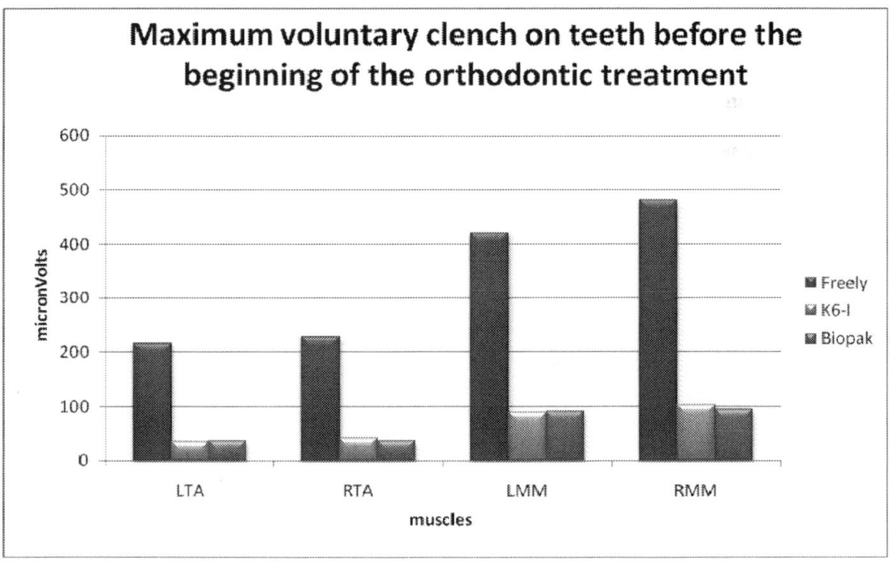

Fig. 2.

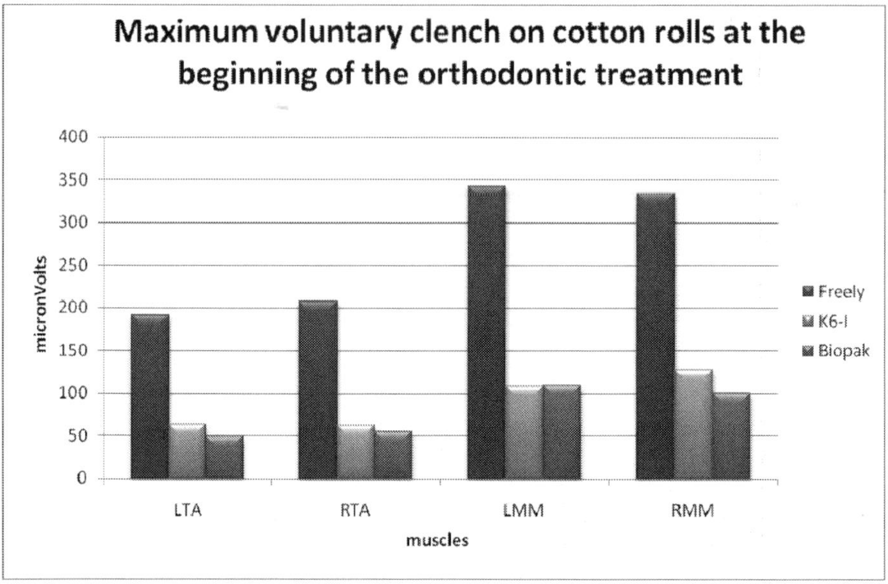
Maximum voluntary clench on cotton rolls at the beginning of the orthodontic treatment
micronVolts
400
350
300
250
200
150
100
50
0
LTA
RTA
LMM
RMM
muscles
Freely
K6-I
Biopak

Fig. 3.

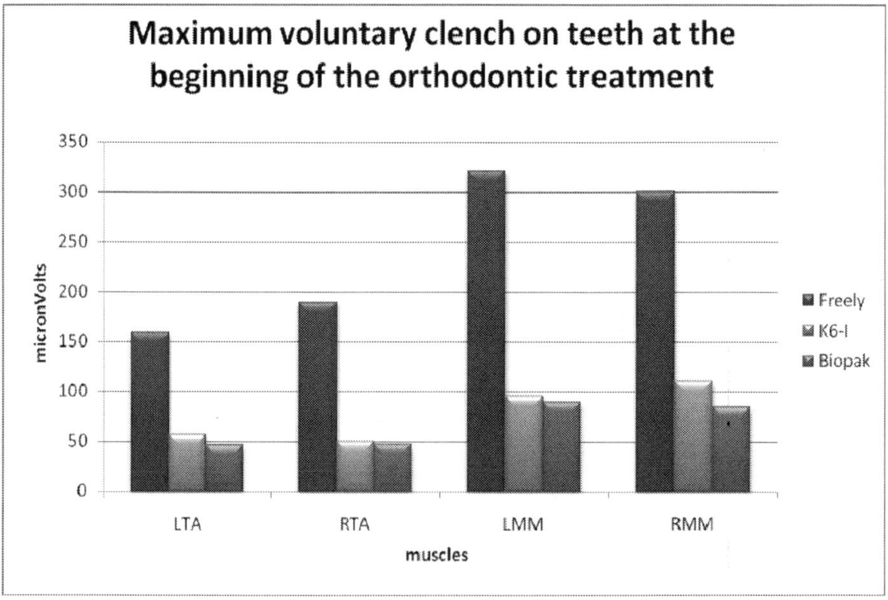
Maximum voluntary clench on teeth at the beginning of the orthodontic treatment
micronVolts
350
300
250
200
150
100
50
0
LTA
RTA
LMM
RMM
muscles
Freely
K6-I
Biopak

Fig. 4.

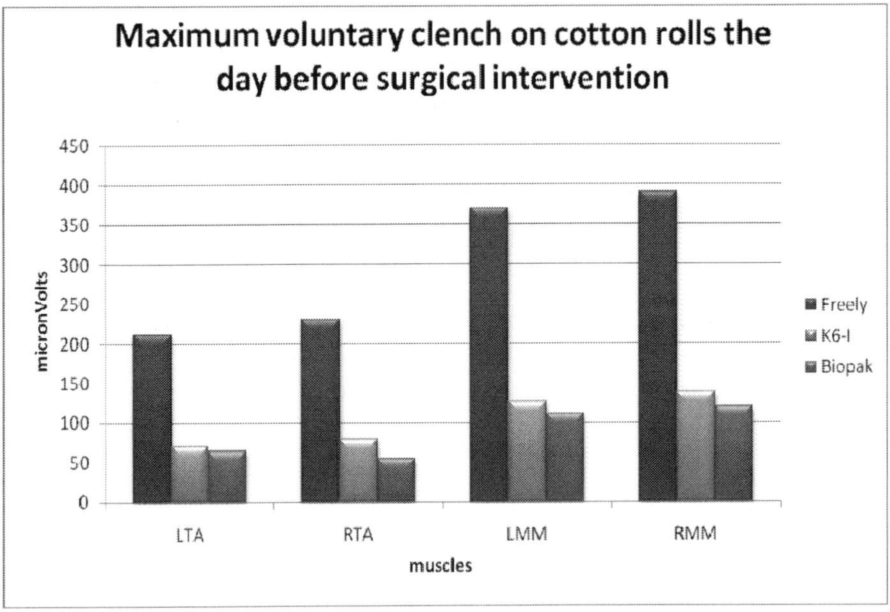
Maximum voluntary clench on cotton rolls the day before surgical intervention
450
400
350
300
250
200
150
100
50
0
micronVolts
LTA
RTA
LMM
RMM
muscles
Freely
K6-I
Biopak

Fig. 5.

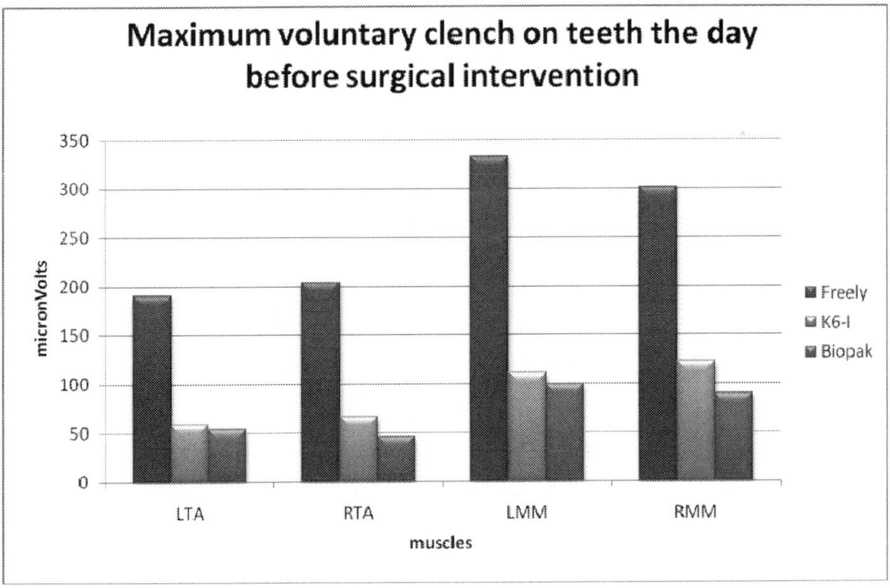
Maximum voluntary clench on teeth the day before surgical intervention
350
300
250
200
150
100
50
0
micronVolts
LTA
RTA
LMM
RMM
muscles
Freely
K6-I
Biopak

Fig. 6.

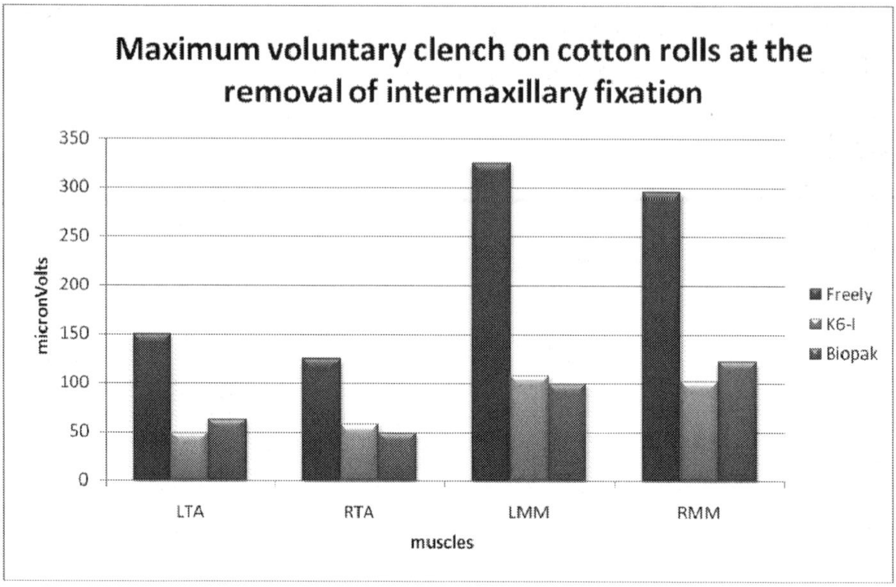
Maximum voluntary clench on cotton rolls at the removal of intermaxillary fixation
350
300
250
200
150
100
50
0
micronVolts
Freely
K6-I
Biopak
LTA
RTA
LMM
RMM
muscles

Fig. 7.

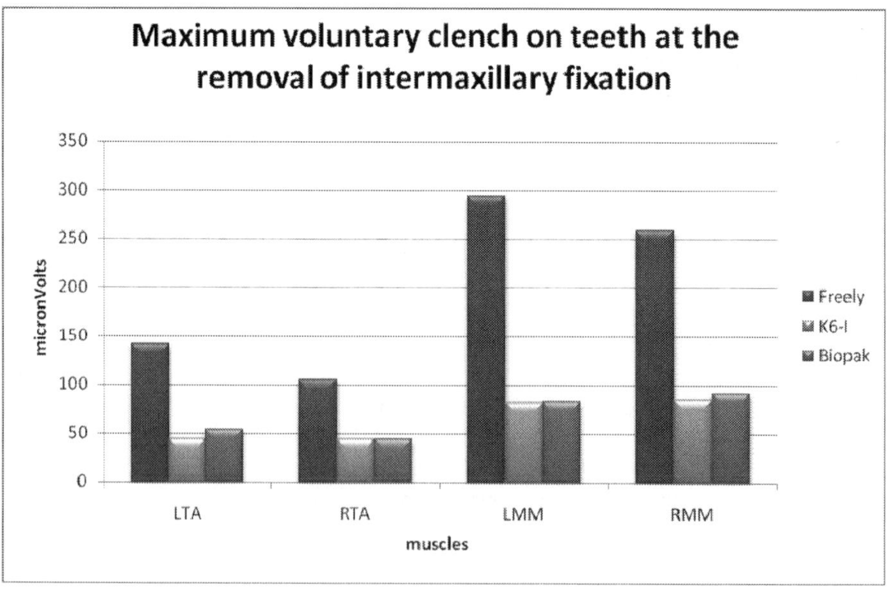
Maximum voluntary clench on teeth at the removal of intermaxillary fixation
350
300
250
200
150
100
50
0
micronVolts
Freely
K6-I
Biopak
LTA
RTA
LMM
RMM
muscles

Fig. 8.

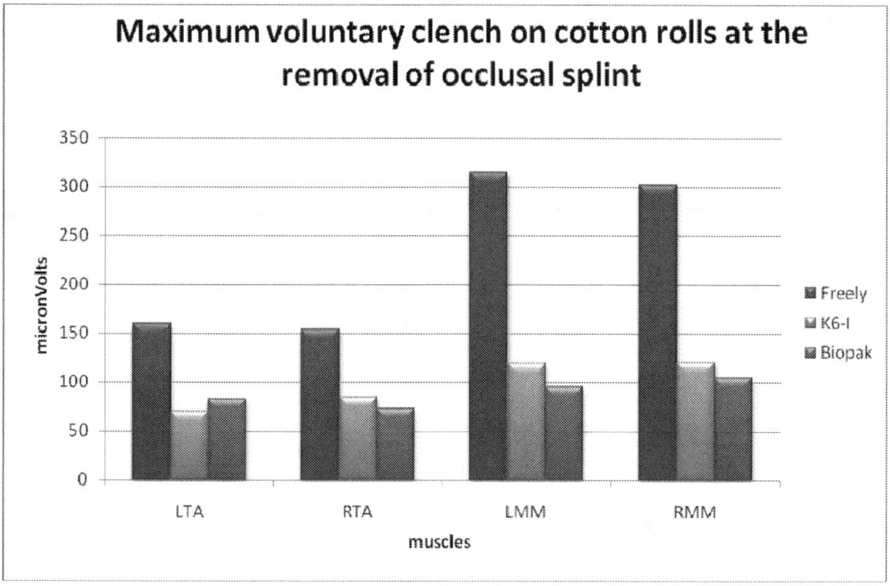
Maximum voluntary clench on cotton rolls at the removal of occlusal splint
350
300
250
200
150
100
50
0
micronVolts
LTA
RTA
LMM
RMM
muscles
Freely
K6-I
Biopak

Fig. 9.

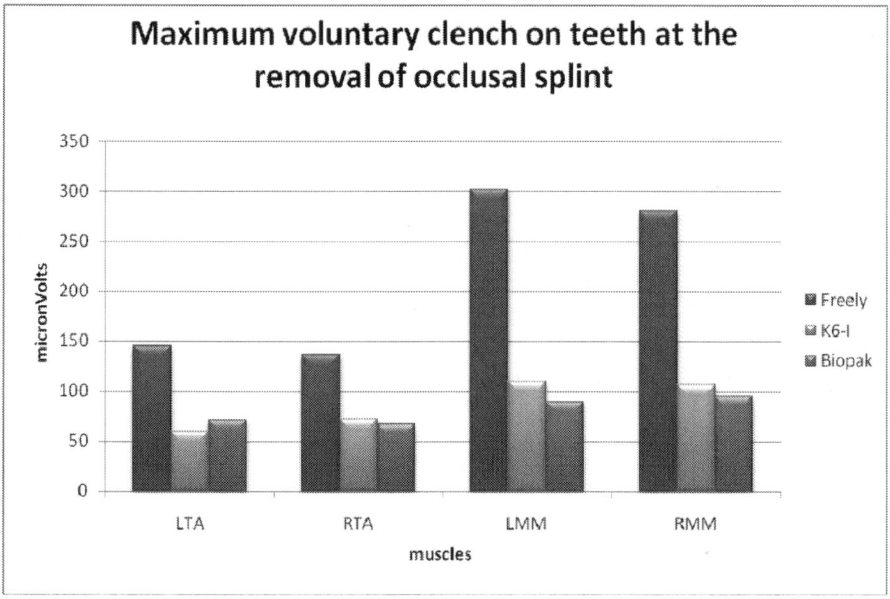
Maximum voluntary clench on teeth at the removal of occlusal splint
350
300
250
200
150
100
50
0
micronVolts
LTA
RTA
LMM
RMM
muscles
Freely
K6-I
Biopak

Fig. 10.

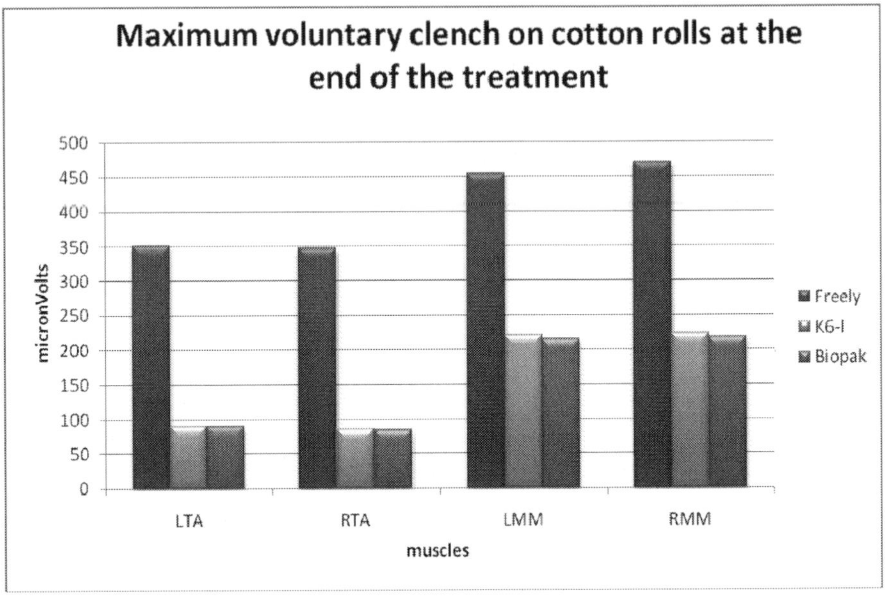
Maximum voluntary clench on cotton rolls at the end of the treatment
microVolts
500
450
400
350
300
250
200
150
100
50
0
LTA
RTA
LMM
RMM
muscles
Freely
K6-I
Biopak

Fig. 11.

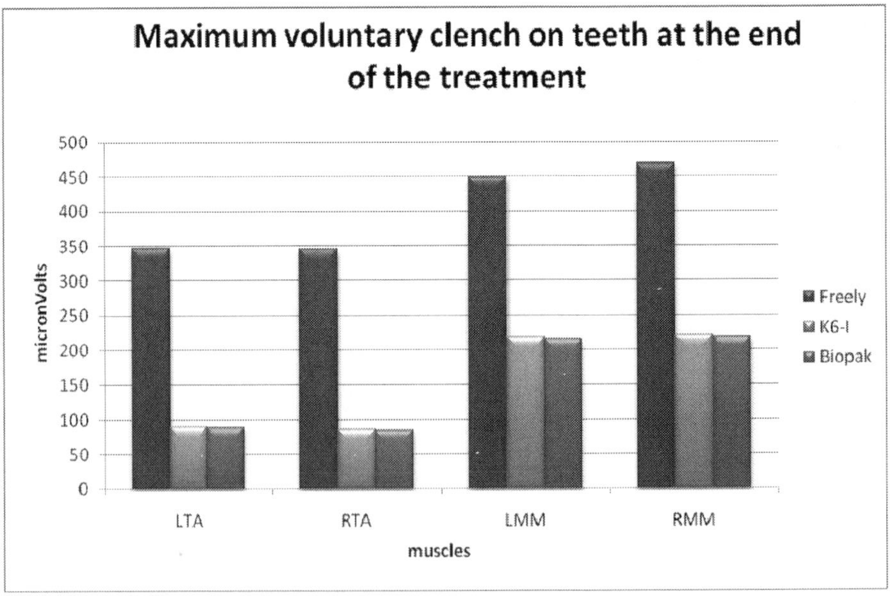
Maximum voluntary clench on teeth at the end of the treatment
micronVolts
500
450
400
350
300
250
200
150
100
50
0
LTA
RTA
LMM
RMM
muscles
Freely
K6-I
Biopak

Fig. 12.

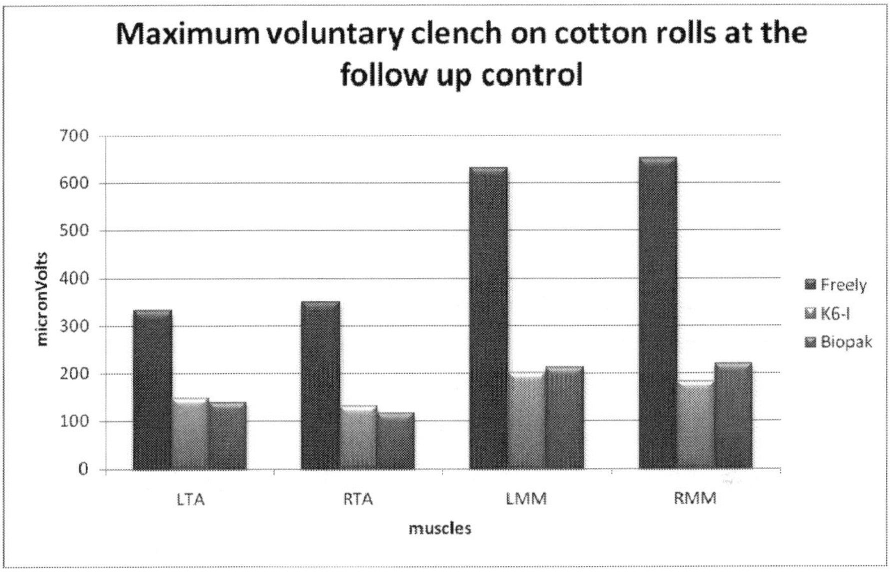

Fig. 13.

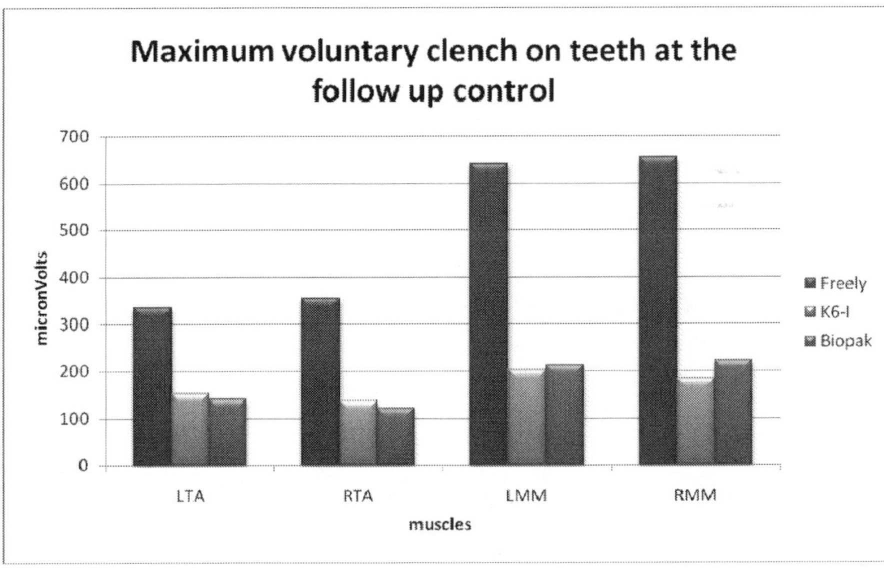

Fig. 14.

Fig. 1-14. Maximum voluntary clench on cotton rolls and on teeth during the different phases of the treatment.

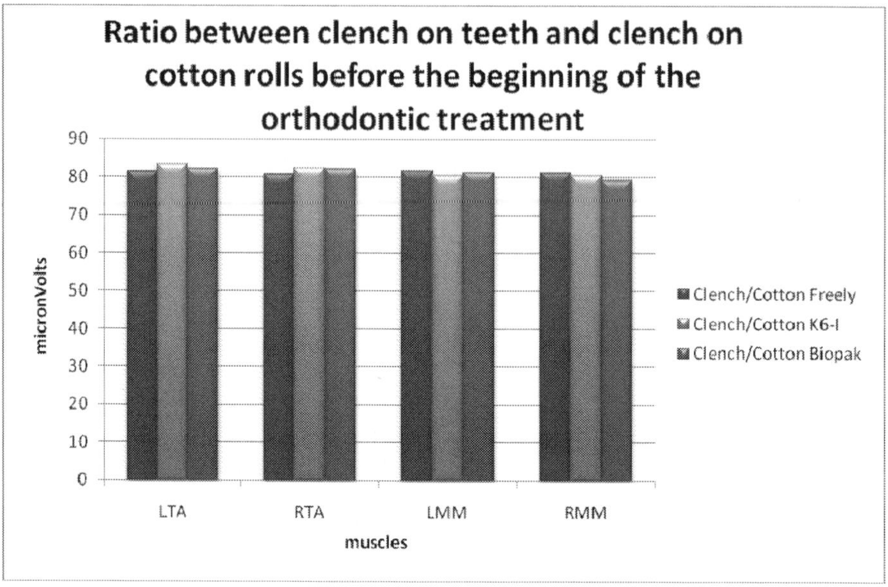
Ratio between clench on teeth and clench on cotton rolls before the beginning of the orthodontic treatment
90
80
70
60
50
40
30
20
10
0
microVolts
LTA
RTA
LMM
RMM
muscles
Clench/Cotton Freely
Clench/Cotton K6-I
Clench/Cotton Biopak

Fig. 15.

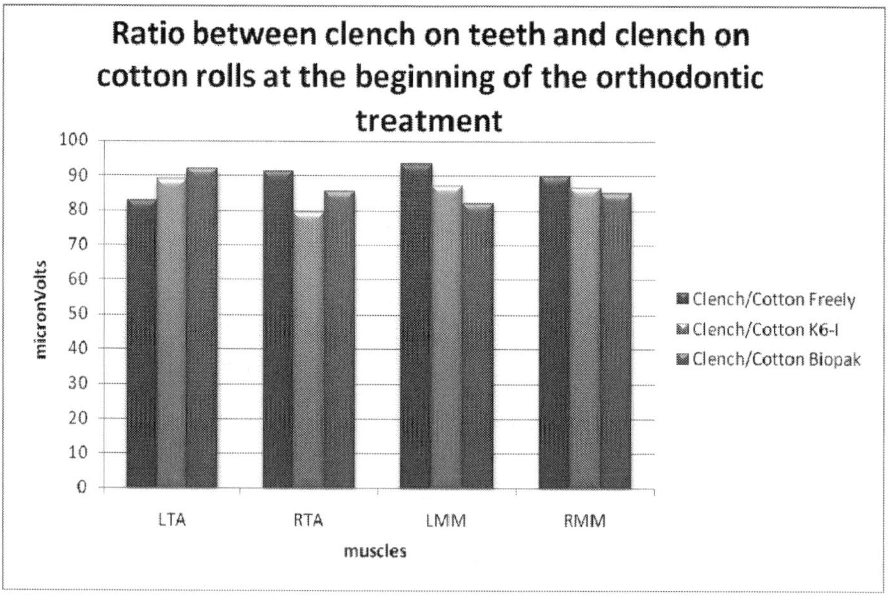
Ratio between clench on teeth and clench on cotton rolls at the beginning of the orthodontic treatment
100
90
80
70
60
50
40
30
20
10
0
microVolts
LTA
RTA
LMM
RMM
muscles
Clench/Cotton Freely
Clench/Cotton K6-I
Clench/Cotton Biopak

Fig. 16.

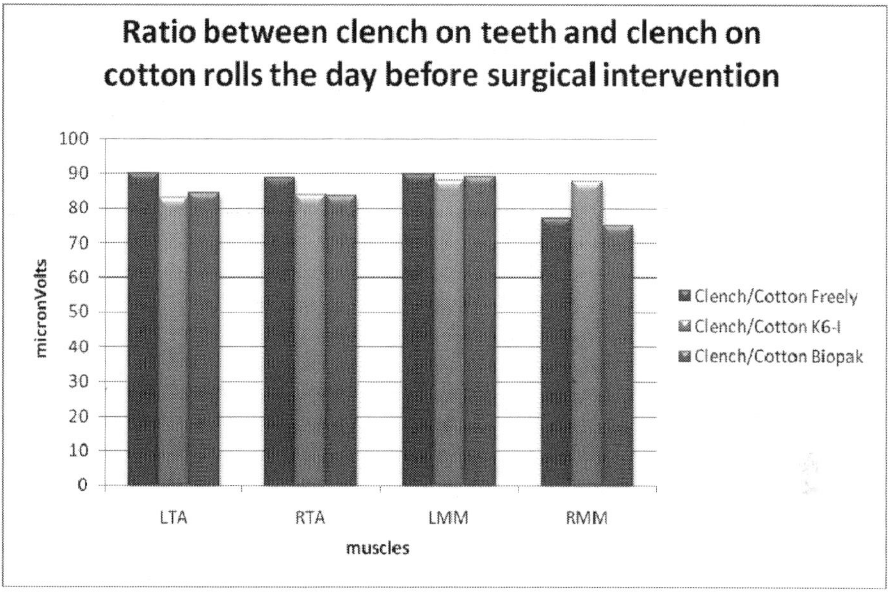
Ratio between clench on teeth and clench on cotton rolls the day before surgical intervention
100
90
80
70
60
50
40
30
20
10
0
micronVolts
LTA
RTA
LMM
RMM
muscles
Clench/Cotton Freely
Clench/Cotton K6-I
Clench/Cotton Biopak

Fig. 17.

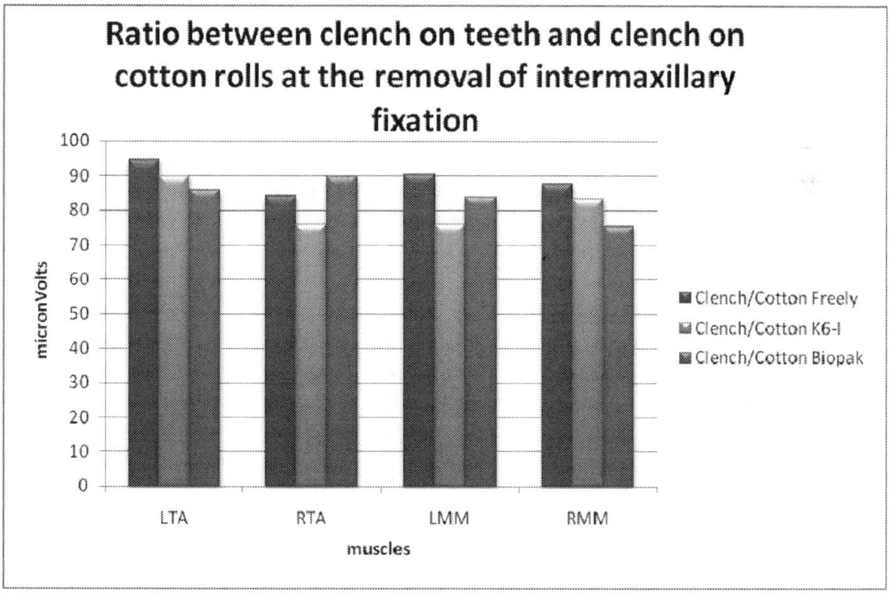
Ratio between clench on teeth and clench on cotton rolls at the removal of intermaxillary fixation
100
90
80
70
60
50
40
30
20
10
0
micronVolts
LTA
RTA
LMM
RMM
muscles
Clench/Cotton Freely
Clench/Cotton K6-I
Clench/Cotton Biopak

Fig. 18.

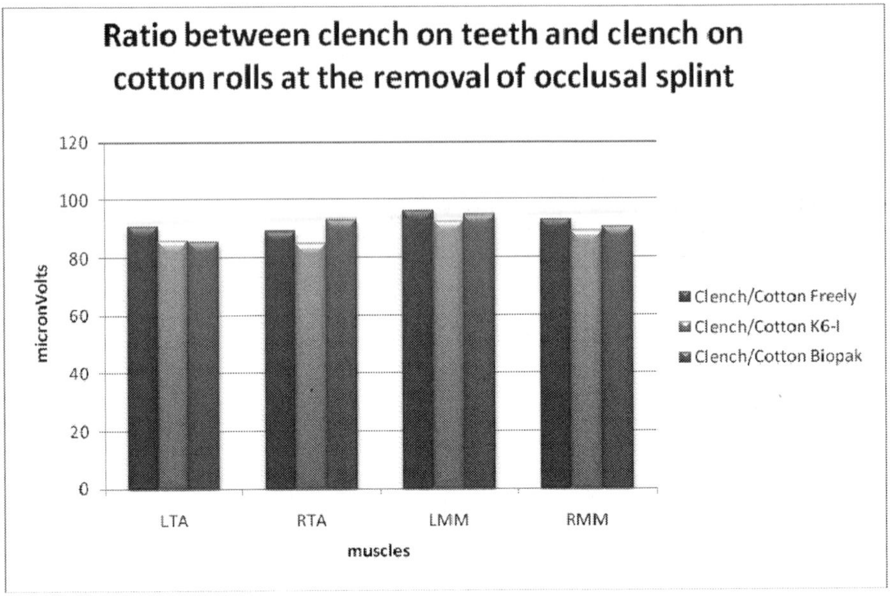
Ratio between clench on teeth and clench on cotton rolls at the removal of occlusal splint
120
100
80
60
40
20
0
micronVolts
LTA
RTA
LMM
RMM
muscles
Clench/Cotton Freely
Clench/Cotton K6-I
Clench/Cotton Biopak

Fig. 19.

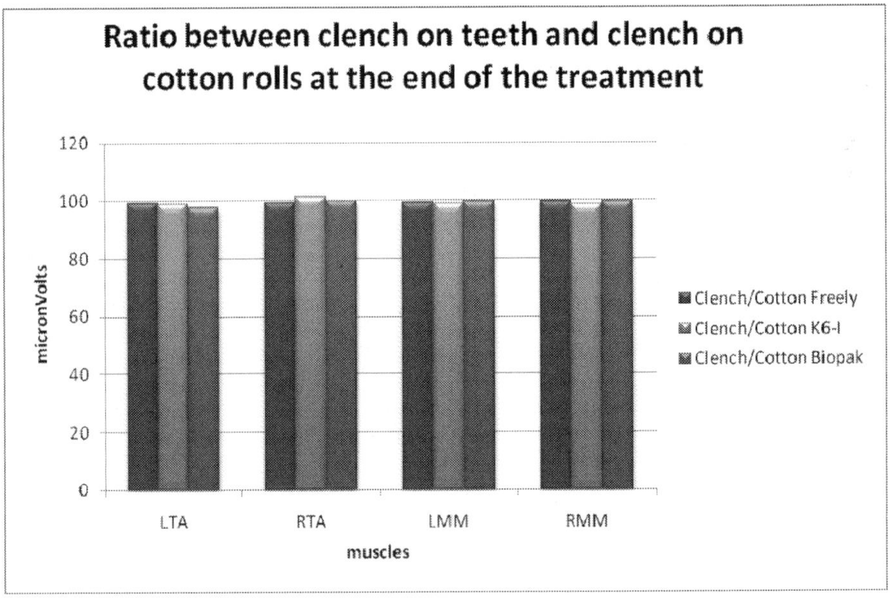
Ratio between clench on teeth and clench on cotton rolls at the end of the treatment
120
100
80
60
40
20
0
micronVolts
LTA
RTA
LMM
RMM
muscles
Clench/Cotton Freely
Clench/Cotton K6-I
Clench/Cotton Biopak

Fig. 20.

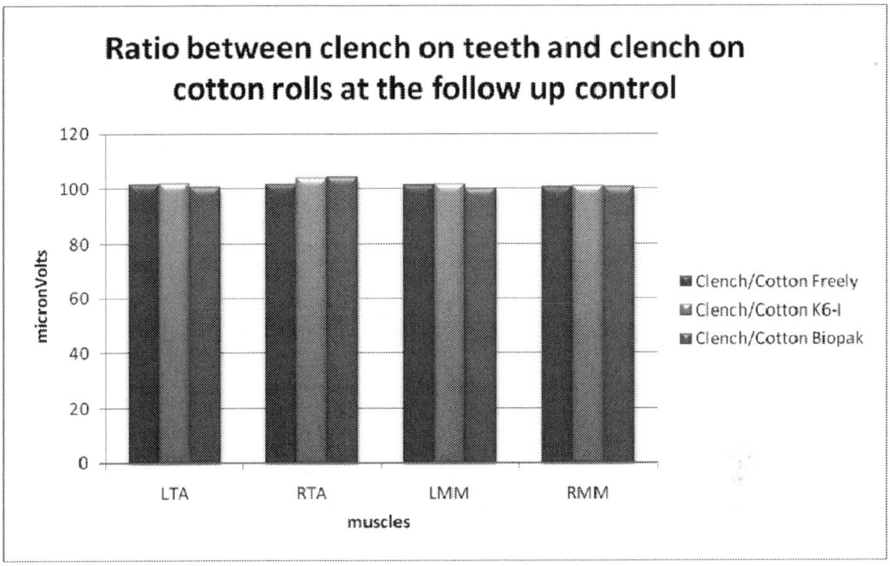

Fig. 21.

Fig. 15-21. Ratio between maximum voluntary clench on cotton rolls and on teeth during the different phases of the treatment.

4. Discussion

The instruments have been planned through different principles, they are based on different ideas and they have different aims.

The protocol studied for Freely by Ferrario et al has been organized in order to obtain the maximum of reproducibility because it is based on a standardized methods which allows to evaluate real percent data.[6]

Following this protocol, micronVolt in maximum voluntary clench on teeth and on cotton rolls were not considered in order to avoid false evaluations.[6]

Besides, this protocol consists in evaluating tests executed in clench on teeth and in comparing them with the ones executed on cotton rolls, in order to obtain percent data with a higher degree of reliability because of the override of every kind of interference due to a non correct position in electrodes or to other external variables.

K6-I electromyograph was projected based on different principles and it does not do this calculation. Besides, ratio between maximum voluntary clenac on teeth and on cotton rolls have been calculated manually in order to obtain data comparable with Freely.

Moreover, the instruments are calibrated in different way and they use different amplifiers and signal filters.

Besides, comparing micronVolt values registered on both instruments in the same time, huge differences can be underlined, but comparing their percent values obtained from clench/cotton ratio similar data can be obtained.

This indicate that the micronVolt muscle activity is different from the two instruments but their percent values are similar and both electromyographs can be overlapped.

Expecially, in this study in patients in orthodontic-surgical therapy, values obtained by the instruments are more similar in the phases which preceed the orthodontic surgical therapy and at the end of the treatment.

In the immediate postsurgical phase, patients have an instable occlusion and there is a lower reproducibility of the measurements.

Lots of differences between skeletal class II and skeletal class III patients have been evidenced by the analysis of the data obtained.

The IMPACT index, which underlines the muscular force expression in time, is definitely major in skeletal class II patients than in skeletal class III patients almost in all treatment phases.

Such difference is statistically significative. Only at the end of the treatment does not a statistically significative difference between the different groups persist.

The activity of the four muscular fasciae, expressed in micronVolt, is definitely major in skeletal class II than in skeletal class III subjects at the beginning of the treatment.

This difference, statistically significative, tends to disappear in the successive phases.

These results have been obtained both on the exercises with cotton rolls between the arches and in clench, with both the electromyographic systems.

As regards mandibular kinesiology, the maximum mandibular opening movement is wider in skeletal class III patients in all the treatment phases, except for the end of the therapy.

The protrusive movement is always major in skeletal class II patients. This gap is reduced at the end of the therapy, but it does persist.

Statistically significative differences about right and left lateral movements have not been evidenced.

By a comparison of the temporal muscle PERCENT OVERLAPPING COEFFICIENT [POC] index it has been underlined that in the initial phases the muscular activity presents a reduced neuromuscular equilibrium. Skeletal class II patients are particularly uncompensated at the beginning of the treatment. After the start of the orthodontic therapy the POC index improves but the value, which isn't included in the physiological range, is constant up to the surgical operation. In the last part of the surgical orthodontic treatment the POC index improves and at the end of the treatment it is included in the physiological range. Skeletal class III patients present in the pre-surgical phases values close to the physiologic limit and improve only at the end of the treatment. Values are physiologic at the end of the treatment.

Skeletal class II patients present a major harmony in the temporal muscle activity compared with skeletal class III patients. The masseter muscle POC index presents a light reduction of the overriding range of the muscular activity after the appliance cementing. This value improves up to the end of the treatment, when the POC index is similar in all skeletal class.

As regards POC medium progressive improvement of the value between the first acquisition made at the beginning of the treatment until the end of the fix orthodontic therapy can be noticed.

Class II patients are more overriding than class III patients at the beginning of treatment. At the end of treatment POC values underline a sufficient neuro-muscular equilibrium, yet there is a difference of about two points of percentage between the classes (the index is slightly better for class II patients).

The progressive improvement of POC indexes in all classes shows that orthodontic treatment tends to develop a major equilibrium among different muscular activities.

As regards POC index a similar progress to skeletal class II and III patients has been noticed even in small samples, hence the insertion of the value of skeletal class I patients in the relative figures.

TORS index shows similar values in skeletal class II and III patients, without the attainment performed at the beginning of the treatment; data remain higher than the normal value [considered equal to 10%] during the period of the orthodontic treatment, at the end of the treatment the TORS value is nearly normal.

The ASIMMETRY index which shows the side of prevalence has an opposite course between the two classes, that is, while for class III patients it diminishes up to the attainment performed in the final part of the orthodontic post-surgical treatment where it starts to increase again, class II patients have an opposite response, nevertheless values are still quite normal.

About the index of TORQUE, class II patients tend to have an occlusal prior centre of mass [negative value], in order to become positive in post-surgical attainments and to arrange themselves close to zero at the end of the treatment. In class III patients the index always remains positive [posterior contact] and it always remains in the range of normality; at the end of the treatment the value is close to zero.

TORQUE index has an alternating course in both classes, its values are quite normal.

The ability in developing force in time in the test on cotton rolls shows a course in part superposable between the two skeletal classes, the decrease of the force up to the level of the attainments performed after the beginning of the orthodontic therapy and after the surgical operation it remains constant, in order get back to the previous values at the end of the treatment. Also the course of the IMPACT in the test of the greatest clench shows a similar response, but not completely superposable between two skeletal classes; nevertheless the decreases of the value of IMPACT up to the level of the surgical operation are still confirmed.

The IMPACT values %*sec highlighted by the two classes show a partial superposable course, with the exclusion of the attainment performed after the beginning of the orthodontic therapy in class II patients where the value tends to diminish, while it increases in class III patients. Finally all the values are quite normal [100 ± 15%*sec] but for the attainment performed after the period of intermaxillary block. At the end of the treatment values are slightly inferior than 100%*sec.

Observing more data of class II and III patients, it has to be noticed that the first group develops a minor muscular activity in comparison to the second group, nevertheless in the other levels class II patients develop a major electric energy, during all the orthodontic fixed treatment, the same observations can be noticed for IMPACT indexes µV*sec. This factual information could be connected to the reduced number of subjects who have an attainment in the initial phase, and it could be the same for attainments performed at the end of the treatment. Considering the afore said things and observing the index of medium POC, there's to notice that even if on the one hand skeletal class III develop a major clench force, it is always true that these result balance than class II patients [medium POC class II patients =80%; class III patients=78%] and the program connected to the electromyography Freely results more important and bases itself on data got from formulas instead from relative values.

Lots of differences between open and deep skeletal bite patients have been underlined by the analysis of the electromyographic data obtained at the beginning of the treatment.

The impact value and muscular activity in micronVolt analysis shows a major muscle activity in deep bite patients than in deep bite ones.

These results have been obtained with both the electromiographic systems.

The following authors too proved that high angle cases were associated with weaker musculature than low angle patients: Möller (1966), Sassouni (1969), Ingerval et al (1974), Bakke (1991), Kayukawa (1992), Farronato (1992) and Bong Kuen Cha (2007). [27-33]

Ahlgren et al. (1973, 1985) proved a positively correlation between the mandibular plane angle (SNGoMe) and the temporal muscle activity (TMA).[34,35] Moller and Ingervall obtained opposite results.[36,37]

Ueda et al (1998) proved that vertical craniofacial morphology is positively correlated with temporal muscle activity (TMA) and negative correlated with masseter muscle activity (MMA).[11]

Fogle et al. (1995) obtained opposite results. They proved that a correlation between craniofacial morphology and masticatory function doesn't exist. The only correlation is between muscle function and patients age.[38] The differences existing between the two groups at the beginning of the treatment, statistically significative, tend to disappear at the removal of the fix orthodontic appliance confirming the orthodontic surgical treatment's corrective role in according to Santoro's study.[39]

Furthermore, before the starting of the fix orthodontic therapy, patients present a compensatory equilibrium to disgnatia. During successive phases electromyographic and electrognatographic continue worsening according to Oliver et al (1985), Proffith et al (1989), Brown et al (1991) and Thomas et al (1995). They improve in post surgical orthodontic phase only.[40-43]

At the end of the orthodontic surgical treatment electromyographic values improve and reach optimal values.

Mandibular movement rehabilitation needs more time than the muscular one even if it is satisfactory and constant too.

At the end of the treatment maximum mandibular opening is still less than the preoperatory one.

No statistically significative differences between the two groups have been highlighted about mandibular kinesiology.

5. Conclusion

This study confirms that the functional rehabilitation in patients in orthodontic-surgical treatment occurs in a good way and in a good time.

The functional evaluation in patients during orthodontic-surgical therapy is an important element to reduce as much as possible a incorrect neuromuscular activity that can cause a relapse; it also helps clinicians to follow treatment phases and to control the results obtained.

6. References

[1] Serrao G. Relation between vertical facial morphology and jaw muscle activity in healthy young man. Prog Orthod 2003;4:45-51.

[2] Farronato G. Aesthetic in Ortodontic surgery. Rivista Italiana di chirurgia maxillo-facciale 2003;14(3):123-6.

[3] Avis V. The significance of the angle of the mandible: an experimental and comparative study. Am J Phys Anthropol 1961;19:55-61.

[4] Watt DG. The effects of the physical consistency of food on the growth and development of the mandible and the maxilla of the rat. Am J Orthod 1951;37(12):895-928.

[5] Ferrario VF. The effects of a single intercuspal interference on electromyographic characteristics of human masticatory muscles during maximal voluntary teeth clenching. J Craniomandib Pract 1999;17:184-8.

[6] Ferrario VF. The use of surface electromyography as a tool in differentiating temporomandibular disorders from neck disorders. Man Ther 2007;12(4):372-9.

[7] Jankelson B. Kinesiometrik instrumentation: a new technology. JADA 1975;90:834-40.

[8] Jankelson B. The physiology of the sthomatognatic system. JADA 1953;46:375-86.

[9] Jankelson. Physiological aspects of masticatory muscle stimulation the myomonitor. Quintessence Int Dent Dig 1972;3(12):57-62.

[10] Jankelson B. The intherited methodology of occlusion. Calif Dent Ass meeting San Francisco 1976;10:1-3.

[11] Ueda HM, Ishizuda Y, Miyamoto N, Morimoto N, Tanne K: Relationship between masticatory muscle activity and vertical craniofacial morphology. Angle Orthod 68:233-238,1998.

[12] Sforza C, Peretta R,Grandi G, Ferronato G,Ferrario VF. Soft Tissue Facial Planes and Masticatory Muscle Function in Skeletal Class III Patients Before and After Orthognathic Surgery Treatment. J Oral Maxillofac Surg 66:691-698,2008.

[13] Throckmorton GS, Ellis E III, Bushang PH. Morphologic and biomechanical correlates with maximum bite forces in orthognathicsurgery patients. J Oral Maxillofac Surg 58:515,2000.

[14] Precious DS, Goodday RH, Bourget L, Skulsky FG. Pterygoid plate fracture in Le Fort I osteotomy with and without pterygoid chisel: a computed tomography scan evaluation of 58 patients. J Oral Maxillofac Surg 51(2):151-3,1983.

[15] Dean JS, Throckmorton GS, Ellis E 3rd, Sinn DP. A preliminary study of maximum voluntary bite force and jaw muscle efficiency in pre-orthognathic surgery patients.J Oral Maxillofac Surg 50(12):1284-8,1992.

[16] Thomas GP, Throckmorton GS, Ellis E III, Sinn DP. The effects of orthodontic treatment on isometric bite forces and mandibular motion in patients before orthognathic surgery. J Oral Maxillofac Surg 53:673–678,1995.

[17] Proffit WR, Turvey TA, Fields HW, Phillips C. The effect of orthognathic surgery on occlusal force. J Oral Maxillofac Surg 47:457–463,1989.

[18] Braun S, Bantleon HP, Hnat WP, Freudenthaler JW, Marcotte MR, Johnson BE. A study of bite force. Part 2. Relationship to various cephalometric measurements. Angle Orthod 65:373–377,1994.

[19] Bertelè GP: Trattamento ortodontico-chirurgico. Dental Cadmos 4:13,1989.

[20] Farronato G, Maspero C, Giannini L, Farronato D. Occlusal splint guides for presurgical orthodontic treatment. Journal of clinical orthodontics 9:508-12,2008.

[21] Farronato G, Maspero C, Paini L, Farronato D. Sistematica di programmazione ortodontica-pre chirurgica. Mondo Ortodontico 3:197-202,2004.

[22] Finn RA, Throckmorton GS, Bell WH, Legan HL. Biomechanical considerations in the surgical correction of mandibular deficiency.correction of mandibular deficiency. J Oral Surg 38:257–263,1980.

[23] Van den Braber W, Van der Bilt A, Van der Glas H, Rosenberg T, Koole R. The influence of mandibular advancement surgery on oral function in retrognathic patients: a 5-year follow-up study. J Oral Maxillofac Surg 64(8):1237-40,2006.

[24] Athanasiou AE, Toutountzakis N, Mavreas D, Ritzau M, Wenzel A. Alterations of hyoid bone position and pharyngeal depth and their relationship after surgical

correction of mandibular prognathism. Am J Orthod Dentofacial Orthop 100(3):259-65,1991.

[25] Kobayashi T, Honma K, Shingaki S, Nakajima T: Changes in masticatory function after orthognathic treatment in patients with mandibular prognathism 39(4):260-5,2001.

[26] Tatsumi H, Takada K, Hiraki T, Sakuda M, Minami K, Mori Y, Sugahara T, Sakuda M. A cephalometric electromyographic and kinesiographic appraisal of a patient with mandibular prognathism and anterior openbite malocclusion before and after surgical orthodontic therapy a case report. Osaka Daigaku Shigaku Zasshi 35(2):618-32,1990.

[27] Möller E. The chewing apparatus. Acta Physiol 1966; 69: 571-4.

[28] Ingervall B, Thilander B. Relation between facial morphology and activity of the masticatory muscles. J Oral Rehabil 1974; 1: 131–147.

[29] Bakke M, Michler L. Temporalis and masseter muscle activity in patients with anterior open bite and craniomandibular disorders. Scand J Dent Res 1991 Jun; 99(3): 219-28.

[30] Kayukawa. Malocclusion and masticatory muscle activity: a comparison of your types of malocclusion. J Clin Pediatr Dent 1992; 16(3): 162-77.

[31] Farronato G, Giannì AB, Bianchini R. Problematiche ortognatodontiche funzionali ed open-bite dentario contributo elettromiografico (emg) ed elettrognatografico (egg). Ortognatodonzia Italiana 1992; 3(1):307-321.

[32] Bong K.C, Chun-Hi K, Seung-Hak B. Skeletal Sagittal and Vertical Facial Types and Electromyographic Activity of the Masticatory Muscle. Angle Orthodontist 2007: 77(3): 463-470.

[33] Sassouni V. A classification of skeletal facial types. Am J Orthod 1969; 55: 109-114.

[34] Ahlgren JG, Ingervall BF, Thilander BL. Muscle activity in normal and postnormal occlusion. Am J Orthod. 1973;64: 445–456.

[35] Ahlgren J, Sonesson B, Blitz M. An electromyographic analysis of the temporalis function of normal occlusion. Am J Orthod 1985;87:230–239.

[36] Ingervall B. Facial morphology and activity of temporal and lip muscles during swallowing and chewing. Angle Orthod 1976; 46: 372–380.

[37] Möller E. The chewing apparatus. Acta Physiol 1966; 69: 571-4.

[38] Fogle LL, Glaros AG. Contributions of facial morphology age and gender to EMG activity under biting and resting conditions a canonical correlation analysis. J Dent Res 1995; 74: 1496–1500.

[39] Santoro F, Maiorana C. Il trattamento ortodontico-chirurgico delle disgnazie. Milano: Ariesdue; 1998.

[40] Thomas GP, Throckmorton GS, Ellis E III, Sinn DP. The effects of orthodontic treatment on isometric bite forces and mandibular motion in patients before orthognathic surgery. J Oral Maxillofac Surg 1995; 53: 673–678.

[41] Proffit WR, Turvey TA, Fields HW, Phillips C. The effect of orthognathic surgery on occlusal force. J Oral Maxillofac Surg 1989; 47: 457–463.

[42] Brown DF, Moerenhout RG. The pain experience and psychological adjustment to orthodontic treatment of preadolescents, adolescents and adults. Am J Orthod Dentofac Orthop 1991; 100: 349-56.

[43] Oliver RG, Knapman YM. At Attitudes to orthodontic treatment. Br J Orthod 1985; 12: 179-88.

19

Surgical Orthodontic Treatment of Class III Malocclusions

Paolo Ronchi[1] and Alberto Guariglia[2]
[1]Maxillo-Facial Unit, St. Anna Hospital, Como,
[2]Private Practice, Milan,
Italy

1. Introduction

The correction of dental malocclusions has always had a dual goal, functional and aesthetic. Normal stomatognathic functioning associated with satisfactory facial aesthetics must inevitably have significant repercussions on a patient's general state of health. The physical health of patients with severe malocclusion may be altered or compromised in various ways; if the problem is such as to significantly reduce masticatory capability there may be repercussions on the digestive tract or, in some cases, impossibility of chewing certain types of food. Marked dentoskeletal malposition may cause problems with speech or induce respiratory deficiency in the upper airways.

If teeth are irregular, protruded or crowded it is more difficult to maintain good oral hygiene, with a consequent increased predisposition to caries, and periodontal problems may become severe. Some conditions also predispose to an increased probability of developing temporomandibular joint pain and/or dysfunction (Laskin et al 1986, White & Dolwich, 1992).

Nevertheless, we believe that the aesthetic aspect of severe malocclusion with its related psycho-social impact is more important than the correlated physical problems, above all in modern society. The positive effect of having an attractive face on an individual's mind-frame are clear, in terms of self confidence and self respect; and on the other hand it is quite probable that a subject with a severe dentoskeletal alteration may develop such a significant lack of self-confidence, or even depression of varying severity. Thus the cornerstone for valid treatment must be to combine good functionality and satisfactory aesthetics.

In recent years, increasing numbers of patients elect to undergo orthodontic-surgical treatment to correct severe malocclusion not susceptible to simple orthodontic solution: currently this type of alteration is defined as dentofacial anomaly or dentofacial deformity.

But who should be given orthodontic-surgical treatment in class III patients? The most immediate and the simplest reply to this question, but also the most banal one, is that orthodontic-surgical treatment is necessary whenever orthodontics alone is insufficient to resolve the problem. In reality, this response is both inexact and insufficient, and furthermore it conceals a severe risk: that of beginning exclusive orthodontic treatment only to realize, after treatment is underway, the impossibility of achieving a good final result. This may leave the patient in a dramatic and irreversible situation. Thus the response must be both more complete and more complex (Ronchi, 2005).

In cases of severe malocclusion with dentoskeletal discrepancy there are generally only three possible therapeutic options: modification of growth; camouflage through dental compensation; surgical repositioning of the bony bases.

With regard to growth, it is obvious that the fundamental parameters we must consider are age, gender, type of malocclusion and skeletal involvement in the defect. Clearly, age and gender impose precise limits with regard to the timing of any orthopedic-functional treatment. Furthermore, at present there is reasonable consensus on two fundamental points. Firstly, growth may be modified favorably only in some types of patient, which rather limits this approach: the maxilla or the mandible may be stimulated to grow by a few additional millimeters (much more difficult to limit growth by the same amount) than would have occurred naturally. Thus it is not possible to obtain significant transformations. Secondly, during all orthopedic-functional treatment the teeth inevitably also move in the direction of the correct occlusal relation. This tooth movement, which may be called "dental compensation for skeletal discrepancies" hinders complete orthopedic-skeletal correction and introduces some elements of dental camouflage.

In our view, we may deduce from these considerations, for example, that in Class III, orthopedic treatment only plays a role in cases of slight isolated maxillary hypodevelopment with no mandibular protrusion and without any significant vertical alteration. In all other cases treatment should be postponed until the end of growth, when surgical correction will be applied.

Concerning the purely orthodontic treatment, with regard to subjects in whom growth is complete, it is clear that there is a lot of contingent difficulties relating to tooth movement: periodontal conditions, bone support, morphological and structural characteristics of the alveolar bone in which the teeth must move, patient collaboration and compliance. Furthermore, these camouflage corrections, even if possible from the theoretical and technical standpoints, are not always associated with improvement in facial aesthetics. In reality dental camouflage only leads to an effective improvement of aesthetics in a few situations. More frequently it has no significant influence on facial aesthetics, as in purely orthodontic correction of Class III cases.

We are now in a position to give a rather more complete reply to the above question: in a subject during growth, malocclusion may be considered too severe to be corrected without the help of surgery when the changes to growth that can be achieved with dentofacial orthopedics for that type of condition are not sufficient to ensure an optimal result from the functional and aesthetic standpoints. In an adult with dentoskeletal discrepancy, surgery is the only sure treatment option if the dental defect cannot be corrected by orthodontics alone or if dental camouflage would involve technical or periodontal contraindications, or would not produce a marked aesthetic improvement (Ronchi, 2005).

We may therefore reasonably say that the great majority of adult Class III patients require orthodontic-surgical treatment, chiefly in order to provide an optimal solution to their aesthetic problems.

Lastly, we must consider that the improvement that has come about in surgical techniques over recent years has undoubtedly helped to decrease surgery-related complications and to improve patients' post-operative progress. We may therefore assume that indications to orthodontic-surgical treatment of dentoskeletal discrepancies will continue to increase, above all in the interest of patients. However, we must not forget that all such treatment is always elective, though it is also in part therapeutic and in part preventive; that it involves at the same time and with equal importance both aesthetics and functionality; and that fundamentally it must contribute to improving the quality of life for our patients from the psychological and physical standpoints. This is the approach and the philosophy that must always guide the physician in his or her work and in his or her treatment choices.

2. Clinical features

Clinical examination of a patient with Class III malocclusion, as indeed with all types of dentofacial anomaly, must be extremely thorough; it must analyze occlusion and, above all, must carefully evaluate the morphological characteristics of the face. This type of anomaly cannot and must not only be examined in the sagittal direction, since frequently transverse or vertical alterations exist that are so significant as to influence the treatment plan. Clinical examination of the face takes time and is of particular importance. The face should be evaluated from the front, in profile and in three-quarters profile (Figure 1,2,3,4,5).

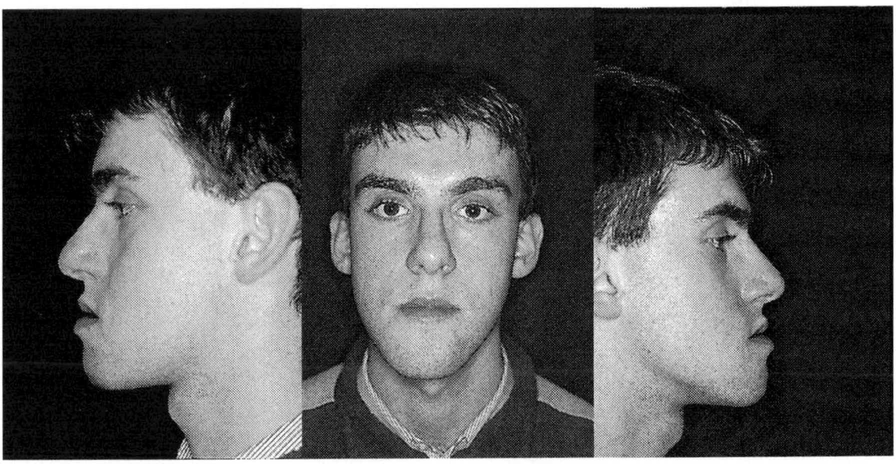

Figs. 1, 2, 3. Front and profile (left and right) of the patient

For simplicity data may be transcribed onto the medical record only for the frontal view and profile, but the evaluation must always be as complete as possible (we must remember that the patient always sees him or herself from the front or in three-quarters profile, almost never in profile!). The clinical examination should begin from the top, proceeding from forehead to neck. The following should be considered: hairline, frontal eminences, palpebral fissures, intercanthal distance, prominence or otherwise of the cheek-bones, thickness of the cheeks and of the soft tissues in general. Particular attention must be paid in these patients to the sub-orbital area, also evaluating the characteristics of the infraorbital rim and determining the presence or otherwise of scleral exposure on looking forwards (Figure 6).

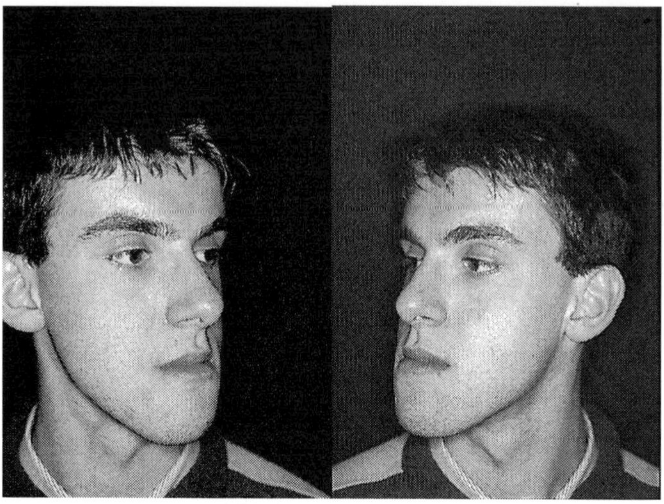

Figs. 4, 5. Three quarter view of the patient (right and left)

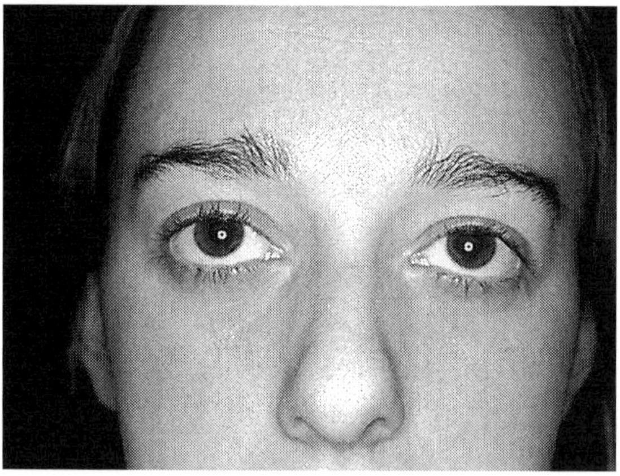

Fig. 6. Tipical example of scleral show

The nose, the central structure of the face, is of great importance in the clinical examination: glabella, dorsum, hump if any, characteristics of the tip, the columella and the opening of the nares should all be carefully examined. The width of the alar base should be measured, both the maximum distance and that at the point of insertion on the upper lip, and their mobility during speech and smiling should also be observed. Lastly, anterior rhinoscopy can reveal any deviation of the septum and the presence of endonasal synechia. The lips must also be examined both at rest and in movement, evaluating shape, thickness and muscle tone, as well as the shape and characteristics of the prolabium and of the Cupid's bow, any hypertrophism of the frenulae, labial competence or incompetence (obviously this is evaluated with the lips completely relaxed with no contraction, see Figure 7,8).

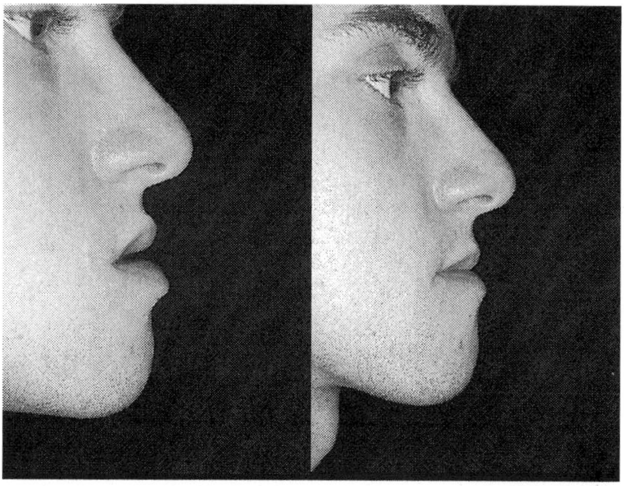

Figs. 7,8. Incompetent lips : contraction of the mentalis muscle during lip closure is evident

Particular attention should be paid to the relationship between lips and teeth and between lips and gingiva, both at rest and when smiling, considering tooth exposure and gummy smile, if any (Figure 9).

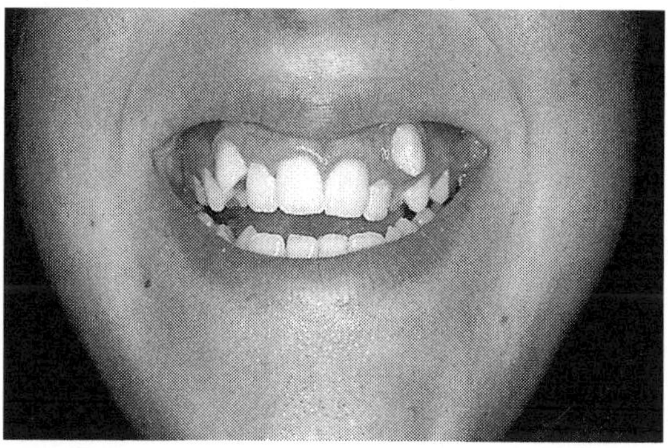

Fig. 9. Tipical gummy smile

Lastly, the nasolabial angle and the paranasal areas must be evaluated and examined for depressions as well as the naso-genial fold, which in some cases may be highly accentuated (Figure 10).

With regard to the clinical examination of the lower third of the face, the overall shape of the mandible should be evaluated, considering the characteristics and position of angles of the mandible, the shape and symmetry of the chin, the presence and extent of the labiomental fold; it is also important to evaluate the shape and characteristics of the angle between neck and chin and the soft tissues beneath the chin (thickness, tone, hypertrophy, excess of soft or adipose tissue) . The endoral examination must only in part be dedicated to the inter-arch relationship (Figure 11).

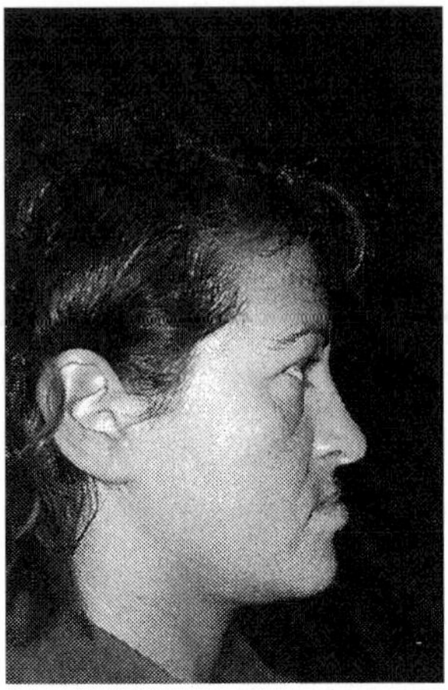

Fig. 10. Depression in paranasal areas

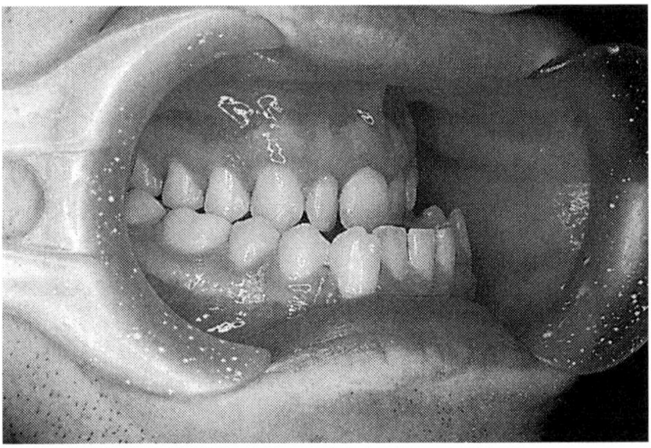

Fig. 11. Tipical example of class III malocclusion

In practice the most significant aspect in this connection consists in quantifying the negative over-jet evaluated at the incisal level; any anterior open bite should also be evaluated. Right from the first examination it is necessary to become used to seeing the two arches independently, since this is the way they will be treated and prepared for definitive surgical correction. The presence and number of teeth must be evaluated, any cases of agenesis, presence of tooth rotation, extent of crowding. The periodontal condition above all of the lower incisors must be carefully evaluated (Figure 12), these being the critical points in the treatment plan for these patients.

Simple clinical examination can reveal the presence and extent of dental compensation at this level. The quality and quantity of adherent gingiva must be evaluated, as must any pockets, the characteristics of the frenulum linguae and of the frenulum labii inferioris.

Lastly, true macroglossia (a very rare condition) must be determined, alongside the presence of undesirable habits and/or swallowing abnormalities.

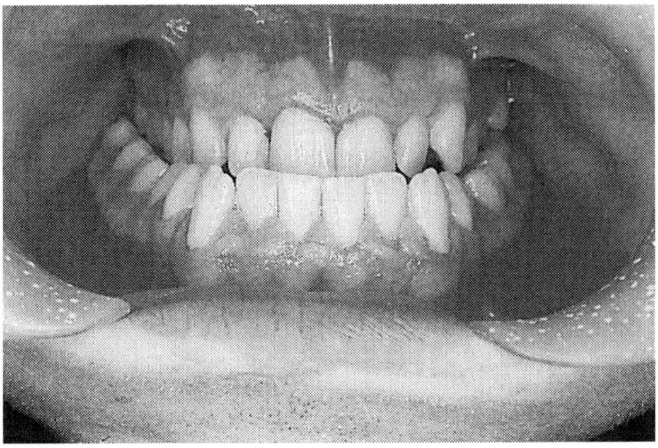

Fig. 12. Lower incisors and their periodontal evaluation

Radiological examination including full panoramic orthopantomography completes the clinical examination of the tooth arches, providing useful elements concerning the presence of any impacted teeth and on the inclination and direction of tooth roots.

3. Cephalometry

An enormous amount has been written on the question of cephalometric analysis in dentofacial anomalies, from Schwarz (1954) analysis of the profile to the more recent and sophisticated analyses by Arnett & Bergman (1993) , via intermediate contributions from Fish & Epker (1980) , and Ricketts (1961). In reality each of these analyses reflects its author's philosophy and intentions, privileging skeletal relationships or those of the soft tissues according to taste.

Cephalometric analysis on a radiograph taken in lateral projection is without doubt an excellent method to study the relationships between skeletal structures and between these and the soft tissues and teeth. It is useful for orthodontic planning of any extractions and consequent choice of anchorage, and it is also a useful tool to verify orthodontic treatment that has been performed in function of profilometric changes. Cephalometry must not however be used as the primary component in diagnosis.

The primary aim of treatment is not to bring cephalometric values within the normal range, but rather to make facial esthetics attractive and to allows a good chewing function, regarding muscular balance and tmj movements. Nevertheless, reaching these two goals is not extremely simple and easy to interpret.

In our opinion cephalometric analysis, in the sphere of orthodontic-surgical treatment, must be extremely simple and easy to interpret, both in the diagnostic phase and during treatment planning; it must also always and constantly be related and integrated with aesthetic clinical examination, and in the case of a discrepancy (always possible!) between the two evaluations, the one that is most useful to achieve our specific aesthetic or functional goal must be followed, on the merits of the individual case.

Cephalometric analysis includes angular and linear skeletal measurements, measurement of the relationship between bony bases and the base of the skull, measurement of soft tissues and/or aesthetic evaluations, dentobasal and dentoskeletal relationships, in all cases respecting the concepts of simplicity and pragmatism given above.

Lateral radiographs must be taken with the teeth in centric relation and the lips in the rest position. The centric relation is always used except in those cases in which there is a marked discrepancy between centric relation and habitual relation. In this case two radiographs are taken, one in centric relation and the other in the habitual position: on that taken in centric relation the sagittal relationship between maxilla and mandible is determined, whereas that taken in the habitual relation is used to measure the vertical dimensions.

In our analysis, the values are subdivided into five groups: maxilla, mandible, vertical parameters, dental parameters and soft tissues.

With regard to the bony bases, we take into consideration three angular measurements to evaluate their position three-dimensionally, and a linear anthropometric measurement to determine length and development. Evaluation of soft tissues, as also that of the vertical dimension, follows the indications given by Fish & Epker (1980) , in their turn taken from Ricketts (1961) analysis (Fig. 13, 14, 15, 16). Nevertheless, all strictly cephalometric and geometric considerations must always be integrated and compared with clinical and aesthetic considerations, and in the case of any discrepancy the surgeon's or the orthodontist's experience and intuition must, as the case merits, privilege clinical diagnosis or cephalometric analysis. Frequently, the final decision will be based on aesthetic considerations.

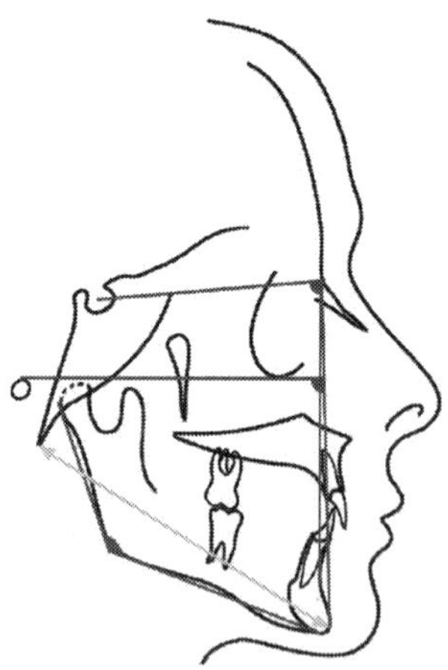

Fig. 13. Mandibular angular (red) and linear parameters (green)

For the mandible the reference values in cephalometric analysis consist of three angular and one linear measurement

The first angle is the angle SNB; the normal value is 80+-2° in men and 78+-2° in women. As in the case of the maxilla, this value is confirmed by the angle at which the Frankfurt plane meets the line N-Pog. The latter value is 89+-3°. These values enable us to determine the antero-posterior position of the mandible.

The linear distance measured from the line joining the basion and the pogonion provides further confirmation concerning size and position of the mandible.
The last measurement taken into consideration is the gonial angle. This value, normally in the range 130+-7°, gives useful indications both for evaluation of the sagittal position of the mandible and, when related to vertical parameters, in studying vertical anomalies and open bite.

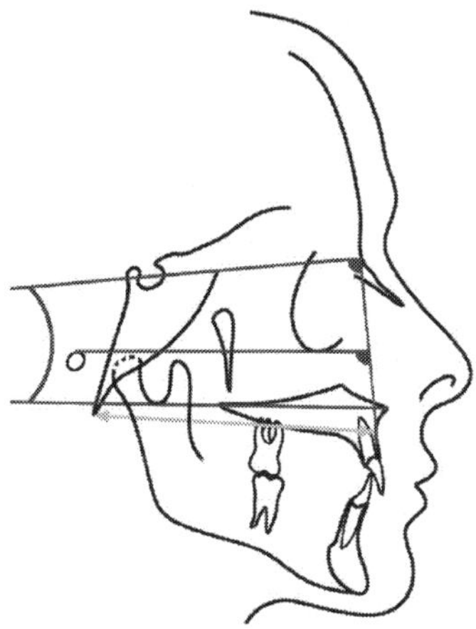

Fig. 14. Maxillary angular (red) and linear parameters (green)

The maxilla is analyzed in relation to the base of the skull in the sagittal and vertical sense by determining three angles and one linear measurement: the angle SNA, the angle Frankfurt/Na, the craniospinal angle, plus the length of the line Ba-A .

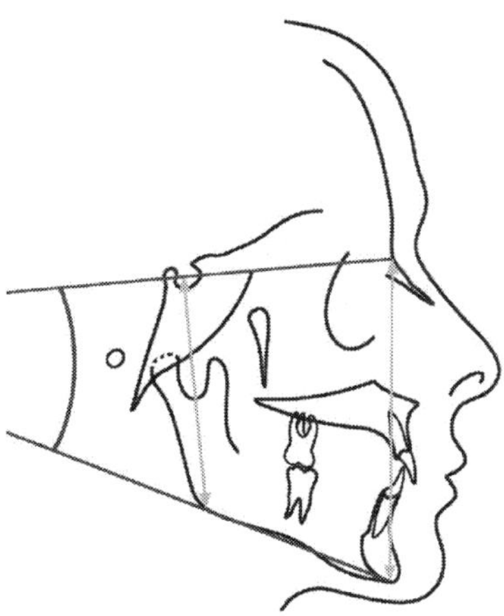

Fig. 15. Vertical angular (red) and linear parameters (green)

The angle SNA, whose normal value is in the range 82+-2° in men and 80+-2° in women, can be to some extent conditioned by the inclination of the plane SN, therefore another angular value is also taken into consideration, that at which the Frankfurt plane meets the line passing through NA. This latter value is normally 90+-3°. This value indicates the antero-posterior position of the maxilla and aids interpretation of dentoskeletal anomalies.
The craniospinal angle (that between the bispinal plane and the plane SN) indicates the position of the maxilla with regard to the base of the skull and may reveal any rotation of the maxilla clockwise or anti-clockwise; this evaluation is very important in diagnosing and planning treatment for open bite (normal value 10+-3°).
Lastly, the antero-posterior position of the maxilla and its sagittal development are confirmed by measuring the line Ba-A, that is the distance between the basion and point A. This value is normally 94+-6 mm in men and 88+-4 mm in women.
The vertical dimension, from the skeletal standpoint, is studied by measuring the angle between the mandible and the base of the skull and the relationship between anterior and posterior vertical dimensions. The angle Go-Me/SN is equal to 32+-4°; wider or narrower values of this angle objectively indicate the presence of open bite or deep bite.
The relationship between anterior and posterior vertical dimension is determined by measuring the segments S-Go and N-Me. This ratio is normally 62+-3%. This parameter enables us to establish with some accuracy whether the subject is normo-, hyper- or hypo-divergent.

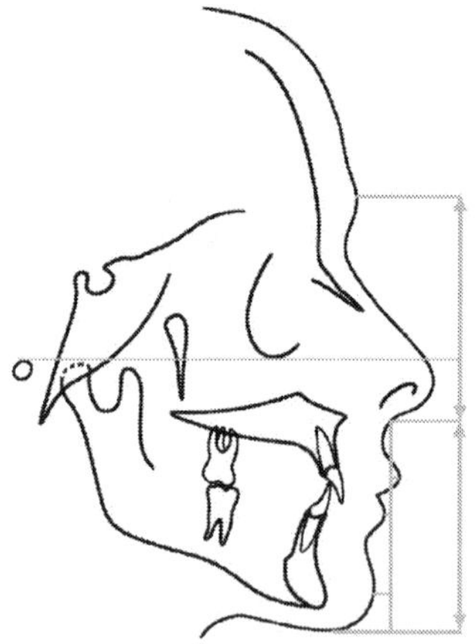

Fig. 16. Linear parameters (green) for the soft tissues

Different types of profilometric analysis have been proposed for the soft tissues . Figure 16 illustrates the analysis method we use, which is extrapolated from analyses by Fish & Epker (1980) and uses the perpendicular to the Frankfurt plane.
In the first instance we observe the ratio between the median third and the lower third, that is between the glabella-subnasale and subnasale-soft tissue menton distances. This ratio is normally 1:1.
We then measure the length of the upper lip, joining the subnasale to the stomion. The normal value is 22+-2 mm in men and 20+-2 mm mm in women; below these values the subject is said to have a short upper lip.

Another reference value in studying the soft tissues is the inter-labial distance. This is measured as the distance between the stomion of the upper lip and the stomion of the lower lip, obviously with the lips in the rest position. Normal values vary from 0 - 3 mm, although higher values are now also accepted, up to 5 mm . Values above 5 mm indicate incompetent lips.

There are also three values that indicate the antero-posterior position of the soft tissues, lips and chin. In this connection we measure the distance from the stomion of the upper and that of the lower lip to a straight line passing through the subnasale perpendicular to the Frankfurt plane. For the upper lip, normal values are between –2 and +2 mm; for the lower lip between –4 and 0 mm. The distance from the same line to the soft tissue pogonion indicates the position of the chin; normal values are between –6 and -2 mm. Naturally, all these numerical evaluations must be related to the overall aesthetics of the face.

On the contrary, where cephalometric analysis has an irreplaceable, almost a dogmatic, value is with regard to the position and inclination of the maxillary and mandibular incisors; their inclination with regard to their respective bony bases must always be rigorously sought and achieved: 109° to the bispinal plane for the maxillary incisors, and 90° to the mandibular plane (Go-Me) for the mandibular incisors.

In the case of significant rotational movements of the maxilla, inclination of the maxillary incisor to the S-N plane must also be taken into consideration; this situation comes about above all in cases of open bite. Compromise solutions over the position of the incisors with respect to their bone bases should only be contemplated where periodontal problems limit the possible orthodontic movement.

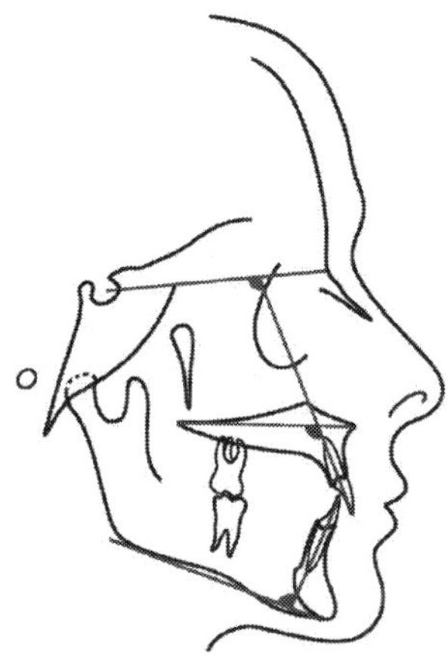

Fig. 17. Angular parameters (red) for maxillary and mandibular incisors

As we have already said, the study of dental relationships is undoubtedly the most important component of cephalometric analysis. These are the only values that, with rare exceptions, must always be brought within the normal range. The cephalometric analysis of the relationships between the incisors and their respective bony bases is the true guide for planning pre-surgical orthodontic treatment, and substantially is the fulcrum of orthodontic decompensation. These values also guide us in the need for any tooth extractions and the choice of anchorage.

As far as the maxillary incisors are concerned, the tooth axis normally forms an angle of 109+-5° with the bispinal plane, and this value must always be respected. The primary task of orthodontic treatment is to bring these values within the normal range. It is known that in cases of dentoskeletal anomaly, the teeth tend to move to compensate for the malocclusion, in an attempt to achieve contact. Thus it is almost normal to find an increased value of this angle in Class III subjects.

Another very important value is the angle the axis of the maxillary incisor forms with the cranial base. The normal value is 103+-2°, and this serves as a point of reference in cases of surgical rotation of the maxilla to correct open bite. In these cases, obviously the bispinal plane also changes, so that a comparison of the two values enables us to modulate the extent of movement of the maxillary incisors.

Another important value that may be considered in the spatial evaluation of the maxillary incisors is the distance between the perpendicular to the Frankfurt plane passing through point A and the most anterior point of the crown of the maxillary incisor. This value is 4 mm.

The same may be said for the mandibular incisor, whose axis forms an angle of 90+-5° with the mandibular base Go-Me. A decrease in this angle is almost always found in Class III subjects, as a compensatory factor for malocclusion.

These are the only cephalometric values that must almost always be normalized, hence the importance of orthodontic planning, because these values will guide us in sagittal movements and in the choice of any necessary extractions to achieve good orthodontic decompensation.

4. Pre-surgical orthodontic treatment

4.1 General principles

Pre-operative orthodontic treatment must aim to obtain two ideal arches capable of being coordinated, with each tooth in the correct position, always treating the two arches separately, and always bearing in mind the goals of the subsequent surgical repositioning.

In order to correctly approach pre-operative orthodontic treatment, careful study of the casts is fundamental. Initially they must be analyzed separately: the shape of the arch (parabolic, triangular, square), the extent of crowding, tooth rotation and the curve of Spee must be evaluated.

Only after this preliminary examination should the relationship between the two arches be examined. It is sufficient initially to position the casts manually with the molars in Class I occlusion, so as to evaluate discrepancies between the two arches that impede their co-ordination and to gain the first general indications concerning the requirements and goals of pre-operative orthodontic treatment (Figure 18). After this first brief and general indication, the first thing to be examined is the position of the maxillary and mandibular incisors, and any crowding. The entire orthodontic treatment plan will be developed from these evaluations as will be explained in detail successively.

With regard to the type of equipment and techniques to be used, we believe that standard equipment and the simplest and most widely used orthodontic techniques are preferable. Brackets cemented directly onto the teeth are perfectly acceptable even for orthodontic-surgical treatment.

Ceramic brackets may be used in the anterior maxillary sector, from canine to canine, whereas metallic attachments are always preferable in the mandibular arch.The first and second molars must always be banded.

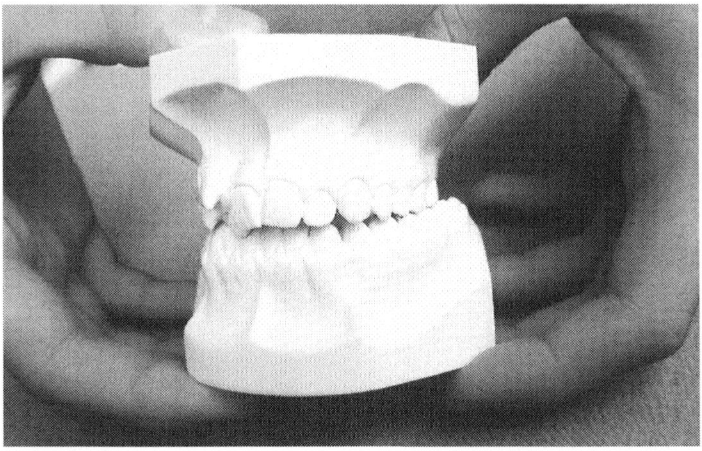

Fig. 18. Preliminary evaluation of arches coordination by positioning the casts in molars class I relationship (see 4.1 general principles)

With regard to the height at which to cement the brackets, on the mandibular arch they must be placed 0.5 - 1 mm more apically than normal to allow for intra-operative and immediate post-operative requirements.

The goals and basic concepts of orthodontic preparation may be subdivided thus: *position of incisors, transverse coordination, dental midlines, symmetry of canines, curve of Spee* (Ronchi, 2005). We will analyze each aspect separately.

4.2 Position of incisors

As we have already said, this is an essential point in all orthodontic-surgical treatment and should probably be considered one of its key points.

Restoration of the correct inclination of the incisors versus their respective bony bases thus becomes a condition "sine qua non" in pre-operative orthodontic treatment. Reference parameters for correct evaluation are exclusively of the cephalometric type. The most suitable and reliable cephalometric values are the inclination of the maxillary incisors on the bispinal plane and that of the mandibular incisors on the mandibular plane (generally Go-Men).

Restoration of the correct position of the incisors, also defined as decompensation, together with correction of any crowding, of necessity dictate whether or not tooth extractions will be required. Normally, mild to moderate crowding of the mandibular arch can be resolved through vestibularization of the incisors without requiring extraction. In general, crowding of 2-3 mm per hemiarch can be resolved in this way; in most cases, correction of the inclination of the incisors is achieved simply by using increasingly heavy square or rectangular archwires. Obviously, in calculating spaces to correct crowding, the starting position and the planned final position of the mandibular incisors must be taken into consideration. In more severe crowding, above 4 mm per hemiarch, the first or second premolars are extracted, depending on whether the crowding is more marked in the anterior or posterior arch sectors . In some situations, tooth condition (extensive carries, root-canal therapy) may dictate extractions.

Similar considerations apply to the maxillary incisors. Since in a high percentage of cases they are markedly vestibularized, decompensation at this level requires an amount of space that can often only be gained by extracting the first premolars. Whether or not therapeutic extraction of premolars is planned obviously conditions the final molar relationship: if extractions are limited to the maxillary arch the final molar relationship will be Class II; if no teeth are extracted, or if they are extracted from both arches, the final molar relationship will be Class I. Therapeutic extractions of the mandibular first premolars in Class III of necessity also involves extracting the maxillary first or second premolars.
The orthodontic procedures required to prepare these patients for surgery (extraction of upper teeth but frequently not of lower teeth, Class II elastics) are thus the exact opposite of corrective orthodontic treatment, and thus produce a temporary worsening of the situation. It is therefore essential to explain this temporary worsening of the functional and aesthetic situation to the patient.

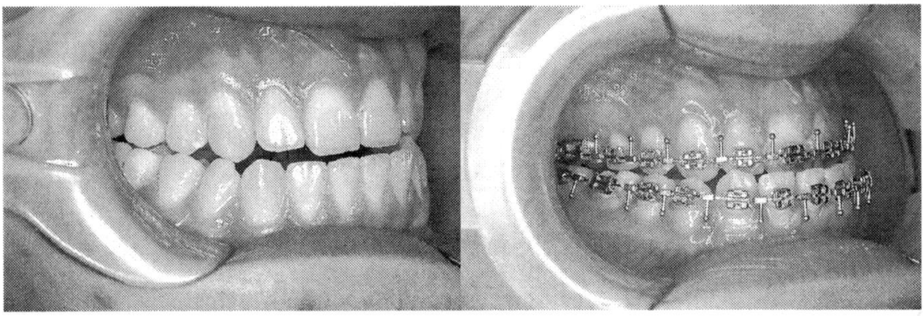

Figs. 19, 20. Decompensation of mandibular incisors

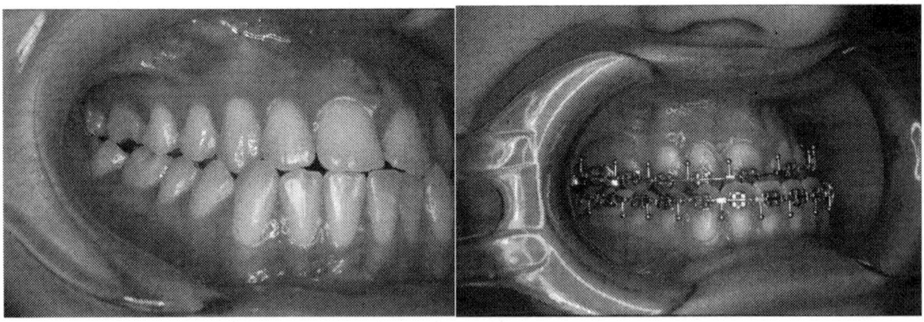

Figs. 21, 22. Decompensation of maxillary incisors by premolars extraction

4.3 Transverse coordination

With regard to this aspect, two fundamental concepts must be taken into account: how to evaluate any lack of transverse coordination, and how to correct it.
As we already said, right from the start of treatment we must become accustomed to looking at each arch independently, so that the transverse relationship must be evaluated on each plaster cast singly, and never on the endoral clinical examination. Furthermore, this step

must only be done after having decided on any premolars destined for extraction, and thus after having established what the molar relationship will be at the end of treatment (molar Class I or Class II). At this point, simply by taking hold of the plaster casts and placing the molars in the planned final relationship, we have a clear view of the transverse relationship and of any need to correct it (Figure 20).

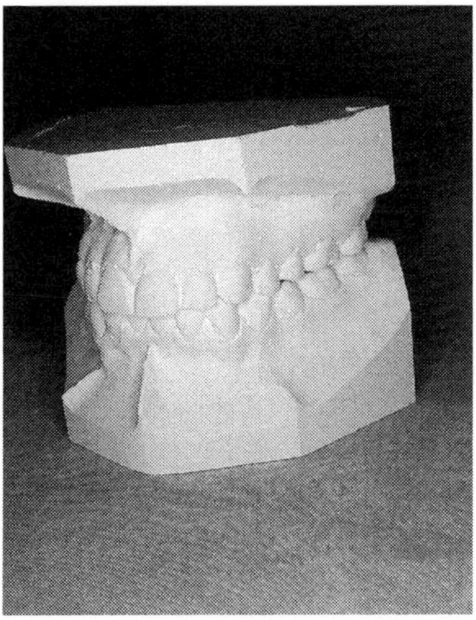

Fig. 23. Evaluating the casts in a Class I relationship shows an acceptable transverse coordination

In Class III an apparent contraction of the maxilla frequently resolves spontaneously simply through sagittal displacement of the bony bases.

In cases in which there is true contraction of the maxilla, the extent of the required expansion must be established, as well as deciding how it can best be achieved. A basic concept is to apply approximately 20% over-correction of the transverse defect; if the transverse deficiency, as measured on the plaster casts, is 3 mm, then orthodontic expansion should be 4 mm.

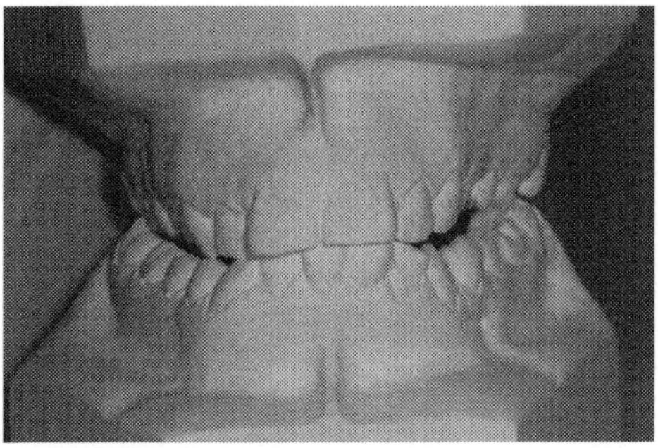

Fig. 24. Evaluating the casts in a Class I relationship shows a true narrowness of the maxillary arch

Even in a patient who has completed growth, expansion of up to 4 mm can generally be obtained orthodontically (through expansion arches, palato-vestibular torque in posterior sectors, Quad-Helix). For values above 4 mm, on the contrary, orthopedic approaches are necessary, such as disjunction of the palatine suture. This procedure may easily be performed in patients up to 16 years of age with the classic palatal torque expansion device cemented onto premolars and molars. Surgically-assisted expansion, which employs osteotomy lines similar to those of the Le Fort I osteotomy, is always necessary above the age of 18 years. In patients between the ages of 16 and 18, the choice of orthopedic or surgically-assisted expansion must take into consideration the patient's skeletal structure (subjects with large bones and with clinical or radiographic signs that growth is complete); in some cases, evaluation of the carpal index; the radiographic appearance of the suture; in any case, for expansions above 8 mm; lastly, cases of failed purely orthopedic expansion.

Once expansion has been achieved, the expansion device must be kept in place for approximately four months. Fixed appliance therapy must follow immediately: the two steps must always take place in a single appointment to avoid the risk of early relapse.

In general, if rapid palatal expansion is required, it should be the first procedure of the entire pre-operative treatment.

4.4 Dental midlines

The concept that must guide the orthodontist and surgeon through all planning and operative phases is that, once treatment is completed, the two dental midlines must coincide not only with one another, but must of necessity fall on the facial midline axis. By "facial midline axis" we mean the axis drawn perpendicular to the bipupillar line, in cases of clinical evaluation, or the axis drawn perpendicular to the line that joins the fronto-zygomatic suture, in the case of postero-anterior cephalometric evaluation. Furthermore, the point that characterizes the mental symphysis must also coincide with the facial midline axis. A discrepancy of 1 mm between the two dental midlines and the facial midline axis may be tolerated

Thus, the ideal and theoretical goal of all pre-operative orthodontic treatment is that the maxillary dental midline coincide with the facial midline axis and that the mandibular dental midline must coincide with the line of mental symphysis; unfortunately, in some cases insuperable orthodontic limits make this impossible.

Concerning the maxilla, initial deviation of the dental midline above 3 mm, requires in general surgical repositioning of the maxilla; the same, in the mandible, when the initial deviation of dental midline is more than 3 mm from symphyisis line, a compensatory genioplasty with lateral translation must be planned.

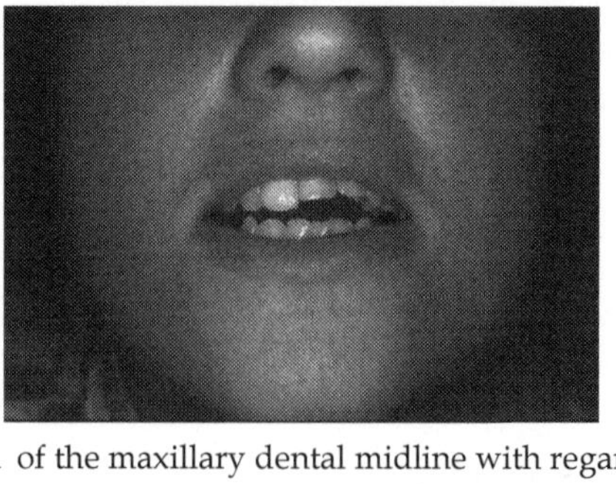

Fig. 25. Evident deviation of the maxillary dental midline with regard to tha facial axis

In case where maxillary osteotomy alone is planned, it is mandatory that orthodontic preparation of mandibular arch perfectly center mandibular dental midline to the facial axis; and the same, when mandibular osteotomy alone is planned, it is necessary that maxillary dental midline exactly coincide with the facial axis. In case when bimaxillary osteotomy is planned, the superimposition of dental midlines and facial axis will be achieved surgically.

4.5 Symmetry of canines

The position of the canines constitutes another key point in pre-operative orthodontic treatment. It is imperative that these teeth occupy a symmetrical position in the two arches. Indeed, an asymmetrical position of the canines would inevitably cause lateral deviation or some form of dentofacial asymmetry.

Thus symmetry of the canines must be obtained through suitable mesio-distal or disto-mesial orthodontic tooth movement. In cases of accentuated asymmetry, strategic unilateral extraction of the premolars may be necessary to achieve this goal correctly.

4.6 Curve of spee

Analysis and management of the curve of Spee in pre-operative orthodontic treatment is of particular strategic importance. First of all it must be remembered that in Class III cases with mandibular dental compensation and tendency to covered bite there is often an accentuated mandibular curve of Spee. The decompensation of the mandibular incisors and leveling of the corresponding tooth arch automatically bring about a flattening of this curve; nevertheless the flattening must not be complete and some curvature, which we could define as physiological, must be maintained in order to simplify management of occlusion immediately post-surgery. Maintenance of some curvature of the mandibular arch enables post-surgical occlusion to be obtained with a slight over-bite (2-3 mm) that facilitates immediate post-surgery physiotherapy and helps to control any tendency to relapse in subsequent weeks and months.

The maintenance of curve of Spee on the inferior arch, associated with an anterior over-bite, necessarily implies, as an inevitable corollary, that the position of the brackets on the mandibular teeth must be 0.5-1 mm more apical than normal positions used in orthodontics, at the least from the first premolars forwards.

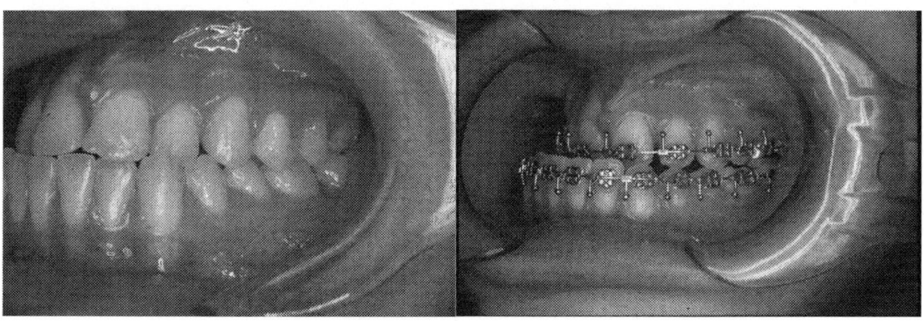

Figs. 26,27. Correction of curve of Spee

In patients with associated anterior open bite, maintaining or increasing curve of Spee must be further exasperated to obtain an over-bite of 3 mm. The position of the mandibular brackets must also be adequate for this purpose. Furthermore, the curvature of the maxillary arch must be maintained and perfectly adapted to the mandibular arch, carefully avoiding creating any posterior lateral open bite, which would bring a high risk of post-operative relapse. Frequently, in patients with anterior open bite, the mandibular curve of Spee is initially flat or even inverse, and pre-operative orthodontic treatment must of necessity recreate a "physiological" curve of Spee.

4.7 New aesthetic appliances

New invisible appliances, like lingual tecnique and Invisilign, propagate in orthodontic field in the last years, to get a better compliance and satisfaction out of patients.

Lingual technique may involve some difficulties in pre-surgical treatment, during models analysis, because, in particular in superior arch, brackets could interfere with a correct occlusion and cause precontacts with the inferior arch.

Furthermore, in any case, during surgical and post-surgical phases vestibular appliances are necessary to make an intermaxillary temporary fixation or to positioning post-surgical occlusal elastic guide. Since a kind of appliance both vestibular and lingual is not thinkable, replace lingual tecnique with vestibular one, or prepare a vestibular device easily compatible with the lingual one, become unavoidable. Indeed, bars, in this case, are hardly to position and to manage.

In the following pictures we show an illustrative case.

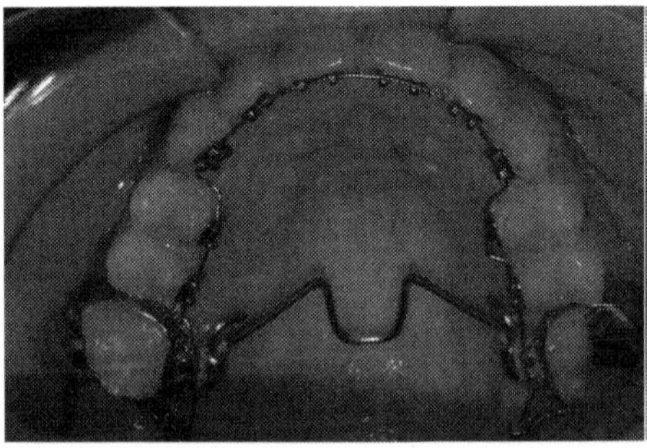

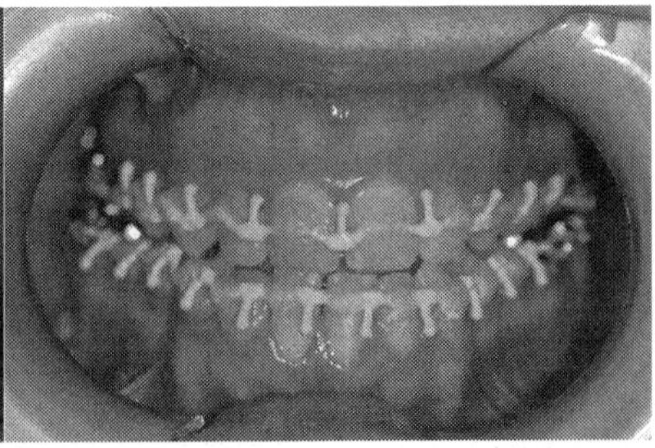

Figs. 28, 29. Example of lingual tecnhique

Invisilign treatment has certainly less difficulty, but dental movements with this technique may be limited, especially regarding extrusion, rotation and torque of the teeth. So, this kind of device is indicated in selected cases, and is it often necessary to change the technique into the traditional full-brackets vestibular appliance in the last phases of the presurgical orthodontic treatment.

However, if we want to make use of this tecnique for all the treatment length, and if that is possible from the orthodontic point of view, we have to use bars during surgical and immediatly post-surgical phases and, most important, a perfect surgical occlusion, without precontacts, is mandatory, because elastic occlusal guide has more effect on bars than on dental arches.

In the following pictures we show an illustrative case.

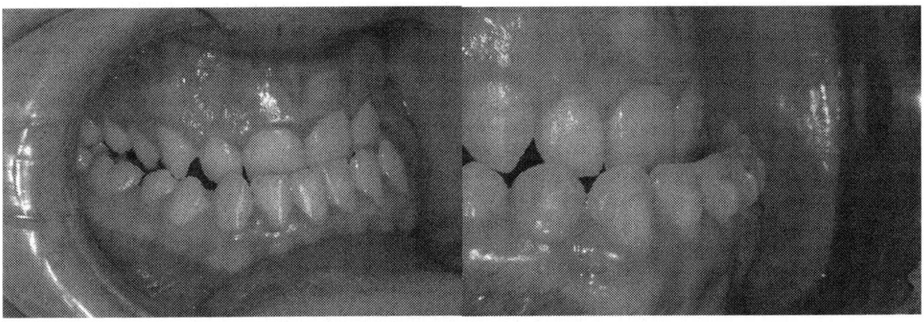

Figs. 30, 31. Full preoperative orthodontic treatment with Invisalign

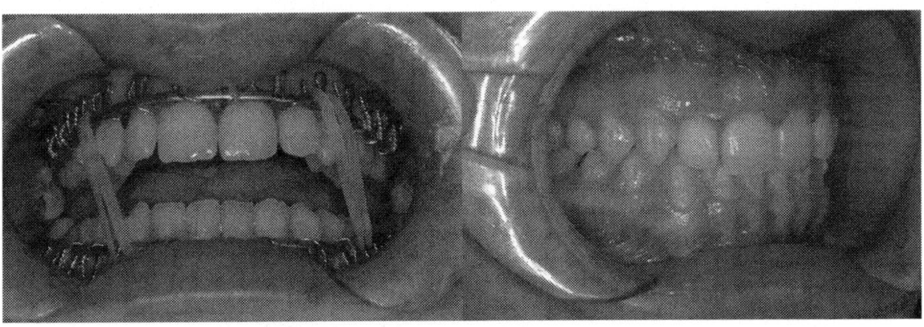

Figs. 32, 33. Immediate post-surgical phase with bars, and final occlusal result

5. Surgical procedure selection

Furthermore, surgical correction of Class III cases must always be postponed until growth is completed and thus, in general terms, not before 18 years of age for women and 19 or 20 for men. Surgical correction that is done too early can easily lead to a relapse due to residual mandibular growth.

The choice of surgical procedure to correct Class III cases essentially takes into account aesthetic evaluation in the three planes of space: sagittal, vertical, and transverse. It must answer the following question: which is more appropriate, a maxillary osteotomy, a mandibular osteotomy or a double jaw operation? Cephalometric analysis of skeletal structures takes second place after aesthetic considerations; if skeletal values are in agreement with the surgical approach selected on aesthetic grounds, so much the better; if not, then aesthetic evaluation should always dominate.

From the sagittal standpoint, the parameters that indicate advancement of the maxilla with Le Fort I osteotomy are: flattening of the paranasal areas, accentuated naso-genial fold, moderate flattening of the cheek-bones, obtuse nasolabial angle, maxillary prolabium little in evidence, prominent nose with some degree of hump and tip tilted downwards

Where a larger increase at the middle third is necessary, Bell's high osteotomy may be taken into consideration, because this provides greater filling at the cheek-bones (Bell et al, 1988)

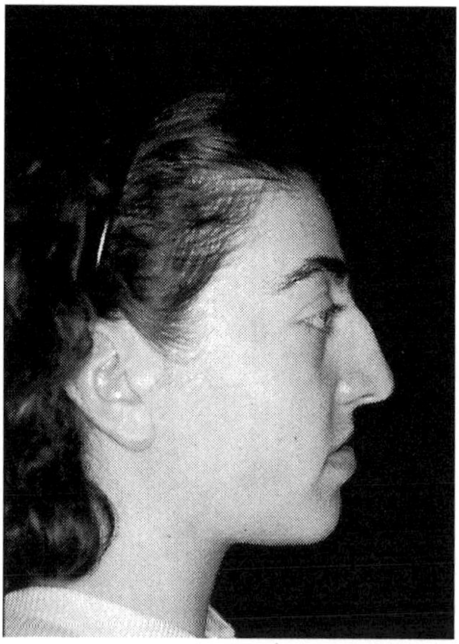

Fig. 34. Tipical case in wich is indicated an advancement Le Fort I ostetomy

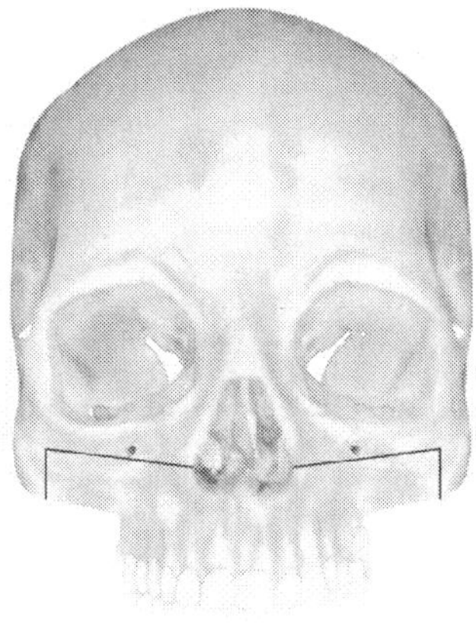

Fig. 35. High Le Fort I osteotomy according by Bell

In cases of severe hypoplasia of the middle third of the face, with flattening of the inferior orbital rim and scleral exposure, a maxillo-malar osteotomy may be employed (Keller & Sather 1987). However, this type of osteotomy only affords limited vertical or transverse movement and thus indications are specific: anomaly that is solely antero-posterior, normal or decreased vertical dimension, maxillary dental midline coinciding with the median axis of symmetry or at most deviated by 2 mm. In other cases, where this type of osteotomy cannot be adopted, the best alternative is the classic Le Fort I osteotomy associated with implantation of alloplastic material or lipofilling in the sub-orbital area.

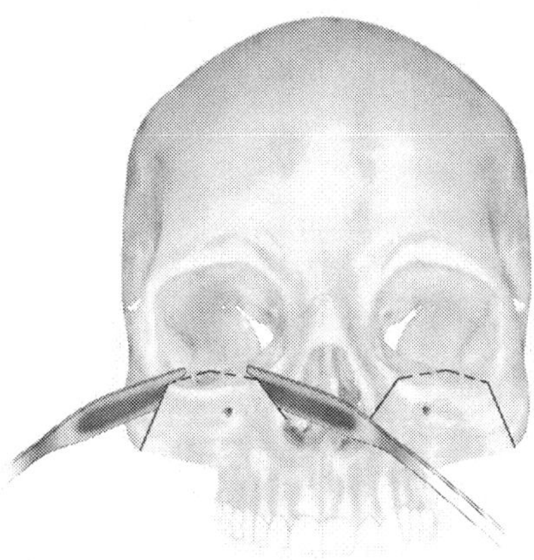

Fig. 36. Intraoral maxillo-malar osteotomy

In few selected cases, a true anterior position of the mandible and chin requires a mandibular set back alone. In this case it is necessary that cheek, nose and superior lip have a good balance. However, correction of Class III cases with mandibular osteotomy alone should be limited to clinical situations with negative over-jet not above 3-4 mm.
Indeed, marked mandibular setback may produce excess soft tissue beneath the chin, which is negative from the aesthetic standpoint, and cause a reduction of posterior airway space, with possible tendency to develop an OSAS in the future (Riley et al, 1987).

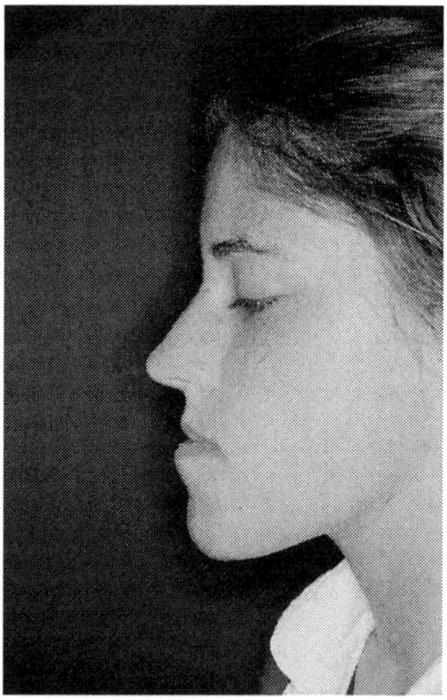

Fig. 37. Tipical case in wich is indicated a mandibular set back alone

In a great number of patients, for larger amount of initial over-jet, double jaw osteotomy should otherwise be preferred because it guarantees in these cases greater skeletal and muscular stability, a less stretching of the pterygomasseteric sling, and in order to avoid excessive bi-protrusion.

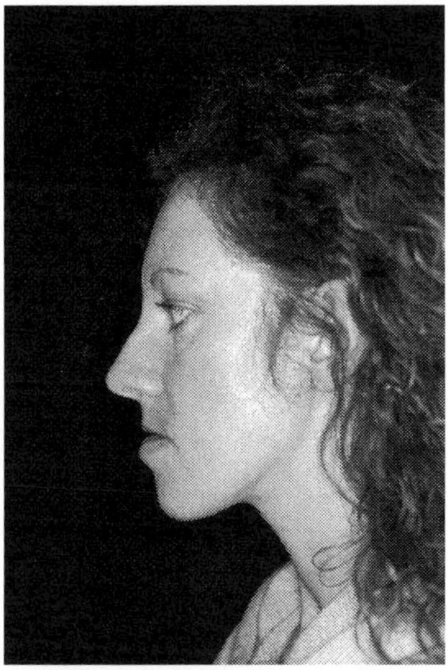

Fig. 38. Tipical case in wich a double osteotomy is indicated

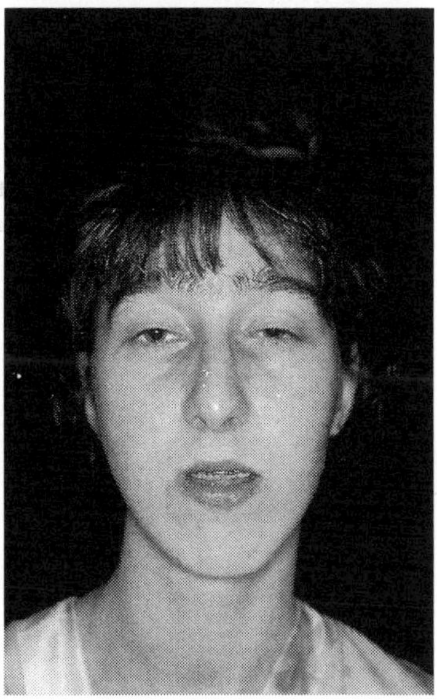

Fig. 39. Tipical case in wich is indicated a bimaxillary osteotomy with superior repositioning of the maxilla

With regard to the vertical dimension, the fundamental parameters to take into consideration are: relationship between lips and teeth, gummy smile if present, labial competence or incompetence, and the ratio between middle and lower thirds of the face. A

vertical excess of the maxilla with labial incompetence, gummy smile and excessive tooth exposure tends to indicate repositioning the maxilla superiorly.
On the contrary, in a small percentage of cases characterized by little vertical development and insufficient tooth exposure (short face) repositioning the maxilla downward is indicated. If, on the contrary, the vertical excess is exclusively in the lower third, genioplasty with vertical reduction will be required.
With regard to transverse dimensions, these concern both the occlusal relationship and aesthetic parameters. From the occlusal standpoint, transverse discrepancy should be corrected, as we have already seen, during pre-operative orthodontic treatment. Only in some particular cases may segmental maxillary osteotomy, in two or more pieces, be taken into consideration. However, the transverse changes that can be obtained with these types of osteotomy are fairly limited: 4 - 5 mm with regard to maxillary expansion and this limitation is due to the fact that the palatine fibro-mucosa is not elastic (Proffit et al, 1996).
With regard to aesthetics, the fundamental parameter in the transverse dimension is the ratio between the bi-zygomatic and the bi-gonial widths. In Class III cases there is usually a reduced bi-zygomatic width, and various methods exist to achieve an increase in this measurement, as lipofilling or biomaterial implants.
With regard to correction of the mandibular angles, this may quite easily be done endorally by remodeling with a pear-shaped bur, or through otsteotomy and resection with an angled saw.

6. Post-operative orthodontic treatment

In the first post-operative weeks, the active and passive physiotherapy is essential: active mandibular movements, again guided by elastics, are gradually increased. Normally, over a 2-week period, the patients achieve a substantial degree of mandibular opening, about 3.0 to 3.5 mm, and the physiotherapy is complete at about 4 to 6 weeks.
After the physiotherapy phase is finished, the patient may begin the final orthodontic treatment. The goal is to achieve occlusal relationships that we might define as ideal, in terms of canine class, molar class and coincidence of the dental midlines. In practice, in this phase some simple orthodontic maneuvers will suffice, such as closing any small residual diastemas, correcting a slight lateral cross-bite, perfecting intercuspidation, optimizing over-jet and over-bite.
Obviously the duration of the final orthodontic phase depends on the degree of preparation achieved during pre-surgical treatment. In most cases, however, two or three months will suffice.
Retention, in orthodontic-surgical treatment, serves the dual purpose of stabilizing tooth relationships and contributing to skeletal stability, although in our opinion this latter point depends to a greater extent on other factors, such as correct condylar position and condition of the musculature. It is, however, important to stress that good dental retention contributes to maintaining the final occlusion that was achieved surgically, guaranteeing occlusal stability, which will surely have positive repercussions on the final stability in the widest sense. In general, the methods used for retention are those used in traditional orthodontics rather than in surgical treatment.
Fixed retainers are normally preferred, applied to the mandibular and maxillary anterior sectors, in cases of high risk of dental relapse in these areas (resolution of tooth crowding without extraction, decompensation). In some cases, especially at the maxillary arch, it may be indicated to use removable retention plates of various types, for example to be worn at night, partly to guarantee stability of orthodontically and orthopedically corrected transverse relations.

7. Clinical cases

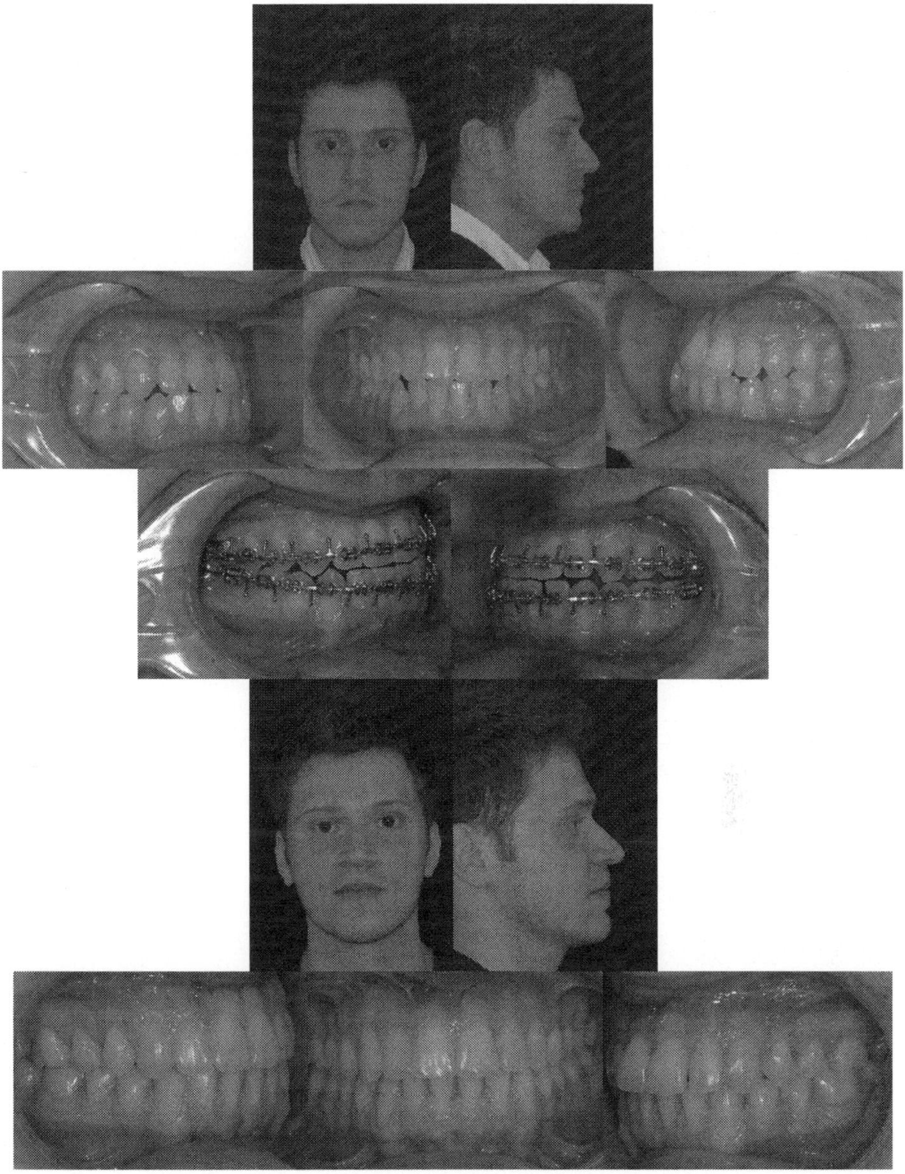

Case 1. Class III deformity with maxilla hypoplasia. Presurgical orthodontic treatment with Invisalign and vestibular brackets just on surgical phases. Surgical correction with Le Fort I maxillary osteotomy. Result two years later.

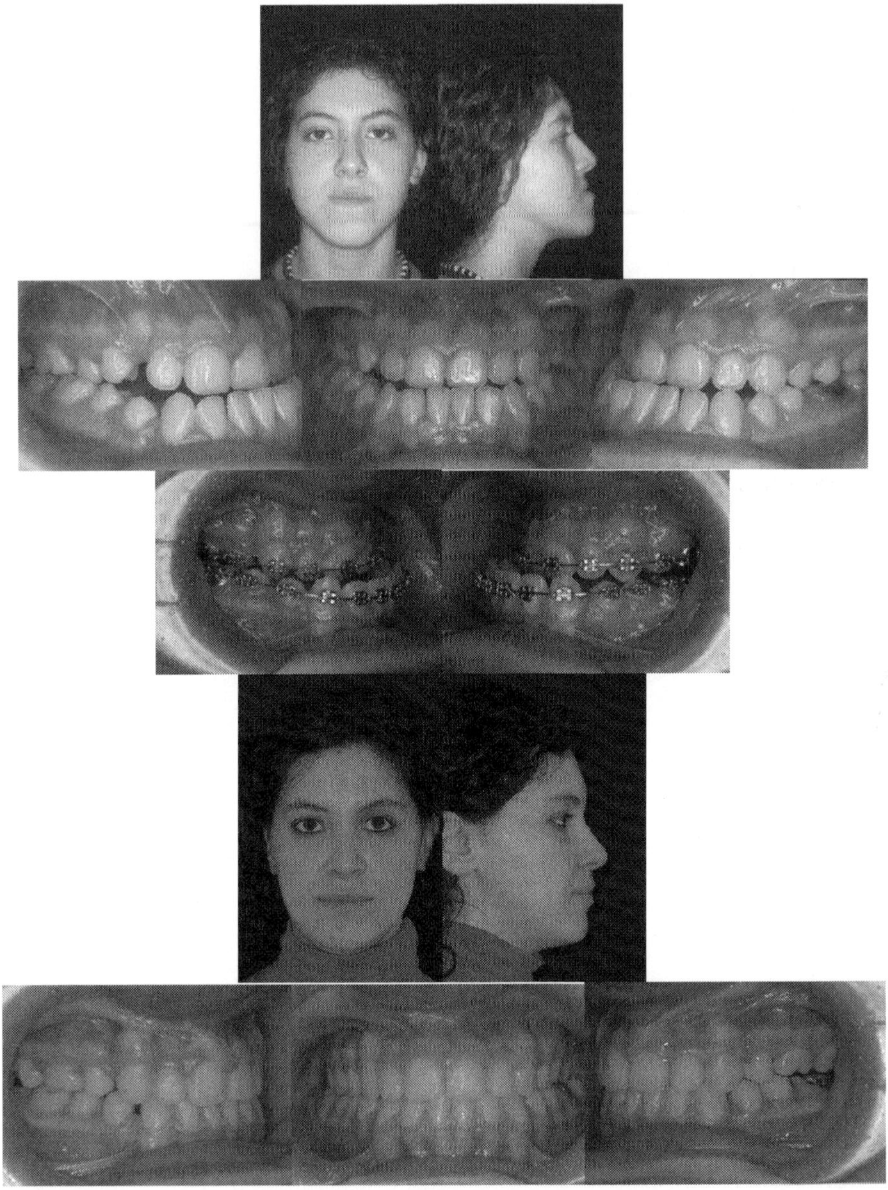

Case 2. Class III deformity. Presurgical orthodontic treatment with fixed appliance and decompensation of superior and inferior incisors, extraction of 14 and 24. Surgical correction with bimaxillary osteotomy (Le Fort I maxillary osteotomy and mandibular set back.) Result six years later

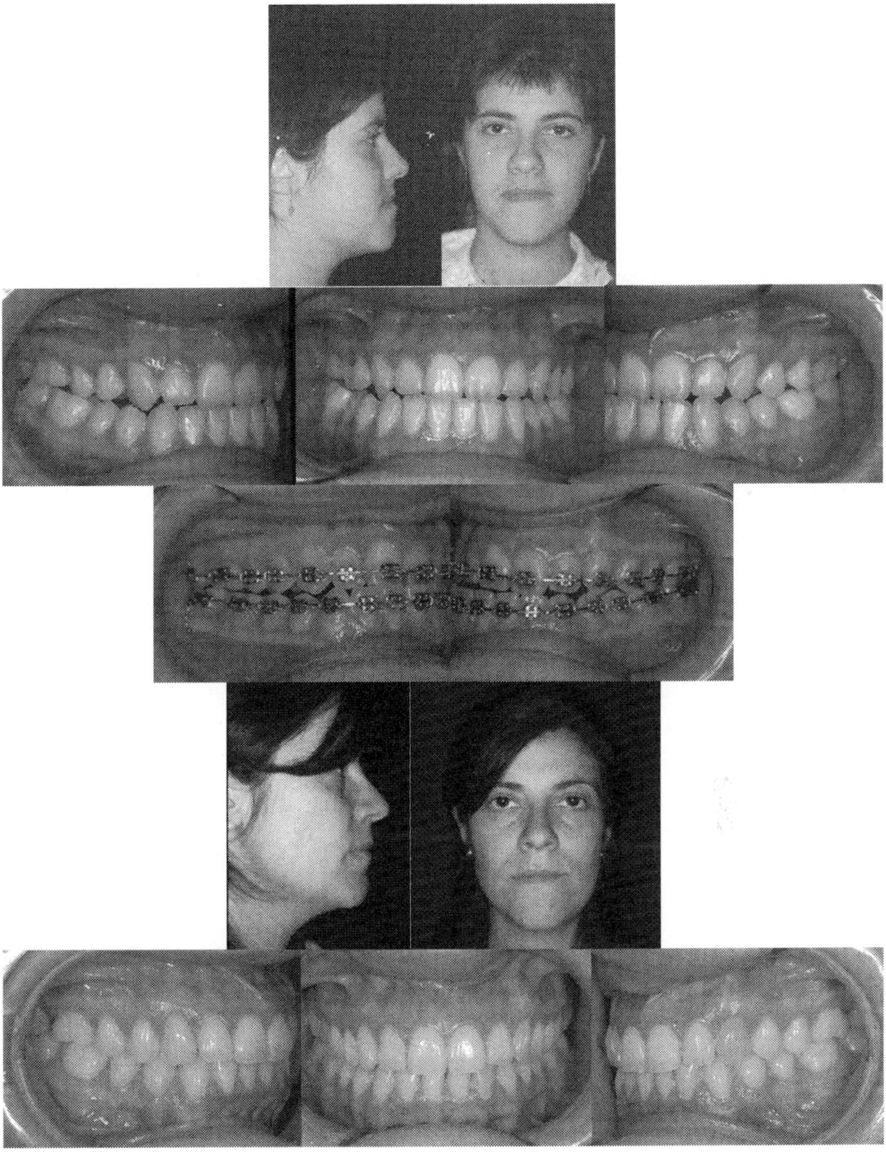

Case 3. Class III deformity. Presurgical orthodontic treatment with fixed appliance and decompensation of mandibular incisors. Surgical correction with mandibular set back alone. Result ten years later.

8. References

Arnett G.W., Bergman R.T. (1993) : Facial keys to orthodontic diagnosis and treatment planning. Part I *Am. J. Orthod. Dentofac. Orthop.* Vol. 103, pp. 299-312

Bell W.H., Mannai C., Luhr H.G. (1988) : Art and science of the Le Fort I downfracture. *Int.J.Adult. Orthod. Orthognath.Surg.* vol. 1, pp. 23-52

Fish L.C., Epker B.N. (1980) : Surgical-orthodontic cephalometric prediction tracing *J. Clin. Ortod.* vol. 14, pp. 36-52

Keller E.E., Sather A.H. (1987): Intraoral quadrangular Le Fort II osteotomy. *J.Oral. Maxillofac. Surg.* Vol. 45, pp. 223-232

Laskin B.M., Ryan W.A., Greene C.S. (1986) : Incidence of temporomandibular symptoms in patients with major skeletal malocclusions: a survey of oral and maxillofacial surgery training programs *Oral. Surg. Oral. Med. Pathol.* vol. 61, pp. 537-541

Proffit W.R., Turvey T.A., Phillips C. (1996) : Orthognathic surgery : A hierarchy of stability *Int J Adult. Orthod. Orthognath. Surg.* vol. 11, pp.191-204.

Ricketts R.M. (1961) : Cephalometric analysis and synthesis *Angle Orthont.* vol. 31, pp. 141-156

Riley R.W., Powell N.B., Guilleminault C., Ware W. (1987) : Obstructive sleep apnea syndrome following surgery for mandibular prognathism. *J. Oral Maxillofac. Surg.* vol. 45, pp. 450-452

Ronchi P. : (2005) : *Orthodontic Surgical Treatment of Dentofacial Anomalies. An Integrated Estthetic Functional Approach.* Ed. Quintessence Publishing, ISNB 9708-0-86715-397, New Malden

Schwarz A.M. (1954) : Ueber eckzahnverlagerung und ihre Behebung *Fortchr-Kieferorthop* vol. 15, pp. 119-112

White C.S., Dolwick F. (1992) : Prevalence and variance of temporomandibular disfunction in orthognathic surgery patients. *Int.J. Adult. Orthod. Orthognath Surg* vol. 7, pp. 7-14

Part 5

Research

20

Does Comtemporary Orthodontics Comply with Universal Logic?

Hicham Khayat
Maitrise Universitaire en Orthodontie et Orthopédie Dento-Faciale
Diplôme Universitaire de Prothèse et de Réhabilitation Maxillo-Faciale
Diplôme Universitaire d'Implantologie Chirurgicale Orale et Maxillo-Faciale
Certificat post-universitaire de Radiologie Tridimensionnelle Dento-Maxillo-Faciale
Head of Polyclinique Dentaire Casablanca's Global care department
Morocco

1. Introduction

Contemporary orthodontic practice is segmented into schools and methods. These divisions within the specialty lay bare the lack of consensus on such fundamental issues as the conduct of the diagnosis, the design of a treatment plan or the fundamentals of appliance's mechanics!
Such a situation would not be acceptable in any other medical discipline. Our purpose is to highlight a few inconsistencies responsible for this situation, under the harsh lights of philosophy and history of medicine.

2. Clinic

In the late eighteenth century, a new concept of Mankind takes place. Along with the development of sciences, the growing accumulation of knowledge boosted by the advances in printing, and an improved flow of knowledge. By grouping the patients in the same place-the hospital, initially a "mourroir"[1], a place where sicks were taken to die, the society, aiming to prevent epidemics, has extracted the patients from their own personal conditions, their homes and their family care; Thus Reducing the variability of forms of the same "disease" mainly related to the terrain; Thus making possible the observation of similarities in different patients. And finally society has created the conditions giving rise to another view, another thought: A new method based on the observation of symptoms and signs, the methodical and comprehensive grouping and consolidation of these "clinical signs"in "tables". This method took place although no one claimed to have built it and deeply contrasted with the previous discurses. The clinical method, that is to say modern medicine was born. It is constituted as a way of thinking opposed to the archaic medical practice. By "Clinique", was meant a "rationalist methodology" of medicine.
This original meaning has been forgotten over time. Many doctors today confuse it with office. This confusion may reflect the fact that in his genealogy, the clinic combines the knowledge, the Sick and the Institutions. As Michel Foucault has shown, its foundations are local, political and institutional factors. When the fundamentals changes, knowledge changes and sometimes loses. The doctors have forgotten the meaning of the Clinic. They

have forgotten his former discoveries. Worse, doctors have forgotten that they have forgotten, willing to remember no more than the incompressible know-how mandatory to exercise: the technique.

As the clinic was established to accommodate the new, it disintegrates as it is no more than preserving what is already known, a repetition of what is already certain. Moreover, today, among the fundamental basis of contemporary orthodontics, medical marketing in all its forms, plays an increasingly important role.

Any theory always vanishes at the patient's bedside. The first premise of the clinical method is the perfect match between the visible and the expressible. Recovery without rest between the visible and the expressible. This is the logic of Condillac, the vision of a talking eye. With the clinical method, the eye finally cleared of chimeras is ready to welcome the new. And to describe it. Appoint to recognize. Recognize to treat. Probabilistic reasoning will appear and anatomopathology will assign a seat to evil in the very thickness of the living. But the Clinic which is whole based on this unprecedented relationship between vision and language should not be reduced to the systematic collection of signs already described. The "look" of the clinician, in any discipline is, and has to be the basis of any progress. Based on what is known as certain, with an extensive multi-disciplinary vocabulary, the true clinician will find the key point without losing his way gazing to everything and measuring everything. The eye must keep its edge. Beware of habits and systems. Reject the blinders of theory. Stay acute in order to detect the different, the new and the subtle.

3. Care givers and the principle of rationality

In preclinical times, men and women took over the health of their community, claiming to enjoy a mythical rationality[2]. The witch healers from prehistoric times invoked the devil. The priests of ancient times interceded for the patient with the divine (Serapis in Egypt, Apollo and Aesculapius in Greece ...). But the church abhorred blood: *Ecclesia abhorret a sanguine*. The monks of the Middle Ages are striving to console the sick: Question: Why does God allow us to endure such terrible evils? Answer: Because it is expedient for His glory and for the good of our soul. God is purifying its elected. He is not a judge who punishes. He is a father who corrects and chastises his beloved sons. And thus, the evils become great assets.The doctors were, mostly, members of the clergy and therefore unable to practice surgery. Surgery is thereby relegated to a lower rank in society, mainly performed by tooth-pullers, fairground merchants or barbers. They will become our ancestors, the "barber-surgeons", after a long conflict with the organized, educated and Latin-speaking body of physicians. With the clinical method and the more predictable and reproducible therapeutic results it provides, the care giver becomes a scientist. Accused yesterday of *mentir comme un arracheur de dents* (NDLT: "lying like a tooth-puller") dentists today aspires to an evidence-based practice.

Contemporary Orthodontics is a living example of the decline of the clinic. For many renowned authors, performing a diagnostic is no more than obtaining senseless measures compared to meaningless tables the only justification for which being the fact that everyone uses them. It rejects the individual in a face or a smile, while the clinic was established to the contrary from the individual, to welcome the new far from any dogmatic closure.

Treatments are standardized. As the barber who only deals with bleeding, we simply perform the same techniques reported by few measures and a programmable frame of mind, moving away from the path of Hippocrates who was attached to the observation and despised any form of system.You have to observe and to look askew. As mentioned by

Michel Foucault, "Looking askew" is a productive intellectual tactic, a must for clinical way of thinking. This is an invitation to observe from a novel standpoint, the intellectual processes by which we assess the functional or aesthetic situation of our patients and transform it into a good outcome through our diagnosis and our treatment.

4. Seeing, knowing, treating

Looking askew is the condition of birth of new thinking and relevant mind processes. Learning to see better, to see differently, learning to describe better. This is the only approach that always has and can still allow the emergence of better paradigms in phase with the up-to-date knowledge and cutting-edge technologies. See the subject but also its further investigations. Open to all vocabularies of modern dentistry and more broadly to any exact and universal knowledge.

5. Measuring, calculating, executing

In contrario, the "ready to wear thought system", and its inconsistencies, violate the fundamental clinical postulate, veiled the eyes of the practitioner, format his vocabulary and confine his arguments. The technique comfortably installs the practitioner in a robot status from witch that may be difficult to break free. Retreating into its certainties, abdicating critical sens and without curiosity about the fundamentals, the practitioner takes the risk of falling into dogmatism. The speech, the challenges and promises of the Clinic are threatened with extinction in the furrows of the technique and repetition.Today, orthodontic diagnosis is often based on a "fetishist" methodology : The dimensional statistical cephalometry.
Implicitly, this assumes that there is a cephalometrical numerical standard, a geometric "ideal" [3]canvas which can serve as an *étalon* to establish a diagnosis, develop a treatment plan and express a prognosis. This contradicts the morphological and biological variability of living organisms. The majority of cephalometric analysis authors has cautioned against the misuse of their own indicators and have sometimes confessed to their arbitrairy. Nevertheless, the ease of the method, compatible with delegation and mass-practice orthodontics has assured its wide spreading among doctors and scholars. In the other hand, a relevant vision of the human head brought by architectural analysis does exists. Here, the clinician's eye look at the pillars, beams, arches and voids that form a functional structure, lively and full of meaning: The scene and spectacle of oral and facial function.
Once and for all, our purpose is not to condemn cephalometry. It keeps sens as a comparative or statistical tool, but to warn against shortcuts ang this kind of magic thinking that transforms a few integers without any clinical signification into a diagnostic panacea. Warn against The Mismeasure of Man. Againt this "eugenic" Violence of caregivers, forcing life-wide "cases" into narrow "boxes".The difference is enormous between a physician who takes the time to observe and one who "reads" labels, pasted on a radiological shadow.The aesthetics, which occupies a central place in the pattern of consultation and the therapeutic purpose is rarely the subject of academic teaching in our specialty. Straight lines, disastrous shortcuts of hurry thinking[4], hides the faces. Blind clinician Eyes.

6. Recipes instead of thinking

We see the tooth moving but, in reality,it is the socket that moves. Mechanics is the essence of orthodontic treatment. The resulting forces at the periodontal interface multiplied by the amount of tooth displacement is a mechanical energy than is expressed in joules. Thus, for an equal outcome, the best treatment, the most respectful, may well be that which minimizes the total energy transmitted to the periodontal tissues, labile but delicate. Periodontium, as a biological entity, is blind to the endless sophistications of our self-ligating or heat-memory fireworks. Only count the pressures that stimulate or otherwise degrade it. Primum non nocere.Basically, a force is an active ingredient, similar to a pharmacological molecule. The analogy is fruitful since the application point and direction of a force, as the tropism of a molecule, determines the target tissue. The intensity of a force equals to the dosimetry and the duration of exposure to the setting time. In the state of the art, and unusually for orthodontics, we accept that overdosing, over-treatment or bad prescription are not the key poiny.The debate focuses mainly on "ideal" bracket "information", easy opening, easy closing, etcetera. Magic thinking again. Marketing as the foundation of the clinic.Mechanics is an exact science, fortunately, as every day our lives depends on it. Nevertheless, it is never treated seriously. The vast majority of orthodontic literature figures are senseless from a "mechanical" point of view. Several authors have based upon physicists mechanics and contributed to the successful rationalization of orthodontic's mechanics. Their universal input does not enjoy the same penetration in the professional body that the ready to wear technique. They offen have nothing to sale and therefore no communication budget !

Sapere aude! Dare to think, "cried Emmanuel Kant to his contemporaries to help them break free of the intellectual minority[5]. The field of the unthought in orthodontics is much wider than one might think at first sight. The advent of evidence-based orthodontics in the soil of fetishism and inconsistencies of the specialty is problematic. A cure of common sense is highly indicated . "Common sense is the best shared thing in the world, for everyone thinks he is so well equipped that even those who are hardest to satisfy in everything else do not usually want to have more than they do. And as the diversity of our opinions do not come from what some are more reasonable than others, but only that we conduct our thoughts in various ways, and do not consider the same things "[6]

7. Conclusion

Turning his back on exact sciences and universal knowledge, the contemporary orthodontic practice is locked into normalized and similar techniques. Major Clinical issues are sinking in the furrows of repetition. In this context, the research is often a daily checking of what is already known. Innovations are too often minor improvements of what is already used. It will be interesting to retrieve all the subversive potential of the true Clinical method. Subversive in the truest sense, which is put in reverse, move things, violate the order things establish between themselves, and finally overcome them. It is urgent to move away from dogmatic closure. There hides the promises of the clinic.

8. References

[1] Foucault M, Naissance de la Clinique] XXXX

[2] Lebrun S] Se soigner autrefois] Médecins, saints et sorciers au XVII° et XVIII° siècles] Histoire.

[3] Gould S.J] The Mismeasure of Man] New York] WW Norton.

[4] Sabot P] L'Expérience, le savoir et l'Histoire dans les premiers écrits de Michel Foucault] Archives de Philosophie 2006 ;69 :285-303.

[5] Kant I] Was ist Aufklarung ? Berlinische Monatschrifte, 1784.

[6] Desccartes R] Le discours de la méthode] 1637.

21

The Artificial Intelligence Approach for Diagnosis, Treatment and Modelling in Orthodontic

Kazem Bahaa[1], Garma Noor[2] and Yousif Yousif[3]

[1]Mechatronics Eng. Dept., Baghdad University,
[2]Orthodontic Dept., Dentistry College, Baghdad University,
[3]Ministry of Higher Education and Scientific Research/ R&D Department, Baghdad
Iraq

1. Introduction

The discipline, science, and art of orthodontics are concerned with the face and ability to modify its growth. Orthodontists achieve their goals by manipulating the craniofacial skeleton, with particular emphasis on modifying the dentoalveolar region, external orthopedic forces are applied that mirror some techniques used in medical orthopedics. Most treatments, however, focus on modifying the occlusion and controlling dentoalveolar development and abnormal facial growth, thus, enormous amounts of designs and techniques invented in the diagnostic and treatment domains aiming at boolean etiological identification and optimized strategies of solution delivered. A valid problem assessment enables health providers to determine treatment need and priority, and as health care moves toward more stringent financial accountability. the inventory of the computer and its implementation in different medical field was of great interest, this interest are even greater with the artificial intelligence introduction (AI).

The best definition for the phrase "AI" calls for formalization of the term "intelligence". Psychologist and cognitive theorists are of the opinion that intelligence helps in identifying the right piece of knowledge at the appropriate instances of decision making [1,2].The phrase "AI" thus can be defined as the simulation of human intelligence on a machine. Thus, AI alternatively may be stated as a subject dealing with computational models that can think and act rationally [3-7].

The subject of AI spans a wide horizon. It deals with the various kinds of knowledge representation schemes, different techniques of intelligent search, various methods for resolving uncertainty of data and knowledge, diffrent schemes for automated machine learning and many others. Among the application areas of AI, we have Expert systems, Game-playing, and Theorem-proving, Natural language processing, Image recognition, Robotics and many others. This chapter aims at bringing the insight of interest to the conjugation relatively recently happened between orthodontics discipline and AI subject.

2. Introduction to AI

The subject of AI was originated with game-playing and theorem-proving programs and was gradually progressed with theories from a number of parent disciplines. As a young discipline of science, the significance of the topics covered under the subject changes considerably with time. The subject of AI has been enriched with a wide discipline of knowledge from Philosophy, Psychology, Cognitive Science, Computer Science, Mathematics and Engineering. Thus in fig.1, they have been referred to as the parent disciplines of AI.

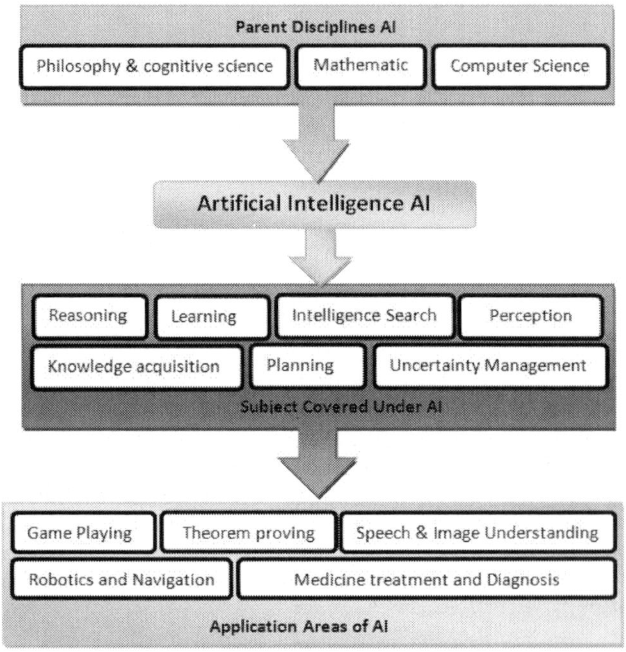

Fig. 1. Parent disciplines of AI

2.1 Artificial neural nets

Neural networks are composed of simple elements operating in parallel. These elements are inspired by biological nervous systems. As in nature, the network function is determined largely by the connections between elements. You can train a neural network to perform a particular function by adjusting the values of the connections (weights) between elements , fig. 2. Commonly neural networks are adjusted, or trained, so that a particular input leads to a specific target output. Such a situation can be shown as follows: there, the network is adjusted, based on a comparison of the output and the target, until the network output matches the target. Typically many such input/target pairs are needed to train a network [7,8]. One type of network sees the nodes as 'artificial neurons'. These are called Artificial Neural Networks (ANNs). Natural neurons receive signals through synapses located on the dendrites or membrane of the neuron. When the signals received are strong enough (surpass a certain threshold), the neuron is activated and emits a signal though the axon. This signal might be sent to another synapse, and might activate other neurons.

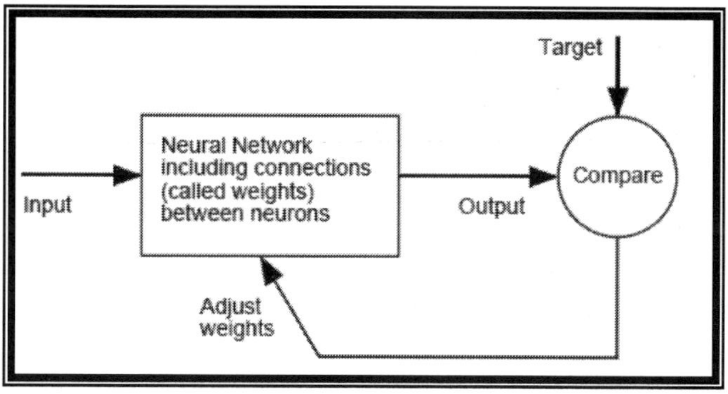

Fig. 2. Basic operation of ANN [9]

An interconnected assembly of simple processing elements, units or nodes, whose functionality is loosely based on the animal brain. The processing ability of the network is stored in the inter unit connection strengths, weights, obtained by a process of adaptation to, or learning from, a set of training patterns.

The benefits of using the neural network can be summarized as follows [10]:

1. Nonlinearity: an artificial neuron can be linear or non-linear a neural netmade up of interconnection of non-linear neurons, is itself non-linear, note that even linear function could be modeled by non-linear neurons, while the inverse can't be done.
2. Input and output mapping: usual learning process of neural network carried out in a popular paradigm of learning called learning with teacher "supervised learning" here modification of synaptic weights of a neural network done by applying set of labeled training samples, each sample consist of a unique input signal and a corresponding desired response. The previous samples could be arranged in different manners so the network constructing an input output mapping for the problem.
3. Adaptively: neural networks have a built in capability to adapt their synaptic to change in the surrounding environment. This could be done by retraining of the model or make the network changes itssynaptic weights in real time and this will be useful for pattern classification, signal processing, and control application.
4. Fault tolerance: a neural network, implemented in hard ware form, has the potential to be inherently fault tolerance, or capable of robust control. For example if a neuron or its connecting links are damaged and due to the nature of distributed information in neural network, this damage little effect on network response.

Neural Network Architecture: A neuron is an information-processing unit that is fundamental to the operation of a neural network. The block diagram of fig. 3 shows the model of a neuron, which forms the basis for designing (artificial) neural network.

The neuronal model of fig. (3) also includes an externally applied bias, denoted by (bk). The bias (bk) has the effect of increasing or lowering the net put of the activation function, depending on whether it is positive or negative, respectively [11], fig 4 shows common types of activation functions.

In mathematical terms:

$$f(x) = \left(\sum_{j=1}^{n} w_{jk} x_j + b_k \right) \quad (1)$$

Where f (w,x,b)) is the activation function.

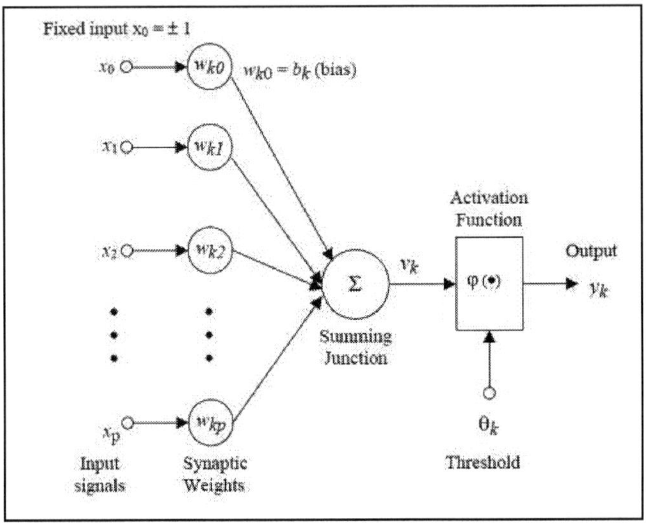

Fig. 3. Nonlinear model of a neuron

In general , there are four basic types of activation functions:

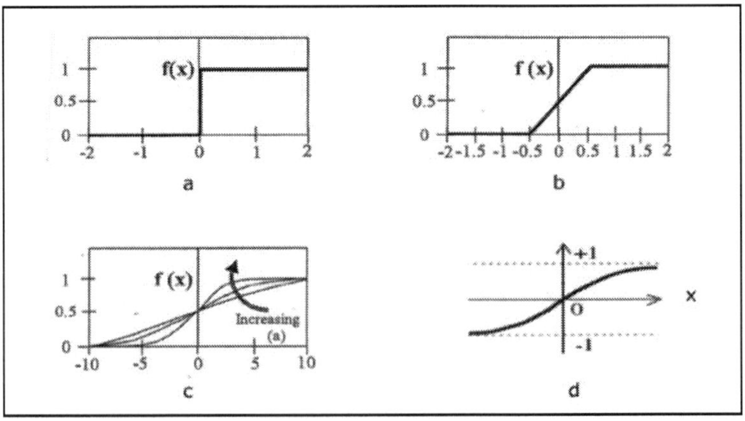

Fig. 4. Activation Functions

The management of neurons into layers and the connection patterns within and between layers is called the net architecture. The manner in which the neurons of a neural network are structured is intimately linked with the learning algorithms used to train the network [11]. Fig (5) shows different closes of network architecture

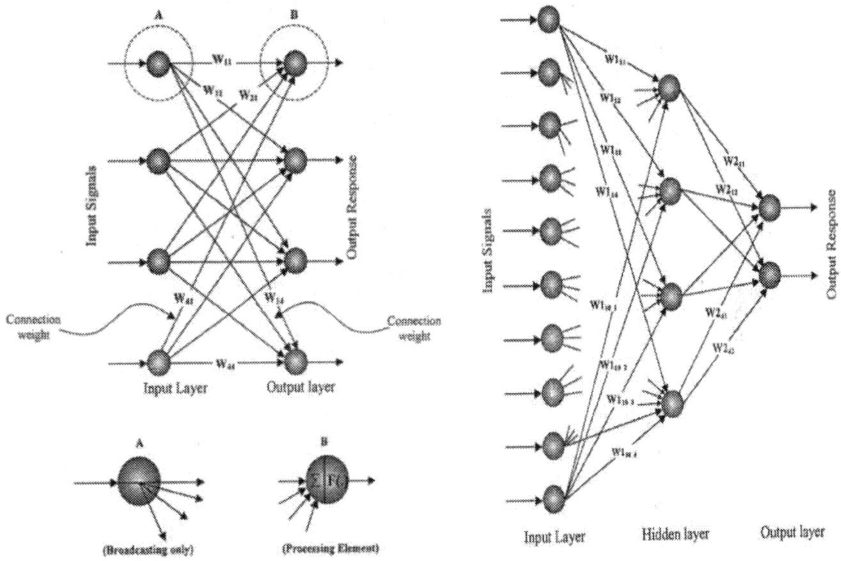

Fig. 5.a. Single-Layer Feedforward Networks b. Multilayer Feedforward Networks

2.2 Genetic algorithms

A genetic algorithm (GA) is a search heuristic that mimics the process of natural evolution. This heuristic is routinely used to generate useful solutions to optimization and search problems. Genetic algorithms belong to the larger class of evolutionary algorithms (EA), which generate solutions to optimization problems using techniques inspired by natural evolution, such as inheritance, mutation, selection, and crossover.In a genetic algorithm, a population of strings (called chromosomes or the genotype of the genome), which encode candidate solutions (called individuals, creatures, or phenotypes) to an optimization problem, evolves toward better solutions. Traditionally, solutions are represented in binary as strings of 0s and 1s, but other encodings are also possible. The evolution usually starts from a population of randomly generated individuals and happens in generations. In each generation, the fitness of every individual in the population is evaluated, multiple individuals are stochastically selected from the current population (based on their fitness), and modified (recombined and possibly randomly mutated) to form a new population. The new population is then used in the next iteration of the algorithm. Commonly, the algorithm terminates when either a maximum number of generations has been produced, or a satisfactory fitness level has been reached for the population. If the algorithm has terminated due to a maximum number of generations, a satisfactory solution may or may not have been reached.

Genetic algorithms find application in bioinformatics, phylogenetics, computational science, engineering, economics, chemistry, manufacturing, mathematics, physics and other fields.
A typical genetic algorithm requires:

- a genetic representation of the solution domain,
- a fitness function to evaluate the solution domain.

A standard representation of the solution is as an array of bits. Arrays of other types and structures can be used in essentially the same way. The main property that makes these genetic representations convenient is that their parts are easily aligned due to their fixed size, which facilitates simple crossover operations. Variable length representations may also be used, but crossover implementation is more complex in this case. Tree-like representations are explored in genetic programming and graph-form representations are explored in evolutionary programming.[12]
The fitness function is defined over the genetic representation and measures the quality of the represented solution. The fitness function is always problem dependent. For instance, in the knapsack problem one wants to maximize the total value of objects that can be put in a knapsack of some fixed capacity. A representation of a solution might be an array of bits, where each bit represents a different object, and the value of the bit (0 or 1) represents whether or not the object is in the knapsack. Not every such representation is valid, as the size of objects may exceed the capacity of the knapsack. The fitness of the solution is the sum of values of all objects in the knapsack if the representation is valid, or 0 otherwise. In some problems, it is hard or even impossible to define the fitness expression; in these cases, interactive genetic algorithms are used.
Once we have the genetic representation and the fitness function defined, GA proceeds to initialize a population of solutions randomly, then improve it through repetitive application of mutation, crossover, inversion and selection operators as shown in fig 6.

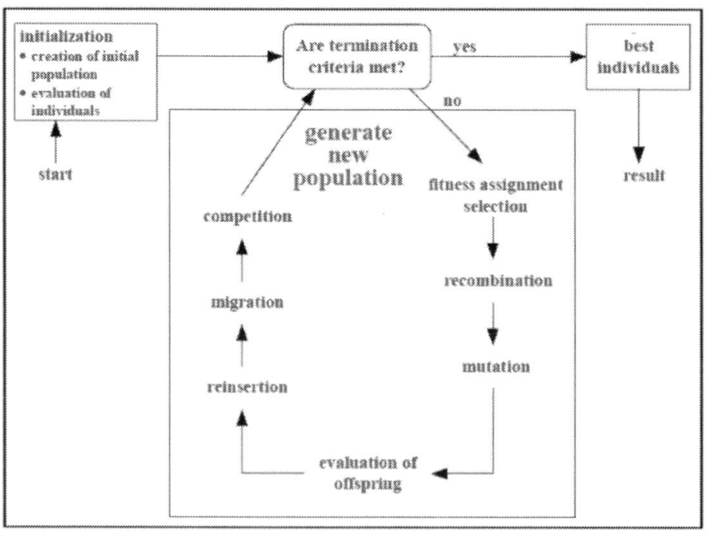

Fig. 6. Structure of an extended multi-population evolutionary algorithm

2.3 Fuzzy logic

Fuzzy logic [13] deals with fuzzy sets and logical connectives for modeling the human-like reasoning problems of the real world. A fuzzy set, unlike conventional sets, includes all elements of the universal set of the domain but with varying membership values in the interval [0,1]. It may be noted that a conventional set contains its members with a value of membership equal to one and disregards other elements of the universal set, for they have zero membership.

Fuzzy Sets and Crisp sets: The very basic notion of fuzzy systems is a fuzzy (sub)set. In classical mathematics we are familiar with what we call crisp sets. For example, the possible interferometric coherence g values are the set X of all real numbers between 0 and 1. From this set X a subset A can be defined, (e.g. all values $0 \leq g \geq 0.2$). The characteristic function of A, (i.e. this function assigns a number 1 or 0 to each element in X, depending on whether the element is in the subset A or not) is shown in fig7.[14]

The elements which have been assigned the number 1 can be interpreted as the elements that are in the set A and the elements which have assigned the number 0 as the elements that are not in the set A.

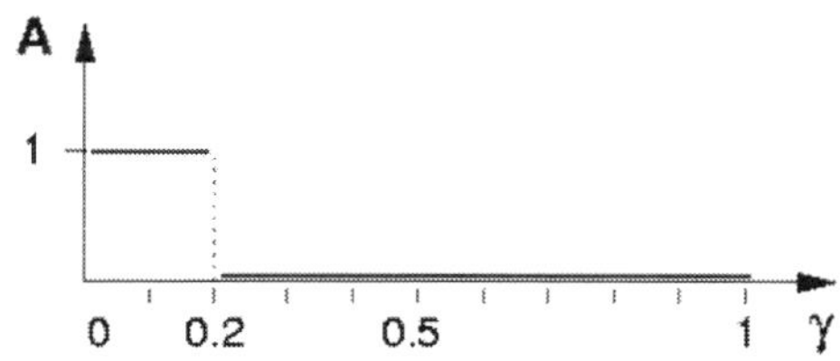

Fig. 7. Characteristic Function of a Crisp Set

This concept is sufficient for many areas of applications, but it can easily be seen, that it lacks in flexibility for some applications like classification of remotely sensed data analysis. For example it is well known that water shows low interferometric coherence g in SAR images. Since g starts at 0, the lower range of this set ought to be clear. The upper range, on the other hand, is rather hard to define. As a first attempt, we set the upper range to 0.2. Therefore we get B as a crisp interval B=[0,0.2]. But this means that a g value of 0.20 is low but a g value of 0.21 not. Obviously, this is a structural problem, for if we moved the upper boundary of the range from g =0.20 to an arbitrary point we can pose the same question. A more natural way to construct the set B would be to relax the strict separation between low and not low. This can be done by allowing not only the crisp decision Yes/No, but more flexible rules like " fairly low". A fuzzy set allows us to define such a notion. The aim is to use fuzzy sets in order to make computers more 'intelligent', therefore, the idea above has to be coded more formally. In the example, all the elements were coded with 0 or 1. A straight way to generalize this concept, is to allow more values between 0 and 1. In fact, infinitely many alternatives can be allowed between the boundaries 0 and 1, namely the unit interval I = [0, 1].

The interpretation of the numbers, now assigned to all elements is much more difficult. Of course, again the number 1 assigned to an element means, that the element is in the set B and 0 means that the element is definitely not in the set B. All other values mean a gradual membership to the set B.

This is shown in Fig. 8. The membership function is a graphical representation of the magnitude of participation of each input. It associates a weighting with each of the inputs that are processed, define functional overlap between inputs, and ultimately determines an output response. The rules use the input membership values as weighting factors to determine their influence on the fuzzy output sets of the final output conclusion.

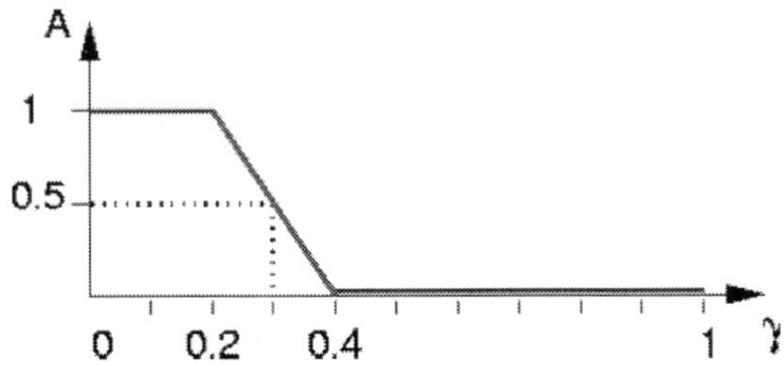

Fig. 8. Characteristic Function of a Fuzzy Set

Operations on fuzzy sets: We can introduce basic operations on fuzzy sets. Similar to the operations on crisp sets we also want to intersect, unify and negate fuzzy sets. In his very first paper about fuzzy sets [14], L. A. Zadeh suggested the minimum operator for the intersection and the maximum operator for the union of two fuzzy sets. It can be shown that these operators coincide with the crisp unification, and intersection if we only consider the membership degrees 0 and 1. For example, if A is a fuzzy interval between 5 and 8 and B be a fuzzy number about 4 as shown in the fig. 9.

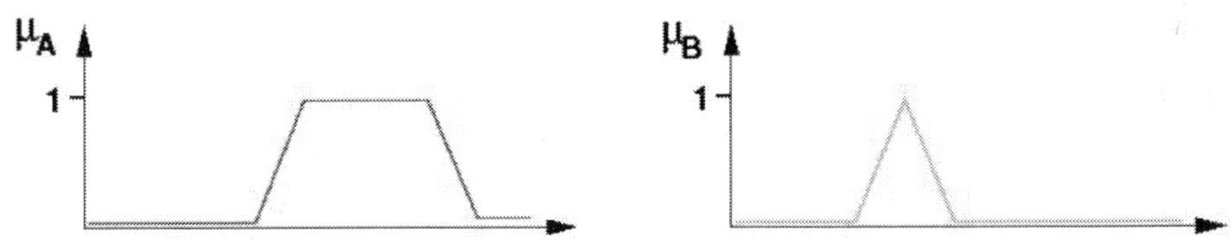

Fig. 9. Example fuzzy sets

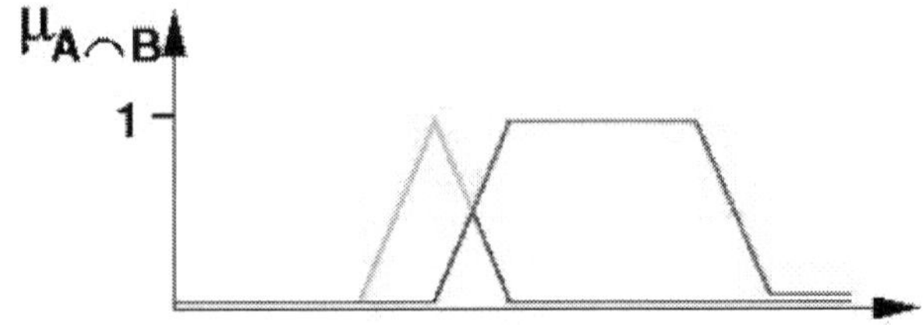

Fig. 10. Example: Fuzzy AND

In this case, the fuzzy set between 5 and 8 AND about 4 is set between 5 and 8 OR about 4 is shown in fig 11, and the the NEGATION of the fuzzy set A is shown in fig 12.

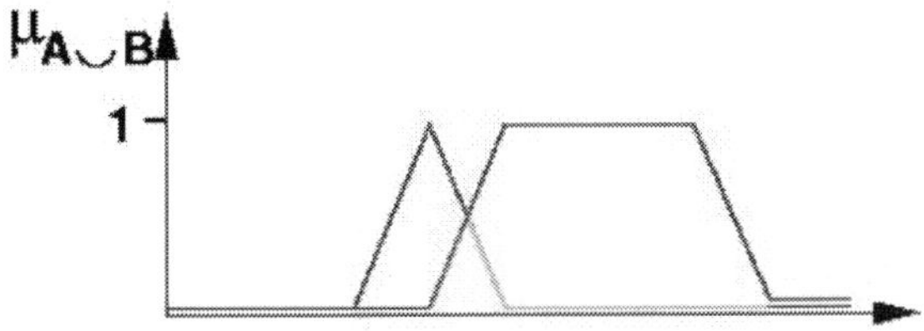

Fig. 11. Example: Fuzzy OR

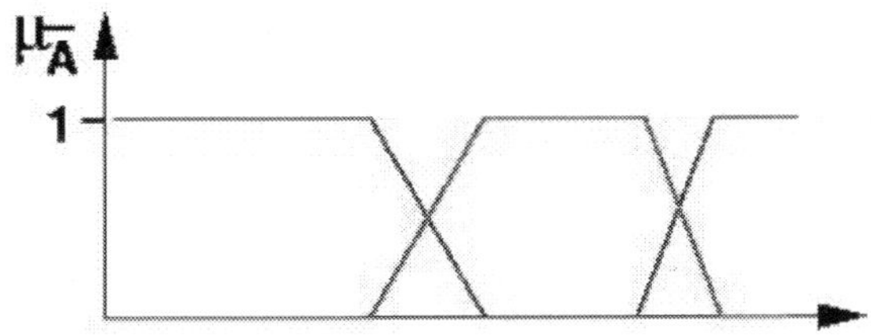

Fig. 12. Example: Fuzzy NEGATION

Fuzzy Classification: Fuzzy classifiers are one application of fuzzy theory. Expert knowledge is used and can be expressed in a very natural way using linguistic variables , which are described by fuzzy sets Now the expert knowledge for this variables can be formulated as a rules like
IF feature A low AND feature B medium AND feature C medium AND feature D medium THEN Class = class4
The rules can be combined in a table calls rule base [14]

R#	Feature A	Feature B	Feature C	Feature D	Class
1:	Low	Medium	Medium	Medium	Class 1
2:	Medium	high	Medium	Medium	Class 2
3:	Low	Medium	Medium	Medium	Class 3
4:	low	Medium	Medium	Medium	Class 1
5:	Medium	Medium	Medium	Medium	Class 4
...:	...	...	...	...	...
N:	Low	High	Medium	Low	Unknown

Linguistic rules describing the control system consist of two parts; an antecedent block (between the IF and THEN) and a consequent block (following THEN). Depending on the system, it may not be necessary to evaluate every possible input combination, since some may rarely or never occur.[14].

By making this type of evaluation, usually done by an experienced operator, fewer rules can be evaluated, thus simplifying the processing logic and perhaps even improving the fuzzy logic system performance. The inputs are combined logically using the AND operator to produce output response values for all expected inputs. The active conclusions are then combined into a logical sum for each membership function. A firing strength for each output membership function is computed. All that remains is to combine these logical sums in a defuzzification process to produce the crisp output. e.g for a for the rule consequents for each class a so-called singleton or a min-max interference can be derived which is the characteristic function of the respective set . e.g. For the input pair of H = 0:35 and _ = 30 the scheme below (see Fig 14.) would apply.

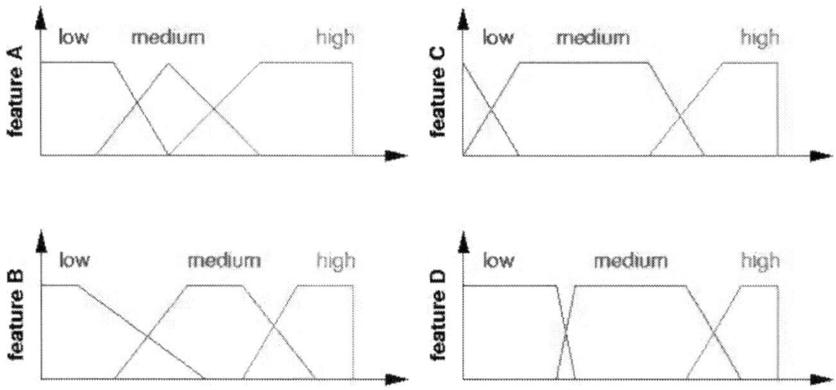

Fig. 13. Example: Linguistic Variables

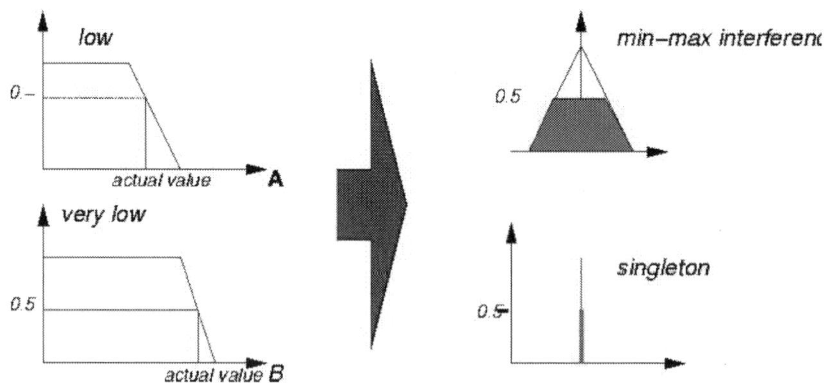

Fig. 14. Interference for rule IF H very low AND a low THEN Class = class 1

The fuzzy outputs for all rules are finally aggregated to one fuzzy set. To obtain a crisp decision from this fuzzy output, we have to defuzzify the fuzzy set, or the set of singletons. Therefore, we have to choose one representative value as the final output. There are several heuristic methods (defuzzification methods), one of them is e.g. to take the center of gravity of the fuzzy set as shown in fig 15., which is widely used for fuzzy sets. For the discrete case with singletons usually the maximum-method is used where the point with the maximum singleton is chosen.

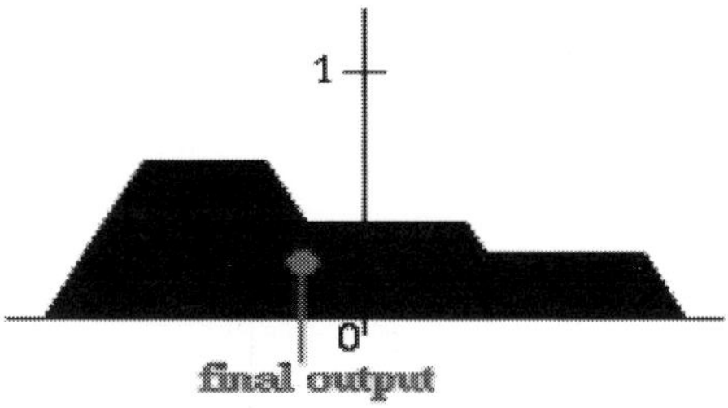

Fig. 15. Defuzzification using the center of gravity approach

3. Applications of AI techniques

Almost every branch of science and engineering currently shares the tools and techniques available in the domain of AI. However, we mention here a few typical applications, [15-20].
Expert Systems: An expert system consists of a knowledge base, database and an inference engine for interpreting the database using the knowledge supplied in the knowledge base.
Image Understanding and Computer Vision: A digital image can be regarded as a two-dimensional array of pixels containing gray levels corresponding to the intensity of the reflected illumination received by a video camera .
Navigational Planning for Mobile Robots: Mobile robots, sometimes called automated guided vehicles (AGV), are a challenging area of research where AI finds extensive applications. The navigational planning problem persists in both static and dynamic environments.
Speech Understanding: the main problem is to separate the syllables of a spoken word and determine features like amplitude, and fundamental and harmonic frequencies of each syllable. The words then could be identified from the Extracted features by pattern classification techniques.
Scheduling: In a scheduling problem, one has to plan the time schedule of a set of events to improve the time efficiency of the solution.
Intelligent Control: In process control, the controller is designed from the known models of the process and the required control objective. When the dynamics of the plant is not completely known, the existing techniques for controller design no longer remain valid. Rule-based control is appropriate in such situations.
System Modeling and Optimization:
Optimization methods have been applied over years to generate solutions that solely maximize performance. In order to assess the performance variance of a solution, a few near optimal solutions are selected and studied under assumed stochastic parametric variations via simulation. There are reports on the use AI guide or bias search strategies. A new evolutionary algorithm that is capable of generating robust optimal solutions for constrained robust design problems.

3.1 Using AI for medical applications

The implementation of human intelligence in scientific equipment has been the subject of scientific research for a long time and of the medical research in the last decades. In the 1950's computer simulation of biological neural network was first introduced. In 1943 McCullogh and Pitts stated the definition of the first artificial neuron. In parallel with the evolution of computer technology, modeling of increasingly complicated neural functions and activity of simple neural clusters was defined. Mathematical models that could be applied for practical applications were developed between 1982 and 1987 based on the works of Hopfield [21], Kohonen [22] and Rummelhart and McLelland [23]. The advantage of neural networks over conventional programming lies in their ability to solve problems that do not have an algorithmic solution or the available solution is too complex to be found. Neural networks are well suited to tackle problems that people are good at solving, such as prediction and pattern recognition. Neural networks have been applied within the medical domain for clinical diagnosis [24-26], image analysis and interpretation[27,28] signal analysis and interpretation [29] and drug development [30]..

Functional division of neural network applications in medicine; Papik et al, 1998) [31]:

1. Modelling: Simulating and modelling the functions of the brain and neurosensory organs.
2. Signal processing: Bioelecric signal filtering and evaluation.
3. System control and checking: Intelligent artificial machine control and checking based on responses of biological or technical systems given to any signals
4. Classification: Interpretation of physical and instrumental findings to achieve more accurate diagnosis.
5. Prediction: Neural network provide prognostic information based on retrospective parameter analysis.

Fuzzy logic [11] has been applied to dental and medical sciences n3(Sims-Williams et al, 1987) in order to construct systems that can infer precise recommendations for solving problems that have uncertain properties [32-36] .Brown et al. (1991) [37] applied fuzzy logic to solve orthodontic problems in an expert system, designed to provide advice for treatment planning of Class II division 1 malocclusions. They reported that their system produced more acceptable treatment plans than those used by general dental practitioners. Similarly, Tanaka et al. (1997) [36] applied fuzzy reasoning to their computer-assisted diagnostic system for ultrasonography for the purpose of providing a diagnostic aid for unskilled clinicians.(head gear)

4. Using AI for orthodontics

Many researchers intended to capture the outlines matching between pleasing smile and harmonically face. Usually the challenging face the orthodontist to figure out the orthodontic problems, there diagnosis and environment of origin keeping away distracting factors. The traditional regime for diagnosis include multiple steps for orthodontic problem identification , these steps generally categorized according to three sources (1) multiple questioning records including chief complaint, patient's dental and medical history; (2) clinical examination of the patient; and (3) assessment of diagnostic records, including dental casts, radiographs, and facial and intraoral images [38].

It is mandatory to contextualize data have been driven. All the data base collected gathered in an elaborate process to achieve the most appropriate treatment planning, treatment plan is the second challenge facing the orthodontist, the enormous variation in dental malocclusion gathered with different facial pattern and the presence of large number of available treatment modalities, all these leading the decision process in orthodontics to challenging area even to the experienced orthodontist. Often more than one treatment plan can successfully resolve an orthodontic problem, and as a consequences form these two interrelated orthodontic processes (diagnosis and treatment plan) the treatment can be customized , orthodontic books and articles are profound with researches discussing protocols for decision making process regarding orthodontic problem definition and treatment option. Thus our chapter attempt to bring the insight to the invention of the artificial intelligence as a system aid in the essential orthodontic steps namely; diagnosis, treatment plan and treatment optimization.

4.1 Diagnosis using expert system

Expert system (ES) is an important branch of the field of artificial intelligence (AI).. ES is a computer program system that processes knowledge and information, which is composed primarily of a knowledge base and an inference machine. ES simulates the decision making and working processes of experts and solves actual problems in the field of a single specialty[39]. Generally, in a medical or dental expert system, a set of knowledge base is derived from experienced clinicians and represents their knowledge, which can be used for clinical consultations [40,41].With this type of system, uncertainty is a major problem in decision making because non-evidence-based knowledge has to be represented mathematically. Poon et al [42] were the first to use a new approach to knowledge acquisition known as Ripple-Down Rules in Dentistry to develop an ES in clinical orthodontics. This system comprises a knowledge base of 680 rules. Investigators found that such an ES has potential as an interactive advisory tool and is applicable in clinical orthodontic situations.

Hammond et al [43] pointed out in a review that traditional rule-based expert systems had some limitations when applied to orthodontic diagnosis and treatment planning. These limitations may be avoided by using a case-based system, which is a particular type of ES that uses a stored data bank of previously treated cases to provide knowledge for use in solving new treatment problems. Hammond et al [44] also investigated the application of this method in the field of orthodontic diagnosis and treatment planning. A case base of 300 cases was entered into a case based ES shell. A test set of 30 consecutive cases then was used to test the diagnostic capacity of the system. The computer-generated treatment plan matched the actual treatment plan in 24 of the 30 cases. In another work by Lux et al [45] the growth of 43 orthodontically untreated children was analyzed by lateral cephalograms taken at the ages of 7 and 15. For the description of craniofacial skeletal changes, the concept of tensor analysis and related methods were applied. Through the use of an ANN, namely, self-organizing neural maps (SOM), resultant growth data were classified, and relationships of the various growth patterns were monitored. This type of network provided a frame of reference for classifying and analyzing previously unknown cases with respect to their growth pattern, Brickley et al [46] concluded that ANN expert systems may be trained with clinical data only and therefore can be used in cases where "rule-based" decision making is not possible. This is the case in many clinical situations. ANN therefore may become important decision-making tools within dentistry, we'll discuss one of these expert systems;

An expert orthodontic index:

A valid initial assessment enables health providers to determine treatment need and priority, an accurate final diagnostic assessment assists patients and orthodontists to conclude if a worthwhile improvement is achieved. Orthodontists have developed several occlusal indices during the past few decades to evaluate treatment need, complexity, and success. Among the developed indices, Peer Assessment Rating (PAR) is one of the most common ones that is used to evaluate the quality of treatment. Richmond et al [47] developed PAR in 1992 to create consistency and standardization in assessing orthodontic treatment outcome. It is a weighted summation of health traits that influence the malocclusion. It summarizes data about the misalignment in a single score that reflects deviation from the ideal occlusion. The treatment success can then be evaluated by comparison of the pre- and post-treatment PAR scores. In spite of its extensive use, PAR suffers from several limitations. In summary, PAR is constrained by its strict linear mathematical expression with fixed coefficients, while a non-linearity may enhance the subjective opinions of orthodontists more accurately. Different versions of PAR index have been developed in order to improve the weighting system by using traditional regression techniques, but they are still restricted by the non-adjustable linear coefficient. A fuzzy index was developed by Zarei A.et al in 2007[48] using neural network with fuzzy approach . Zarei et al in 2009 [49] improved the quality of fuzzy index using union rule configuration. Further, an intelligent system that represent orthodontists' visual perception in assessing patients was developed.

Panel of orthodontists with randomized patients' files, each of which contained their data prior to treatment, during treatment progress, and at the end of treatment. profiles of 560 cases of malocclusion was used by the panel of orthodontist . each profile includes clinician's assessment that based on cephalometric tracing interpretations, visual perception, and clinical appearance. The panel assessed the cases using a visual analog scale. A visual analog scale is one of the most common measurement scales used in health care research and has also been used in dental studies [50].

Modeling was used for the identification of the expert system using the input-output data. Sugeno models [51] are good candidates for situations when a desired action can not necessarily be described verbally by experts. Therefore, Sugeno models provide a good way to model clinicians' assessment when using numerical data. a set of input-output data to first identify the fuzzy system for this collection of data and then optimize this model by adjusting the parameters. Input to this fuzzy inference model includes five variables that orthodontists associate with assessment of treatment outcome, The input variables for this model include the following linear and angular cephalometric measurements; overjet, ANB angle, Lower Incisor to Mandibular Plane angle (LI-MnPI), SNB angle and Upper Incisor to Sella Nasion angle (Ul-SN),while the output parameter is the arithmetic mean of the panel's assessments. Subtractive clustering to identify the rule base was performed, clustering of data forms the basis of many system modeling algorithms.

Neural networks were utilized to learn the characteristics of the data and selected the parameters of input and output membership functions to best reflect those characteristics. The parameters of membership functions are modified during the learning process to minimize the fitness function. The adjustments of these parameters are facilitated by a gradient vector, which provides a measure of how well the fuzzy inference system is modeling the data. Optimization of the parameters of the initial model with respect to training data by minimizing the sum of the squared difference between actual and desired outputs. Fig 16 depicts the performance of the model in predicting the assessment for training and testing patterns. It is evident from this figure that the model assessment is very close to the panel assessment for most of the patterns.

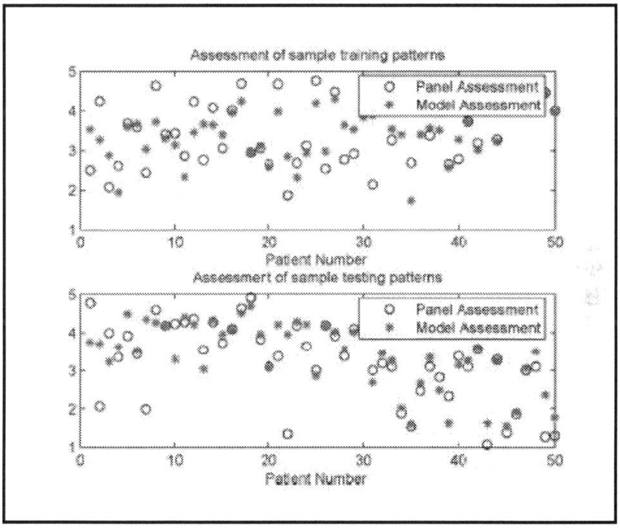

Fig. 16. Comparison of the panel assessment and the model assessment [49]

a Neuro-Fuzzy Assessment Index that is highly correlated with clinicians' opinion were successfully produced. neural network and fuzzy logic had been used for assessing orthodontic treatment outcome and developed a robust and realistic model that has a flexible interpretation of data. Applying Subtractive Clustering technique avoided the combinatorial explosion of rules in our model. hybridization of neural network and fuzzy logic improved the quality of the orthodontic index.[52].

Cephalometrics Analysis

Cephalometric analysis is a useful diagnostic tool to determine facial type and prediction of growth pattern, enabling clinician to determine facial disharmonies in order to centralize therapeutic measures during treatment and modify facial growth.

According to Graber and Vanarsdall [38], the commonly used radiographic views are:

Lateral or profile cephalograms: used to study anteroposterior and vertical relationships.

Frontal or postero-anterior celphalograms: used to evaluate the transversal and vertical relationships in the frontal plane. Submentovertex or basal cephalograms: used to the balance in transversal plane.

Two approaches may be used to perform a cephalometric analysis: a manual approach, and a computer- aided approach. The manual approach is the oldest and most widely used. It consists of placing a sheet of acetate over the cephalometric radiograph, tracing salient features, identifying landmarks, and measuring distances and angles between landmark locations. The other approach is computer-aided. Computerized cephalometric analysis uses manual identification of landmarks, based either on an overlay tracing of the radiograph to identify anatomical or constructed points followed by the transfer of the tracing to a digitizer linked to a computer, or a direct digitization of the lateral skull radiograph using a digitizer linked to a computer, and then locating landmarks on the monitor.[42-44].

Afterwards, the computer software completes the cephalometric analysis by automatically measuring distances and angles. The evolution from full manual cephalometrics to computer assisted-cephalometric analysis is aimed at improving the diagnostic ability of cephalometric analysis through errors reduction and time saving. Computerized or computer-aided, cephalometric analysis eliminates the mechanical errors when drawing lines between landmarks as well as those made when measuring with a protractor. However, the inconsistency in landmark identification is still an important source of random errors both in computer-aided digital cephalometry and in manual cephalometric analysis.[45-47] taking into account the imprecise, inconsistent, and paracomplete data inherent to the analytical process. There have been efforts to automate cephalometric analysis with the aim of reducing the time required to obtain an analysis, improving the accuracy of landmark identification and reducing the errors due to clinicians' subjectivity.

In an automated cephalometric analysis a scanned or digital cephalometric radiograph is stored in the computer and loaded by the software. The software then automatically locates the landmarks and performs the measurements for cephalometric analysis. The challenging problem in an automated cephalometric analysis is landmark detection, given that the calculations have already been automated with success. The first attempt at automated landmarking of cephalograms was made by Cohen in 1984,[53] ,followed by more studies on this topic. Automatic identification of landmarks has been undertaken in different ways that involve computer vision and artificial intelligence techniques.

The automated approaches can be classified into four broad categories, based on the techniques, Leonardia R et al[54] mentioned these categories with techniques examples for each approach recorded by different authors:

1. Image filtering plus knowledge-based landmark search; [55-58]
2. model- based approaches [59-64]
3. soft-computing approaches [65-68]
4. hybrid approaches. [69-73]

the relative advantages and disadvantages of these technical approaches used in the automated identification of cephalometric landmarks; Image filtering plus knowledge-based landmark search are list in table 1.

The informational importance of the cephalometric analysis was accompanied by many unnegligible sites of imprecision, this significant degrees of vagueness, and even inconsistency, was also making clinical application of the cephalometric data interpretation and driven information of less effective values than expected by the clinicians. to interpret how cephalometric variables behave in a complete contextualized scenario. Many trials was made to extract the ability of artificial intelligent techniques as favorable interpretational tool for the usual inconsistency of biological information. As a matter of fact artificial intelligence (AI) theories or techniques have few and recent applications in craniofacial biology, specifically in clinical application of cephalometrics, the multiple discussed studies was successfully produced at the level of researches taking in to account that the systems described in the literature are not accurate enough to allow their use for clinical purposes as errors in landmark detection were greater than those expected with manual tracing, therefore; most of these methods have not been adopted in clinical practice [53]. The inconsistency of the informational driven cephalometric data gave the authors an additional challenging interface to overcome both cephalometric and modeling techniques inconsistencies, and yields sequential attempts of automated cephalometric analysis; we'll discuss some of these attempts in details hoping the enrichment of reader information of artificial intelligent approach for this diagnostic tool;

Techniques	Advantages	Disadvantages
Image filtering plus knowledge-based landmark search	Easy to implement Image filtering techniques are well studied and a large number are available By encoding proper anatomical knowledge better accuracy	Can fail to capture morphological variability in the radiographs Filtering results are highly dependent on image quality and intensity level Sensitive to noise in the image. Not all landmarks lie on edge and, moreover, the edges or curve are often unclear.
Model-based approach	Is invariant to scale, rotation, and translation (the structure can be located even if it is smaller or bigger than given model). Accommodates shape variability	Needs models that must be created by averaging the variations in shape of each anatomical structure on given set of radiographs. Model deformation must be constrained and is not always precise Cannot be applied to partially hidden regions Sensitive to noise in image.
Soft-computing or learning approach	Accommodates shape variability. Tolerant to noise. Techniques are well studies. Large selection of software tools available.	Results depend on the training set. Difficult to interpret some results. A number of network parameters, such as topology and number of neuron must be determined empirically.

Table 1. Technical approaches used to automatically identify cephalometric landmarks and their advantages and disadvantages [54].

Abe [74] and Mario et al [75]mentioned important limitations that conventional cephalometric holds, mostly due to the fact that the cephalometric variables are not assessed under a contextualized scope and carry on important variation when compared to samples norms. Because of that, its clinical application is subjective. Also discordance between orthodontists about diagnosis and treatments it is not uncommon, due to the inevitable uncertainties involved in the cephalometrics variables, and both suggest that this is a perfect scenario to evaluate the paraconsistent neural network capacity to perform with uncertainties, and inconsistencies in a practical problem.

Abe [74] develops an expert system in his work to support orthodontic diagnosis, the system based on the paraconsistent approach. Paraconsistent artificial neural network (PANN) was introduced in the Bulletin of Symbolic Logic [74], In the structure proposed the inferences that were based upon the degrees of evidence (favorable and unfavorable) of

abnormality for cephalometrics variables, which may have infinite values between "0" and "1", the suggested PANN refined in Abe [74] work to produce an expert system to support orthodontic diagnosis, which may have infinite values between "0" and "1". Therefore, the system may be refined with more or less outputs, depending upon the need. Such flexibility allows that the system can be modeled in different ways, allowing a finer adjusting. The system requires measurements taken from the head lateral radiography of the patient that will be assessed. The precision of the system increase as much as data is added.
Another work was made by Mario et al [75] to overcome these interpretational shortcomings, once again suggesting the contribution of Mathematics to Biology, better translating natural phenomena. Moreover, single correlations are insufficient for the assessment of facial patterns as many variables must be simultaneously considered in order to establish patterns. And once again the paraconsistent logic suggested as a model for detection and treatment of contradictions, enriching the use of soft mathematics tools in biology. research intends to test such model, it is reasonable to expect that the proposed model can well detect inconsistencies and better interpret craniofacial morphology [75], the cephalometric diagnostic model used logical states which represented in figure 7.

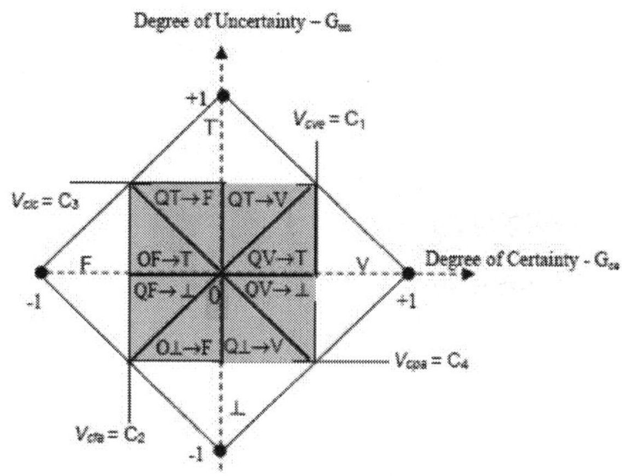

Fig. 17. Logical states: extreme and nonextreme states [75]

PANN

PANN was introduced in the *Bulletin of Symbolic Logic* (10). Its basis leans on paraconsistent annotated evidential logic Eτ(10). Let us present it briefly. The atomic formulas of the logic Et are of the type
$p(\mu, \lambda)$, where $p(\mu, \lambda)$, $\in[0, 1]^2$ and [0, 1] is the real unitary nterval (p denotes a propositional variable).The $p(\mu, \lambda)$, can be intuitively read: "It is assumed that p's favorable i.evidence is μ and contrary evidence is λ. Thus,

- $p(1.0, 0.0)$ can be read as a true proposition;
- $p(0.0, 1.0)$ can be read as a false proposition;
- $p(1.0, 1.0)$ can be read as an inconsistent proposition;
- $p(0.0, 0.0)$ can be read as a paracomplete (unknown) proposition;
- $p(0.5, 0.5)$ can be read as an indefinite proposition.

In the PANN, the main aim is to know how to determine the certainty degree concerning a proposition, if it is False or True. Therefore, the model took the certainty degree Gce into account. The uncertainty degree Gun indicates the "measure" of the inconsistency or paracompleteness [78]. If the certainty degree is low or the uncertainty degree is high, it generates an indefinition; the basic scheme is shown in Fig. 18.

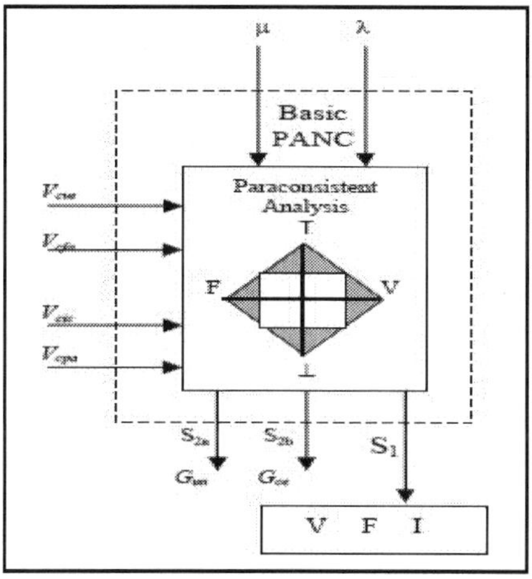

Fig. 18. The basic steps of a paraconsistent artificial neural cell

The model suggested by Mario et al [75] utilize selected set of cephalometric variables based on expertise (Figs. 9 a and b). These cephalometric variables are usually collected by experts [79] through characteristic points in a cephalometric X-ray.
The selected cephalometric variables feed the PANN in the following three units: Unit I, considering the anteroposterior discrepancy; Unit II, considering vertical discrepancy; and Unit III, taking into account dental discrepancy (see Fig. 20).

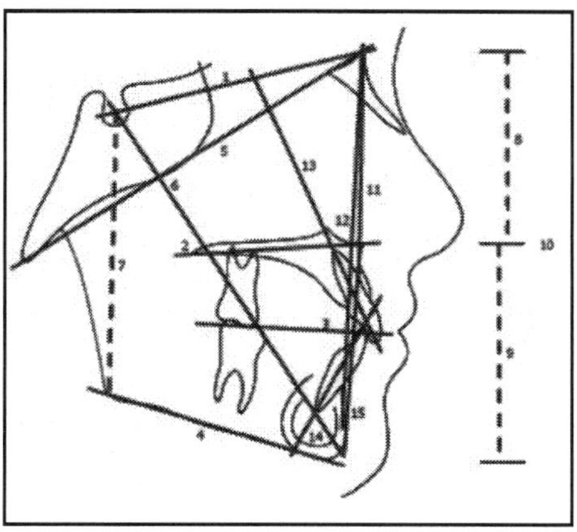

Fig. 19. a Cephalometric Variables [73]

(1. Basion 2. Sella 3. Nasion 4. Posterior Nasal Spine 5. Anterior Nasal Spine 6. Inter-Molars 7. Inter-Incisors 8. Gonion 9. Menton 10. Gnathion 11. A Point 12. B Point 13. Pogonion 14. Incisal Edge - Upper Incisor 15. Apex - Upper Incisor 16. Incisal Edge - Lower Incisor 17. Apex - Lower Incisor)

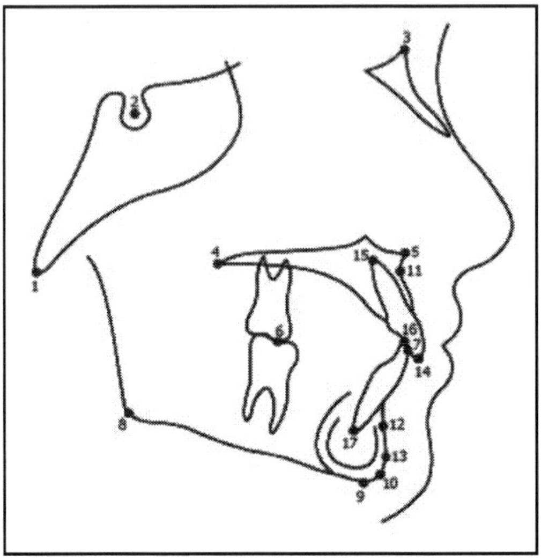

Fig. 19. b Proposed Cephalometric Analysis [73]

1. Anterior Cranial Base 2. Palatal Plane (PP) 3. Oclusal Plane (OP) 4. Mandibular Plane (MP) 5. Cranial Base 6. Y Axis 7. Posterior Facial Height 8. Anterior Facial Height - Median Third 9. Anterior Facial Height - Lower Third 10. Anterior Facial Height 11. SNA 12. SNB 13. Long Axis - Upper Incisor 14. Long Axis - Lower Incisor 15. A Point - Pogonion Line Wits: distance between the projections of the A and B Points on the occlusal plane.

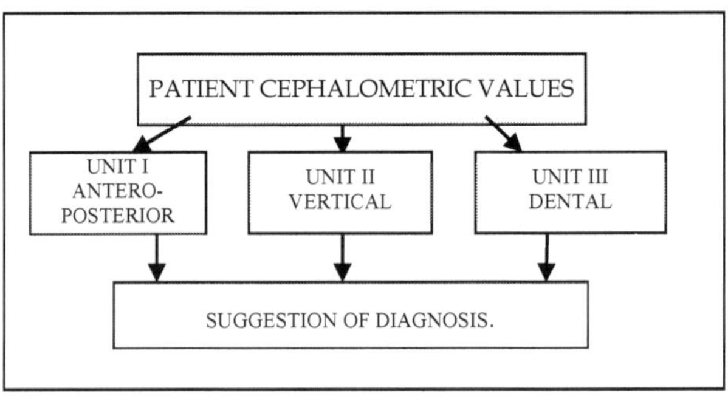

Fig. 20. Functional macroview of the paraconsistent artificial neural network architecture used by Mario et al [75]

Each unit has the specific following components, as shown in Fig 21:

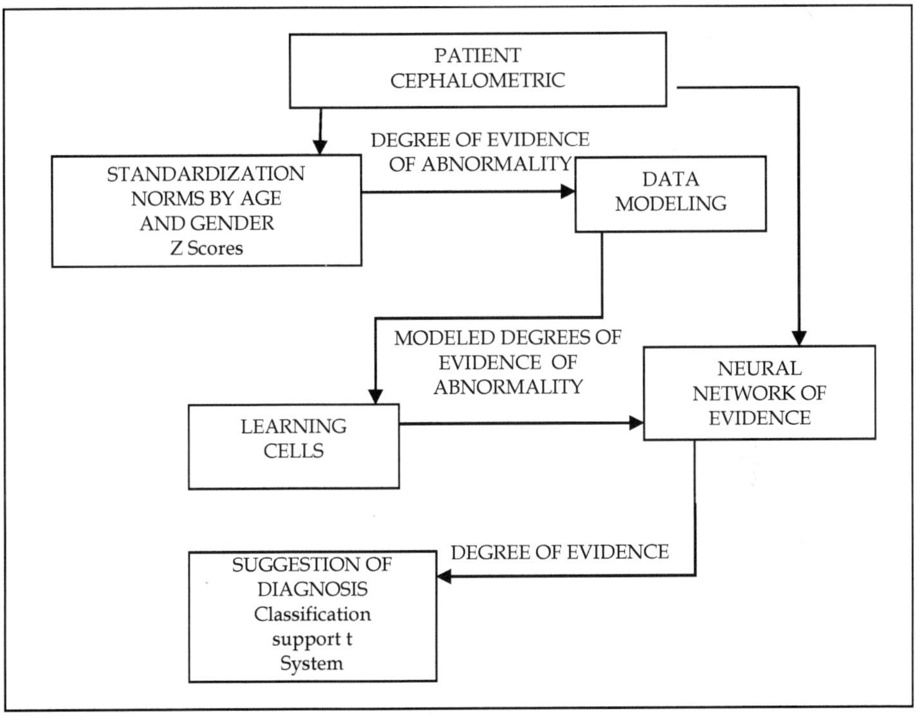

Fig. 21. Functional microview of the structure of each unit represented in Fig. 20 [75]

Tanikawa C etal [80] studied the reliability of a system that performs automatic recognition of anatomic landmarks and their surrounding anatomic structures in which the landmarks are located on lateral cephalograms using landmark-dependent criteria unique to each respective landmark. Recently, a system that recognizes general grayscale images using an automated psychologic brain model [81] has been developed.ie, a hardware-friendly algorithm to accomplish real-time recognition by recalling a set of modeled data that is mathematically described using a finite number of traits and previously stored in the system. This system employs a new technique called the projected principal edge distribution (PPED) as a means for extracting features from an image, and it has been confirmed that the system demonstrates robust performance in recognizing images, including cephalograms [82-84]. Although experiments have suggested the efficacy of the system in recognizing images, it remains uncertain whether such a system will detect conventionally used landmarks with high precision. On the other hand, as mentioned before, that topographic variations exist in humans' subjective judgments of cephalometric landmarks, and the shapes and size of the variances are unique to each landmark [85]. Mathematical formulation of these landmark-dependent variations in measurement would be help researchers to evaluate objectively the reliability of the automatic cephalogram recognition system.

Tanikawa C et al [80] system incorporates two major tasks: the "knowledge-generation" (system learning) phase and the "recognition" phase. In the knowledge generation phase, image data extracted from learning asamples are converted into PPED vectors consisting of 64 variables that feature contours of the anatomic structures [81,82,83] .From these vectors, template vectors, i.e., the principal information for identifying the landmarks, are generated using a generalized Lloyd algorithm [86] for each landmark, which are stored in the system as the system's knowledge. During the recognition phase, the system is designed to perform pixel- by-pixel film scanning with template-matching operations between PPED vectors that are generated from an input film and template vectors stored on the system. The system recognizes the most matched position as a landmark position. schematic representation can be seen in fig 22.

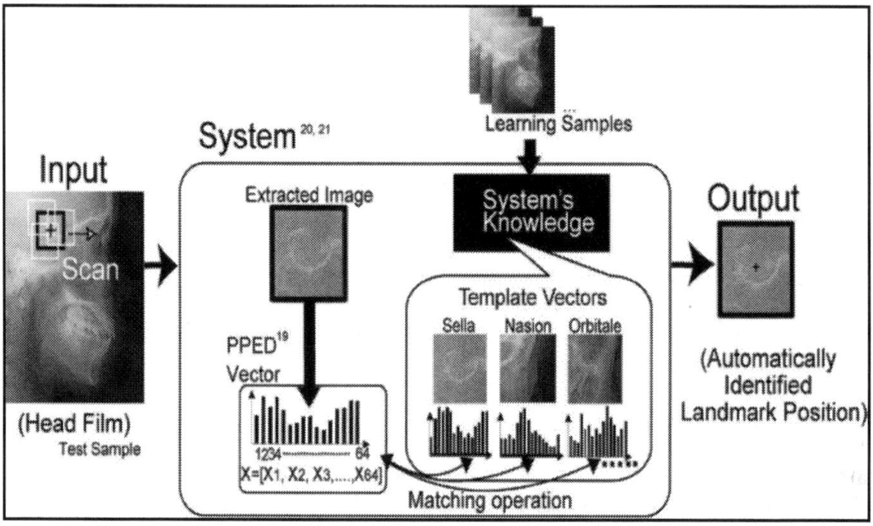

Fig. 22. Schematic representation for automatic recognition of anatomic landmarks [80]

To evaluate the system's performance reliability, scattergrams that designated errors for manual landmark identification when 10 orthodontists identified a landmark on 10 cephalograms were obtained according to the method reported by Baumrind and Frantz [85]. Confidence ellipses with a confidence limit of α were developed for each landmark from the scattergram, the system was evaluated using confidence ellipses with α =.01 In short, when a system-identified point was located within a confidence limit of α = .01, the landmark identification was judged to be successful.

To evaluate the accuracy of the landmark identification provided by the systems and if system's definition of a landmark position is clinically acceptable, it has been a critical issue in testing the performance reliability of such systems. Three major methods for such an evaluation have been employed so far. In the first method, an individual orthodontist makes a visual judgment as to whether or not the system's recommendation is acceptable [87] The second approach involves describing mean recognition errors, i.e., the mean distance between the point provided by an orthodontist(s) and the point determined by the system [88,89]. The third method is to examine whether the system-identified landmark is located in a circle with a 2-mm radius [88-93], see fig13.

The fiducial zones established by the panel of experienced orthodontists are considered valid for evaluation of the ability of the automatic recognition system to recognize anatomic features. With the incorporation of the rational assessment criteria provided by confidence ellipses, the proposed system was confirmed to be reliable. The system successfully recognized anatomic features surrounding all the landmarks. The mean success rate for identifying the landmark positions was 88% with a range of 77% to 100%.

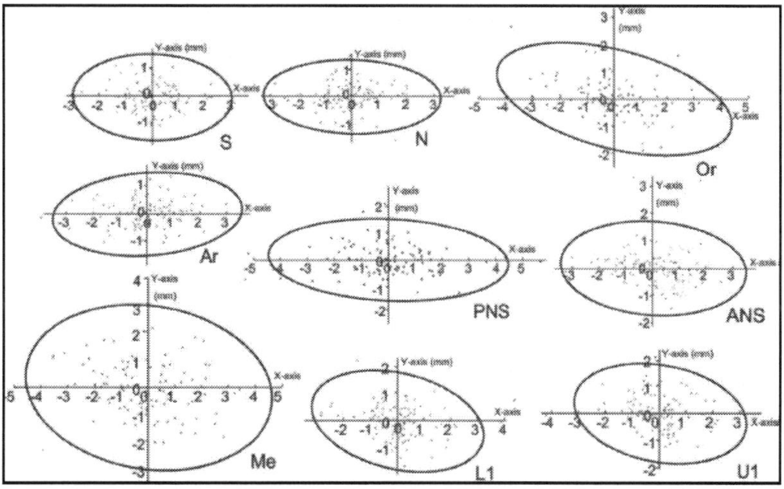

Fig. 23. Confidence ellipses obtained for cephalometric landmarks. Black points indicate coordinate values of landmarks identified by 10 orthodontists on 10 cephalograms. The black lines designate confidence ellipses with α=01. Origin indicates the best estimate; x-axis, the line that passes through the origin and is parallel to the line S-N; and y-axis, the line that is perpendicular to the x-axis through the origin. [80].

In 2011 Banumathi A et al suggested [94] Another diagnostic model, Artificial intelligence role in dentofacial deformities diagnosis was discussed. The dentist must be familiar with morphological and functional maturity also oral surgeon and the orthodontist should be able to relate this knowledge to specific clinical problems such as skeletal mealocclusion and craniofacial anomalies. This understanding should influence the selection, planning and timing of treatment for patients who require orthognathic surgery. And the decision forming through the available choices, whether accepting the underlying deformity and taking the camouflage treatment as a choice or maybe surgical correction is the sole solution could be offered, of course full awareness of patient psychological aspects, underlying skeletal and\or dental malrelations and specific age, all should be taken into account. Cephalometric analysis was of important priority in deciding the acceptance and selection of appropriate orhognathic surgery for the underlying case. the diagnostic model was proposed by Edge sharpening of various bones in the lateral view of the face in cephalometric image referred to preprocessing, this is achieved through a histogram equalization process. From the literature, histogram equalization is enough to improve the contrast of the cephalometric image [95]. The edge features are then extracted from the enhanced cephalometric image and they are classified as landmark and non landmark points using Support vector machine technique. Finally, angles between various landmark points are calculated to find out the deformities in the dento-facial growth. Banumathi A. et al [94] used in this study the Projected Principal Edge Distribution (PPED) vectors as a system for medical image recognition, and was used also in image recognition system dicussed above described by Tanikawa C et al [80], as this techniques proved to provide better results.

4.2 Planning of treatment using AI

Enormous amount of variant subjects lies in the etiological list of orthodontic problems, we'll try at this section to show the artificial intelligent task in the planning of appropriate therapeutic goals can be achieved within certain boundaries for each problem, these boundaries considers the available problematic outcomes and its related factor as the backbone of system modeling and comparing these treatment plan with authors subjective opinions to simulate the treatment plan created by human brain.

Cranifacial Growth modification

Planning of treatment in the field of orthodontics and maxillo-facial surgery is largely dependent on the classification of individual growth of a patient. Work by Lux CJ et al[45] suggested the use of an artificial neural network, namely self-organizing neural maps, the growth of 43 orthodontically untreated children was analyzed by means of lateral cephalograms taken at the ages of 7 and 15. For the description of craniofacial skeletal changes, the concept of tensor analysis and related methods have been applied. Thus the geometric and analytical limitations of conventional cephalometric methods have been avoided, the resultant growth data were classified and the relationships of the various growth patterns were monitored by using an artificial neural network. As a result of self-organization, the 43 children were topologically ordered on the emerging map according to their craniofacial size and shape changes during growth. As a new patient can be allocated on the map, this type of network provides a frame of reference for classifying and analysing previously unknown cases according to their growth pattern. The morphometric methods applied as well as the subsequent visualization of the growth data by means of neural networks can be employed for the analysis and classification of growth-related skeletal changes in general.

Impacted canine

An impacted canine requires a complex therapeutic management, The therapeutic approach to impacted canines is interdisciplinary, with many factors accounting for the final orthodontic and periodontal outcomes. Pretreatment radiographic features of impacted canines—α-angle, d-distance, and sector of impaction according to Ericson and Kurol[96,97]have been shown to be predictive factors for the durations of orthodontic traction and comprehensive orthodontic treatment to reposition the impacted tooth. The more severely displaced the canine with regard to the adjacent maxillary incisors, the longer the orthodontic treatment[98], most investigations evaluated the relationships between factors accounting for treatment outcomes of impacted canines with descriptive statistics or linear regression on a priori identified variables; more recent studies used multilevel statistics to study associations among factors without determining causal relationships [99,100]. The multiple factors affecting the ultimate treatment approaches and duration should be included in the overall AI model. In 2010 Nieri M et al [101] used Bayesian networks (BN) to comprehensive surgical-orthodontic treatment of maxillary impacted canines to evaluate the relative role and the possible causal relationships among various factors affecting the clinical approach to this condition. BN adopt an intermediate approach

between statistics and artificial intelligence. An automatic structural learning algorithm of the BN was used as an explorative statistical technique for detecting possible causal relationships among these variables:
demographic variables (sex and age);
topographic variables (clinical and radiographic): site (buccal or palatal), side (left or right), unilateral or bilateral (patient), a-angle, d-distance,
s-sector; treatment technique (tunnel); duration of traction, duration of treatment;
periodontal variables ; Width of keratinized tissue (KT), from the gingival margin to the mucogingival junction; and Probing depth (PD) measurements. These were evaluated for the treated teeth through the therapeutic course.
In the BN analysis. the metric variables were transformed into binary variables by using the median values as a threshold as shown in fig 24.

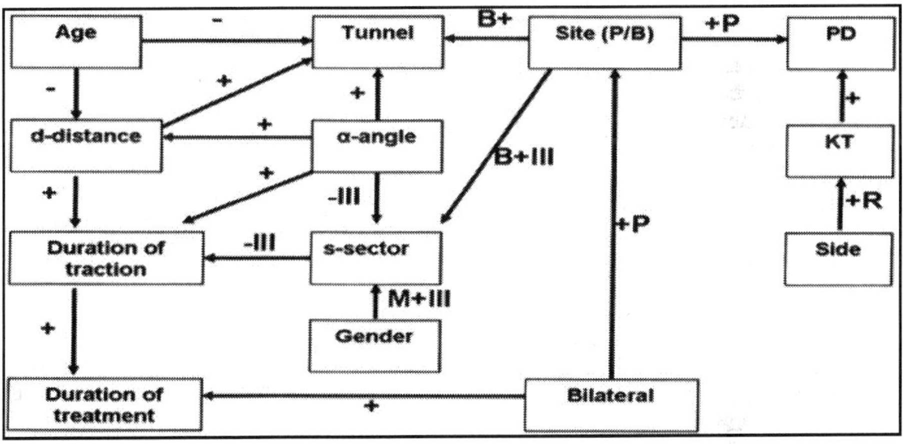

Fig. 24. The graph generated by the structural learning algorithm .P, Palatal; B, buccal; PD, probing depth; KT, keratinized tissue; R, right side; III, sector 3;M, male;1, the variable at the base of the arrow positively influences the variable at the arrowhead,the variable at the base of the arrow negatively influences the variable at the arrowhead, from Nieri M et al [101]

The BN approach confirmed the results of previous investigations on the same population in which the final periodontal outcomes after the surgical-orthodontic repositioning of maxillary impacted canines were unrelated to pretreatment diagnostic variables on the panoramic radiographs [100,102].The application of BN to diagnostic and therapeutic aspects of comprehensive surgical-orthodontic treatment of maxillary impacted canines identified several possible causal relationships among factors affecting the final outcomes of therapy.

Extraction demands in orthodontics

Early in the 20th century the maintaining of intact dentition became an important goal of orthodontic treatment. Angle and his followers strongly opposed extraction for orthodontic purposes. With the emphasis on dental occlusion that followed, however, less attention came to be paid to facial proportions and esthetics at that time. Small jaw size relative to the size of the teeth is an important factor in planning orthodontic therapy, as it implies that a significant percentage of patients will continue to require extractions to provide space for aligning the remaining teeth. for over 100 years it has been a key question in planning orthodontic treatment. In orthodontics, there are two major reasons to extract teeth [103]:

1. to provide space to align the remaining teeth in the presence of severe crowding, and
2. to allow teeth to be moved (usually, incisors to be retracted) so protrusion can be reduced or so skeletal Class II or Class III problems can be camouflaged.

The alternative to extraction in treating dental crowding is to expand the arches; the alternative for skeletal problems is to correct the jaw relationship, by modifying growth or surgery. the majority of patients were treated with extractions to provide enough space for the other teeth. At present there again is great enthusiasm for expanding dental arches, on the theory that soft tissue adaptation will allow the expansion to be maintained, therefore; orthodontic treatments for malocclusion can be classified as extraction treatments and nonextraction treatments. The decision of extraction or not might be challenging and aimed to correct the malocclusion and enhancement of dental and facial appearance.

The decision to extract requires a multiple-factor analysis, which often includes the clinical experiences of the orthodontist. Currently, many multiple-factor analysis methods are available for use. Among these, the most frequently used is the statistical process known as fuzzy grouping analysis. Fuzzy grouping analysis regroups multiple factors based on their closeness in affecting the extraction decision. Classification by this algorithm is applicable to many patients. Xie X et al [39] study construct a decision-making expert system (ES) for orthodontic treatment by using a new approach. The ANN model was constructed to predict whether malocclusion patients between 11 and 15 years old required orthodontic extraction treatment. ANN model had 23 neurons in the input layer and 1 neuron in the output layer; this corresponded to the use of extraction or nonextraction treatments.

The model was implemented using the FORTRAN programming language, which is based on the principle of artificial neural networks. This Back Propagation (BP) ANN employs the error backward propagation learning algorithm. The basic principle of the BP algorithm is the propagation of errors from the output layer backward to the input layer by each layer that "shares" the error with neurons of each layer. Thus the reference errors of each layer of neuron are obtained for use in adjusting the corresponding connection weights, to make the error function diminish as far as possible. To enhance the performance of BP networks, a suitable learning parameter η and momentum parameter ε should be chosen properly. 25indices were selected for screening of subjects. Two of these were nonquantification indices, which included the situation of heredity and protruded anterior teeth uncovered by incompetent lips. Among the quantifiable indices, 5 were derived from cast measurement, 13 from hard tissue cephalometrics, and 5 from soft tissue cephalometrics.

Contributions of the 23 input layer indices to the output layer index were analyzed through the method of neural network data processing. The connection strengths of each neuron in the input layer with each neuron in the hidden layer were used to represent the values of contribution from every input index. The values of a new index F (i) were calculated respectively to represent the contributions. These new indices were ordered by their magnitude, with the largest on top. The new index described the contributions from every input index to the result, as is shown in Table 2. After the data were preprocessed, all input indices were valued at between 0 and 1. the output index was extraction or nonextraction, quantification was processed as 0.99 for "yes" and 0.01 for "no."

Data from the 180 patients-in-training set were used to train the ANN model described above. Data from 20 patients were used to test the accuracy of the ANN model. When $\eta$was chosen as 0.9 and ε as 0.7, and the number of neurons in the hidden layer was 13, the model had a nice learning effect. The 20 test samples proved successful in evaluating factors that affect the decision-making process. The rate of accuracy was 100%, which demonstrated that the constructed ANN could make correct decisions regarding the data of the trained 180 samples. Then, the data of 20 testing set samples that had not been trained were tested, and it demonstrated that the rate of accuracy was 80%. As for the marginal cases.

Input index	F(i)	order
Anterior teeth uncovered by incompetent lips	14042.44	1
IMPA (LI-MP)	11833.00	2
Overjet	6693.52	3
Crowding in the upper dental arch, mm	6135.12	4
Space for correction Sppe's curve, mm	5948.78	5
ANB	5891.38	6
Overbite	5689.83	7
LI-NB	5640.86	8
LL-E plane, mm	4697.43	9
Soft tissue convexity (Ns-Sn-Pos)	4033.89	10
Interincisal angle (UI-LI)	4000.84	11
UI-NA, mm	3967.02	12
Z angle	2872.43	13
Wits, mm	2664.37	14
NLA (Cm-Sn-UL)	2620.67	15
UI-SN	2447.43	16
UL-E plane, mm	2250.07	17
UI-NA	2199.48	18
Heredity	2190.95	19
Crowding in the lower dental arch, mm	2173.83	20
FMIA (L1-FH)	1966.10	21
L1-NB, mm	1520.10	22
FMA (FH-MP)	410.39	23

Table 2. Analysis of Contributions of Every Input Index used inXie X et al [39] expert system

Using AI in selecting the appropriate treatment modalities

a computer-assisted inference model for selecting appropriate types of headgear appliance for orthodontic patients and act as a decision-making aid for inexperienced clinicians was developed by Akgam M.O and Takada K [104] Headgear is mainly used in orthodontic practice to deliver extra-oral forces to the upper dental arch for anchorage purposes, distalizing teeth and/or inhibiting forward maxillary growth. It has three main types, i.e. low, medium, and high-pull describing the direction of force applied to the upper molar teeth in the sagittal plane[105]. The choice of the precise type of headgear may not be difficult when considering its application in 'typical' cases, such as those exhibiting a Class II malocclusion with a deep overbite, large over jet, and a low mandibular plane angle. A problem may arise, however, particularly for orthodontists who have less clinical experience, with 'borderline' or 'marginal' subjects, such as those having a deep overbite, a moderate to severe over jet, and a high mandibular plane angle. This is because decision making in choosing an appropriate headgear type cannot be dealt with in a discrete, but rather a continuous manner, i.e. *fuzzy logic.* the study incorporates three variables, namely, overjet, overbite, and mandibular plane angle, were used as input variables to the system. The mandibular plane angle was defined as the angle formed by the SN and mandibular planes. These variables were obtained from the lateral cephalograms.

For each input variable, three fuzzy sets for the low, medium, and high-pull types of headgear were defined on the basis of the authors' subjective judgment, which included their clinical experience and knowledge of the normative means and standard deviations for each variable. For each fuzzy set, the *fuzzy trapezoid function* was employed to construct membership functions. The fuzzy sets for each variable were determined with an assumption that the remaining two variables took normative values. For ease of understanding and simplicity, a graphic interpretation of the element and membership grade pairs which were created for the low, medium and high-pull types using each input variable is provided in Figures 25,26,27,Geometric mean aggregation was used for the inference, Geometric mean aggregation

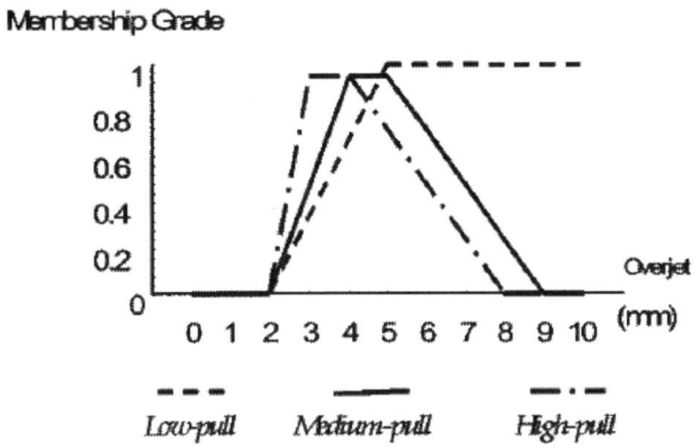

Fig. 25. Plot of membership functions for the input of overjet for each of three sets, i.e. the low-, medium-, and high-pull types of headgear.

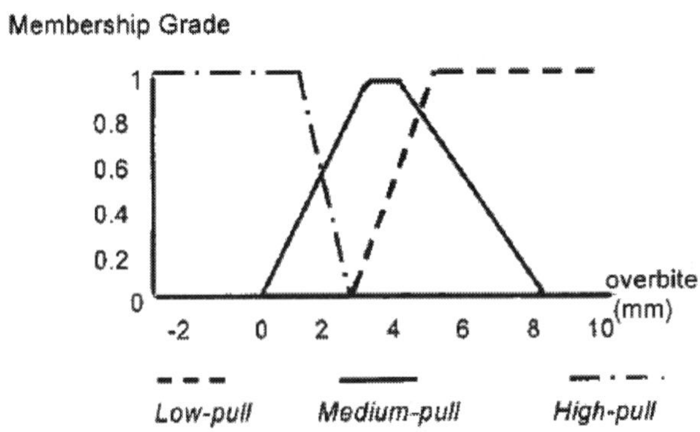

Fig. 26. Plot of membership functions for the input of overbite for each of three sets, . the low-, medium-, and high-pull types of headgear.

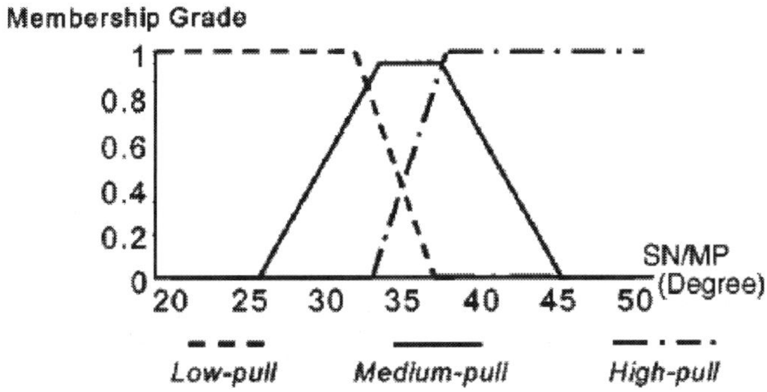

Fig. 27. Plot of membership functions for the input of mandibular for each of three sets, . the low-, medium-, and high-pull types of headgear.

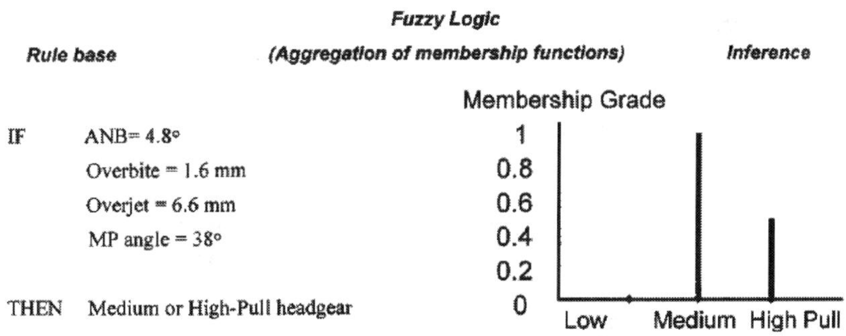

Fig. 28. The computer provides a selection of headgear types in which each choice is accompanied by a membership grades.

was the operation by multiple fuzzy sets were combined to produce single fuzzy set, the inference system was designed to calculate degrees of certainty for the use of each headgear type by means of membership grades fig 28.

The model was designed to calculate the degree of certainty for choosing low-, medium- or high-pull types of headgear. Eight orthodontic experts evaluated the decisions inferred by the system for 85 orthodontic cases. This group of clinicians was satisfied with the system's recommendations in 95.6 percent of the cases. In addition, the majority of the examiners (i.e. equal to or more than six out of eight) were satisfied with the system's recommendations in 97.6 per cent of the cases examined. Thus, the inference system developed was confirmed as being reliable and effective for clinical use in orthodontics.

4.3 The force system design for orthodontic treatments using AI

The most common aspects in the orthodontic treatment of extraction cases are the canine, the incisor and the mass retraction ,tooth retraction during space closure is achieved through two types of mechanics a. Sliding mechanics (friction mechanics) and b. Segmental or sectional mechanics (friction free technique). In the segmented arch technique, frictionless springs are used to attract the segments of teeth on either side of an attraction site , there are different retraction springs that can be used. Many variables affect the force system they could produce; geometry, material, cross section, position, activation distance, etc. Tooth movement and orthopedic changes are the result of an applied force system and the tissue response to it . The force system is currently the major factor that the orthodontist can control to achieve desirable orthodontic tooth movement. Force system generated from complex geometric appliances produce forces and moments, it's important to control not only the magnitude of the force but also the moment to force ratio to produce the desired tooth movement. Force systems originated from orthodontic appliances have been studied by means of static systems for simple springs[106,107]or by experimental method _[108-112], and numerical approaches _[113]_ or by dynamic systems (typodont systems) [114].The numerical methods are the most recent approaches having been merged with the medical area due to computer science, while in the experimental methods, the body of evidence is submitted to mechanical tests, which might determine the force system more accurately- [115]

During an orthodontic space closure, the optimum response, both clinically and histologically, depends on the precision and calibration of the force systems to be used, therefore; a variety of prefabricated and precalibrated orthodontic loops are able to deliver precise and carefully controlled forces was utilized. Attempts to improve the force systems produced by this appliance have resulted in a number of different loop designs. Control of the force systems applied to the teeth is one of the main challenges in orthodontic biomechanics. Thus, the theoretical prediction of the forces and moments produced by the orthodontic appliance is important to control treatment.

It can be seen that if a reliable analytical or numerical method of the closing loop analysis is available, then any orthodontist can use this tool to calculate the characteristics of the closing loops theoretically without resorting to costly and time-consuming experiments. In many previous studies many researchers were developed a mathematical models for simulating the force system produced by orthodontic appliances based on small-deflection linear theory, large-deflection nonlinear theory and finite element methods, the last decade witness the innovative AI modeling using soft computing approaches, The advantage for using a black box of AI elements (like Neural networks, Genetic algorithms) in simulating the force system produced by the orthodontic appliances its ability to capture the real behavior of the orthodontic appliances (spring system).

In this section we will discuss some of the available AI models that can be used in modeling of the effective design for appliances for orthodontic treatment.

5. Force system prediction using artificial neural network

As we mentioned above the retraction loops force system namely, force, moment and moment to force ratio is affected by various parameter, Kazem et al [116] produced an artificial neural network based on an experimental force system evaluation of T-retraction springs, the experimental procedure includes studying the effect of cross section and activation distance on the force system produced by T-retraction springs, Forty T-looped stainless steel arch wires of three different cross sections were used in the testing procedure ,their sizes were(0.018*0.025 in., 0.017*0.025 in., and 0.016*0.022 in.), A new test apparatus specially designed and operated by the researcher [117](Garma NMH) for the measurement of the horizontal forces and the moments of sectional springs is used for teeth retraction, Each one of the already prepared twenty sectional stainless steel T-loop of each group was activated by 1 mm, 2 mm, and 3 mm, respectively, and the readings from load cell outputs were recorded, .

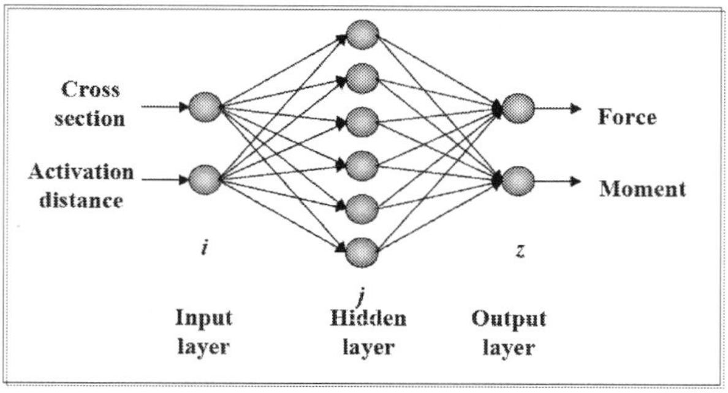

Fig. 29. NN architecture used for the force system modeling

After the results were obtained, they were used in the ANN modeling to evaluate its ability in the prediction process of the T-spring force system. Neural network training can be made more efficient if certain preprocessing steps are performed on the network inputs and targets. Figure 5 illustrates the preprocessing and postprocessing stage in prediction model. The neural network model is organized as a number of input neurons equal to the number of independent variables, which are spring properties (cross section and activation distance), and a number of output neurons equal to the number of dependent variable, which is the force system component (force and moment). Although the number of neurons in the input and output layers is specified depending on the problem, there is no hard and fast rules to specify the number of neurons in the hidden layer. Up to this day, the problem of specifying the optimal number of hidden neurons is an active area of research. Often a trial and error approach is starting with a modest number of hidden neurons and gradually increasing the number if the network fails to reduce its performance index (training error)[118,119]. The simulated annealing technique is used to capture the best weights and biases. The experimental results were used to train and test in neural network; seven measured results were used, from the total of nine, as data sets to train the network. Many neural networks architectures are used to train the data set to produce the least error; the neural network model was trained by using Levenberg - Marquardt Algorithm. many different trial numbers of the hidden layer neurons and types of the activation function were used at each time. Figure show optimized ANN training session. To evaluate the effect of increasing the hidden layer in to two layers on the ANN performance, many trial numbers of the two hidden layers training and accuracy prediction was done with different number of the two layer hidden neurons., the prediction accuracy for the testing patterns is based on the mean absolute percent error .

A network with one hidden layer include 6 neurons trained by Levenberg-Marquardt algorithm showed the best performance indication. Figure (20) shows the resulted network architecture, the network architecture consists of two input neurons (i), and one hidden layers contain six neuron (j) with nonlinear activation function (tangential sigmoid) and two output neurons (z) with linear activation function.

The prediction accuracy of the optimized ANN architecture are illustrated in (table), the mean error of data test set of the force prediction is (5.707%), while for the moment prediction is (4.048%),The multilayer feed forward neural network was successful in mapping the relationship among inputs parameters of the T-spring "cross section and activation distance" and output force system "horizontal force and moment." The successful ANN mapping of the relationship between the spring properties and resultant force system can happen by utilizing other researche\ results, and it would be more beneficial as generalization increased with increasing input data set _spring properties_ in this situation.

Set No.	Actual force (gm)	ANN Prediction	Error %	Moment (gm mm)	ANN Prediction	Error %
1	291.3	299.3	2.7487	1311.11	1301.7	0.7183`
8	375.3	342.8	8.666	2177.14	2016.5	7.3785

Table 3. Test data sets and network prediction after optimization

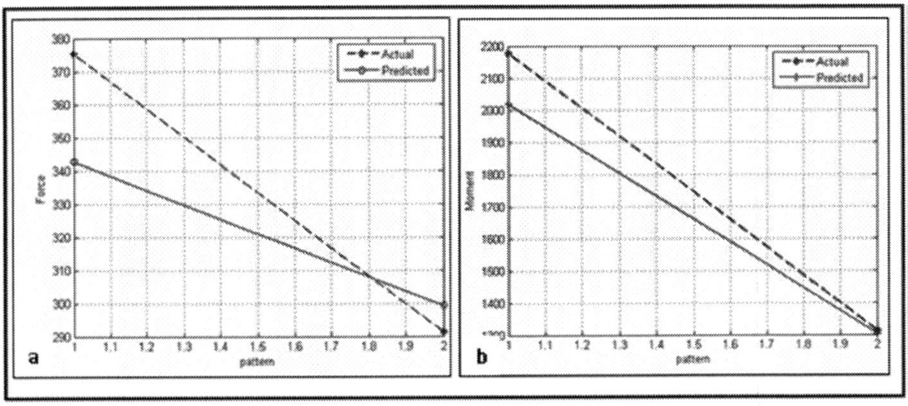

Fig. 30. Predicted and measured data in test set a-force, b- moment.

6. Multi-objective design optimization using GA

The multi-objective optimization is a vector of decision variables which satisfies constraints and optimizes vector functions whose elements represent the objective function. These functions form the mathematical description of performance criteria which are usually in conflict with each other. Hence, the term 'optimizes' means finding such a solution which would give the values of all objective functions acceptable to the designer, Osyczka [120].

The Genetic Algorithm is used in this work to optimize our engineering-orthodontic problem (select the best T-spring dimension and Material to get the required spring stiffness and moment to force ratio); i.e. to obtain an optimal force (spring stiffness) and a (M/H) ratio capable of pure translation together.

The spring design parameters are encoded directly, using real codification, as strings (chromosomes) to be used for GA. For T-spring thirteen parameters should be optimized as shown in the following chromosome:

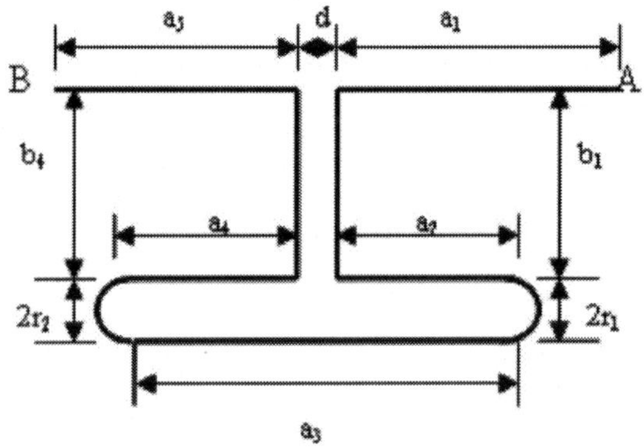

Fig. 31. T-spring Dimensions

$$x = [x_1 x_2, x_3, x_4, x_5, x_6, x_7, x_8, x_9, x_{10}, x_{11}, x_{12}, x_{13}] \quad (2)$$

$$= [a_1, a_2, a_3, a_3, a_4, a_5, b_1, b_3, r_{1,}, r_2, d, t, w, E] \quad (3)$$

Of these variables, a1, a2, a3, a4 ,a5,b1,b3, r1, r2 are real-parameters with specific range (Lmin, Lmax), t and w are discrete variables having the standard cross section dimensions values of orthodontic arch wires, E is a discrete variable having the standard Young's modulus values of orthodontic arch wires.

The two objective optimization problems are as follows [121]:

$$\text{Minimize } f_1(x) = springstiffness(kx) \quad \text{Minimize } f_2(x) = \left|[(M/H) - (M/H)_D]\right| \quad (4)$$

Subjected to

$$g_1(x) = (x_1 + x_2 + x_3 + x_4 + x_5 + x_6 + x_7 + \pi x_8 + \pi x_9 + x_{10}) \geq (L_T)$$

$$g_4(x) = (x_1 + x_5 + x_{10}) \leq (L_T)) \quad (5)$$

$$g_2(x) = (x_6 + 2x_8) \leq (H_T) \quad (6)$$

$$g_3(x) = (x_7 + 2x_9) \leq (H_T) \quad (7)$$

$$g_5(x) = (x_2 + x_5 + x_{10}) \leq (L_T)) \quad (8)$$

$$g_6(x) = (x_2 + x_8 + x_9 + x_4) \leq (x_1 + x_5 + x_{10}) \quad (9)$$

$$g_7(x) = (x_3 + x_8 + x_9) \leq (x_1 + x_5 + x_{10}) \quad (10)$$

$$g_8(x) = x_2 + x_4 + x_{10} = x_3 \quad (11)$$

$$g_9(x) = (x_6 + 2x_8) - (x_7 + 2x_9) \leq \Delta \quad (12)$$

Where the kx and M/H are calaculated using Castigliano's second theorem. (M/H)D is the required moment to force ratio for orthodontic treatment. The nine constraints are chosen to make sure that the produced solutions are within the required total spring dimensions (total length (LT) and total height (HT)). The maximum allowable difference in total height between the left and right end is given by (Δ). We can add any type of design constraint and to be sure that we will converge to some applicable design for the required application.

The presence or absence of a member in the spring structure is determined by comparing the length of the member with the designer defined small critical length, e. If a length is smaller than e, that member is assumed to be absent in the realized T-spring.

Operators in genetic algorithm

A new methodology for the optimization of the design parameters for T-spring arch wire had been developed by Kazem [121]. The proposed analytic model depending on the Castigliano's second theorem with an accurate boundary conditions and geometrical representation provides acceptable results for symmetric and asymmetric spring although it depends on the small deflection theory, in comparison with the results obtained using non-linear FEM. The multi-objective optimization for the spring design parameters is adopted successfully using GA method and the results show that depending on the above methodology, we can make good estimation of the required design parameters for the T-spring. Future work includes improving the analytical model for the spring system depending on the large deflection theorem and also, more inspection is needed by using other evolutionary algorithms like Strength Pareto Evolutionary Algorithm (SPEA) and SPEA 2 that update the ranking and selection criteria used in GA.

The initial population of strings (Real number coding) is generated at random and then the search is carried out among this population. The evolution of the population elements is non-generational, which means that the new replace the worst ones. The main different operators adopted in the GA are reproduction, crossover and mutation.

What concerns the reproduction operator is the successive generations of new strings which are generated based on their fitness values. In this case, a 5-tournament is used to select the strings for reproduction. For the tournament selection, only discrete values can be assigned and for higher range of selection intensity rather than ranking selection. About 50% of the population is lost at tournament size Tour=5. Tournament selection leads to high diversity for the same selection intensity compared to truncation selection [122]. At current search, tournament size less than 5 makes the solution progress slow toward the optimum solution and that which is more than 5 makes solution fall in the local optimum.

With a given probability Pc, the crossover operator adopts the single point technique and, therefore, the crossover point is only allowed between genes or, in other words, the crossover operator cannot disrupt genes. The mutation operator replaces one gene value xt with another one generated randomly with a specified range by a given probability Pm.

According to our knowledge, such an approach has not been tested yet on orthodontic spring optimum design problem.

The size of the mutation step is usually difficult to choose. The optimal step-size depends on the problem considered and may even vary during the optimization process. It is known, that small steps (small mutation steps) are often successful, especially when the individual is already well adapted. However, larger changes (large mutation steps) can, when successful, produce good results much quicker. Thus, a good mutation operator should often produce small step-sizes with a high probability and large step-sizes with a low probability.

Two indices are used to qualify the evolving solution. All indices are translated into penalty functions to be minimized. Each index is computed individually and is integrated in the fitness function evaluation. The fitness function ff adopted for evaluating the candidate solutions is defined after Coello and Christiansen [123]:

$$f_f = \beta_1 f_1 + \beta_2 f_2$$

Where $\beta_1 + \beta_2 = 1$

The optimization goal consists of finding a set of design parameters that minimize ff according to the priorities given by the weighting factors βi (i = 1, 2), where each different set of weighting factors must result in a different solution.

Optimization weight factor (β1, β2)	Spring shape and material for Optimized solution vector (x)	f1			f2		
		GA	From FEM	Error %	GA	From FEM	Error%
(0.75,0.25)	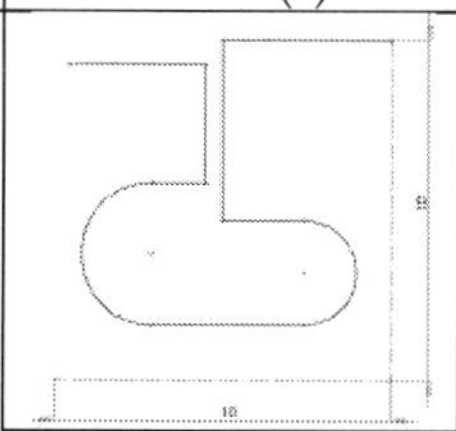 txw=0.40x0.55 E=172,000Mpa	40.32	42.67	-5.8	1.31	1.11	15.2
(0.5,0.5)	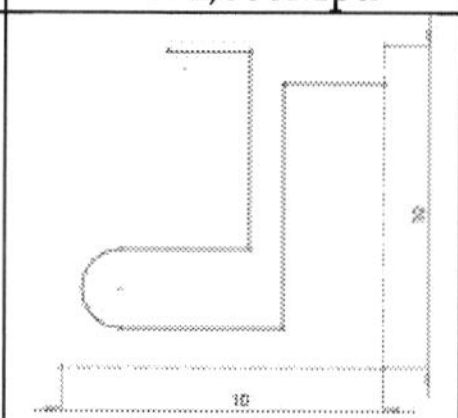 txw=0.40x0.55 E=172,000Mpa	49.11	58.56	-19.2	1.66	1.4	15.6
(0.25,0.75)	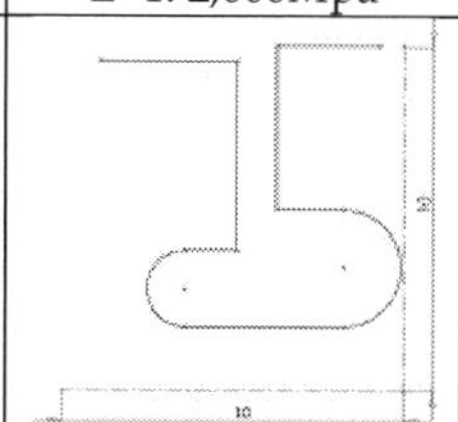 txw=0.482x0.635 E=192,000Mpa	50.29	46.18	8.17	0.61	0.67	-9.8

Table 4. Optimized Solutions for T-Spring design.

The optimized spring geometry and materials produced by GA were modeled by using FEM to calculate the spring stiffness (=f1) and the difference between resultant moment to force ratio and the user specified ratio (=f2) as given in Table 4.

7. Summary

In summary the subject of artificial Intelligence (AI) deals with symbolic processing than numeric computation. Knowledge representation, reasoning, planning, learning, intelligent search and uncertainty management of data and knowledge are the common areas covered under AI. Some of the applications areas of AI are speech and image understanding, expert systems, pattern classification, system optimization and navigational planning of mobile robots, the recent implementation of AI in the medical field and orthodontics was of special concern in this chapter, as the discipline of orthodontics task is to deal with the boolean etiological identification and optimized strategies of solution delivered to treat dentoalveolar and/or facial skeletal malrelation, the AI role used to achieve this task using variant techniques , AI incorporated many trial of changing the techniques used to simulate the clinical situations in the three essential sequences, diagnosis, treatment plan and treatment. The presence of differential problematic orthodontic problems , their origins and the consequence treatment makes the understanding of the AI aspect and its techniques essential to choose the techniques discriminating different problems and subsequent solution. Three aspects of AI;

- Artificial Neural Nets
- Genetic Algorithms
- Fuzzy logic

Artificial intelligence trials with these three techniques in different orthodontic steps yield numerous researches enrich the orthodontic domain with logical and economic tool substitutes the elongated sequential and sophisticated techniques, these trials yet are active area of research and need elaborated studies to reach their ultimate clinical assumption.

8. References

[1] Konar A., Uncertainty Management in Expert Systems using Fuzzy Petri Nets, Ph.D. thesis, Jadavpur,1999.

[2] Newell, A .and Simon, H.A., Human Problem Solving, Prentice-Hall, Englewood Cliffs, NJ, 1972.

[3] Luger, G. F. and Stubblefield, W. A., Artificial Intelligence: Structures and Strategies for Complex Problem Solving, Benjamin/Cummings, Menlo Park, CA, 1993.

[4] Schalkoff, J., Culberson, J., Treloar, N. and Knight, B., "A world championship caliber checkers program," Artificial Intelligence, vol. 53, no. 2-3, pp. 273-289, 1992.

[5] Winston, P. H., Artificial Intelligence, Addison-Wesley, 2nd ed., Reading, MA, 1994.

[6] Newell, A .and Simon, H.A., Human Problem Solving, Prentice-Hall, Englewood Cliffs, NJ, 1972.

[7] Charniak, E. and McDermott, D., Introduction to Artificial Intelligence, Addison-Wesley, Reading, MA, 1985.

[8] E. A. Metzbower , J. J. DeLoach , "*Secondary effects in neural network analysis of the mechanical properties of welding alloys for HSLA shipbuilding steels*" Mathematical

Modeling of Weld Phenomena 6, eds H. Cerjak and H. K. D. H. Bhadeshia, published by Maney, London, 2002. pp. 231-242.

[9] H Demuth,M Beale,M Hagan "*Neural Network Toolbox User's Guide Ver5* " the mathworks ,Inc.,Natick,MA,USA,2006

[10] D. T.Pham and L.Xing "*Neural networks for identification, prediction and control*" Springer publishing company (1997)

[11] Haykan Simon, "*Neural Network - a comprehensive foundation*", prentice Hall, 1999.

[12] Pohlheim, Hartmut, GEATbx: Introduction Evolutionary Algorithms: Overview, Methods and Operators GEATbx version 3.8 (2006)

[13] Zadeh L A 1965 Fuzzy sets. Information and Control 8: 338-353

[14] M. Hellmann, Fuzzy Logic Introduction Laboratoire Antennes Radar Telecom , F.R.E CNRS 2272, Equipe Radar Polarimetrie, Universit´e de Rennes, France

[15] Dean, T., Allen, J. and Aloimonds, Y., Artificial Intelligence: Theory and Practice, Addison-Wesley, Reading, MA, 1995.

[16] Dickmans, E.D., Mysliwetz, B. and Christians, T., "An integrated spatio-temporal approach to vehicles," IEEE Trans. on Systems, Man and Cybernetics, vol. 20, no. 6, Dec. 1990.

[17] Dougherty, E. R. and Giardina, C.R., Mathematical Methods for Artificial Intelligence and Autonomous Systems, Prentice-Hall, Englewood Cliffs, NJ, 1988.

[18] Feigenbaum, E. A. and Feldman, J., Eds., Computers and Thought, McGraw-Hill, New York, 1963.

[19] Haugeland, J., Ed., Artificial Intelligence: The Very Idea, MIT Press, Cambridge, 1985.

[20] Jackson, P., Introduction to Expert Systems, Addison-Wesley, Reading, MA, 1986.

[21] Hopfield JJ. Neural networks and physical systems with emergent collective computational abilities. Proc Nat Acad Sci. 1982; 2554- 2558.

[22] Kohonen T. Self-organised formation of topologically correct feature maps. Biological Cybernetics, 1982; 43: 59-69.

[23] Rummelhart DE, McLelland JL. Parallel distributed processing: Explorations in the microstructure of Cognition. Vol. I. Foundation, MIT Press 1987.

[24] Baxt, W. J., Application of artificial neural network to clinical medicine. Lancet. 346:1135–1138, 1995.

[25] Kocyigit, Y., Alkan, A., and Erol, H., Classification of EEG recordings by using fast independent component analysis and artificial neural network. J. Med. Syst. 32 (1)17–20, 2008.

[26] Silva Lopes H F & Abe J M. , Anghinah R. Application of Paraconsistent Artificial Neural Networks as a Method of Aid in the Diagnosis of Alzheimer Disease J Med Syst (2010) 34:1073–1081

[27] Ventouras, E. M., Monoyou, E. A., Ktonas, P. Y., Paparrigopoulos, T., Dikeos, D. G., Uzunoglu, N. K., and Soldatos, C. R., Sleep spindle detection using artificial neural networks trained with filtered timedomain EEG: a feasibility study. Comput. Methods Programs Biomed. 78 (3)191–207, 2005.

[28] Miller, A., The application of neural networks to imaging and signal processing in astronomy and medicine, Ph.D. thesis, Faculty of Science, Department of Physics, University of Southampton, 1993.

[29] Prado, J. C. A. Constelação fônica e redes neurais artificiais: aplicabilidade na análise computacional da produção da fala (in Portuguese). Ph.D. Thesis. FFLCH—USP; São Paulo, SP, BR; 2007.

[30] Weinstein, J., Kohn, K., and Grever, M., Neural computing in cancer drug development: predicting mechanism of action. Science. 258:447–451, 1992.

[31] Papik K, Molnar B, Schaefer R, Dombovari Z, Tulassay Z, Feher J. Application of neural network in medicine. Med Sci Monit. 1998; 4(3): 538-46.

[32] Sims-Williams J H, Brown I D, Matthewman A, Stephens C D 1987 A computer controlled expert system for orthodontic advice. British Dental Journal 163: 161-166

[33] Mackin N, Sims-Williams J H, Stephens C D 1991 Artificial intelligence in dental surgery: an orthodontic expert system, a dental tool of tomorrow. Dental Update 18: 341-343

[34] Hudson D L, Cohen M E 1994 Fuzzy logic in medical expert systems. IEEE Engineering in Medicine and Biology 3: 693-698

[35] Stephens C D, Mackin N, Sims-Williams J H 1996 The development and validation of an orthodontic expert system. British Journal of Orthodontics 23: 1-9

[36] Tanaka T, Miwa K, Kanda S 1997 Application of fuzzy reasoning in an expert system for ultrasonography. Dentomaxillofacial Radiology 26: 125-131

[37] Brown I D, Adams S R, Stephens C D, Erritt S J, Sims-Willianis J H 1991 The initial use of a computer controlled expert system in the treatment planning of Class II division 1 malocclusion. British Journal of Orthodontics 18: 1-7

[38] Graber TM, Vanarsdall RL. Orthodontics: Current principles and techniques. 2nd ed. St. Louis: Mosby, 1994.

[39] Xie X; Wang L; Wang A. Artificial Neural Network Modeling for Deciding if Extractions Are Necessary Prior to Orthodontic Treatment Angle Orthod. 2010;80:262–266.

[40] Stheeman S E, Van der Stelt P F, Mileman P A 1992 Expert systems in dentistry past performance—future prospects. Journal of Dentistry 20: 68-73

[41] Takada K, Sorihashi Y, Akcam M O 1998 Orthodontic treatment planning: its rationale for inference. In: Carels C, Willems G (eds) The future of orthodontics. Leuven University Press, Belgium, pp. 203-211

[42] Poon KC, Freer TJ. EICO-1: an orthodontist-maintained expert system in clinical orthodontics. Aust Orthod J. 1999; 15:219–228.

[43] Hammond RM, Freer TJ. Application of a case-based expert system to orthodontic diagnosis and treatment planning: a review of the literature. Aust Orthod J. 1996;14:150–153.

[44] Hammond RM, Freer TJ. Application of a case-based expert system to orthodontic diagnosis and treatment planning. Aust Orthod J. 1997;14:229–234.

[45] Lux CJ, Stellzig A, Volz D, Jäger W, Richardson A, Komposch G. Department of Orthodontics, Dental School, University of Heidelberg, Germany. Growh dev.aging. A neural network approach to the analysis and classification of human craniofacial growth. 1998:(6) 295-106

[46] Brickley MR, Shepherd JP, Armstrong RA. Neural networks: a new technique for development of decision support systems in dentistry. J Dent. 1998;26:305–309.

[47] S. Richmond, WC. Shaw, KD. O'Brien, lB. Buchanan, R. Jones ,CD. Stephens, CT. Roberts, M. Andrews, "The development of the par index (peer assessment rating): reliability and validity," European J of Orthodontics, vol. 14, no. 2, pp. 125-129, 1992.

[48] Zarei A, El-Sharkawi M, Hairfield M. An intelligent system for assessment of orthodontic treatment outcome using fuzzy union rule configuration. in Proc. lASTED, May 2007, 428-433.

[49] Zarei A, Hairfield M, Mirsaeidghazi SS. A Novel Neuro-Fuzzy Assessment Index for Orthodontics. IEEE Xplore. 2009;3493-3497.
[50] Vieira A, Lawrence H, Limeback H, Sampaio F, and Grynpas M. A visual analog scale for measuring dental fluorosis severity. American Dental Association, vol. 136, pp. 895-901, 2005.
[51] Takagi T and Sugeno M. Fuzzy identification of systems and its applications to modeling and control, IEEE Trans. Systems, Man. And Cybernetics, 1985;15: 116-132,.
[52] Jyh-Shing Roger Jang and Chuen-Tsai Sun, Neuro-fuzzy and control. in Proc. IEEE.1995; 83(3): 378-406.
[53] Cohen AM, Ip HH, Linney AD. A preliminary study of computer recognition and identification of skeletal landmarks as a new method of cephalometric analysis. Br J Orthod. 1984;
[54] Leonardi R, Giordano D, Maiorana F, Spampinato C. Automatic cephalometric analysis. Angle Orthod. 2008;78:145-15.
[55] Parthasarathy S, Nugent ST, Gregson PG, Fay DF. Automatic landmarking of cephalograms. Comput Biomed Res.1989;22:248-269.
[56] Tong W, Nugent ST, Jensen GM, Fay DF. An algorithm for locating landmarks on dental X-rays. Conference proceedings: 11th Annual International Conference of the IEEE Engineering in Medicine and Biology Society. IEEE 1989(2): 552-554.
[57] Forsyth DB, Davis DN. Assessment of an automated cephalometric analysis system. Eur J Orthod. 1996;18:471-478.
[58] Ren J, Lid D, Feng D, Shao J. A knowledge-based automatic cephalometric analysis method. Conference proceedings: 20th International Conference of the IEEE Engineering in Medicine and Biology Society. IEEE 1998;20(2):723-727.
[59] Cardillo J, Sid-Ahmed MA. An image processing system for locating craniofacial landmarks. IEEE T Med Imaging. 1994; 13:275-289.
[60] Rudolph DJ, Sinclair PM, Coggins JM. Automatic computerized radiographic identification of cephalometric landmarks. Am J Orthod Dentofacial Orthop. 1998;113:173- 179.
[61] Hutton TJ, Cunningham S, Hammond P. An evaluation of active shape models for the automatic identification of cephalometric landmarks. Eur J Orthod. 2000;22:499-508.
[62] Romaniuk B, Desvignes M, Revenu M, Deshayes MJ. Shape variability and spatial relationships modeling in statistical pattern recognition. Pattern Recogn Lett. 2004;25: 239-247.
[63] Saad AA, El-Bialy A, Kandil AH, Sayed AA. Automatic cephalometric analysis using active appearance model and simulated annealing. GVIP 05. Conference proceedings: InterAUTOMATIC
[64] CEPHALOMETRIC ANALYSIS 151 Angle Orthodontist, Vol 78, No 1, 2008 national Conference on Graphics, Vision and Image Processing, 2005 Dec 19-21, Cairo, Egypt (2005). ICGST; 2005.
[65] Innes A, Ciesielski V, Mamutil J, Sabu J. Landmark detection for cephalometric radiology images using pulse coupled neural networks. In: Arabnia H, Mun Y, eds. Conference proceedings: IC-AI '02, International Conference on Artificial Intelligence, 2002 June 24-27, Las Vegas, Nevada. CSREA Press; 2002;2:511-517.
[66] Chakrabartty S, Yagi M, Shibata T, Cauwenberghs G. Robust cephalometric identification using support vector machines. Conference proceedings: ICME '03,

International Conference on Multimedia and Expo, 2003 Jul 6-9. IEEE 2003;III:429-432. 32.

[67] Ciesielski V, Innes A, Sabu J, Mamutil J. Genetic programming for landmark detection in cephalometric radiology images. Int J Knowl Based Intell Eng Syst. 2003;7:164-171.

[68] El-Feghi I, Sid-Ahmed MA, Ahmadi M. Automatic localization of craniofacial landmarks for assisted cephalometry. Pattern Recognit. 2004;37:609-621.

[69] Liu J, Chen Y, Cheng K. Accuracy of computerized automatic identification of cephalometric landmarks. Am J Orthod Dentofacial Orthop. 2000;118:535-540.

[70] Grau V, Alcaniz M, Juan MC, Monserrat C, Knoll C. Automatic localization of cephalometric landmarks. J Biomed Inform. 2001;34:146-156. 34.

[71] Yang J, Ling X, Lu Y, Wei M, Ding G. Cephalometric image analysis and measurement for orthognathic surgery. Med Biol Eng Comput. 2001;39:279-284.

[72] Giordano D, Leonardi R, Maiorana F, Cristaldi G, Distefano M. Automatic landmarking of cephalograms by CNNS. Lect Notes Artif Int. 2005;3581:342-352.

[73] Yue W, Yin D, Li C, Wang G, Xu T. Automated 2-D cephalometric analysis on X-ray images by a model-based approach. IEEE Trans Biomed Eng. 2006;53:1615-1623.

[74] Abe JM. Paraconsistent Artificial Neural Networks: an Introduction, Lecture Notes in Artificial Intelligence. Carbonell & J. Siekmann, 2004.

[75] Mario M C, Abe J M., Ortega N R S., Santo Jr M D. Paraconsistent Artificial Neural Network as Auxiliary in Cephalometric Diagnosis. Artificial Organs2010 34(7):E215-E221,Wiley Periodicals, Inc..

[76] Sylvan R, Abe JM. On general annotated logics, with an introduction to full accounting logics. Bull Symb Log 1996;2:118-9.

[77] Mario MC. Modelo de análise de variáveis craniométricas através das Redes Neurais Artificiais Paraconsistentes. PhD thesis, University of São Paulo, 2006.

[78] Da Silva Filho JI, Abe JM. Fundamentos das Redes Neurais Paraconsistentes—Destacando Aplicações em Neurocomputação, (in Portuguese) Editôra Arte & Ciência: ISBN 85-7473-045-9. 2001;247.

[79] Ricketts RM. Cephalometric analysis and synthesis. AngleOrthod 1961;31:141-56.

[80] Tanikawa C, Yagi M, Takada K. Automated Cephalometry: System Performance Reliability Using Landmark-Dependent Criteria. Angle Orthod. 2009;79:1037-1046.

[81] Shibata T. Intelligent VLSI systems based on a psychologicalbrain model. Proc IEEE Int Sym on Intelligent Signal

[82] Yagi M, Shibata T. An image representation algorithm compatible to neural-associative-processor-based hardware recognition systems. IEEE Trans Neural Netw. 2003;14(5):1144-1161.

[83] Levy-Mandel AD, Venetsanopoulos AN, Tsotsos JK. Knowledge- based landmarking of cephalograms. Comput Biomed Res. 1986;282-309.

[84] Takada K, Yagi M, Tanikawa C. Dependable systems for decisions in clinical dentistry-how electronics implements what dentists know. Proc Int Sym on Advanced Electronics for Future Generations, "Secure-Life Electronics" for Quality Life and Society. 2005 Oct 11-12, Tokyo, Japan. 2005:15- 21.

[85] Baumrind S, Frantz RC. The reliability of head film measurements. 1. Landmark identification. Am J Orthod. 1971; 60:111-127

[86] Fujita K, Takada K, QianRong G, Shibata T. Patterning of human dental arch wire blanks using a vector quantization algorithm. Angle Orthod. 2002;72:285-294.

[87] Levy-Mandel AD, Venetsanopoulos AN, Tsotsos JK. Knowledge- based landmarking of cephalograms. Comput Biomed Res. 1986;282–309.

[88] Rudolph DJ, Sinclair PM, Coggins JM. Automatic computerized radiographic identification of cephalometric landmarks. Am J Orthod Dentofacial Orthop. 1998;113:173- 179.

[89] Romaniuk B, Desvignes M, Revenu M, Deshayes MJ. Shape variability and spatial relationships modeling in statistical patter recognition. Pattern Recogn Lett. 2004;25: 239–247.

[90] Grau V, Alcaniz M, Juan MC, Monserra C, Knoll C. Automatic localization of cephalometric landmarks. J Biomed Inform. 2001;34:146–156.

[91] Ciesielski V, Innes A, Mamutil J. Genetic programming for landmark detection in cephalometric radiology images. Int J Knowl Base Intell Eng Syst. 2003;7:164–171.

[92] Giordano D, Leonardi R, Maiorana F, Cristaldi G, Distefano ML. Automatic landmarking of cephalograms by cellular neural networks. Lect Notes Artif Int. 2005;3581:342–352.

[93] Yue W, Yin D, Wang G, Xu T. Automated 2-D cephalometric analysis on X-ray images by a model-based approach. IEEE Trans Biomedical Eng. 2006;53:1615–1623.

[94] Banumathi A, Raju S. , Abhaikumar V. Diagnosis of Dental Deformities in Cephalometry Images Using Support Vector Machine J Med Syst (2011) 35:113–119

[95] Romaniuk, B., Desvignes, M., Robiaille, J., Revenu, M., Deshayes, M. J., Augmented reality and semi automated landmarking of cephalometry radiographs. Comput. Anal. Images Patterns, 9th International Conference CAIP 2001. 410–418, 2001. Sep 5–7

[96] Ericson S, Kurol J. Radiographic assessment of maxillary canine eruption in children with clinical signs of eruption disturbance. Eur J Orthod 1986;8:133-40.

[97] Ericson S, Kurol J. Early treatment of palatally erupting maxillary canines by extraction of the primary canines. Eur J Orthod 1988; 10:283-95.

[98] Stewart JA, Heo G, Giover KE, Williamson PC, Lam EWN, Major PW. Factors that relate to treatment duration for patients with palatally impacted maxillary canines. Am J Orthod Dentofacial Orthop 2001;119:216-25.

[99] Crescini A, Nieri M, Buti J, Baccetti T, Mauro S, Pini Prato GP. Short- and long-term periodontal evaluation of impacted canines treated with a closed surgical-orthodontic approach. J Clin Periodontol 2007;34:232-42.

[100] Crescini A, Nieri M, Buti J, Baccetti T, Pini Prato GP. Pre-treatment radiographic features for the periodontal prognosis of treated impacted canines. J Clin Periodontol 2007;34:581-7.

[101] Nieri M, Crescini A, Rotundo R, Baccetti T, C Pierpaolo, Pratoe GPP. Factors affecting the clinical approach to impacted maxillary canines: A Bayesian network analysis. Am J Orthod Dentofacial Orthop 2010;137:755-62.

[102] Crescini A, Nieri M, Buti J, Baccetti T, Pini Prato GP. Orthodontic and periodontal outcomes of treated impacted maxillary canines. Angle Orthod 2007;77:571-7.

[103] Proffit W R, Fields H W, Sarver DM,Contemporary orthodontics. Mosby Elsevier,4th ed., 2007.

[104] Akgam M. O, Takada K. Fuzzy modelling for selecting headgear types. European Journal of Orthodontics.2002(24):99-106.

[105] Williams J K, Cook P A, Isaacson K G, Thorn A R Fixed orthodontic appliances—principles and practice.1996, Wright, Oxford

[106] Braun, S., and Garcia, J. L., 2002, "The Gable Bend Revisited," Am. J. Orthod. Dentofacial Orthop., 122, pp. 523–527.

[107] Choy, K., Pae, E., Park, Y. C., and Burstone, C. J., 2002, "Controlled Space Closure With Statically Determinate Retraction System," Angle Orthod., 72, pp. 191-198.

[108] Solonche, D. J., Burstone, C. J., and Vanderby, R., 1977, "A Device for Determining the Mechanical Behavior of Orthodontic Appliances," IEEE Trans. Biomed. Eng., BME-24, pp. 538–539.

[109] Nagerl, H., Burstone, C. J., Beacher, B., and Messenburg, D. K., 1991, "Center of Rotation With Transverse Forces," Am. J. Orthod. Dentofacial Orthop., 99, pp. 337–345.

[110] Braun, S., Sjursen, R. C., and Legan, H. L., 1997, "On the Management of Extraction Sites," Am. J. Orthod. Dentofacial Orthop., 112, pp. 645–655.

[111] Siatkowski, R. E., 1997, "Continuous Arch Wire Closing Loop Design, optimization, and Verification Part I," Am. J. Orthod. Dentofacial Orthop., 112, pp. 393–402.

[112] Ferreira, M. A., 1999, "The Wire Material and Cross Section Effect on Double Delta Closing Loops Regarding Load and Spring Rate Magnitude: An In Vitro Study," Am. J. Orthod. Dentofacial Orthop., 115, pp. 275–282.

[113] Raboud, D. W., Faulkner, M. G., Lipsett, A. W., and Haberstock, D. L., 1997,"Three Dimensional Effects in Retraction Appliance Design," Am. J. Orthod. Dentofacial Orthop., 112, pp. 378–392.

[114] Rhee, J., Chu, Y., and Row, J., 2001, "A Comparison Between Friction and Frictionless Mechanics With a New Type Simulation System," Am. J. Orthod. Dentofacial Orthop., 119, pp. 292–299.

[115] Ferreira, M. A., Oliveira, F. T., Ignacio, S. A., and Borges, P. C., 2005, Experimental Force Definition System for a New Orthodontic Retraction Spring," Angle Orthod., 75_3_, pp. 368–377.

[116] Kazem B. I, ; Ghaib N. H;. Garma N. M. H., "Experimental Investigation and Neural Network Modeling for Force System of Retraction T-Spring for Orthodontic Treatment"; Journal of Medical Devices ,ASME, Vol 4, 2010, pp 021001-1-7.,

[117] Garma N. M. H., An experimental and artificial neural network prediction of cross section and activation distance effect on T-spring force system. Master's thesis. Department of orthodontics, Baghdad.

[118] Sukthomya, W., and Tannock, J., 2005, "The Training of Neural Networks to Model Manufacturing Processes," J. Intell. Manuf., 16_1_, pp. 39–51.

[119] Yousif, K. Y., Daws, K. M., and Kazem, B. I., 2008, "Prediction of Friction stir welding Characteristics Using Neural Network," Jordan Journal of Mechanical and Industrial Engineering _JJMIE_, 2_3_, pp. 151–155.

[120] Osyczka, A., 1985, "Multicriteria Optimization for Engineering Design," in Design Optimization, J. S. Gero, ed., Academic, New York, pp. 193–227.

[121] Bahaa I Kazem "Multi-Objective Optimization for the Force System of Orthodontic Retraction Spring Using Genetic Algorithms ";Journal of Medical Devices ,ASME, Vol 3, 2009, pp 041006-1-7.,

[122] Pohlheim, H., 2004, "GEATbx Introduction Evolutionary Algorithms: Overview, Methods and Operators," Version 3.5a, July 2004, http:// www.geatbx.com

[123] Coello, C. A., and Christiansen, A. D., 2000, "Multiobjective Optimization for Trusses Using Genetic Algorithms," Comput. Struct., 75, pp. 647–660.

22

Biomechanics of Tooth-Movement: Current Look at Orthodontic Fundamental

Joanna Antoszewska[1] and Nazan Küçükkeleş[2]
[1]*Wroclaw Medical University,*
[2]*Marmara University,*
[1]*Poland*
[2]*Turkey*

1. Introduction

Numerous methods of efficient orthodontic tooth-movement have been described in the literature for over 100 years, since Edward Hartley Angle had introduced foundations of malocclusion treatment (fig. 1). In such long term, different treatment philosophies have been permanently encountering beginning from Tweed[1] and his extraction concept versus

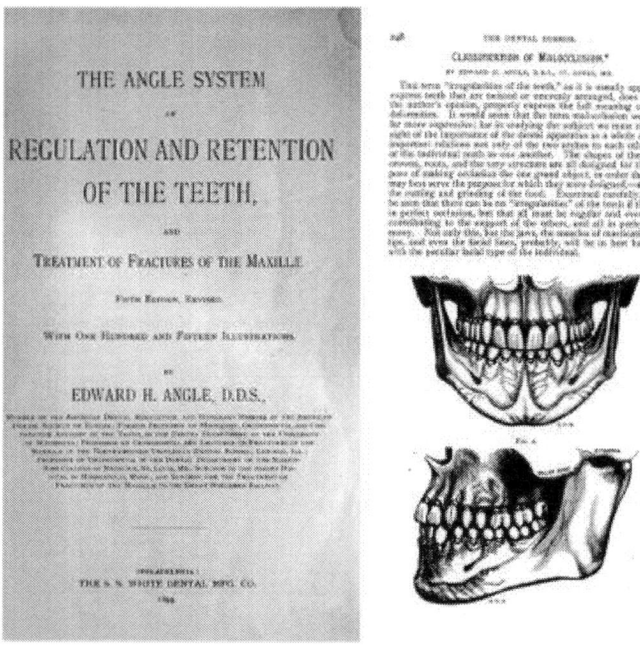

Fig. 1. Beginning of former century: philosophy proposed by the father of Orthodontic School, E.H. Angle

orthopedic functional expansion approach of acknowledged masters, such as: Andresen, Bimler, Klammt, Fränkel, Stockfish or Balters[2] (fig. 2a, b). Numerous appliances and techniques have been designed to accomplish treatment goals assumed by advocates and followers of both schools, especially challenging in adults who more and more frequently seek orthodontic care. Evidence based efficiency of sliding mechanics[3] and segmented technique[4-11] mostly related to the space closure (fig. 3a-c), maxillary enlargement in different skeletal configurations: class III[12-25] or II[26-28] prior to mandibular advancement or distalization of maxilla[29-46] are approaches of choice in non-extraction protocol.

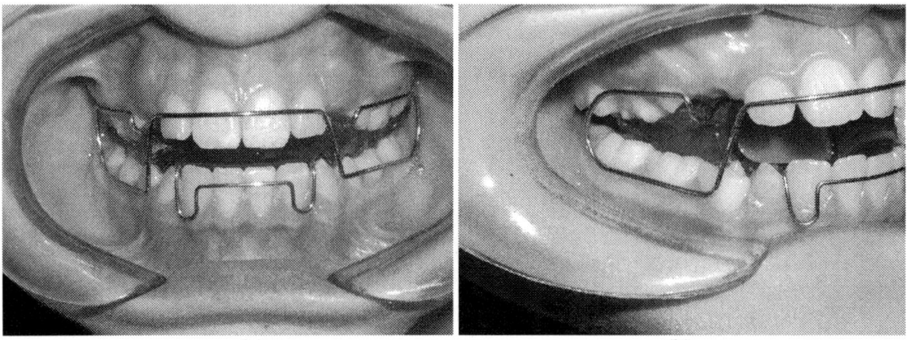

(a) (b)

Fig. 2. Balters' bionator in situ: a) en face view, b) right side

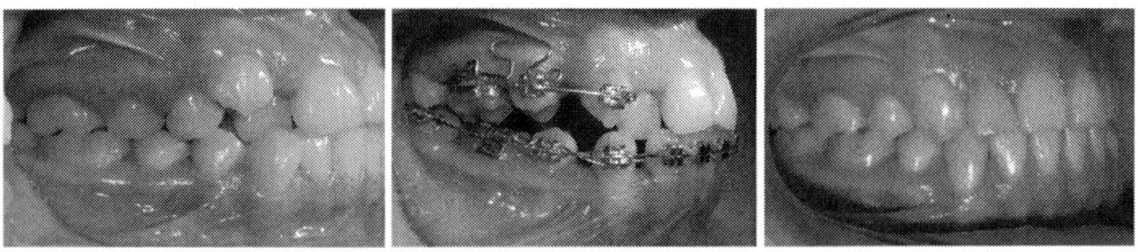

(a) (b) (c)

Fig. 3. Space closure with T-loop segmented archwire: a) initial occlusion, right side, b) T-loop in situ, c) final occlusion, right side

Independently on the treatment plan calling either for reduction of teeth number or dental arch expansion and despite modern and sophisticated orthodontic appliance or technique, even the most currently performed dental movements base on Newton's 3rd law established already in 1687: *to every action there is always opposed an equal reaction or the mutual actions of two bodies upon each other are always equal, and directed to contrary parts*[47]. Such fundamental enlightened orthodontist - beyond the shadow of the doubt - that any teeth-anchored desired movement produced the undesired one and the latter was to be carefully predicted thus fully controlled (fig. 4a, b). Meticulous evaluation of moments and forces resulting from planned tooth displacement[48-51], unavoidable for "orthodontic-driven" and efficient tooth-movement, initiated development of biomechanics: pure physics transferred into the oral cavity (fig. 5a-c, 6a-c). The concept resulted in deliberate anchorage reinforcement: increase of resistance of fulcrum located either in on teeth or skeletal structures[52].

Anchorage may be reinforced utilizing: a) extra-oral skeletal structures, b) teeth and intra-oral skeletal structures.

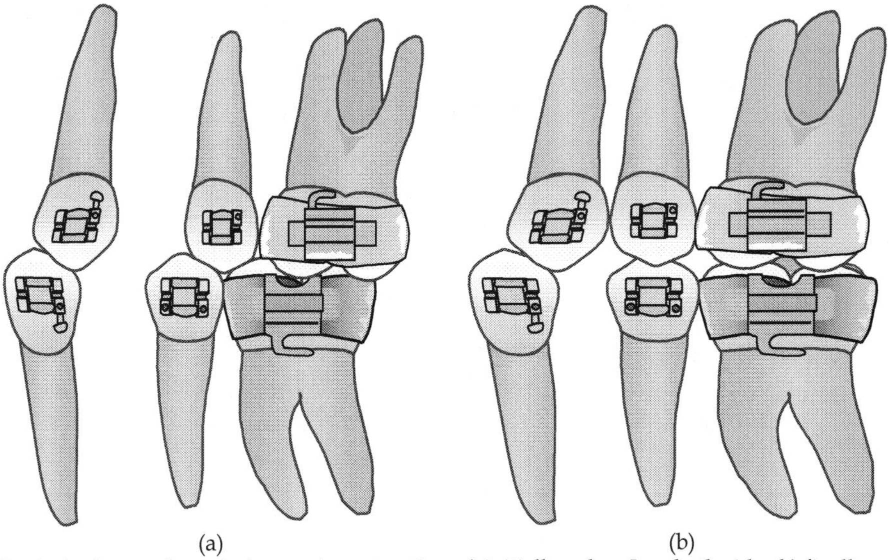

Fig. 4. Anchorage loss during canine retraction: a) initially - class I on both sides b) finally - cusp to cusp relationship due to mesial displacement of upper molars

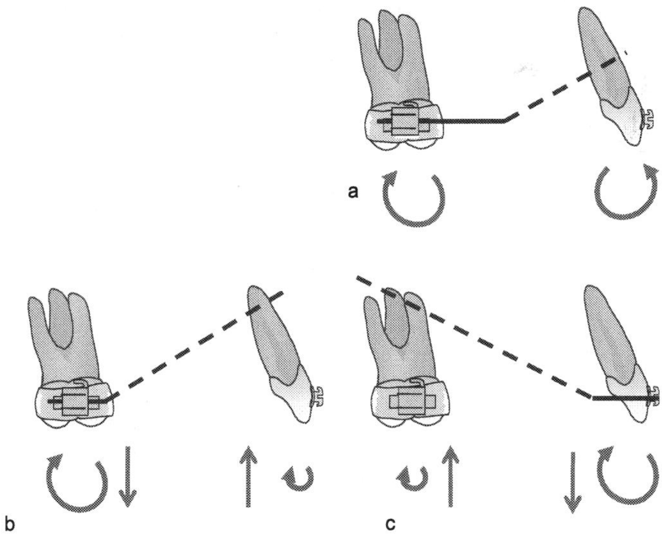

Fig. 5. Force vectors and moments displacing teeth in sagittal-vertical plane, depending on localization of the archwire bending between canine and 1st molar (provided there are no brackets on premolars): a) middle of the distance, b) close to 1st molar, c) close to a canine

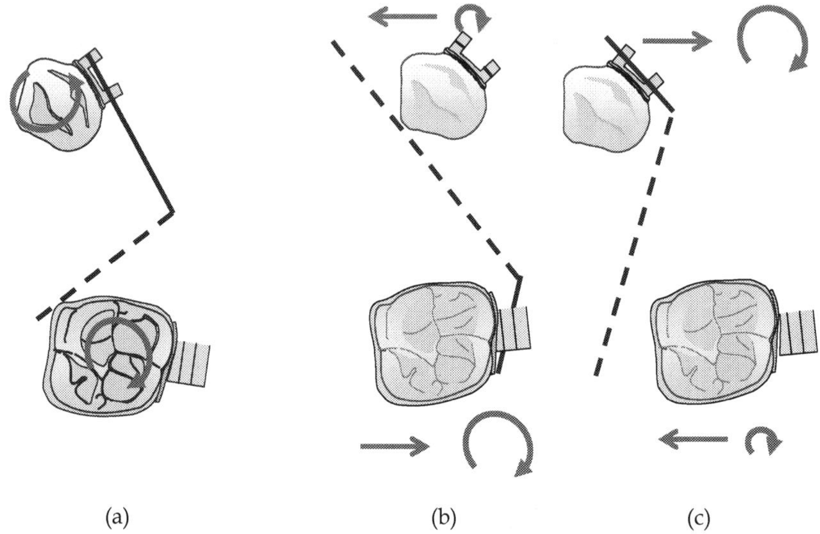

Fig. 6. Force vectors and moments displacing teeth in occlusal plane, depending on localization of the archwire bending between canine and 1st molar (provided there are no brackets on premolars): a) middle of the distance, b) close to 1st molar, c) close to a canine

a. Extra-oral appliances

Headgear - known already in 19th century allows orthodontic reacting forces pass through cranium and back bone: immobile structures, thus absolute anchorage is achieved. Position of external arms of the face bow dictates line force, in other words: enable precise prediction of the desired direction of tooth-movement[53] (fig. 7a-c). In order to adjust the line force, molar center of resistance must be established first. According to Schmuth et al.[54] such location may be easily predicted in several steps: 1) the face-bow, after adjustment of internal arms must lie flat on the surface, 2) reference points must be marked on external arms, 3 mm mesially to the ends of internal ones, 3) once the face-bow has been inserted in to the headgear tubes, next reference points must be marked 8 mm above the previous ones, on the patient's skin (fig. 8). Precisely designed headgear (fig. 9a-c) is mainly applied for correction of class II; nevertheless it may also be used for correction of class I with crowding in both jaws, in combination with fixed mechanics (fig. 10).

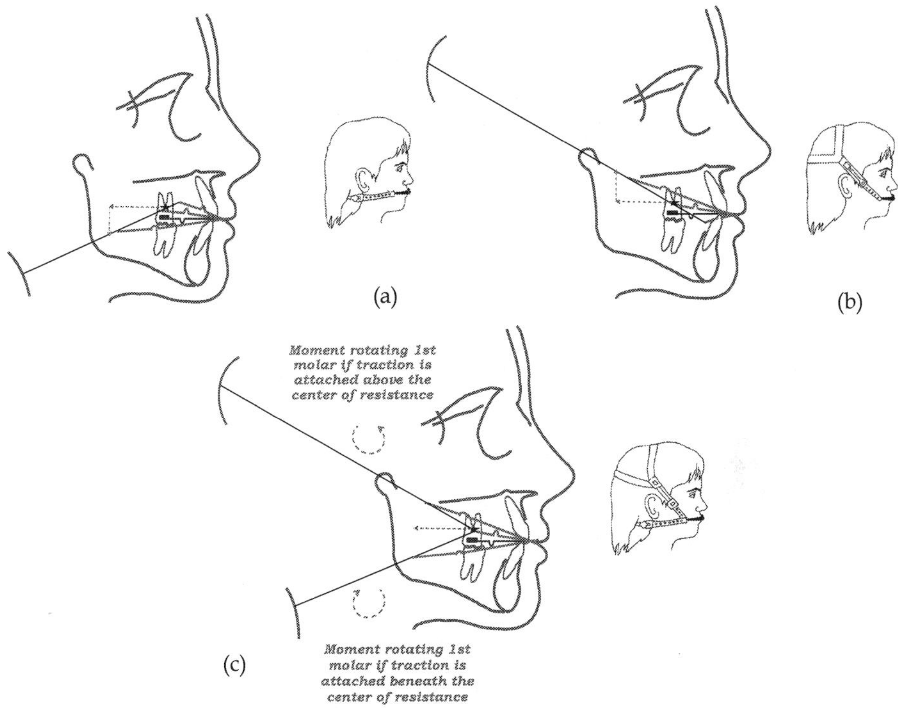

Fig. 7. Headgear - force vectors depending on position of external traction: a) low-pull, b) high-pull ; c) combi-pull; note that elimination of molar rotating moments depends on either the length as well as on angulation of face bow external arms

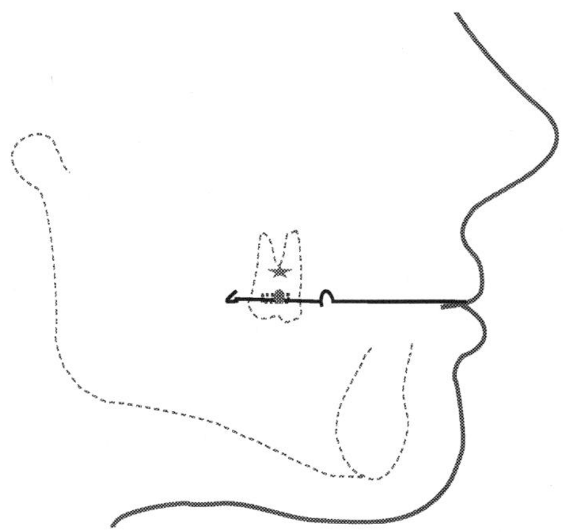

Fig. 8. Headgear adjustment: marking the center of molar resistance (asterisk) on patient's skin

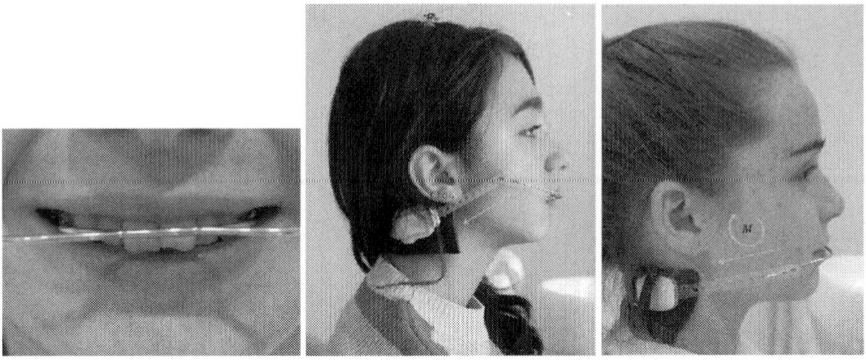

(a) (b) (c)

Fig. 9. Low pull headgear adjusted for class II treatment: a) en face view: position of face bow: it does not lean against lips, b) lateral view - external arms of the face bow bent up, c) external arms of the face bow bent down; note the direction of force line (⟶) and moment (M) rotating molar.

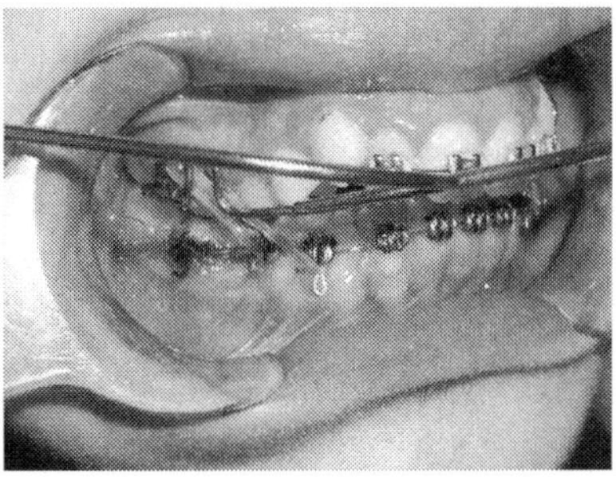

Fig. 10. Headgear combined with fixed appliances: intermaxillary class III traction forces lower canine distally

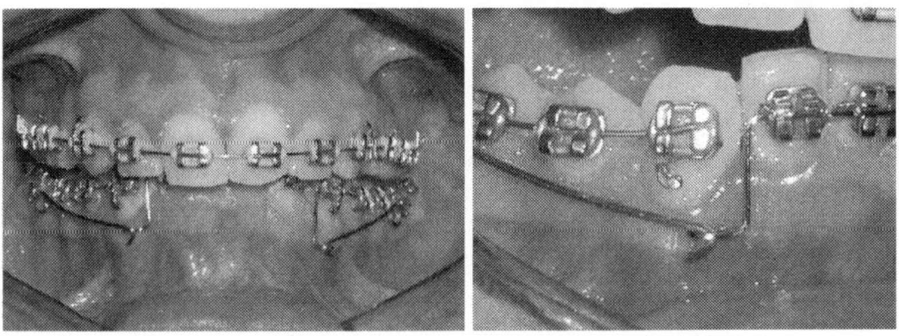

(a) (b)

Fig. 11. Intrusion arch according to Burstone a) en face, in situ, b) connection of cantilever with front segment

Current mathematic calculations of forces couneracting reactive ones resulting from the front teeth movement are presented by Braun[55]. Burstone's intrusion arch (fig. 11a, b) while intruding upper incisors with the 50 g of force, simultaneously extrudes molars with the same force value. To prevent the latter phenomena, high-pull headgear is to be worn 8 hours per day. It is illustrated with the formula: F_1 x 8h = 50 g x 24h, where F_1 = 150 g is a vertical component of the force produced by high-pull traction (fig. 12). However net force

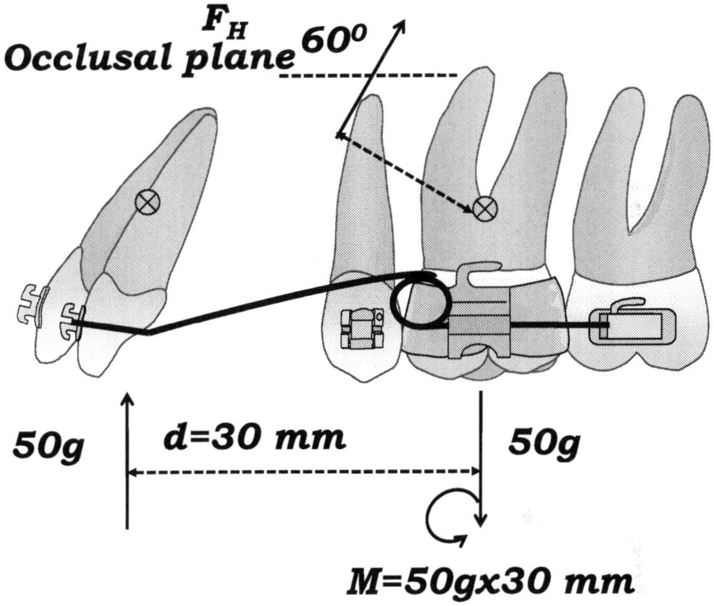

Fig. 12. Biomechanics of incisor intrusion with Burstone's cantilever. Source: Joanna Antoszewska (2009) Wykorzystanie tymczasowego zakotwienia kortykalnego w leczeniu zaburzeń zgryzowo-zębowych. Wrocław : Akad. Med., 5; 111 s. (Rozprawy Habilitacyjne Akademii Medycznej we Wrocławiu). ISBN 978-83-7055-489-7

vector is inclined 60^0 to the occlusal plane, therefore net force value (F_H) equals: $F_H = F_1/\sin 60^0$ = 173 g. Furthermore, in order to compensate side effect of Burstone's cantilever - moment inclining molars distally - stripes of high-pull headgear must be attached at the certain distance (D) from the center of molar resistance, thus inclining molars mesially: 50 g x 24h x 30 = 173 g x 8h x D, so D = 26,01 mm. Another example: retraction of front teeth with the 200 g of force simultaneously displaces molars mesially (fig. 13). Horizontal force reinforcing anchorage (F_2) and originating from the low-pull headgear worn 10 hours per day equals 480 g (200 g x 24 h = F_2 x 10 h). Consequently, since the net force vectors of either high-pull as well as low-pull headgears are inclined to the occlusal plane, their efficient force values equal 627 g ($480/\cos 40^0$) and 679 g (480 g$/\cos 45^0$) respectively.

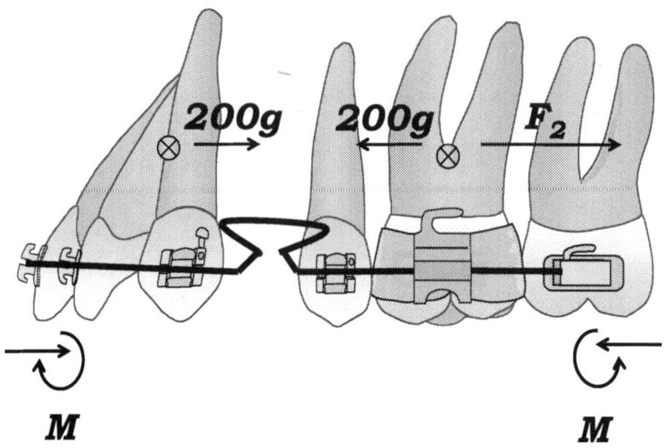

Fig. 13. Biomechanics of controlled space closure. Source: Joanna Antoszewska (2009) Wykorzystanie tymczasowego zakotwienia kortykalnego w leczeniu zaburzeń zgryzowo-zębowych. Wrocław : Akad. Med., 5; 111 s. (Rozprawy Habilitacyjne Akademii Medycznej we Wrocławiu). ISBN 978-83-7055-489-7

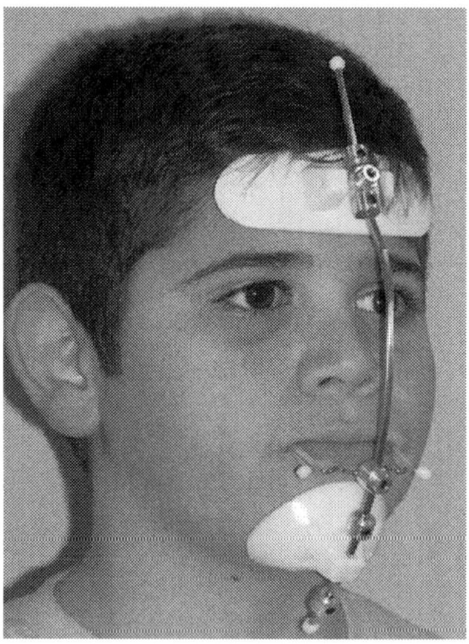

Fig. 14. Face mask

Nevertheless, despite so precise calculations, biologic response is inadequate to the expected one. As reported by Melsen and Bosch[56] when an orthodontic force is applied to a tooth, the cells of periodontal ligaments are differentiated into active osteogenic and osteoclastic cells. As a result, both periodontal ligaments and the adjacent bone exhibit increased cellular activity facilitating tooth movement, therefore headgear - if worn intermittently - is incapable of efficient anchorage reinforcement.

Face mask applied in class III treatment as orthodontic and orthopedic traction (fig. 14) is anchored on a forehead and a chin. Since mandible is a moving structure, therewith its response is unpredictable in terms of mathematic calculations, although efficient clinically. Nevertheless, as anchorage control is also achieved intermittently, all the displacements are resultants of the desired movements and transient collapses.

b. Teeth anchored appliances

Teeth anchored appliances are generally the most popular ones widely used for anchorage reinforcement. Rapid maxillary expander (fig. 15) is an appliance designed to correct transverse discrepancy in class III cases. Nance button - mounted in maxilla and supporting class II correction with eg. repelling magnets[57], superelastic springs[58-60], jones-jig appliance[61-62], pendulum appliance introduced by Hilgers[63] (fig. 16a, b) or Keles slider®[64] (fig. 17) - utilizes hard palate, therefore its efficiency is highly dependent on palatal morphology[65] (fig. 18a, b).

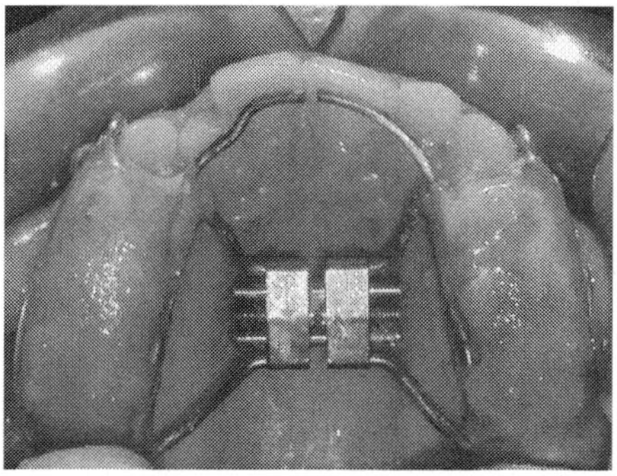

Fig. 15. Rapid maxillary expander

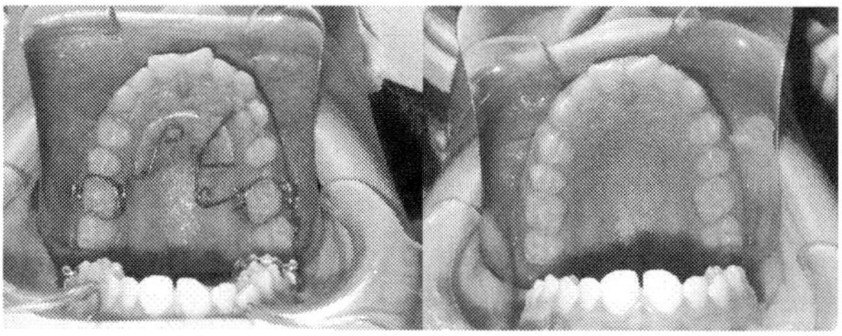

(a) (b)

Fig. 16. Pendulum appliance: a) inter-dental spaces gained after unilateral activation, b) final symmetric positionof upper molars

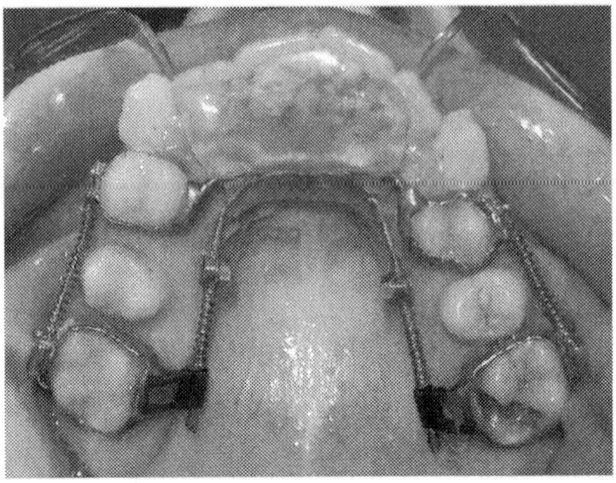

Fig. 17. Keles slider®. Source: Mavropoulos A, Sayinsu K, Allaf F, Kiliaridis S, Papadopoulos MA, Ozlem Keles AO. Noncompliance unilateral maxillary molar distalization. Angle Orthod 2006,3:382-7

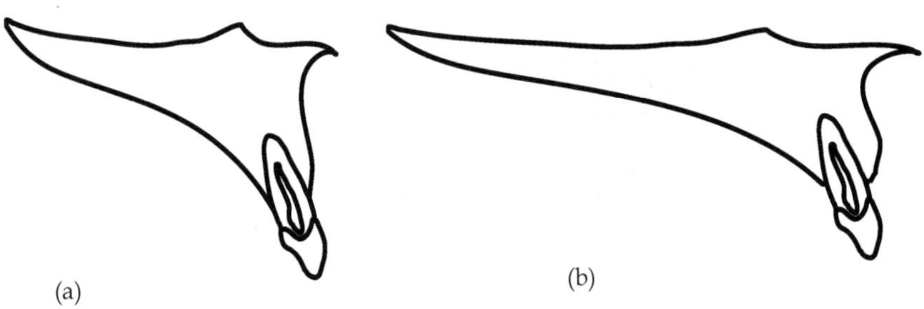

Fig. 18. Palatal morphology: a) steep vault and b) flat vaults, respectively favoring and incumbering Nance-button settling. Source: Joanna Antoszewska (2009) Wykorzystanie tymczasowego zakotwienia kortykalnego w leczeniu zaburzeń zgryzowo-zębowych. Wrocław : Akad. Med., 5; 111 s. (Rozprawy Habilitacyjne Akademii Medycznej we Wrocławiu). ISBN 978-83-7055-489-7

On the other hand, bi-maxillary appliances such as Herbst hinge[66] , Carrière distalizer®[67], jasper-jumper[68] (fig. 19a, b), MALU (fig. 20) or Forsus® (Fig. 21a, b), designed for advancement of mandible in young adolescents with concave profile (fig. 22), are dependent on initial teeth-positions. In other terms, protrusion of lower incisors permits functional treatment of class II, since their further flaring is the adverse, unavoidable effect of mandibular forward displacement.

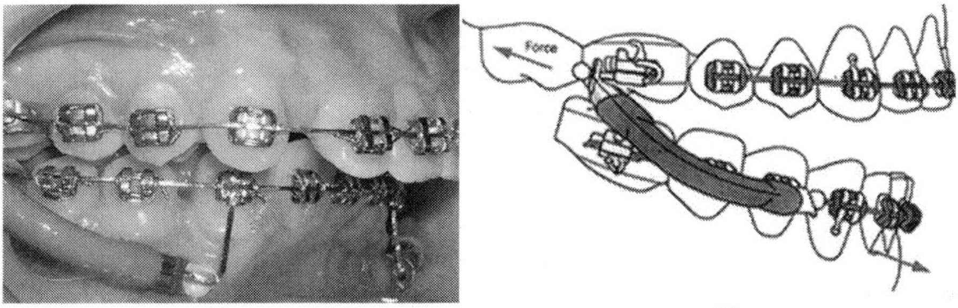

(a) (b)

Fig. 19. Jasper-jumper a) in situ, b) scheme of delivered force vectors. Source: Küçükkeleş N, Ilhan I, Orgun IA. Treatment efficiency in skeletal Class II patients treated with the jasper jumper. Angle Orthod 2007;77:449-56

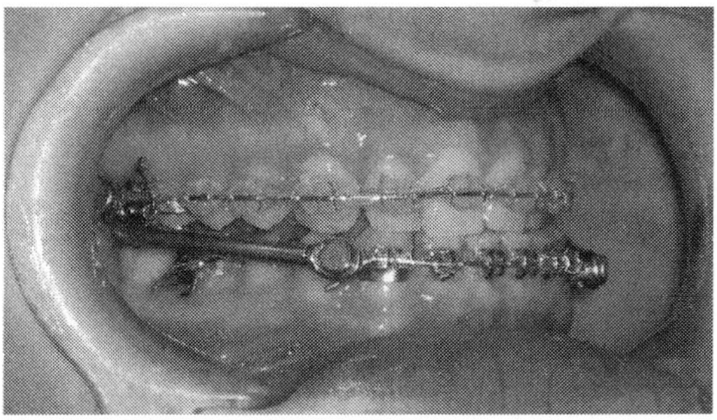

Fig. 20. MALU

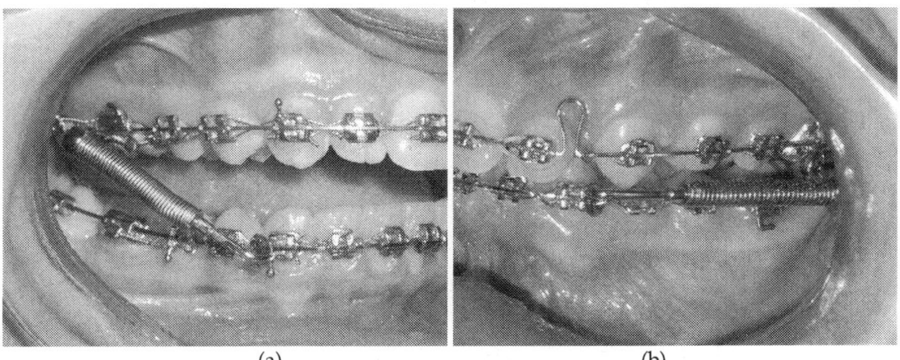

(a) (b)

Fig. 21. Forsus appliance in situ: a) during mouth opening, b) after mouth closure; note transient class III (over-correction of class II) evident on canines and molars

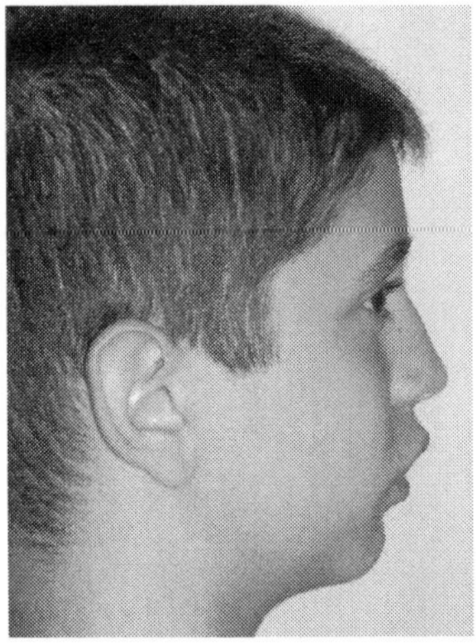

Fig. 22. Concave facial profile of young adolescent - indication for mandibular forward displacement

Evaluating appliances settled on the teeth it may be stated that their biomechanics bases on paradigm that larger overall surface of the roots composing anchor unit is resistant to the orthodontic forces displacing individual tooth (fig. 23). It sounds logic, however this concept is totally opposite to the very interesting one presented by Mulligan and well grounded in terms of biomechanics[69]. The author proved that the undesired molar mesialization during

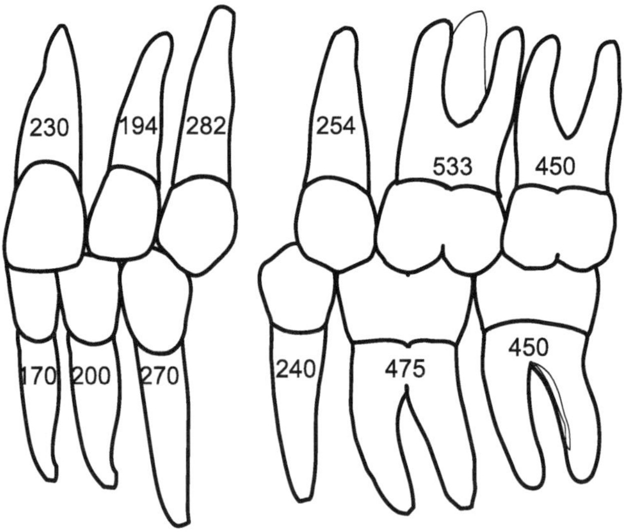

Fig. 23. Periodontal surfaces of each tooth. Source: Proffit W. Contemporary Orthodontics

extraction space closure is independent on periodontal surface of the anchor unit. The only mattering factors are: a) the resilience of the archwire the teeth move along and b) inter-bracket distance from canine to 1st molar. According to this theory, tip-back closest to the mesial margin of a molar-tube rotates anchor tooth-crown distally, whereas magnitude of either force as well as moment acting on canine depend on its distance ("d") from the tip-back bend . If the "d" distance is larger than 2/3 of the inter-bracket distance (fig. 24a), both teeth are subjected to rotating moments of different magnitudes, however of the same direction; thus net rotating moment responsible for anchorage not only has the maximal value, but acts in the direction of canine desired displacement. If the "d" distance equals 2/3 of inter-bracket distance (fig. 24b), although moment rotating favorably exists, however it is not increased with the moment rotating canine distally. Further decrease of the "d" distance" generates rotating moments of the same magnitudes, but of the opposite directions (fig. 24c), uprighting canine root and maintaining molar sagittal position. If such biomechanical standard is embraced, excluding 2nd premolar from the appliance increases the wire resilience and generates higher rotating moments of favorable directions (fig 25a) than including 2nd premolar into the anchor unit (fig. 25b). In other terms, on the contrary to the generally accepted concept, Mulligan's theory proves that decreasing periodontal surface of anchor unit may serve as better anchorage reinforcement.

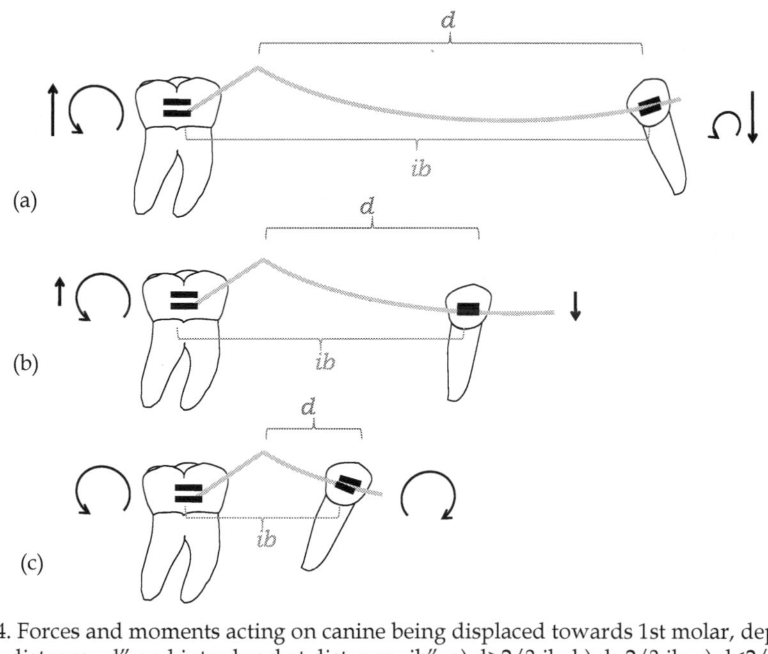

Fig. 24. Forces and moments acting on canine being displaced towards 1st molar, dependent on the distance „d" and inter-bracket distance „ib": a) d>2/3 ib, b) d=2/3 ib, c) d<2/3 ib; note that together with canine distalization (decreasing „d" distance) force value diminishes and moment direction changes after passing a „0" point. Direction of moment acting on canine results from archwire resilience and the distance from 1st molar

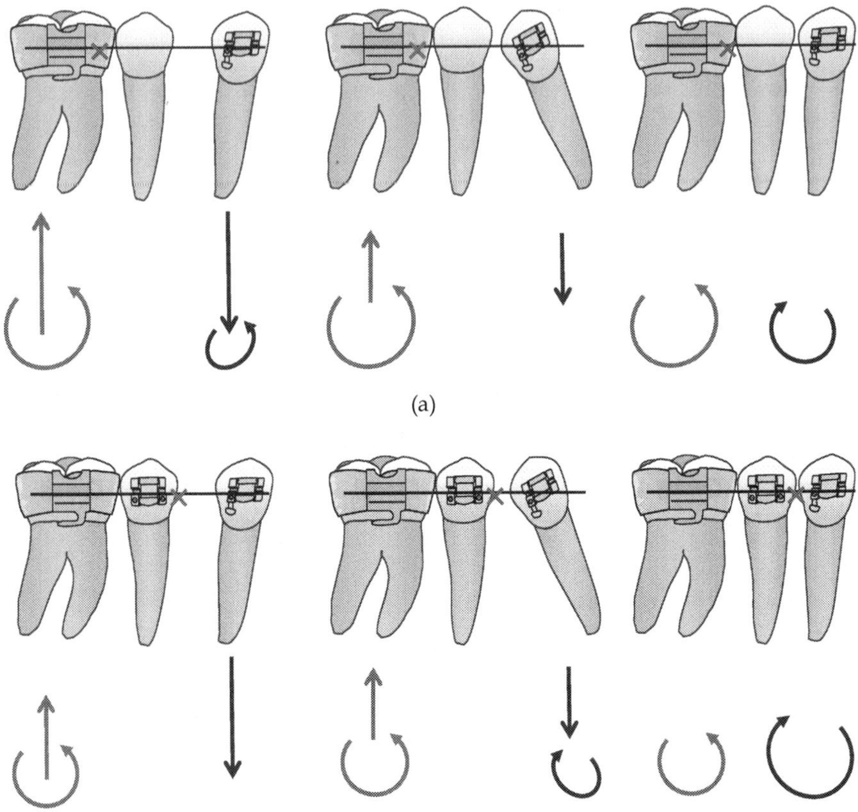

(a)

(b)

Fig. 25. Mulligan's concept: biomechanics of canine distalization if 2nd premolar is: a) excluded from the appliance, b) included in the appliance; "X"-gable bend, moments and forces acting on molars are marked in red, moments and forces acting on canines are marked in blue

2. Current look

Reasons of all the elaborated deliberations are scientifically supported: numerous research upon efficiency and efficacy of conventional anchorage [70-82], directly or indirectly confirm the poorness of their reliability. Despite high prevalence of the appliances reinforcing anchorage - especially in class II treatment - all hitherto discussed devices have certain disadvantages or could not provide anchorage for vertical tooth-movement[83-84]. Furthermore, in the face of overloading periodontal structures possibly leading to root resorption, tissue necrosis or cortical plate atrophy, extra-dental and intraoral source of anchorage has technically become natural point of clinical interest and evaluation: biocompatible implants.

Experimental study began already in 1945, when Gainsforth and Higley[85] introduced vitallium screws to distalize upper teeth (fig. 26). Since they failed (all screws were lost within approximately 1 month), boom for other animal experiments related to implants as anchorage reinforcement falls around turn of 1970 into 1980, after Brånemark and co-workers' success: osseointegration of prosthetic implant and bone. Factors such as alloys used for implant-manufacturing [86,87] as well as resistance to orthodontic loading with forces originating from fixed mechanics[88,89] differentiated the research material. Since the implants succeeded, they were proclaimed as "having the potential to be used as a source of firm osseous anchorage for orthodontics and dentofacial orthopedics"[90].

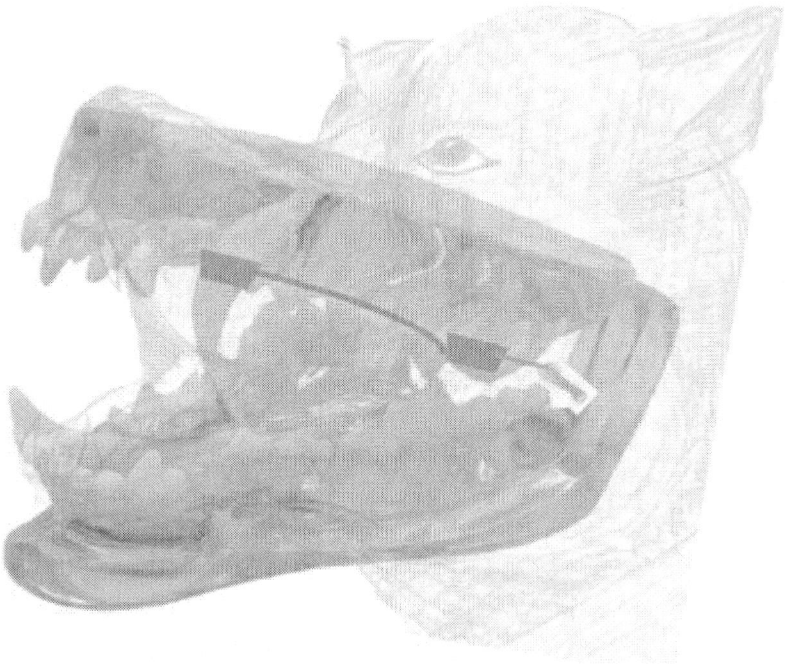

Fig. 26. Study design: Gainsforth and Higley, 1945

Shapiro and Kokich[91] were ones of the pioneers of pre-prosthetic implantation for orthodontic purposes in humans, slowly encouraging other clinicians[92-95]. However, obvious disadvantages of prosthetic implants, such as defeating interadicular placement, complicated surgical procedure associated with insertion, long-lasting osseointegration, biomechanical limitations and high cost were still of a major concern. Such circumstances attracted clinicians' great interest towards "slenderizing" commonly applied screws[96,97] and simplifying their insertion procedures[98] without compromising anchoring properties, thus leading to the development of 21st century orthodontic anchorage: miniscrew implants or TSAD (Temporary Skeletal Anchorage Devices). Their decreased sizes enabled placement in iteradicular spaces of either jaws, for many clinical purposes. Vertical displacements eg. alignment of canted occlusal plane (fig. 27a-c) intrusion of lower incisors (fig. 28a, b) or

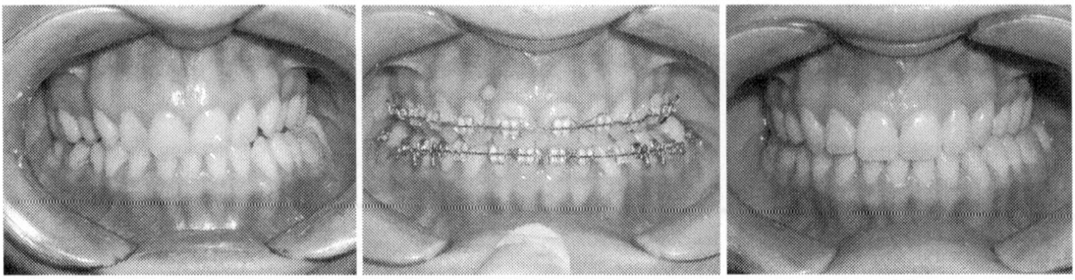

(a) (b) (c)

Fig. 27. Alignment of canted occlusal plane using TSAD: a) initial occlusion, b) TSAD loading mode, c) final occlusion

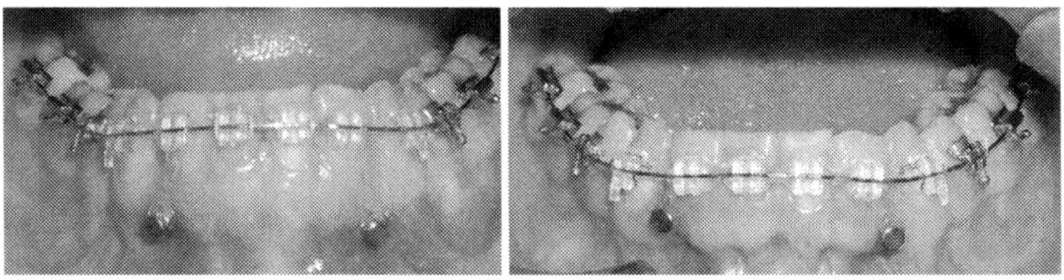

(a) (b)

Fig. 28. Intrusion of lower incisors using TSAD: a) prior to TSAD loading, b) final result

lateral teeth (fig. 29a, b), as well as sagittal ones: protraction of lower molars with either sliding (fig. 30a) or segmented mechanics (fig. 30b) have eventually become facilitated and free of side effects. Clinical efficiency encouraged orthodontist to load TSAD multipurposely eg. applying distalizing and intrusive force on continuous (fig. 31a) or segmented (fig. 31b) archwire, extrusive and intrusive forces simultaneously (fig. 32) or even forces acting in three planes of space at the very same moment (fig. 33).

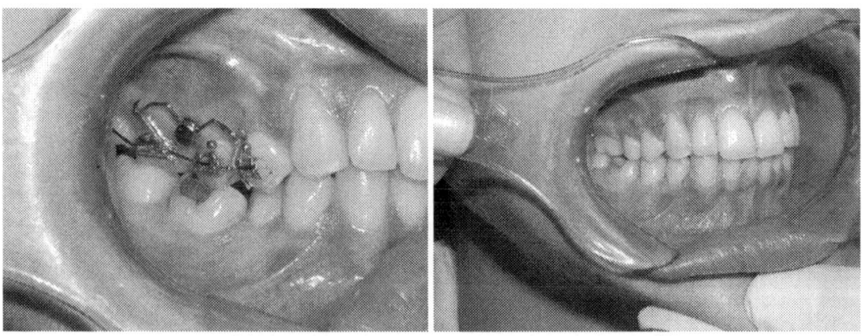

(a) (b)

Fig. 29. Intrusion of upper lateral teeth using TSAD: a) prior to TSAD loading, b) final result

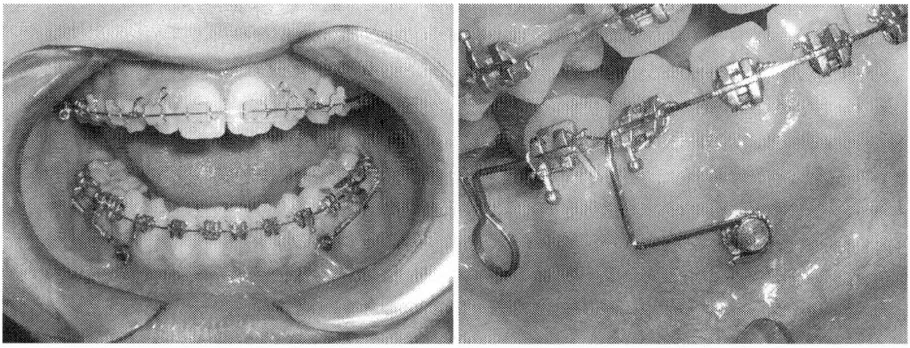

(a) (b)

Fig. 30. Protraction of lower molars using: a) TSAD and sliding mechanics, b) TSAD and segmented archwires

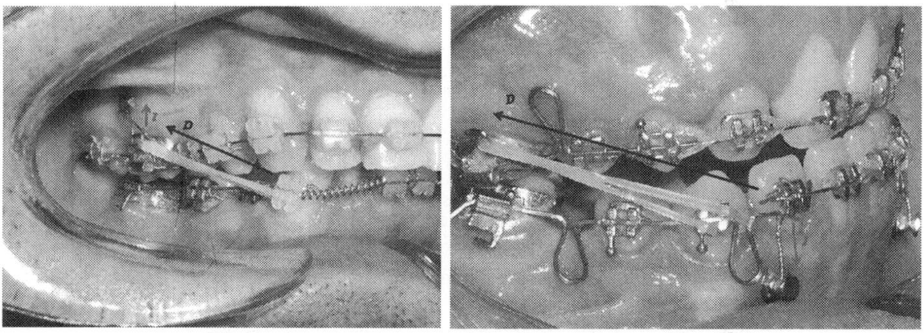

(a) (b)

Fig. 31. Distalizing (D) and intrusive (I) forces on: a) continuous and b) segmented archwires

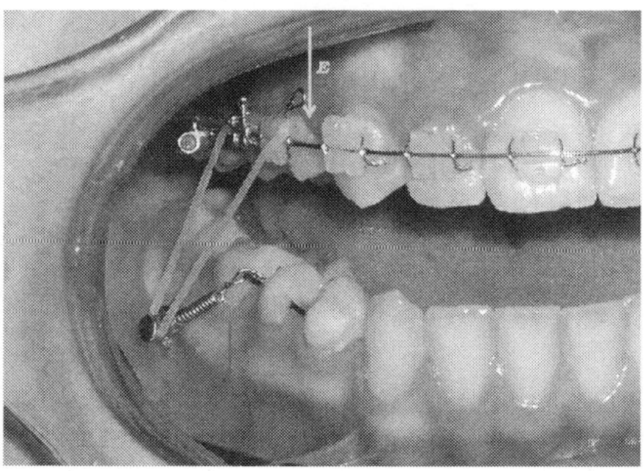

Fig. 32. Extrusive (E) and intrusive (I) forces acting spontaneously

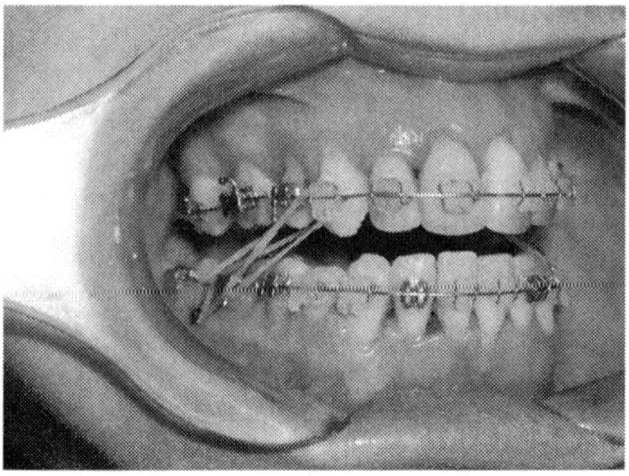

Fig. 33. Transversal, vertical and sagittal forces acting simultaneously

Various practical demands entailed manufacturing and permanent improvement of different miniscrew implant-systems[90,99,100], all the more so that nobody informed about absolute stability (100% success rate) of TSAD. Our routine introducing of the miniscrew implants for anchorage reinforcement in treatment of many types of malocclusion[101-106] allowed us selection of the most versatile and convenient systems: Absoanchor® (Dentos, Daegu, South Corea) and Ortho Easy (Forestadent, Phorzheim, Germany).

Absoanchor® is available as the branch of different diameters, lengths and designs: from 1.2 to 1.6 mm in cross-section, 5 to 12 mm long, cylindrical or tapered, with flat or bracket-like heads, with long, short or no neck. However, in order to make such complex offer less confusing, especially for the beginners we recommend tapered miniscrew implants with small head and convenient hole in the conically-shaped neck; considering lengths and diameters: 6 mm and 1.6 mm in mandible and 8 mm 1.3 mm in maxilla should be chosen for vestibular insertion (fig. 34).

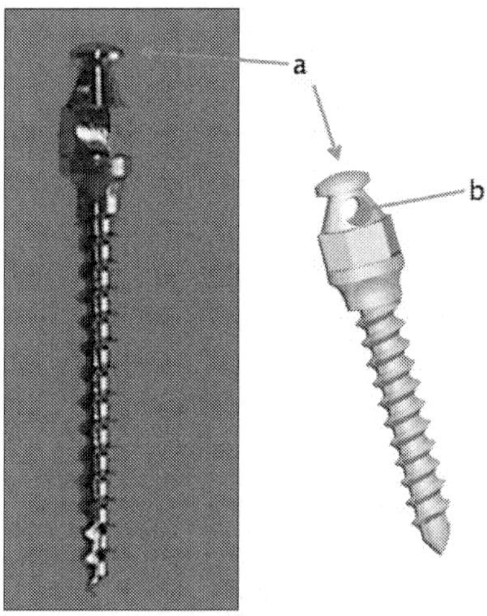

Fig. 34. Absoanchor®: a) small head, b) a hole for utility elements (ligatures, elastomerics)

Ortho Easy pins® are easier to handle: there is only one design available (fig. 35), therefore colour-coded different lengths (pink: 6 mm, violet: 8 mm) simplify the choice dependent on treatment indications and locations in the jaws: short miniscrew implant in mandible, long one in maxilla.

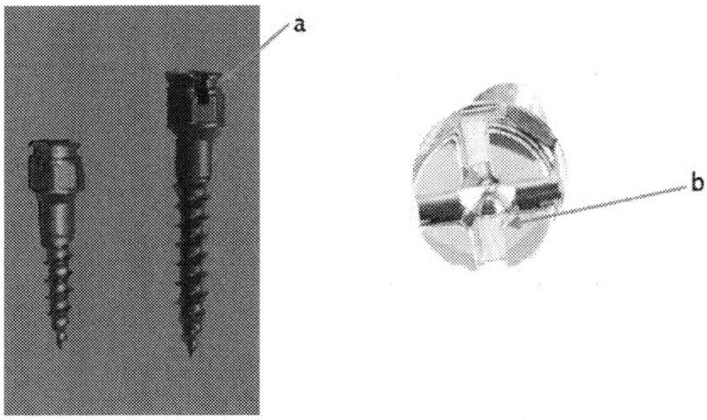

Fig. 35. Ortho Easy pins®: a) undercut facilitating ligating, b) rounded design of slot edges facilitating wire adjustment

Both systems are designed to insert into interadicular space, therefore they may be connected via coil spring with the elements of fixed appliances either bonded to the teeth or attached to the working archwire. It enables loading with forces of mesio-distal direction, so essential in correction of sagittal discrepancies with the vertical component: the most common malocclusions. Direction of the coil spring, dictated by mutual relation of TSAD position and height of attachment (hook) defines the line of force vector (fig. 36a, b).

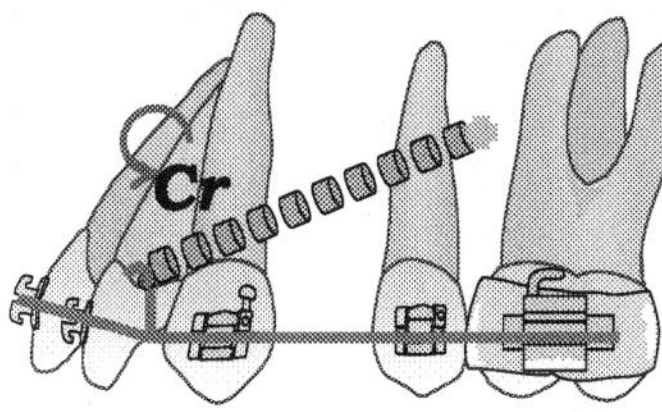

(a)

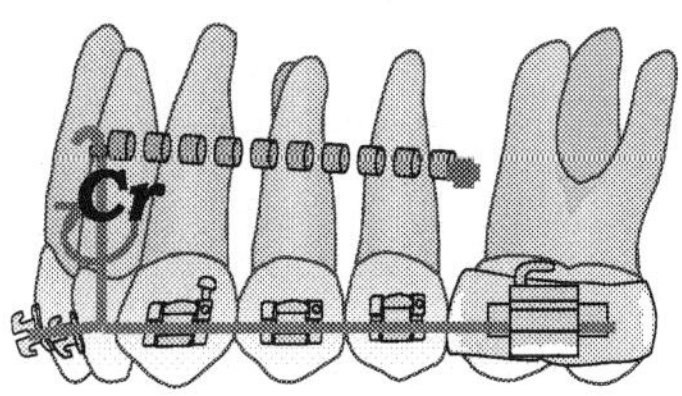

(b)

Fig. 36. Force vectors dependent on mutual relation of TSAD vertical position and height of attachment (hook) on the working archwire: a) rotating moment retruding incisors, b) rotating moment protruding incisors

Forasmuch it is obvious that TSAD position determines biomechanics of orthodontic treatment plan, nobody but orthodontists themselves should insert miniscrew implants. Although there is a myth that bending wires is far beyond the scope of the dentistry, we must not forget we are doctors and if the treatment fails we will be responsible for failures (fig. 37)! The best control is provided by the controller fully aware of the process, thus we would like to encourage our colleagues to become familiar with the details of insertion protocol providing the highest TSAD stability: Wroclaw protocol efficient in 93.43% and obtained after research upon both described TSAD systmes[105-108]. Selection of location for TSAD insertion bases on objective criteria: CT-images at the level of 5 - 7 mm apical of the alveolar crest analyzed by Park et al.[109], visualized the areas of the larger interadicular distances (ID) as well as the ones from the root to the cortical plate (R-CP). According to the provided data, TSAD should be inserted:

1. In maxilla: vestibularly, between central incisors (fig. 38a) or between 2nd bicuspid and 1st molar (fig. 38b) - mean ID = 3.18 mm,
2. In mandible: vestibularly, between 1st and 2nd bicuspids (fig. 39a) - mean ID > 2.20 mm) and between 1st and 2nd molars (fig. 39b) - mean ID = 4.57 mm, mean R-CP = 2.16-5.33 mm; although mean R-CP in mandible progressively increases distally from 1st molar, it is difficult to manipulate in this area, therefore mesial placement seems to be more convenient and still safe.

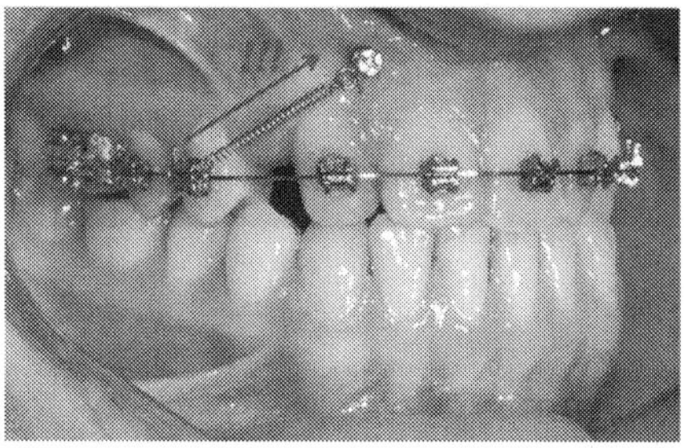

Fig. 37. Improper force vector causing undesired bite opening during planned space closure

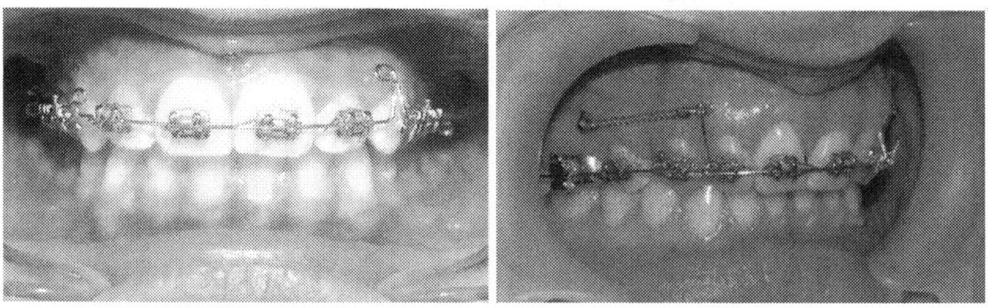

(a) (b)

Fig. 38. Localization of TSAD in vestibulum of maxilla: a) between central incisors, b) between 2nd premolar and 1st molar; note height of the hook together with vertical position of TSAD form the line of force vector passing above the center of incisor resistance, thus forcing them labially during retraction. Source: Joanna Antoszewska (2009) Wykorzystanie tymczasowego zakotwienia kortykalnego w leczeniu zaburzeń zgryzowo-zębowych. Wrocław : Akad. Med., 5; 111 s. (Rozprawy Habilitacyjne Akademii Medycznej we Wrocławiu). ISBN 978-83-7055-489-7

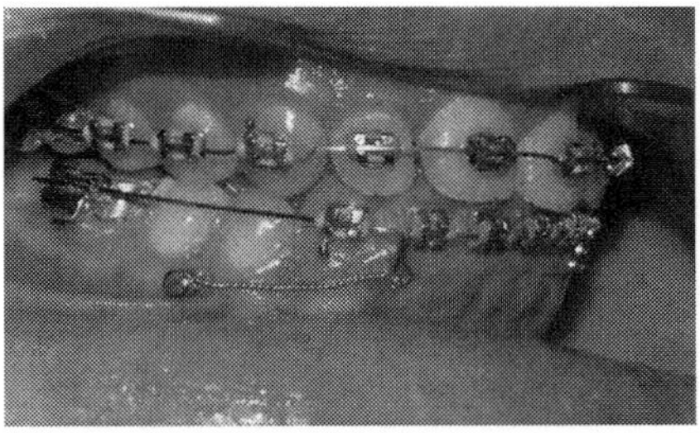
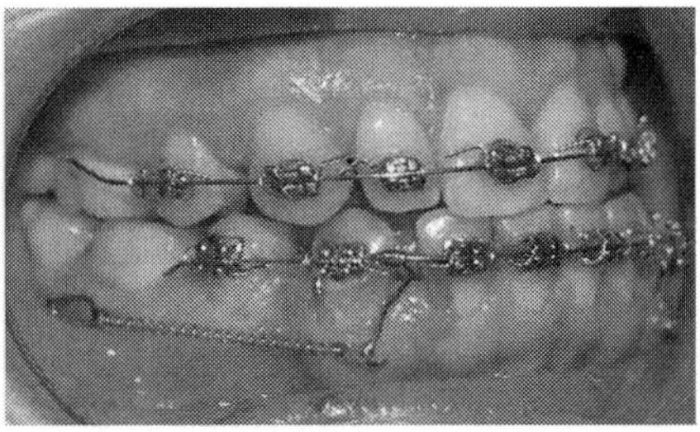

(a) (b)

Fig. 39. Localization of TSAD in vestibulum of mandible: a) between 1st and 2nd bicuspids, b) between 1st and 2nd molars. Source: Joanna Antoszewska (2009) Wykorzystanie tymczasowego zakotwienia kortykalnego w leczeniu zaburzeń zgryzowo-zębowych. Wrocław : Akad. Med., 5; 111 s. (Rozprawy Habilitacyjne Akademii Medycznej we Wrocławiu). ISBN 978-83-7055-489-7

According to this study, palatal ID between 1st and 2nd molars warrants TSAD stability, however Ludwig et al.[99] in contrast report that anterior part of the palatal bone as the best zone for TSAD insertion (fig. 40). Nevertheless, eg. in case of 2 impacted canines, distal part of palate may serve as suitable area securing TSAD stability (fig. 41). Once the location has been selected, local anesthesia is administered and

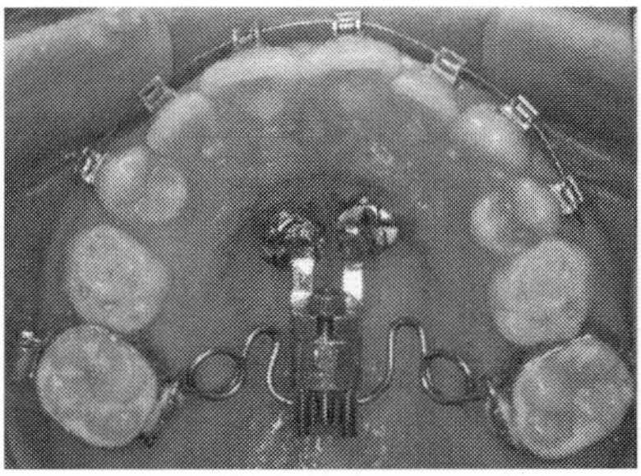
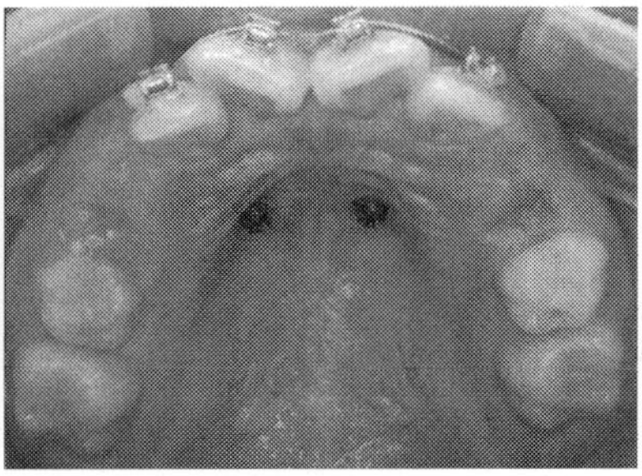

(a) (b)

Fig. 40. Localization of TSAD on palate recommended by Dr. B. Ludwig; picture by the courtesy of Dr. B. Ludwig

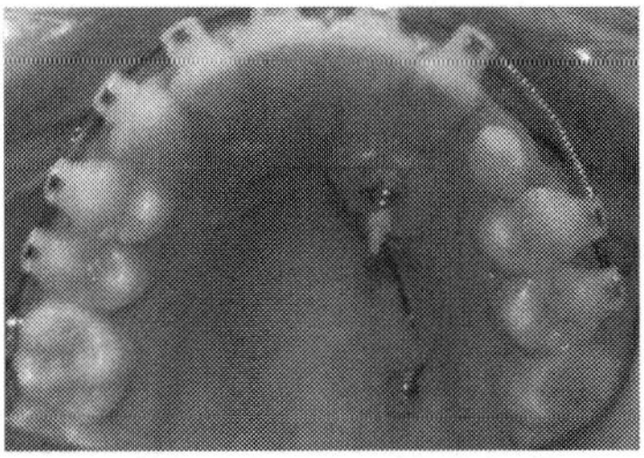

Fig. 41. Localization of TSAD on palate recommended by Prof. Hyo-Sang Park

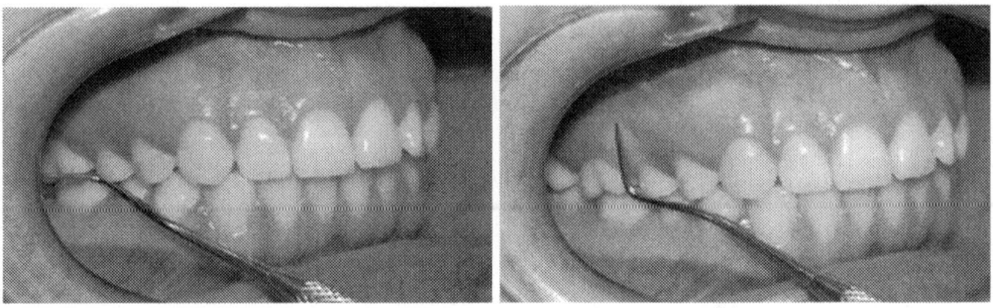

(a) (b)

Fig. 42. Establishing of interadicular position of TSAD: a) initial position of explorer, b) final position of explorer. Source: Joanna Antoszewska (2009) Wykorzystanie tymczasowego zakotwienia kortykalnego w leczeniu zaburzeń zgryzowo-zębowych. Wrocław : Akad. Med., 5; 111 s. (Rozprawy Habilitacyjne Akademii Medycznej we Wrocławiu). ISBN 978-83-7055-489-7

precise determination of TSAD position takes place. It is accomplished with the dental probe initially oriented parallel to the occlusal plane, with the bend tightly pressed between the crowns of the adjacent teeth with (fig. 42a), then rotated 90^0 towards gingiva (fig. 42b): its tip is located directly in the middle of the interadicular distance. Pressing the tip of explorer firmly against gingiva and oral mucosa causes slight indentation and local ischemia of soft tissues serving as the reference for mesio-distal position of the implant. Vertical position is established along the ischemic line. After vertical, short (4 mm) stab incision, wound margins are pushed aside: this incision is mandatory in order to avoid risk of implementation connective tissue into the screw course during TSAD insertion. Subsequently, a pit is made in cortical plate using a round bur oriented perpendicularly to the bone surface , thus followed with a pilot drill angulated at 30-40^0 and 10-20^0 to the root axes in maxilla and mandible respectively (fig. 43a, b). This is a pre-drilling method, less forceful for the alveolar process due to significantly lower insertion torque[110], however more time consuming than self-drilling one.

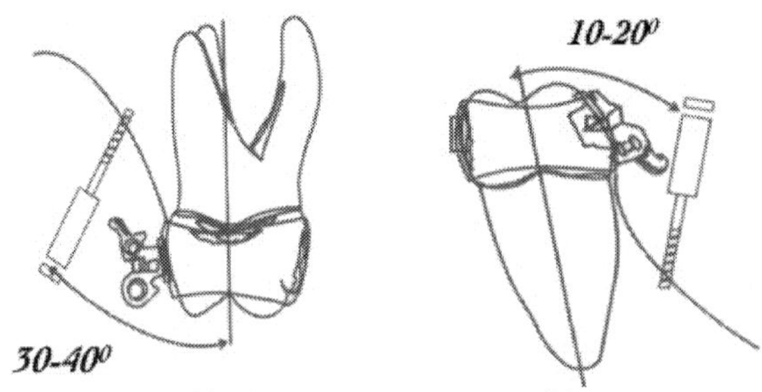

(a) (b)

Fig. 43. Angulation of Absoanchor®: a) in maxilla, b) in mandible. Source: Joanna Antoszewska (2009) Wykorzystanie tymczasowego zakotwienia kortykalnego w leczeniu zaburzeń zgryzowo-zębowych. Wrocław : Akad. Med., 5; 111 s. (Rozprawy Habilitacyjne Akademii Medycznej we Wrocławiu). ISBN 978-83-7055-489-7

Ambidexterity of an operator, utilized in Wroclaw protocol, secures the most accurate view into the insertion area, with no distortion. Drilling with the speed not exceeding 500 rpm requires massive irrigation to avoid overheating of the bone. The miniscrew implant may be

inserted with a manual or engine screw driver, however manual implantation is recommended (especially for the beginners), since during manual insertion orthodontists may notice even minor increase in resistance often related to root contact. If this occurs, it is mandatory to unscrew implant totally and to apply it in a different angulation.
Post-operative inflammation requires no antibiotics[108], however 2-week postponement of loading allows total cease of symptoms.
Periapical radiograms in three projections - perpendicular and two oblique ones to assess root contact recommended by Park[111] are excluded from Wroclaw protocol: one must not neglect neither distortion nor dose protection. In our method, stable position of miniscrew two weeks after insertion indicates no root contact, which allows loading TSAD with initial force value of 50 g, still within primary stability period (fig. 44). This value may be increased accordingly to the treatment needs, after 3 months, up to 180 g per side thus matching data provided by many researchers:

1. forced eruption of impacted tooth: 50g for canine[112] and 80 g for molars[113],
2. intrusion of posterior teeth: 50 g buccolingually per tooth[114], 90 g[115], 100 g[116] or 150-200 g[117],
3. group sagittal movement: 150 g for retraction of 6 front teeth[118] or 180 g[101] for distalization of all upper teeth.

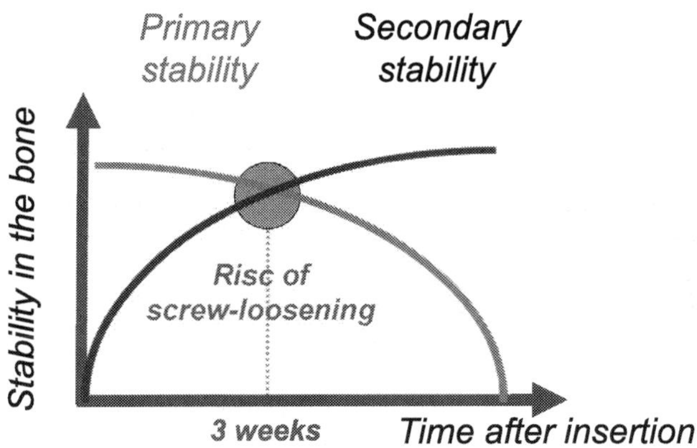

Fig. 44. Diagram illustrating periods of TSAD stability

In serviceable survey of orthodontists[119] evaluation of fear rate before and after TSAD insertion displayed different results. Mean fear level ranked before experiment reached 4.6 and significantly ($p<0.05$) diminished to 3.2 after four trials of TSAD insertion. Factors responsible for fear rate before and after TSAD insertion differed quantitatively and qualitatively (fig. 45). Fear rate before TSAD insertion was mostly associated with risk of injury: dental root (77.14% of clinicians), maxillary sinus (40.00%) or mandibular canal (28.57%). Only few orthodontists submitted other factors such as uncontrolled bur sliding while drilling, breakage of either drill or TSAD, excessive bleeding, soft tissue impaction into the drilled hole, bone necrosis, postoperative complications, and patient's unwilling attitude towards TSAD insertion as well as personal lack of experience. After TSAD insertion, fear rate associated with risk of injury evidently decreased: fear of dental root, maxillary sinus and mandibular canal injuries were submitted by 57.14%, 11.43% and 2.85% of clinicians respectively. Furthermore, spectrum of possibly frightening factors restricted after four trials; besides risk of injury, only uncontrolled bur sliding while drilling remained the fear factor for 2.85% of the surveyed group.

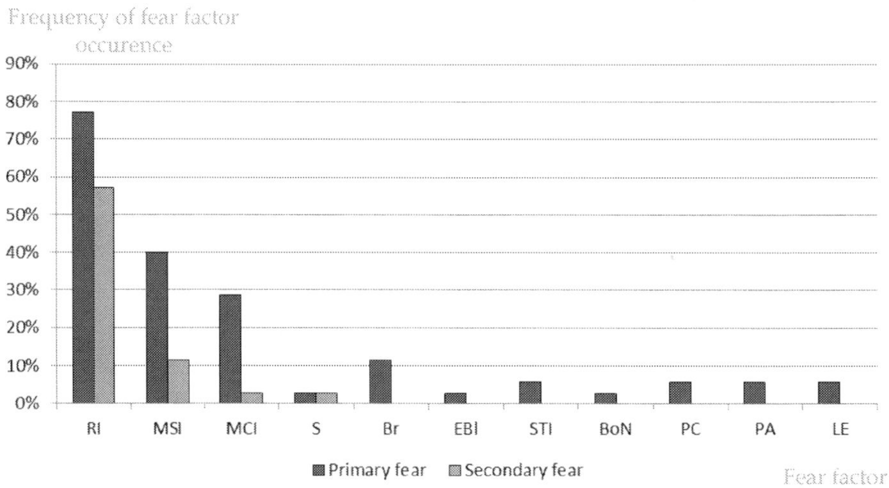

RI - root injury, MSI - maxillary sinus injury, MCI - maxillary canal injury, S - uncontrolled bur sliding while drilling, Br - breakage of either drill or MSI, EBl - excessive bleeding,
STI - soft tissue impaction into the drilled hole, BoN - bone necrosis, PC - postoperative complications, PA - patient's unwilling attitude towards MSI insertion, LE - lack of experience

Fig. 45. Evaluation of fear rate before and after TSAD insertion. Source: Antoszewska J, Trześniewska P, Kawala B, Ludwig B, Park HS. Qualitative and quantitative evaluation of root injury risk potentially burdening insertion of microscrew implants. Korean J.Orthod. 2011;41,2:112-120

Although TSAD are valuable tools for gaining excellent anchorage, especially in non-compliance patients, their stability is still a problem requiring further investigation. The research of Liou et al.[120] has proven that stable TSAD have not kept their initial position during treatment and tipped even 1.5 mm still serving as an excellent anchorage. Nevertheless establishing risk factors of excessive implant mobility impeding orthodontic force application is crucial for treatment success. So far, the list assessing the highest number of parameters related to TSAD failures, based on the Kaplan–Meier product-limit estimate specifies[105]: low position of the line connecting oral commissures (fig. 46), decreased overbite (fig. 47), Angle class III (fig. 48), vertical location in attached gingiva in mandible (fig. 49), right side of mandible between 1st and 2nd molars (fig. 50), lower molars intrusion and class II traction (fig. 51). Clinical parameters favoring failures are also listed: male sex, age < 20, upper midline shift to the right, centered lower midline and, class III on canines - all of them evident already at the clinical examination, therefore easy to manage and control.

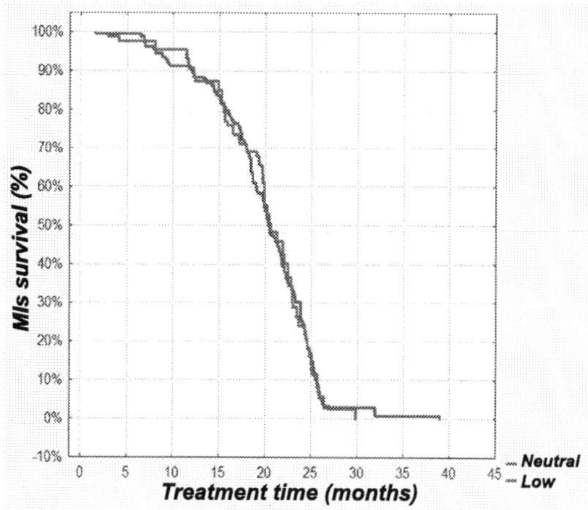

Fig. 46. TSAD stability in relation to position of the line connecting oral commissures: neutral (passing stomion) and low one (beneath stomion). Source: Joanna Antoszewska (2009) Wykorzystanie tymczasowego zakotwienia kortykalnego w leczeniu zaburzeń zgryzowo-zębowych. Wrocław : Akad. Med., 5; 111 s. (Rozprawy Habilitacyjne Akademii Medycznej we Wrocławiu). ISBN 978-83-7055-489-7

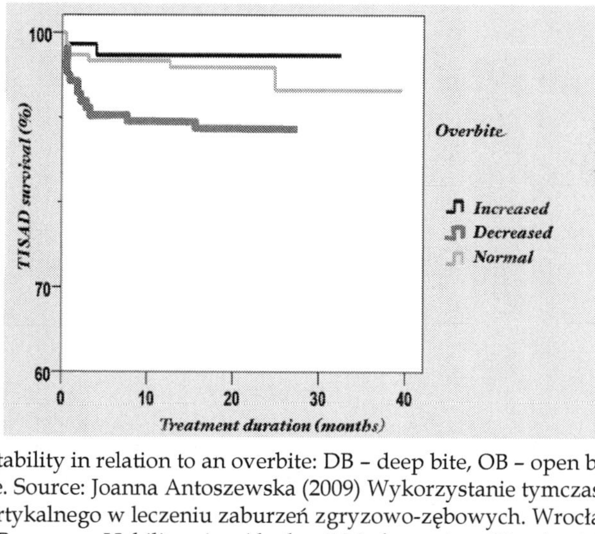

Fig. 47. TSAD stability in relation to an overbite: DB - deep bite, OB - open bite, NOB - normal overbite. Source: Joanna Antoszewska (2009) Wykorzystanie tymczasowego zakotwienia kortykalnego w leczeniu zaburzeń zgryzowo-zębowych. Wrocław : Akad. Med., 5; 111 s. (Rozprawy Habilitacyjne Akademii Medycznej we Wrocławiu). ISBN 978-83-7055-489-7. Source: Antoszewska J, Papadopoulos M, Park HS, Ludwig B. Five-year-experience with orthodontic miniscrew implants: a retrospective investigation of the factors influencing the success rates. Am J Orthod Dentofacial Orthop 2009;136;2:158.e1-158.e10 (on-line), 158-159

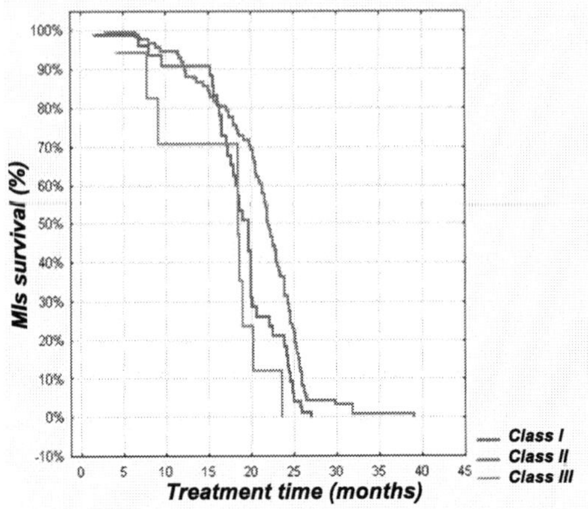

Fig. 48. TSAD stability in relation to the Angle class. Source: Joanna Antoszewska (2009) Wykorzystanie tymczasowego zakotwienia kortykalnego w leczeniu zaburzeń zgryzowo-zębowych. Wrocław : Akad. Med., 5; 111 s. (Rozprawy Habilitacyjne Akademii Medycznej we Wrocławiu). ISBN 978-83-7055-489-7

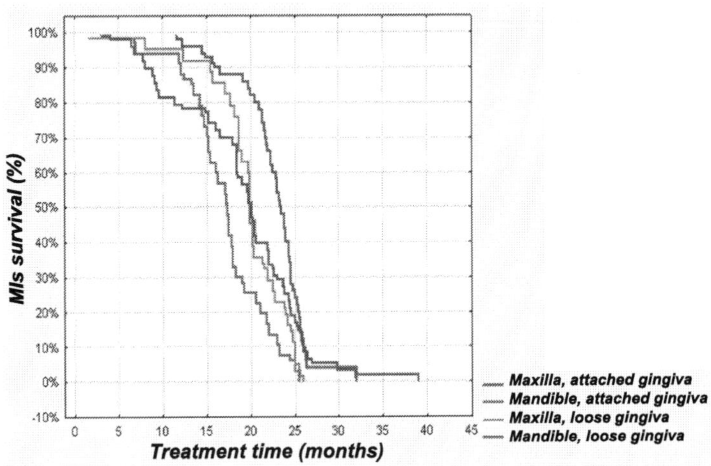

Fig. 49. TSAD stability in relation to its vertical position. Source: Joanna Antoszewska (2009) Wykorzystanie tymczasowego zakotwienia kortykalnego w leczeniu zaburzeń zgryzowo-zębowych. Wrocław : Akad. Med., 5; 111 s. (Rozprawy Habilitacyjne Akademii Medycznej we Wrocławiu). ISBN 978-83-7055-489-7

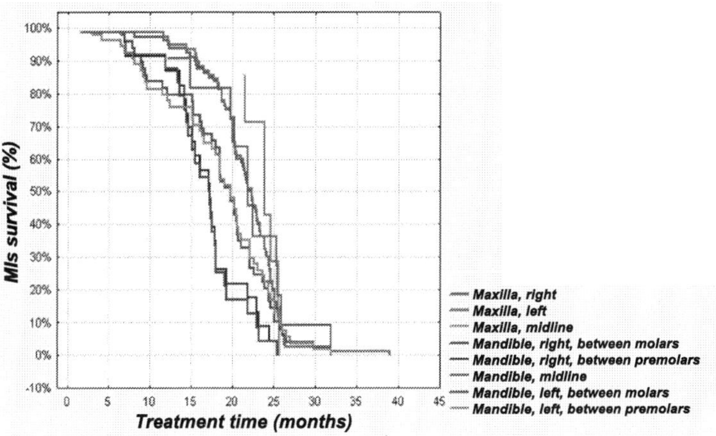

Fig. 50. TSAD stability in relation to its position along the dental arch perimeter. Source: Joanna Antoszewska (2009) Wykorzystanie tymczasowego zakotwienia kortykalnego w leczeniu zaburzeń zgryzowo-zębowych. Wrocław : Akad. Med., 5; 111 s. (Rozprawy Habilitacyjne Akademii Medycznej we Wrocławiu). ISBN 978-83-7055-489-7

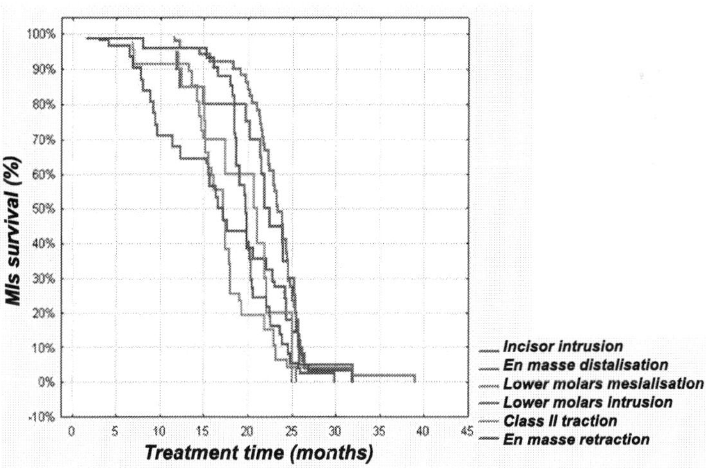

Fig. 51. TSAD stability in relation to orthodontic displacement. Source: Joanna Antoszewska (2009) Wykorzystanie tymczasowego zakotwienia kortykalnego w leczeniu zaburzeń zgryzowo-zębowych. Wrocław : Akad. Med., 5; 111 s. (Rozprawy Habilitacyjne Akademii Medycznej we Wrocławiu). ISBN 978-83-7055-489-7

Considering rate of stability, certainly mini plates prevail over single miniscrew implants, however the former ones demand on more complex surgical protocol[121-126]. Nevertheless, rapid development of orthodontic anchorage design as well as progressively increasing interest of practitioners towards application of mini plates in mostly simple manner already provoked the positive feedback: system addressed to orthodontists only[127-134].
Summing up, miniscrew implants and mini plates increasing popularity among clinicians is quite likely to displace conventional appliances for anchorage reinforcement, therefore "gravity center" of knowledge provided in this chapter has been moved towards details of planning and application of temporary skeletal anchorage devices.

3. References

[1] Tweed Ch. Indications for the extraction of teeth in orthodontic procedure. Am J Orthod Oral Surg. 1944-1945;42:22-45.
[2] Levrini A, Favero L. The masters of functional orthodontics. 2003, Quintessence Publishing, New Malden, Surrey, UK.
[3] McLaughlin RP, Bennett JC, Trevisi H. Systematized orthodontic treatment mechanics. 2001, second edition, Mosby International Ltd.
[4] Gandini LG Jr, Gandini MR, Amaral RM. Continuous torque system with control of the reaction unit. Am J Orthod Dentofacial Orthop. 2010;137:393-5.
[5] Viecilli RF. Self-corrective T-loop design for differential space closure. Am J Orthod Dentofacial Orthop. 2006;129:48-53.
[6] Choy K, Pae EK, Kim KH, Park YC, Burstone CJ. Controlled space closure with a statically determinate retraction system. Angle Orthod. 2002;72:191-8.
[7] Kuhlberg AJ, Burstone CJ. T-loop position and anchorage control. Am J Orthod Dentofacial Orthop. 1997;112:12-8.
[8] Shroff B, Yoon WM, Lindauer SJ, Burstone CJ. Simultaneous intrusion and retraction using a three-piece base arch. Angle Orthod.1997;67:455-61.
[9] Kalra V, Burstone CJ, Nanda R. More on fixed magnetic appliances. Am J Orthod Dentofacial Orthop. 1990;97:27A-28A.
[10] Manhartsberger C, Morton JY, Burstone CJ. Space closure in adult patients using the segmented arch technique. Angle Orthod. 1989;59:205-10.
[11] Burstone CJ. The segmented arch approach to space closure. Am J Orthod. 1982;82:361-78.
[12] Park JH, Cruz C, Alexander RG. An orthodontic/orthopedic correction of the Class III malocclusion in young patients with a modified RPE appliance and a facemask. Int J Orthod Milwaukee. 2010;21:23-6.
[13] Isci D, Turk T, Elekdag-Turk S. Activation-deactivation rapid palatal expansion and reverse headgear in Class III cases. Eur J Orthod. 2010;32:706-15. Epub 2010 May 9.
[14] León-Salazar V, Janson G, de Freitas MR, de Almeida RR, León-Salazar R. Nonextraction treatment of a skeletal Class III malocclusion. Am J Orthod Dentofacial Orthop. 2009;136:736-45.
[15] Hamamci N, Başaran G, Tümen EC, Ozdemir E. Nonsurgical orthodontic treatment of an adolescent girl with Class III malocclusion and asymmetric maxillary narrowing. Am J Orthod Dentofacial Orthop. 2008;134:309-17.
[16] Baccetti T, Rey D, Angel D, Oberti G, McNamara JA Jr. Mandibular cervical headgear vs rapid maxillary expander and facemask for orthopedic treatment of Class III malocclusion. Angle Orthod. 2007;77:619-24.

[17] Pangrazio-Kulbersh V, Berger JL, Janisse FN, Bayirli B. Long-term stability of Class III treatment: rapid palatal expansion and protraction facemask vs LeFort I maxillary advancement osteotomy. Am J Orthod Dentofacial Orthop. 2007;131:7.e9-19.
[18] Kama JD, Ozer T, Baran S. Orthodontic and orthopaedic changes associated with treatment in subjects with Class III malocclusions. Eur J Orthod. 2006;28:496-502. Epub 2006 Jun 13.
[19] Arman A, Ufuk Toygar T, Abuhijleh E. Evaluation of maxillary protraction and fixed appliance therapy in Class III patients. Eur J Orthod. 2006;28:383-92. Epub 2006 May 26.
[20] Liou EJ. Effective maxillary orthopedic protraction for growing Class III patients: a clinical application simulates distraction osteogenesis. Prog Orthod. 2005;6:154-71.
[21] Arslan SG, Kama JD, Baran S. Correction of a severe Class III malocclusion. Am J Orthod Dentofacial Orthop. 2004;126:237-44.
[22] Westwood PV, McNamara JA Jr, Baccetti T, Franchi L, Sarver DM. Long-term effects of Class III treatment with rapid maxillary expansion and facemask therapy followed by fixed appliances. Am J Orthod Dentofacial Orthop. 2003;123:306-20.
[23] Cha KS. Skeletal changes of maxillary protraction in patients exhibiting skeletal class III malocclusion: a comparison of three skeletal maturation groups. Angle Orthod. 2003;73:26-35.
[24] Keles A, Tokmak EC, Erverdi N, Nanda R. Effect of varying the force direction on maxillary orthopedic protraction. Angle Orthod. 2002;72:387-96.
[25] Baccetti T, Franchi L, McNamara JA Jr. Treatment and posttreatment craniofacial changes after rapid maxillary expansion and facemask therapy. Am J Orthod Dentofacial Orthop. 2000;118:404-13.
[26] Lima Filho RM, de Oliveira Ruellas AC. Long-term maxillary changes in patients with skeletal Class II malocclusion treated with slow and rapid palatal expansion. Am J Orthod Dentofacial Orthop. 2008;134:383-8.
[27] Lima Filho RM, Ruellas AC. Long-term anteroposterior and vertical maxillary changes in skeletal class II patients treated with slow and rapid maxillary expansion. Angle Orthod. 2007;77:870-4.
[28] Lima Filho RM, de Oliveira Ruellas AC. Mandibular behavior with slow and rapid maxillary expansion in skeletal Class II patients: a long-term study. Angle Orthod. 2007;77:625-31.
[29] Frye L, Diedrich PR, Kinzinger GS. Class II treatment with fixed functional orthodontic appliances before and after the pubertal growth peak - a cephalometric study to evaluate differential therapeutic effects. J Orofac Orthop. 2009;70:511-27.
[30] Siara-Olds NJ, Pangrazio-Kulbersh V, Berger J, Bayirli B. Long-term dentoskeletal changes with the Bionator, Herbst, Twin Block, and MARA functional appliances. Angle Orthod. 2010;80:18-29.
[31] Chaiyongsirisern A, Rabie AB, Wong RW. Stepwise advancement Herbst appliance versus mandibular sagittal split osteotomy. Treatment effects and long-term stability of adult Class II patients. Angle Orthod. 2009;79:1084-94.
[32] Panigrahi P, Vineeth V. Biomechanical effects of fixed functional appliance on craniofacial structures. Angle Orthod. 2009;79:668-75.
[33] Kinzinger G, Frye L, Diedrich P. Class II treatment in adults: comparing camouflage orthodontics, dentofacial orthopedics and orthognathic surgery - a cephalometric study to evaluate various therapeutic effects. J Orofac Orthop. 2009;70:63-91. Epub 2009 Feb 5.

[34] Sloss EA, Southard KA, Qian F, Stock SE, Mann KR, Meyer DL, Southard TE. Comparison of soft-tissue profiles after treatment with headgear or Herbst appliance. Am J Orthod Dentofacial Orthop. 2008;133:509-14.

[35] Giannasi LC, Magini M, de Oliveira CS, de Oliveira LV. Treatment of obstructive sleep apnea using an adjustable mandibular repositioning appliance fitted to a total prosthesis in a maxillary edentulous patient. Sleep Breath. 2008;12:91-5.

[36] Naini FB, Gill DS, Payne E, Keel B. Medium Opening Activator: design, applications for the management of class II deep overbite malocclusion. World J Orthod. 2007;8:e1-9.

[37] VanLaecken R, Martin CA, Dischinger T, Razmus T, Ngan P. Treatment effects of the edgewise Herbst appliance: a cephalometric and tomographic investigation. Am J Orthod Dentofacial Orthop. 2006;130:582-93.

[38] Kinzinger G, Gülden N, Roth A, Diedrich P. Disc-condyle relationships during class II Treatment with the functional mandibular advancer (FMA). J Orofac Orthop. 2006;67:356-75.

[39] Bass NM. The Dynamax system: a new orthopaedic appliance and case report. J Orthod. 2006;33:78-89.

[40] Shen G, Hägg U, Darendeliler M. Skeletal effects of bite jumping therapy on the mandible - removable vs. fixed functional appliances. Orthod Craniofac Res.2005;8:2-10.

[41] Voudouris JC, Woodside DG, Altuna G, Angelopoulos G, Bourque PJ, Lacouture CY, Kuftinec MM. Condyle-fossa modifications and muscle interactions during Herbst treatment, Part 2. Results and conclusions. Am J Orthod Dentofacial Orthop. 2003;124:13-29.

[42] Voudouris JC, Woodside DG, Altuna G, Kuftinec MM, Angelopoulos G, Bourque PJ. Condyle-fossa modifications and muscle interactions during herbst treatment, part 1: new technological methods. Am J Orthod Dentofacial Orthop. 2003;123:604-13.

[43] Kinzinger G, Ostheimer J, Förster F, Kwandt PB, Reul H, Diedrich P. Development of a new fixed functional appliance for treatment of skeletal class II malocclusion first report. J Orofac Orthop. 2002;63:384-99.

[44] Dolce C, Van Sickels JE, Bays RA, Rugh JD. Skeletal stability after mandibular advancement with rigid versus wire fixation. J Oral Maxillofac Surg. 2000;58:1219-27.

[45] Blomqvist JE, Isaksson S. Skeletal stability after mandibular advancement: a comparison of two rigid internal fixation techniques. J Oral Maxillofac Surg. 1994;52:1133-7.

[46] Sadowsky C, Schneider BJ, BeGole EA, Tahir E. Long-term stability after orthodontic treatment: nonextraction with prolonged retention. Am J Orthod Dentofacial Orthop. 1994;106:243-9.

[47] Newton I. Philosophiae Naturalis Principia Mathematica, 1687, S. Pepys, Reg. Sor. Praeses, London.

[48] Melsen B, Fotis V, Burstone CJ. Vertical force considerations in differential space closure. J Clin Orthod. 1990;24:678-83.

[49] Sifakakis I, Pandis N, Makou M, Eliades T, Bourauel C. Forces and moments on posterior teeth generated by incisor intrusion biomechanics. Orthod Craniofac Res. 2009;12:305-11.

[50] Badawi HM, Toogood RW, Carey JP, Heo G, Major PW. Three-dimensional orthodontic force measurements. Am J Orthod Dentofacial Orthop. 2009;136:518-28.

[51] Cattaneo PM, Dalstra M, Melsen B. Moment-to-force ratio, center of rotation, and force level: a finite element study predicting their interdependency for simulated orthodontic loading regimens. Am J Orthod Dentofacial Orthop. 2008;133:681-9.

[52] Proffit WR, Fields HW Jr., Sarver DM. Contemporary Orthodontics. 2006, Elsevier Health Sciences, Edition 4.
[53] Teuscher UM. An appraisal of growth and reaction to extraoral anchorage. Am J Orthod 1986;89:113-21.
[54] Schmuth GPF, Holtgrave EA, Drescher DISBN: 83-87601-20-9, Czelej, Wydanie 1,
[55] Braun S. Extraoral appliances: a twenty-first century update. Am J Orthod Dentofacial Orthop 2004;125:624-9.
[56] Melsen B, Bosch C. Different approaches to anchorage: a survey and evaluation. Angle Orthod 1997;67;1:23-30.
[57] Steger ES, Blechman AM. Case reports: molar distalization with static repelling magnets. Part II. Am J Orthod Dentofacial Orthop 1995;108:547-55.
[58] Bondemark L. A comparative analysis of distal maxillary molar movement produced by a new lingual intra-arch coil appliance and magnetic appliance. Eur J Orthod 2000;22:683-95.
[59] Dunin-Wilczyńska I. Jednostronna dystalizacja pierwszego trzonowca górnego sprężyną ściśniętą. Ortod. Współcz. 2001;3;2:37-9.
[60] Gulati S, Kharbanda OP, Parkash H. Dental and skeletal changes after intra-oral molar distalization with sectional jig assembly. Am J Orthod Dentofacial Orthop 1998;114:319-27.
[61] Bolla E, Muratore F, Carano A, Bowman SJ. Evaluation of Maxillary Molar Distalization With the Distal Jet: A Comparison With Other Contemporary Methods. The Angle Orthodontist: October 2002, Vol. 72, No. 5, pp. 481-94.
[62] Paul LD, O'Brien KD, Mandall NA. Upper removable appliance or jones jig for distalizing first molars? A randomized clinical trial. Orthod Craniofacial Res 2002;5:238-42.
[63] Hilgers JJ. The pendulum appliance for class II non-compliance therapy. J Clin Orthod 1992;67:249-71.
[64] Keles A. Maxillary unilateral distalization with sliding mechanics. Eur J Orthod 2001;23:507-15.
[65] Roberts-Harry D, Sandy J. Orthodontics. Part 9: anchorage control and distal movement. British Dent J 2004;196;5:255-63.
[66] Pancherz H, Anehus-Pancherz M. The head-gear effect of the Herbst appliance. A cephalometric long-term study. Am J Orthod Dentofacial Orthop 1993;103:510-20.
[67] Carrière L. A new Class II distalizer. J Clin Orthod 2004;38:224-31.
[68] Küçükkeleş N, Ilhan I, Orgun IA. Treatment efficiency in skeletal Class II patients treated with the jasper jumper. Angle Orthod 2007;77:449-56.
[69] Mulligan TF. Common sense mechanics in everyday orthodontics. 2009, CSM Publishing, Phoenix, Arizona, USA.
[70] Lloyd TG, Stephens CD. Spontaneous changes in molar occlusion after extraction of all first premolars: a study of class II/1 cases treated with removable appliances. Br J Orth 1979;6:91-4.
[71] Stephens CD, Lloyd TG. Changes in molar occlusion after extraction of all first premolars: a follow up study of class II/1 cases treated with removable appliances. Br J Orth 1980;7:139-44.
[72] Taner TU, Yukay F., Pehlivanoglu M, Çakirer B. A comparative analysis of maxillary tooth movement produced by cervical headgear and pend-x appliance. Angle Orthod 2003;73:686-91.

[73] Rudge SJ. A simplified method of applying extra-oral anchorage. Br Dent J 1981;152:205-6.
[74] Ghosh J, Nanda RS. Evaluation of intramolar distalization technique. Am J Orthod Dentofacial Orthop 1996;110:639-46.
[75] Byloff FK, Darandeliler MA. Distal molar movement using the pendulum appliance. Angle Orthod 1997;67:249-60.
[76] Bondemark L, Kurol J. Class II correction with magnets and super-elastic coils followed by straight-wire mechanotherapy. J Orofacial Orthop 1998;59:127-38.
[77] Alwali S, Marklund M, Persson M. Apical root resorption of upper first molars as related to anchorage system. Swed Dent J 2000;24:145-53.
[78] Bolla E, Muratore F, Carano A, Bowman J. Evaluation of maxillary molar distalization with the distal jet: a comparison with other temporary methods. Angle Orthod 2002;72:481-94.
[79] Brickman CD, Siha PK, Nanda RS. Evaluation of the jones jig appliance for distal molar movement. Am J Orthod Dentofacial Orthop 2000;118:526-34.
[80] Chiu PP. A comparison of two intraoral molar distalization appliances: distal jet versus pendulum appliance [unpublished master's thesis]. Ann Arbor, Mich: Department of Orthodontics, University of Michigan, 2001.
[81] Langlade M. Clinical distalization with the distalix. World J Orthod 2003;4:215-28.
[82] Paul LD, O'Brien KD, Mandall NA. Upper removable appliance or jones jig for distalizing first molars? A randomized clinical trial. Orthod Craniofacial Res 2002;5:238-42.
[83] Firouz M, Zernik J, Nanda R.: Dental and orthopedic effects of high-pull headgear in treatment of class II division 1 malocclusion. Am J Orthod Dentofacial Orthop 1992;102:197-205.
[84] Ng J, Major P, Flores-Mir C. True molar intrusion attained during orthodontic treatment. Am J Orthod Dentofacial Orthop 2006;130:709-14.
[85] Gainsforth BL, Higley LB. A study of orthodontic anchorage possibilities in basal bone. Am J Orthod Oral Surg 1945;31:406-17.
[86] Sherman AJ. Bone reaction to orthodontic forces or vitreous carbon dental implants. Am J Orthod 1978;74:79-87.
[87] Smith JR. Bone dynamics associated with the controlled loading of bioglass-coated aluminum endosteal implants. Am J Orthod 1979;76:618-36.
[88] Majzoub Z, Finotti M, Miotti F, Giardino R, Cordioli G. Bone response to orthodontic loading of endosseous implants in the rabbit calvaria. Early continuous distalizing forces. Eur J Orthod 1999;21:223-30
[89] Roberts WE, Smith RK, Zilberman Y, Mozsary PG, Smith RS. Osseous adaptation to continuous loading of rigid endosseous implants. Am J Orthod 1984;86:95-111.
[90] Sung J.H., Kyung H.M., Bae S.M., Park H.S., Kwon O.W., McNamara J.A.: Microimplants in orthodontics. Daegu: Dentos 2006.
[91] Shapiro PA, Kokich VG. Use of implants in orthodontics. Dent Clin North Am 1988;32:539-50.
[92] Roberts WE, Nelson CL, Goodacre CJ. Rigid implant anchorage to close a mandibular first molar extraction site. J Clin Orthod 1994;28:693-704.
[93] Block MS, Hoffman DR. A new device of absolute anchorage for orthodontics. Am J Orthod Dentofacial Orthop 1995;107:251-8.
[94] Hong H, Ngan P, Li HG, Qi LG, Wei SHY. Use of onplants as stable anchorage for facemask treatment: a case report. Angle Orthod2005;75:453-60.

[95] Janssesns F, Swennen G, Dujardin T, Glineur R, Malevez C. Use of onplants as orthodontic anchorage. Am J Orthod Dentofacial Orthop 2002;122:566-70.
[96] Creekmore TD, Eklund MK. The possibility of skeletal anchorage. J Clin Orthod 1983;17:266-9.
[97] Kanomi R. Mini-implant for orthodontic anchorage. Int J Clin Orthod 1997;31:763-7.
[98] Costa A, Raffini M, Melsen B. Microscrew as orthodontic anchorage. Int J Adult Orthod Orthognath Surg 1998;13:201-9.
[99] Ludwig B., Baumgaertel S., Bowman S.J.: Mini-implants in orthodontics. Berlin: Quintesence 2008.
[100] Cheol-Ho Paik CH, Park IK, Woo Y, Kim TW. Orthodontic miniscrew implants, clinical applications. 2008 Mosby.
[101] Antoszewska J. Class II division 2 treatment supported by absolute anchorage - case report. Dent. Med. Probl. 2007;44;2:275-80.
[102] Antoszewska J. Mikroimplanty systemu Absoanchor w leczeniu zgryzu otwartego - opis przypadku. Ortod. Pol. 2007;1;1:23-8.
[103] Antoszewska J, Minch L. Literature-based clinical application of microimplants in treatment of different malocclusions. Dent. Med. Probl. 2006 43;1:11-4.
[104] Antoszewska J, Sarul M, Kawala B. Asymetryczna dystalizacja zębów szczęki w oparciu o mikroimplanty Absoanchor. Opis przypadku. Implantoprotetyka 2008;9;4:25-8.
[105] Antoszewska J. Wykorzystanie tymczasowego zakotwienia kortykalnego w leczeniu zaburzeń zgryzowo-zębowych. 2009, Wroclaw Medical University, habilitation thesis ISBN 978-83-7055-489-7.
[106] Antoszewska J, Papadopoulos M, Park HS, Ludwig B. Five-year-experience with orthodontic miniscrew implants: a retrospective investigation of the factors influencing the success rates. Am J Orthod Dentofacial Orthop 2009;136;2:158.e1-158.e10 (on- line), 158-159.
[107] Antoszewska J, Kawala B, Sarul M. Factors affecting stability of orthodontic implants. A Wroclaw method Forum Ortodont. 2010;6,1:5-14.
[108] Antoszewska J, Szeląg J. Pharmacotherapy in orthodontic treatment supported by micro-implants. Pharmacol Rep 2007;59;1:254-6.
[109] Park HS. An anatomical study using CT images for the implantation of micro-implants. Korea J Ortho 2002;32:435-41.
[110] Florvaag B, Kneuertz P, Lazar F, Koebke J, Zöller JE, Braumann B, Mischkowski RA.J Orofac Orthop. Biomechanical properties of orthodontic miniscrews. An in-vitro study. J Orofac Orthop. 2010;71:53-67. Epub 2010 Feb 5.
[111] Park HS. The skeletal cortical anchorage using titanium microscrew implants. Korea J. Orthod. 1999, 29:699-706.
[112] Park HS, Oh YH. Forced eruption of a labially impacted canine using joined micro-implants. J Clin Orthod. 2010;44:108-13; quiz 106.
[113] Janssens F, Swennen G, Dujardin T, Glineur R, Malevez C. Use of an onplant as orthodontic anchorage. Am J Orthod Dentofacial Orthop 2002;122:566-70.
[114] Melsen B, Fiorelli G. Upper molar intrusion. J Clin Orthod 1996;30:91-6.
[115] Kalra V, Burstone CJ, Nanda R. Effects of a fixed magnetic appliance on the dentofacial complex. Am J Orthod Dentofacial Orthop 1989;95:467-78.
[116] Moon CH, Wee JU, Lee HS. Intrusion of overerupted molars by corticotomy and orthodontic skeletal anchorage. Angle Orthod. 2007;77:1119-25.

[117] Park YC, Lee SY, Kim DH, Jee SH. Intrusion of posterior teeth using mini-screw implants. Am J Orthod Dentofacial Orthop 2003;123:690-4.
[118] Park HS, Kwon TG. Sliding mechanics with microscrew implant anchorage. Angle Orthod. 2004;74:703-10.
[119] Antoszewska J, Trześniewska P, Kawala B, Park HS. Qualitative and quantitative evaluation of root injury risk potentially burdening insertion of microscrew implants. Korean J.Orthod. 2011;41,2:112-120.
[120] Liou EJ, Pai BC, Lin JC. Do miniscrews remain stationary under orthodontic forces? Am J Orthod Dentofacial Orthop 2004;126:42-7.
[121] Choi BH, Zhu SJ, Kim YH. A clinical evaluation of titanium miniplates as anchors for orthodontic treatment. Am J Orthod Dentofacial Orthop 2005;128:382-4.
[122] Kärcher H, Byloff FK, Clar E. The Graz implant supported pendulum. A technical note. J Craniomaxillofac Surg 2002;30:87-90.
[123] Sugawara J, Daimaruya T, Umemori M, Nagasaka H, Takahashi I, Kawamura H., Mitani H.: Distal movement of mandibular molars in adult patients with the skeletal anchorage system. Am J Orthod Dentofacial Orthop. 2004;125:130-8.
[124] De Clerck HJ, Cornelis MA, Cevidanes LH, Heymann GC, Tulloch CJF. Orthopedic Traction of the Maxilla With Miniplates: A New Perspective for Treatment of Midface Deficiency. J Oral Maxillofac Surg 2009, 67: 2123-9.
[125] Sugawara J, Aymach Z, Nagasaka DH, Kawamura H, Nanda R. "Surgery first" orthognathics to correct a skeletal class II malocclusion with an impinging bite. J Clin Orthod. 2010;44:429-38.
[126] Nagasaka H, Sugawara J, Kawamura H, Nanda R. "Surgery first" skeletal Class III correction using the Skeletal Anchorage System. J Clin Orthod. 2009;43:97-105.
[127] Kim SH, Kang SM, Choi YS, Kook YA, Chung KR, Huang JC. Cone-beam computed tomography evaluation of mini-implants after placement: Is root proximity a major risk factor for failure? Am J Orthod Dentofacial Orthop. 2010;138:264-76.
[128] Chung KR, Kim SH, Choo H, Kook YA, Cope JB. Distalization of the mandibular dentition with mini-implants to correct a Class III malocclusion with a midline deviation. Am J Orthod Dentofacial Orthop. 2010;137:135-46.
[129] Kim SH, Kook YA, Jeong DM, Lee W, Chung KR, Nelson G. Clinical application of accelerated osteogenic orthodontics and partially osseointegrated mini-implants for minor tooth movement. Am J Orthod Dentofacial Orthop. 2009;136:431-9.
[130] Kim SH, Kook YA, Lee W, Kim I, Chung KR. Two-component mini-implant as an efficient tool for orthognathic patients. Am J Orthod Dentofacial Orthop. 2009;135:110-7.
[131] Chung KR, Kim SH, Kook YA, Kang YG, Sinclair PM. Dental midline correction using two component C-orthodontic mini-implant. Prog Orthod. 2009;10:76-86.
[132] Kim SH, Cho JH, Chung KR, Kook YA, Nelson G. Removal torque values of surface-treated mini-implants after loading. Am J Orthod Dentofacial Orthop. 2008;134:36-43.
[133] Chung KR, Kim SH, Kook YA, Son JH. Anterior torque control using partial-osseointegrated mini-implants: biocreative therapy type I technique. World J Orthod. 2008;9:95-104.
[134] Chung K, Kim SH, Kook Y. C-orthodontic microimplant for distalization of mandibular dentition in Class III correction. Angle Orthod. 2005;75:119-28.

23

Neural Modulation of Orthodontic Tooth Movement

John K. Neubert, Robert M. Caudle, Calogero Dolce, Edgardo J. Toro,
Yvonne Bokrand-Donatelli and L. Shannon Holliday
University of Florida College of Dentistry
United States of America

1. Introduction

Millions of people worldwide have orthodontic therapy for the treatment of dental malocclusions, craniofacial disorders, and simply to improve their appearance. However, orthodontic treatment has several major problems, including the long time braces must be worn, the pain involved during treatment, and the need to wear retainers to prevent relapse. Orthodontics could be improved. Understanding the mechanisms involved with orthodontic tooth movement represents a first step toward this goal. Improvements in the practice of orthodontics would have an immediate and significant impact on the millions of individuals undergoing orthodontic treatment worldwide.

Orthodontic tooth movement can be thought of as an interaction of mechanical force on biological tissue (Krishnan and Davidovitch, 2006; Wise and King, 2008). Much progress in orthodontics has involved finding better means to apply mechanical force to teeth. While advances have been made regarding the mechanics and materials used in orthodontics, there has been a relative plateau in the overall treatment outcomes. For example, a moderately difficult case still requires an average of 18-36 months for treatment, no different than 50 years ago. It is apparent that discoveries relating to biological manipulations may provide a path for significantly improving orthodontic practice.

It is thought that enhancing the speed of orthodontic tooth movement could be accomplished if bone remodeling occurred at an accelerated rate in the alveolar bone associated with the teeth being moved. While this has not been formally demonstrated in the clinic, animal studies strongly support this notion. For example, orthodontic tooth movement in a mouse model was accelerated by overexpressing Receptor Activator of Nuclear Factor Kappa B-Ligand (RANKL) (Kanzaki et al., 2006). RANKL promotes the formation and bone resorptive activity of osteoclasts, the specialized cells charged with bone resorption (Hofbauer and Heufelder, 2001). Conversely, inhibitors of osteoclast formation and activity including osteoprotegerin (OPG), integrin inhibitors, bisphosphonates and inhibitors of matrix metalloproteinases all slowed tooth movement (Holliday et al., 2003; Dolce et al., 2003; Kanzaki et al., 2004; Dunn et al., 2007). Although these studies showed that it is possible to manipulate the speed at which orthodontic tooth movement proceeds by altering osteoclast activity, the specific agents tested to date are probably inappropriate for orthodontic use in the clinic as there would be too much danger of off target effects. Such risks are unacceptable for orthodontic procedures. Although orthodontics as currently practiced is imperfect, it is quite effective. Moreover, children are the most common patients in the orthodontic clinic; for biological manipulations to enhance orthodontics to be contemplated, they must be very safe.

Biological manipulation might be useful in orthodontics to prevent relapse. It is possible that enhancers of bone formation rates might be used to remodel alveolar bone to reduce incidence of relapse and minimize the use of retainers. In this case, it is possible that uncoupled stimulators of bone formation (ie regulation that stimulates bone formation without corresponding bone resorption) might prove ideal. As will be described below, modulators of sclerostin signaling, or other regulators of the Wnt-signaling pathway, are obvious candidates for this application (Paszty et al., 2010; Moester et al., 2010).

Pain is accepted as a necessary off target effect of orthodontics, and is typically treated using common non-prescription pain medications like acetaminophen. For theoretical reasons acetaminophen, which acts centrally, is considered better than ibuprophen or aspirin, which act on prostaglandins locally (Simmons and Brandt, 1992; Kehoe et al., 1996; Walker and Buring, 2001). After an initial period of discomfort (a few days) pain goes away until the next activation of the appliance. The initial activation is usually considered the most painful. In general, orthodontic pain has been considered manageable and acceptable to patients, or at least to the patient's parents, as a necessary component of orthodontic treatment. For this reason, despite its widespread use, relatively little effort has been expended to identify ways to reduce orthodontic pain. Interestingly, as more adults are undergoing orthodontic treatment, more attention has been paid to means for relieving orthodontic pain.

It is thought that pain can be reduced by modifying orthodontic procedures, particularly by using lighter forces to cause less damage and inflammation. Treatment of orthodontic pain is complicated by the fact that tooth movement may require inflammation, triggered by mechanical damage to tissues of the periodontal ligament (PDL) and associated alveolar bone, which is caused by the application of orthodontic force. Efforts to reduce the inflammation either by reducing force or by using local anti-inflammatory agents may compromise the process of tooth movement (Simmons and Brandt, 1992; Kehoe et al., 1996; Walker and Buring, 2001). In fact, there are very few studies that objectively address any of these questions in humans or even in animal models (Bergius et al., 2000; Giannopoulou et al., 2006; Eversole, 2006). For example, there currently are no animal models for studying levels of orthodontic force compared with levels of pain and the amount of tooth movement. Without proper studies, opinions on pain in orthodontics are now based largely on anecdotal evidence.

Orthodontic tooth movement is more complicated than simply applying force, causing mechanical damage and inflammation, followed by bone resorption as part of the response to inflammation and damage. Orthodontic tooth movement requires the presence of a functional PDL (Krishnan and Davidovitch, 2006; Wise and King, 2008). Ankylosed teeth do not move regardless of the amount of force applied to the tooth, or the amount of inflammation induced. The precise mechanisms by which the PDL transduces force to stimulate bone resorption to allow for movement of a tooth through bone are still mysterious. For example, it is known that RANKL is expressed at higher levels on the pressure side of a tooth, but the mechanism supporting the increased RANKL expression is not known.

Recent data demonstrate previously unsuspected links between the neural system and bone remodeling and offer potential strategies for improving orthodontic treatment. Taking advantage of these opportunities requires understanding in greater detail how the neural system is involved in the regulation of orthodontic tooth movement. Neurons and the bone cells involved in the remodelling required for orthodontic tooth movement share numerous molecular components and it *may be possible to identify agents that can at the same time increase the speed of orthodontic tooth movement while reducing pain*. Recent studies have indicated for example that the transient receptor potential (TRP) vanilloid 1 receptor (TRPV1), a key receptor in pain sensing, is also is expressed in osteoclasts (Rossi et al., 2009; Rossi et al., 2011). TRPV1 is the receptor for capsaicin, the ingredient in red chili peppers that produces burning sensations (Caterina, 2007). Capsaicin and other TRPV1 agonists have been shown to stimulate osteoclast formation (Rossi et al., 2009). From this it is plausible that a single agent, an appropriate agonist of TRPV1, may be able to both relieve orthodontic pain and significantly reduce the time required for orthodontic procedures. Capsaicin is already a FDA-approved treatment for clinical pain and a number of studies have indicated that it is

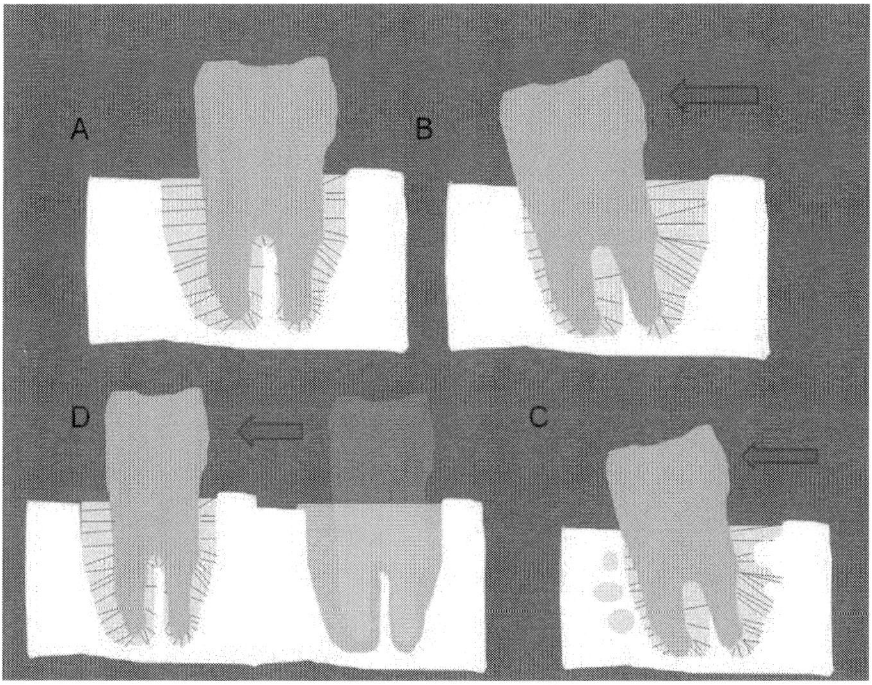

Fig. 1. Orthodontic tooth movement initiates with application of force (B) that compresses the PDL on the pressure side of the tooth, or stretches the periodontal ligament on the tension side. This leads to resorption on the pressure side and bone formation on the tension side (C) which accommodates the repositioning of the tooth (D). Goals of manipulation of tooth movement with bioactive agents include increasing the rate of tooth movement, reducing pain, and preventing relapse

effective in the reduction of pain measures for subjects suffering from arthritis, post-herpetic and diabetic neuropathies (Peikert et al., 1991; McCarthy and McCarty, 1992; Tandan et al., 1992; Watson et al., 1993; Caterina, 2007). As such, an adapted approach might be feasible in the clinic using capsaicin, or other agonists of TRPV1, to easily and safely facilitate the goal of improving orthodontic outcomes.

In summary, opportunities exist for improving orthodontic treatment by enhancing orthodontic tooth movement, preventing relapse, and reducing pain associated with orthodontic procedures (Figure 1). Recent advances in understanding neuromodulation of bone remodeling present new means to affect all of these parameters, perhaps by using the same therapeutic molecule. To examine this in greater detail we will first briefly consider the essential elements of the regulation of bone remodeling, then examine connections between bone cells and neurons.

2. Bone remodeling

Bone remodeling can be thought of simply as a dialog between two cell types, osteoclasts and osteoblasts (Figure 2)(Martin et al., 2009). Osteoclasts are cells of the hematopoetic lineage that are specialized for bone resorption (Teitelbaum, 2007). Osteoblasts are mesenchymal and are specialized for bone formation (Askmyr et al., 2009). Although this is an oversimplification, for example T-cell are known to directly stimulate osteoclast formation and bone resorption (Weitzmann and Pacifici, 2005), and osteocytes are primary regulators of osteoblast bone formation (Winkler et al., 2003; Moester et al., 2010), it is clear

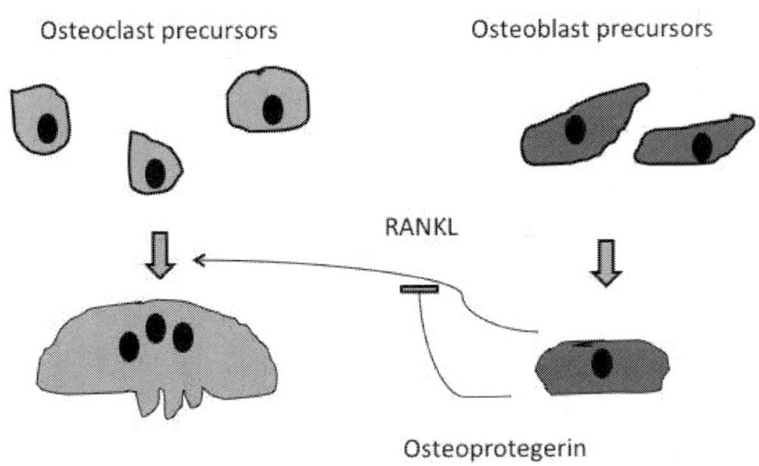

Fig. 2. RANKL produced by osteoblasts stimulates osteoclast formation and osteoclast bone resorption. Osteoprotengerin is also produced by osteoblasts and serves as a competitive inhibitor of RANKL. The humanized monoclonal antibody, denosumab, functions like osteoprotegerin.

that a major element of the regulation of bone remodeling is through expression by osteoblasts of RANKL. This stimulates its receptor, RANK, present on the surface of osteoclast precursors and osteoclasts, which induces osteoclast differentiation, survival and bone resorptive activity (Burgess et al., 1999; Kong et al., 1999). Osteoprotegerin, also produced by osteoblasts, serves as a competitive inhibitor of RANKL and by doing so reduces bone resorption (Hofbauer et al., 2004). Neural regulation of bone remodeling must occur within the constraints of this regulatory system.

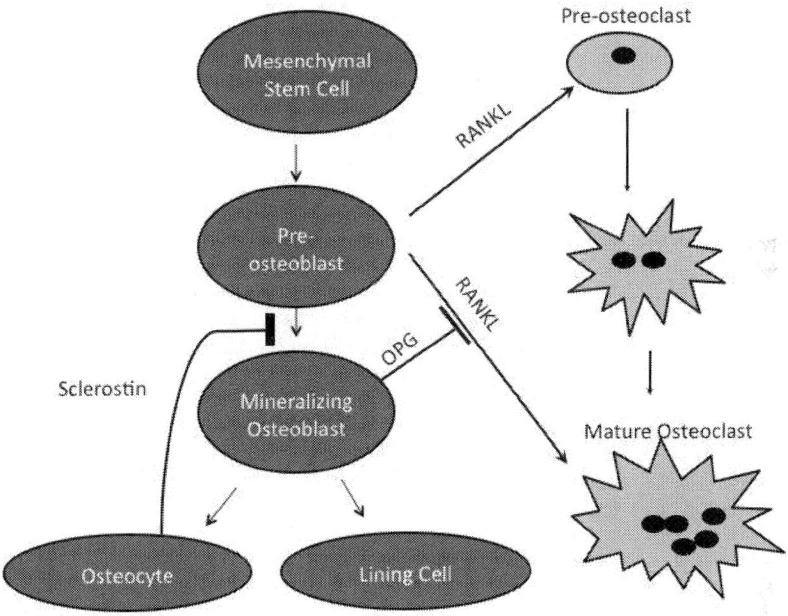

Fig. 3. Sclerostin is thought to inhibit differentiation of osteoblasts from a stage where they promote osteoclastic bone resorption to a stage where they form bone.

RANKL is a tumor necrosis factor (TNF)-related type II transmembrane protein expressed by osteoblasts, T-cells and a few other cell types (Xing et al., 2005). There was great excitement in the bone field in the late 1990s with the demonstration that RANKL was the long sought osteoclast differentiation factor (Lacey et al., 1998). Since the initial reports, this basic finding has been supported by a host of studies (Xing et al., 2005). RANKL binds its receptor RANK to stimulate osteoclast formation and activity. It also binds OPG, which resembles RANK but lacks a transmembrane domain, and serves as a soluble competitive inhibitor. Overwhelming evidence indicates the vital importance of this triad in bone remodeling and has led to the paradigm shown in Figure 2. With the discovery of RANKL came efforts to utilize inhibitors of RANKL in the development of pharmaceutical agents that inhibit osteoclast activity. Recently an anti-RANKL antibody-based pharmaceutical

(Denosumab) was generated by Amgen and approved as an anti-osteoporotic agent (Trade name Prolia) and for bone cancer (Xgeva) (Lewiecki, 2010; Castellano et al., 2011; Baron et al., 2011).

Sclerostin has recently been identified as a vital regulator of bone formation (Moester et al., 2010). Sclerostin is a controller of the Wnt-signaling pathway, which is crucial for modulating bone remodeling (Baron et al., 2006; Kubota et al., 2009). Sclerostin is thought to block the transition of osteoblasts from a step along their differentiation pathway where they produce RANKL, but do not form bone, to a point where they do not produce RANKL (or produce more osteoprotegerin) and do form bone (Figure 3)(Paszty et al., 2010). Thus higher levels of sclerostin will favor bone resorption and lower levels will favor bone formation. Taking advantage of this paradigm, efforts are underway to transition a humanized monoclonal antibody inhibitor of sclerostin to the clinic for the treatment of osteoporosis (Lewiecki, 2011). Sclerostin is one of several molecules that influence osteoblast activity by regulating the Wnt-signaling pathway (Baron et al., 2006).

3. Central control of bone remodeling

During the past decade evidence has accumulated that has shown that levels of bone remodeling and final bone structure is regulated in the central nervous system (Elefteriou, 2008; Wong et al., 2008; Karsenty and Oury, 2010). Three different mechanisms will be discussed in some detail, regulation through leptin signaling, neuropeptide Y and cannibanoid receptors. It is postulated that central regulation of bone remodeling represents a link with bone remodeling and energy metabolism (Karsenty and Oury, 2010). Leptin release by the hypothalamus for example has been shown to regulate both bone remodeling and insulin secretion (Baldock et al., 2002; Takeda, 2008; Kalra et al., 2009; Confavreux et al., 2009; Baldock et al., 2009; Qin et al., 2010; Zengin et al., 2010). Leptin is a 16 kD adipose-derived protein hormone, which plays a key role in regulating energy intake and expenditure. It has a major role in controlling appetite and metabolism.

Evidence suggests that leptin-regulated neural pathways control both bone formation and bone resorption. Mice lacking the gene encoding leptin (*ob/ob*) are obese and have higher bone mass than normal and higher rates of bone remodeling (Elefteriou et al., 2005). Intracerebroventricular infusion of leptin into the mice, under conditions where little or no leptin leaked into general circulation, led to normalization of both rates of bone remodeling and bone mass (Elefteriou et al., 2005). This strongly supported the idea that leptin regulates bone remodeling through a central relay, and this mode of regulation is vitally important in maintaining bone (Kalra et al., 2009; Karsenty and Oury, 2010).

The leptin receptor is expressed on three types of hypothalamic neurons, although its expression in the brain is not restricted to hypothalamic neurons (Karsenty and Ducy, 2006; Kalra et al., 2009). The three neurons in the hypothalamus are the arcuate nucleus, the ventromedical hypothalamic nucleus, and paraventricular nuclei. Lesioning of the arcuate nucleus using two independent strategies did not affect bone mass directly, or alter the ability of infusion of leptin to affect bone mass (Takeda and Karsenty, 2008). In contrast, lesioning ventromedical hypothalamic nuclei neurons in wild type animals resulted in a high bone mass/high bone turnover phenotype similar to that observe in the *ob/ob* mice. Infusion of leptin failed to normalize the bone phenotype in either lesioned wild type mice or the *ob/ob* mice (Guidobono et al., 2006). Taken together, these data suggested that the ventromedical hypothalamic nucleus neurons are required for leptin-dependent central regulation of bone remodeling.

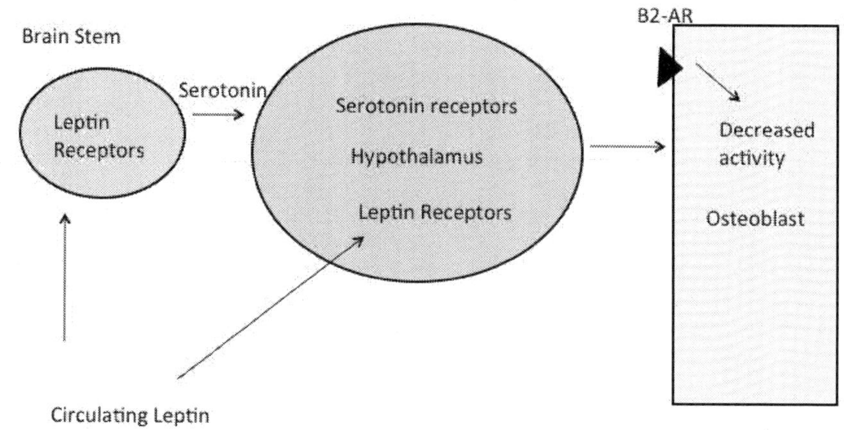

Fig. 4. Leptin stimulates receptors in the brain stem and hypothalamus leading to stimulation of β2 adrenergic receptors in osteoblasts which decrease the activity of osteoblasts

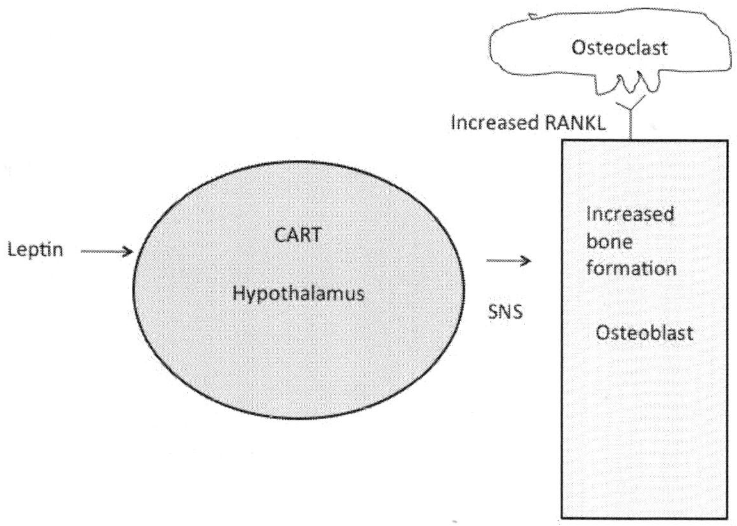

Fig. 5. Leptin stimulates cocaine- and amphetamine- regulated transcript expression which acting through the sympathetic nervous system to stimulate both increased bone formation by osteoblasts and increased resorption by osteoclasts

How then is this regulation mediated? One route is through dopamine β-hydroxylase, an enzyme required for the production of norepinepherine and epinephrine (Figure 4) (Yadav and Karsenty, 2009; Yadav et al., 2009). Mice lacking dopamine β-hydroxylase have a similar bone phenotype to the *ob/ob* mice, and leptin infusion of these mice failed to normalize bone parameters. Only one adrenergic receptor is expressed in osteoblasts, β2 adrenergic receptor. Mice lacking one or both copies of the β2 adrenergic receptor developed a high bone mass phenotype, and leptin infusion into mice lacking the β2 adrenergic receptor decreased fat mass but did not normalize the bone parameters (Yadav and Karsenty, 2009; Yadav et al., 2009).

Another mechanism by which leptin mediates bone remodeling is via the cocaine- and amphetamine- regulated transcript (CART), a neuropeptide precursor protein (Figure 5) (Elefteriou et al., 2005). The level of CART expression in the hypothalamus and peripheral organs including the pancreas and adrenal glands is tied to levels of leptin. Simply, CART expression is stimulated by leptin, and osteoclastic resorption decreases in relation to the amount of CART expressed. This action of CART is mediated through osteoblasts; CART represses RANKL expression of osteoblasts and thus reduces osteoclast formation and bone resorption (Elefteriou et al., 2005).

Neuromedin U is a neuropeptide expressed in hypothalamic neurons and in the small intestine has also been also been implicated as a component of the leptin regulatory pathway (Figure 6) (Sato et al., 2007). Although its receptor is not detected in bone cells, knockout of neuromendin U leads to a high bone mass phenotype. Treatment of leptin deficient mice with neurmedin U resulted in partial rescue of the high bone mass pheneotype suggesting that neuromedin U is downstream of leptin in the bone remodeling regulatory pathway.

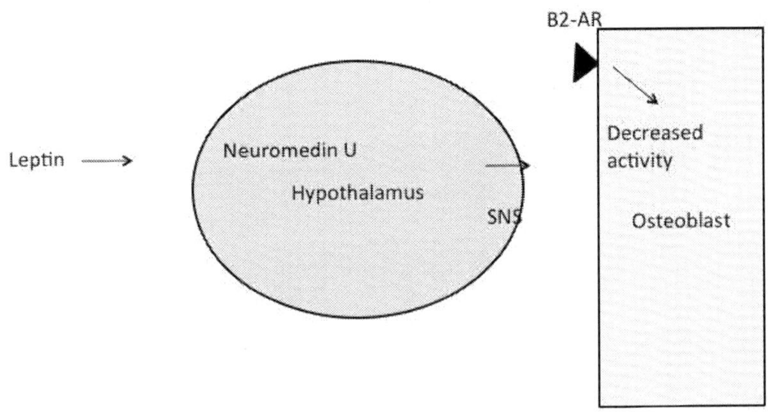

Fig. 6. Leptin also signals through the hypothalamus using a pathway involving neuromedin U and the sympathetic nervous system leading to stimulation of β2 adrenergic receptor which decreases bone formation

Taken together this suggested that leptin regulates bone remodeling through several pathways. Although caution must be exercised in translating these results to humans, they suggest a number of ramifications for humans with respect to orthodontic procedures. First, alterations in elements of this signaling pathway, for example single nucleotide polymorphisms (SNPs) in one or more the genes encoding elements of the pathway may have consequences for the general rate and efficacy of orthodontic procedures in an individual. For example, an SNP in β2 adrenergic receptor that increases signaling from the receptor may be associated with higher than normal bone mineral density, and increased rates of tooth movement.

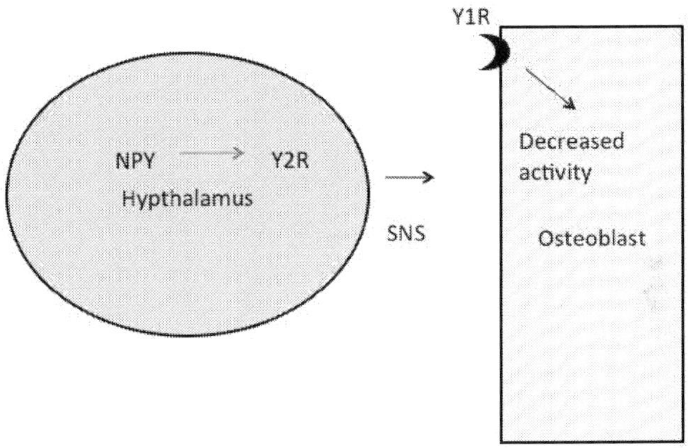

Fig. 7. Neuropeptide Y signals through Y2R receptors in the hypothalamus and Y1R receptors in osteoblasts to decrease osteoblast activity

Secondly, direct local stimulation of osteoblasts in the alveolar bone associated with specific teeth with β2 adrenergic receptor agonists might both enhance rates of tooth movement and increase the speed of bone formation at the tension side of the tooth, perhaps reducing the tendency to relapse. However, care would have to be taken in manipulating these pathways because of the associations of the adrenergic systems with cardiovascular diseases (Saini-Chohan and Hatch, 2009). In addition, a recent study indicated that SNPs in the β2 adrenergic receptor are associated with heterotypic ossification, which is associated with higher rates of fractures. Moreover, recent studies of bisphosphonate-associated oral osteonecrosis suggests that the condition is actually osteosclerosis, and may result from disorganization of normal bone remodeling rather than blocking of the process (Chiu et al., 2010; Treister et al., 2010). *While perturbation in normal bone remodeling on the surface may have favorable outcomes, great care must be taken due to the complexity of bone formation and remodeling which can lead to unexpected adverse consequences.*

Neuropeptide Y, a neurotransmitter that is widely expressed in both central and peripheral nervous systems, has been shown to regulate bone remodeling (Baldock et al., 2007; Baldock et al., 2009)(Figure 7). Knockout mice of either the neuropeptide Y1 or Y2 receptors yielded a high bone mass phenotype with enhanced osteoblast activity (Baldock et al., 2009). Neuropeptide Y receptors are, like the leptin receptor, expressed by cells of the hypothalamus. Knockout of Y2 in the hypothalamus is sufficient to induce a high bone density phenotype. However, knockout of Y1 in the hypothalamus did not alter bone homeostasis (Baldock et al., 2002; Baldock et al., 2007).

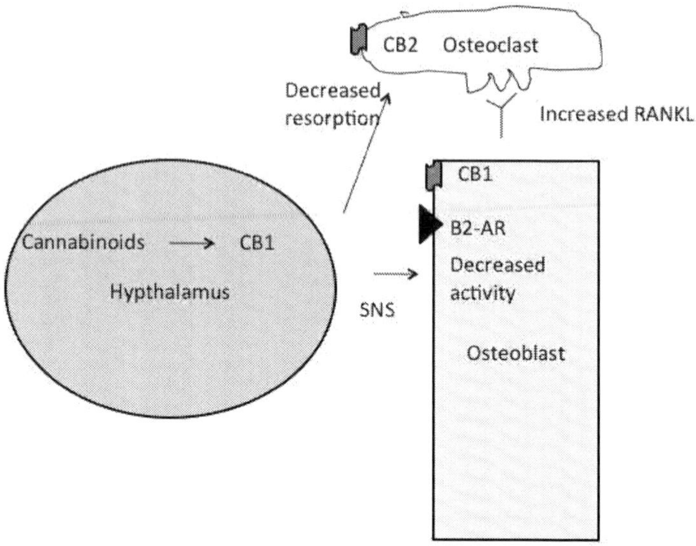

Fig. 8. Cannabinoid stimulate a central response that leads to decreased bone formation. The CB2 receptor of osteoclasts reduces osteoclast activity, but CB1 stimulation increases expression of RANKL which is pro-stimulatory

Recently, the Y1 receptor was knocked out specifically in osteoblasts using a Cre/Lox system (Baldock et al., 2007). It was shown that osteoblast specific knockout of Y1 was sufficient to increase bone mass and enhance bone remodeling. These data indicated that neuropeptide Y signaling could have a role in both central and local neural control of bone remodeling.

Neuropeptide Y signaling has been linked to food intake and like leptin, there are links between neuropeptide Y signaling and obesity (Munoz and Argente, 2002; Feletou and Levens, 2005). Neuropeptide Y receptors are found on pre- and post-synaptic neurons. Presumably activation of the receptors is tied to behavioral changes leading to alterations in food consumption. Whether it is possible to take advantage of neuropeptide Y signaling to influence bone remodeling associated with orthodontic applications is not clear, but most likely, means would have to be devised to deliver agonists locally.

A third route by which bone remodeling can be regulated centrally in through endocannabinoid signaling, which has been shown modulate bone remodeling through central and peripheral cannabinoid receptors(Davenport, 2005; Rossi et al., 2009) (Figure 8). Cannabinoid receptors are a class of G protein coupled membrane receptors. The cannabinoid receptors CB1 and CB2 play a key role in the maintenance of bone mass and are expressed on osteoblasts, osteoclasts and osteocytes. Deficiency in the hypothalamic receptor CB1 in mice has been shown to accelerate age-dependent osteoporosis. Agonists of CB2 reduce bone loss after ovariectomy in rodent models while increasing the thickness of the cortical bone. This makes CB2 a potential target for agents designed to modulate bone remodeling.

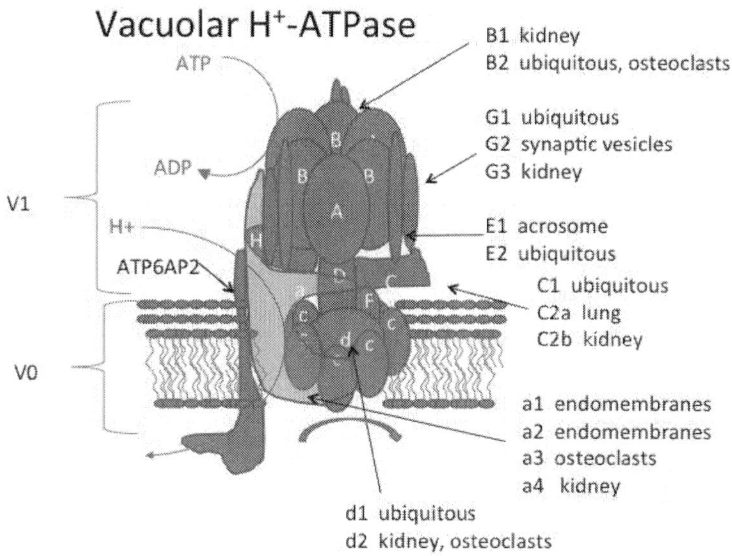

Fig. 9. V-ATPases are ubiquitously-expressed and are composed of many subunits. Some subunits are present in multiple isoforms. Osteoclasts, for example, contain the "housekeeping" isoforms of subunit a (a1, and a2) and the also express the a3 subunit which is required for bone resorption. ATP6AP2 (the prorenein receptor) links bone resorption to rennin/angiotensin signalling.

4. Common molecular features shared by neurons and bone cells

4.1 Specialized machinery for acidification

Evidence has emerged that osteoclasts share a number of molecular features with neural cells. These include the specialized use of vacuolar H^+-ATPase (V-ATPase), chloride channel protein 7 (CLC-7), which work in coordination in order to properly acidify compartments (Schaller et al., 2005; Hinton et al., 2009).

The V-ATPase is a multisubunit enzyme (11-13 subunits) that is expressed in all cells and is required for "housekeeping" acidification of vesicular compartments including lysosomes, late endosomes, compartments of uncoupling receptor and ligand, elements of the golgi, and phagosomes (Hinton et al., 2009). Certain specialized cell types express both the housekeeping subset of V-ATPases, and in addition, an additional subset that is involved in the specialized function of the cell type (Figure 9).

Osteoclasts, which are specialized to resorb bone, are a clear and well-characterized example of a cell type that uses V-ATPases for a specialized function (Blair et al., 1989; Holliday et al., 2005). Osteoclasts express normal housekeeping V-ATPases (Toyomura et al., 2003). In addition, they express a large subset that is destined for the plasma membrane of resorbing cells. When an osteoclast contacts activation signals associated with the bone surface, the specialized subset of V-ATPases is transported to a subdomain of the plasma membrane called the ruffled plasma membrane or ruffled border (Blair et al., 1989). These V-ATPases then use ATP hydrolysis to pump protons against an electrochemical gradient to acidify an extracellular resorption compartment (Figure 10).

Different subsets of V-ATPases are distinguished by isoforms of particular subunits. Some subunits are present in only a single form and are present in all V-ATPases no matter what their function. Others have multiple isoforms that are derived from different genes. For example, there are four isoforms of the a subunit (a1-a4). Subunits a1 and a2 are found in the housekeeping V-ATPases. The a3-subunit has been identified at high levels in osteoclasts, pancreatic beta cells, kidney epithelial cells and microglia (Li et al., 1999; Smith et al., 2001; Sun-Wada et al., 2006; Serrano et al., 2009). The a4 subunit is restricted to epithelial cells of the kidney (Stover et al., 2002).

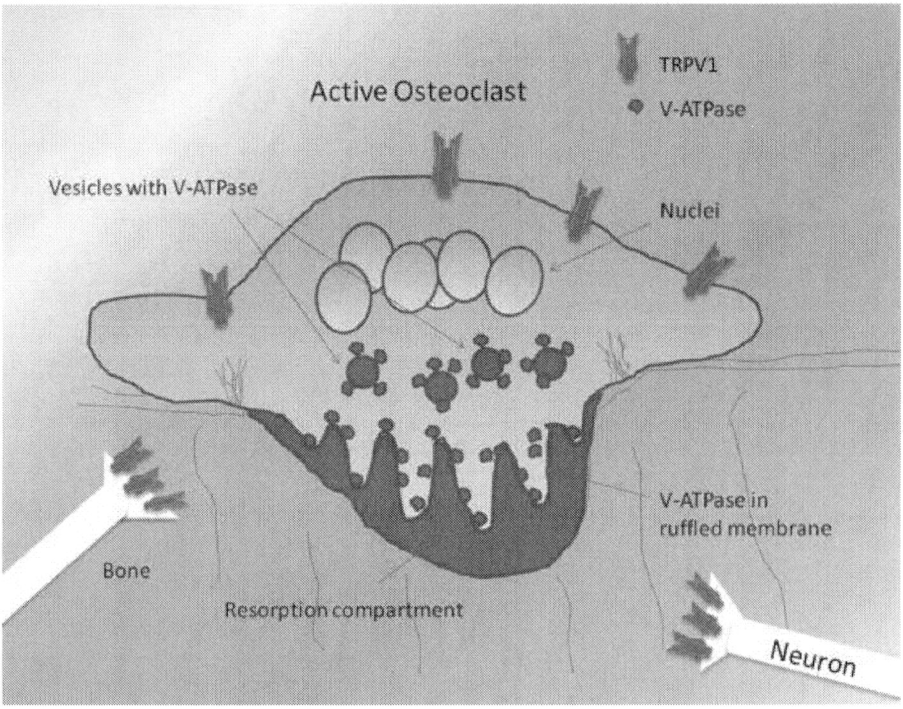

Fig. 10. Osteoclasts insert V-ATPases into the plasma membrane is a region known as the ruffled border. V-ATPases pump protons into the resorption compartment lowering the pH, which is crucial for bone resorption. TRPV1 is expressed on both osteoclasts, where agonists are proresorptive, and on neurons, where agonists reduce pain. This makes it possible that a single therapeutic agent can both increase the rate of tooth movement (which requires increased osteoclastic resorption) and reduce pain associated with orthodontic procedures.

Like osteoclasts, neurons also express subsets of V-ATPases that are utilized for specialized purposes (Moriyama et al., 1992). Neurons are thought to utilize V-ATPases to generate a driving force to power loading synaptic vesicles with neurotransmitters. In addition, there is considerable evidence that a subunit is intimately involved in mediating the fusion of synaptic vesicles with the plasma membrane to allow dumping of neurotransmitters into the synaptic cleft (Hiesinger et al., 2005; Di et al., 2010).

Among the most exciting recent findings was the demonstration that a V-ATPase accessory protein, the pro-renin receptor (PRR, also known as ATP6AP2) forms a vital scaffold between V-ATPase and the Wnt-signaling pathway (Cruciat et al., 2010). Without PRR, mineralization was blocked in a mouse model. Whether PRR is also found in osteoclasts is not known, and whether the recent demonstration that PRR is found in the hypothalamus suggests that it may be another molecule by which central regulation of bone remodeling might occur remains to be explored (Takahashi et al., 2010). In this case, the primary known function of PRR is its involvement in renin-angiotensin signaling which is related to blood pressure and cardiac activity (Nguyen, 2011).

Along with sharing specialized functions of V-ATPases, both neurons and osteoclasts require the voltage-gated chloride channel CLC-7. This channel is thought to open to reduce voltage across membranes produced by the activity of electrogenic V-ATPases. Mutations in CLC-7 lead to both osteopetrosis and neurodegeneration (Kornak et al., 2001; Kasper et al., 2005)

4.2 Sensing receptors shared by neurons and osteoclasts

Both bone remodeling and sensory pain pathways share common inflammatory mediators, including TNF-α, prostaglandins, interleukins, and vasoactive neuropeptides (e.g., substance P), to name a few. Again, specifically targeting the intersection of these pathways may provide unique opportunities for development of innovative therapies related to bone disorders and specifically OTM. The transient receptor potential (TRP) channels is a class of receptors that are involved in sensory and pain processing. For example, The TRP vanilloid 1 receptor (**TRPV1**) is found primarily on neuronal c- and a-δ fiber nociceptors that are responsible for thermal/burning pain. TRPV1 is also a major transducer of inflammatory pain, especially under acidic conditions. Recent work demonstrated that TRPV1 is expressed in human **osteoclasts**, indicating that TRPV1 may promote bone resorption (Rossi et al., 2009; Rossi et al., 2011). Previous work with ultrapotent TRPV1 agonists such as resiniferatoxin (RTX) indicates that inflammatory pain can be eliminated (Neubert, et al. 2008). TRPV1 is activated in response to lowered pH, which is an important regulator of local bone resorption. TRPV1 is expressed on osteoclasts and agonists of TRPV1, capsaicin and resinoferotoxin (RTX), stimulate osteoclast differentiation at concentrations where neuronal pain sensors are not inactivated (Rossi et al., 2009; Rossi et al., 2011). Interestingly, agonists of TRPV1 induce overexpression of the cannabinoid receptor CB2 (Rossi et al., 2009; Rossi et al., 2011). The TRPV1 inhibitor capsazepine was also shown to inhibit both osteoclast and osteoblast differentiation (Idris et al., 2010). Together, this makes TRPV1 a potential integrator between the central nervous system and bone which may be involved in orchestrating both local bone remodeling changes in response to pH and possibly orthodontic force, and augmenting central modulation of bone remodeling. These data suggest that well documented agonists and antagonists of TRPV1 may prove to be ideal agents for manipulation of OTM in ways by which orthodontic practice may be improved. Increased understanding of OTM can also provide insight into mechanisms of bone biology.

Interestingly, agonists of TRPV1 induce overexpression of the cannabinoid receptor CB2 (Rossi et al., 2009; Rossi et al., 2011). Increased understanding of OTM can provide insight into mechanisms of bone biology. For example, this knowledge may have direct implications for the use of TRPV1 agonists in the treatment of pain and bone destruction associated with bone cancer [10] (Figure 10).

5. Summary

Biological manipulation to improve orthodontic procedures is in its infancy, but it appears possible to both improve the speed and efficacy of tooth movement, and to reduce associated discomfort. Proof-in-principle experiments have been performed in animal models but translation to the clinic will require greater understanding of the processes involved. Recent studies uncovering mechanisms by which bone remodeling is controlled by central mechanisms and demonstrating that osteoclasts and neurons share regulatory molecules, although they are used for different purposes, open new avenues for understanding and manipulating orthodontic tooth movement and perhaps simultaneously reducing the discomfort associated with the procedures.

6. References

Wise, G. E. and King, G. J. (2008). Mechanisms of tooth eruption and orthodontic tooth movement. *J. Dent. Res.* 87, 414-434.

Krishnan, V. and Davidovitch, Z. (2006). Cellular, molecular, and tissue-level reactions to orthodontic force. *Am. J. Orthod. Dentofacial Orthop.* 129, 469-32.

Kanzaki, H., Chiba, M., Arai, K., Takahashi, I., Haruyama, N., Nishimura, M. and Mitani, H. (2006). Local RANKL gene transfer to the periodontal tissue accelerates orthodontic tooth movement. *Gene Ther.* 13, 678-685.

Hofbauer, L. C. and Heufelder, A. E. (2001). Role of receptor activator of nuclear factor-kappaB ligand and osteoprotegerin in bone cell biology. *J. Mol. Med.* 79, 243-253.

Dunn, M. D., Park, C. H., Kostenuik, P. J., Kapila, S. and Giannobile, W. V. (2007). Local delivery of osteoprotegerin inhibits mechanically mediated bone modeling in orthodontic tooth movement. *Bone* 41, 446-455.

Kanzaki, H., Chiba, M., Takahashi, I., Haruyama, N., Nishimura, M. and Mitani, H. (2004). Local OPG gene transfer to periodontal tissue inhibits orthodontic tooth movement. *Journal of Dental Research* 83, 920-925.

Dolce, C., Vakani, A., Archer, L., Morris-Wiman, J. A. and Holliday, L. S. (2003). Effects of echistatin and an RGD peptide on orthodontic tooth movement. *Journal of Dental Research* 82, 682-686.

Holliday, L. S., Vakani, A., Archer, L. and Dolce, C. (2003). Effects of matrix metalloproteinase inhibitors on bone resorption and orthodontic tooth movement. *J. Dent. Res.* 82, 687-691.

Moester, M. J., Papapoulos, S. E., Lowik, C. W. and Van Bezooijen, R. L. (2010). Sclerostin: current knowledge and future perspectives. *Calcif. Tissue Int.* 87, 99-107.

Paszty, C., Turner, C. H. and Robinson, M. K. (2010). Sclerostin: a gem from the genome leads to bone-building antibodies. *J. Bone Miner. Res.* 25, 1897-1904.

Kehoe, M. J., Cohen, S. M., Zarrinnia, K. and Cowan, A. (1996). The effect of acetaminophen, ibuprofen, and misoprostol on prostaglandin E2 synthesis and the degree and rate of orthodontic tooth movement. *Angle Orthod.* 66, 339-349.

Simmons, K. E. and Brandt, M. (1992). Control of orthodontic pain. *J. Indiana Dent. Assoc.* 71, 8-10.

Walker, J. B. and Buring, S. M. (2001). NSAID impairment of orthodontic tooth movement. *Ann. Pharmacother.* 35, 113-115.

Bergius, M., Kiliaridis, S. and Berggren, U. (2000). Pain in orthodontics. A review and discussion of the literature. *J. Orofac. Orthop.* 61, 125-137.

Eversole, L. R. (2006). Evidence-based practice of oral pathology and oral medicine. *J. Calif. Dent. Assoc.* 34, 448-454.

Giannopoulou, C., Dudic, A. and Kiliaridis, S. (2006). Pain discomfort and crevicular fluid changes induced by orthodontic elastic separators in children. *J. Pain* 7, 367-376.

Rossi, F., Siniscalco, D., Luongo, L., De, P. L., Bellini, G., Petrosino, S., Torella, M., Santoro, C., Nobili, B., Perrotta, S. et al. (2009). The endovanilloid/endocannabinoid system in human osteoclasts: possible involvement in bone formation and resorption. *Bone* 44, 476-484.

Rossi, F., Bellini, G., Luongo, L., Torella, M., Mancusi, S., De, P. L., Petrosino, S., Siniscalco, D., Orlando, P., Scafuro, M. et al. (2011). The endovanilloid/endocannabinoid system: A new potential target for osteoporosis therapy. *Bone.*

Caterina, M. J. (2007). Transient receptor potential ion channels as participants in thermosensation and thermoregulation. *Am. J. Physiol Regul. Integr. Comp Physiol* 292, R64-R76.

McCarthy, G. M. and McCarty, D. J. (1992). Effect of topical capsaicin in the therapy of painful osteoarthritis of the hands. *J. Rheumatol.* 19, 604-607.

Peikert, A., Hentrich, M. and Ochs, G. (1991). Topical 0.025% capsaicin in chronic post-herpetic neuralgia: efficacy, predictors of response and long-term course. *J. Neurol.* 238, 452-456.

Tandan, R., Lewis, G. A., Krusinski, P. B., Badger, G. B. and Fries, T. J. (1992). Topical capsaicin in painful diabetic neuropathy. Controlled study with long-term follow-up. *Diabetes Care* 15, 8-14.

Watson, C. P., Tyler, K. L., Bickers, D. R., Millikan, L. E., Smith, S. and Coleman, E. (1993). A randomized vehicle-controlled trial of topical capsaicin in the treatment of postherpetic neuralgia. *Clin. Ther.* 15, 510-526.

Martin, T., Gooi, J. H. and Sims, N. A. (2009). Molecular mechanisms in coupling of bone formation to resorption. *Crit Rev. Eukaryot. Gene Expr.* 19, 73-88.

Teitelbaum, S. L. (2007). Osteoclasts: what do they do and how do they do it? *Am. J. Pathol.* 170, 427-435.

Askmyr, M., Sims, N. A., Martin, T. J. and Purton, L. E. (2009). What is the true nature of the osteoblastic hematopoietic stem cell niche? *Trends Endocrinol. Metab* 20, 303-309.

Weitzmann, M. N. and Pacifici, R. (2005). The role of T lymphocytes in bone metabolism. *Immunological Reviews* 208, 154-168.

Winkler, D. G., Sutherland, M. K., Geoghegan, J. C., Yu, C., Hayes, T., Skonier, J. E., Shpektor, D., Jonas, M., Kovacevich, B. R., Staehling-Hampton, K. et al. (2003). Osteocyte control of bone formation via sclerostin, a novel BMP antagonist. *EMBO J.* 22, 6267-6276.

Burgess, T. L., Qian, Y., Kaufman, S., Ring, B. D., Van, G., Capparelli, C., Kelley, M., Hsu, H., Boyle, W. J., Dunstan, C. R. et al. (1999). The ligand for osteoprotegerin (OPGL) directly activates mature osteoclasts. *J. Cell Biol.* 145, 527-538.

Kong, Y. Y., Yoshida, H., Sarosi, I., Tan, H. L., Timms, E., Capparelli, C., Morony, S., Oliveira-dos-Santos, A. J., Van, G., Itie, A. et al. (1999). OPGL is a key regulator of osteoclastogenesis, lymphocyte development and lymph-node organogenesis. *Nature* 397, 315-323.

Hofbauer, L. C., Kuhne, C. A. and Viereck, V. (2004). The OPG/RANKL/RANK system in metabolic bone diseases. *J. Musculoskelet. Neuronal. Interact.* 4, 268-275.

Xing, L. P., Schwarz, E. M. and Boyce, B. F. (2005). Osteoclast precursors, RANKL/RANK, and immunology. *Immunological Reviews* 208, 19-29.

Lacey, D. L., Timms, E., Tan, H. L., Kelley, M. J., Dunstan, C. R., Burgess, T., Elliott, R., Colombero, A., Elliott, G., Scully, S. et al. (1998). Osteoprotegerin ligand is a cytokine that regulates osteoclast differentiation and activation. *Cell* 93, 165-176.

Lewiecki, E. M. (2010). Denosumab--an emerging treatment for postmenopausal osteoporosis. *Expert. Opin. Biol. Ther.* 10, 467-476.

Baron, R., Ferrari, S. and Russell, R. G. (2011). Denosumab and bisphosphonates: Different mechanisms of action and effects. *Bone* 48, 677-692.

Castellano, D., Sepulveda, J. M., Garcia-Escobar, I., Rodriguez-Antolin, A., Sundlov, A. and Cortes-Funes, H. (2011). The role of RANK-ligand inhibition in cancer: the story of denosumab. *Oncologist.* 16, 136-145.

Baron, R., Rawadi, G. and Roman-Roman, S. (2006). Wnt signaling: a key regulator of bone mass. *Curr. Top. Dev. Biol.* 76, 103-127.

Kubota, T., Michigami, T. and Ozono, K. (2009). Wnt signaling in bone metabolism. *J. Bone Miner. Metab* 27, 265-271.

Lewiecki, E. M. (2011). Sclerostin monoclonal antibody therapy with AMG 785: a potential treatment for osteoporosis. *Expert. Opin. Biol. Ther.* 11, 117-127.

Elefteriou, F. (2008). Regulation of bone remodeling by the central and peripheral nervous system. *Arch. Biochem. Biophys.* 473, 231-236.

Karsenty, G. and Oury, F. (2010). The central regulation of bone mass, the first link between bone remodeling and energy metabolism. *J. Clin. Endocrinol. Metab* 95, 4795-4801.

Wong, I. P., Zengin, A., Herzog, H. and Baldock, P. A. (2008). Central regulation of bone mass. *Semin. Cell Dev. Biol.* 19, 452-458.

Confavreux, C. B., Levine, R. L. and Karsenty, G. (2009). A paradigm of integrative physiology, the crosstalk between bone and energy metabolisms. *Mol. Cell Endocrinol.* 310, 21-29.

Kalra, S. P., Dube, M. G. and Iwaniec, U. T. (2009). Leptin increases osteoblast-specific osteocalcin release through a hypothalamic relay. *Peptides* 30, 967-973.

Baldock, P. A., Sainsbury, A., Couzens, M., Enriquez, R. F., Thomas, G. P., Gardiner, E. M. and Herzog, H. (2002). Hypothalamic Y2 receptors regulate bone formation. *J. Clin. Invest* 109, 915-921.

Baldock, P. A., Lee, N. J., Driessler, F., Lin, S., Allison, S., Stehrer, B., Lin, E. J., Zhang, L., Enriquez, R. F., Wong, I. P. et al. (2009). Neuropeptide Y knockout mice reveal a central role of NPY in the coordination of bone mass to body weight. *PLoS. ONE.* 4, e8415.

Qin, W., Bauman, W. A. and Cardozo, C. P. (2010). Evolving concepts in neurogenic osteoporosis. *Curr. Osteoporos. Rep.* 8, 212-218.

Takeda, S. (2008). Central control of bone remodelling. *J. Neuroendocrinol.* 20, 802-807.

Zengin, A., Zhang, L., Herzog, H., Baldock, P. A. and Sainsbury, A. (2010). Neuropeptide Y and sex hormone interactions in humoral and neuronal regulation of bone and fat. *Trends Endocrinol. Metab* 21, 411-418.

Elefteriou, F., Ahn, J. D., Takeda, S., Starbuck, M., Yang, X., Liu, X., Kondo, H., Richards, W. G., Bannon, T. W., Noda, M. et al. (2005). Leptin regulation of bone resorption by the sympathetic nervous system and CART. *Nature* 434, 514-520.

Karsenty, G. and Ducy, P. (2006). The hypothalamic control of bone mass, implication for the treatment of osteoporosis. *Ann. Endocrinol. (Paris)* 67, 123.

Takeda, S. and Karsenty, G. (2008). Molecular bases of the sympathetic regulation of bone mass. *Bone* 42, 837-840.

Guidobono, F., Pagani, F., Sibilia, V., Netti, C., Lattuada, N., Rapetti, D., Mrak, E., Villa, I., Cavani, F., Bertoni, L. et al. (2006). Different skeletal regional response to continuous brain infusion of leptin in the rat. *Peptides* 27, 1426-1433.

Yadav, V. K. and Karsenty, G. (2009). Leptin-dependent co-regulation of bone and energy metabolism. *Aging (Albany. NY)* 1, 954-956.

Yadav, V. K., Oury, F., Suda, N., Liu, Z. W., Gao, X. B., Confavreux, C., Klemenhagen, K. C., Tanaka, K. F., Gingrich, J. A., Guo, X. E. et al. (2009). A serotonin-dependent mechanism explains the leptin regulation of bone mass, appetite, and energy expenditure. *Cell* 138, 976-989.

Sato, S., Hanada, R., Kimura, A., Abe, T., Matsumoto, T., Iwasaki, M., Inose, H., Ida, T., Mieda, M., Takeuchi, Y. et al. (2007). Central control of bone remodeling by neuromedin U. *Nat. Med.* 13, 1234-1240.

Saini-Chohan, H. K. and Hatch, G. M. (2009). Biological actions and metabolism of currently used pharmacological agents for the treatment of congestive heart failure. *Curr. Drug Metab* 10, 206-219.

Chiu, C. T., Chiang, W. F., Chuang, C. Y. and Chang, S. W. (2010). Resolution of oral bisphosphonate and steroid-related osteonecrosis of the jaw--a serial case analysis. *J. Oral Maxillofac. Surg.* 68, 1055-1063.

Treister, N. S., Friedland, B. and Woo, S. B. (2010). Use of cone-beam computerized tomography for evaluation of bisphosphonate-associated osteonecrosis of the jaws. *Oral Surg. Oral Med. Oral Pathol. Oral Radiol. Endod.* 109, 753-764.

Baldock, P. A., Allison, S. J., Lundberg, P., Lee, N. J., Slack, K., Lin, E. J., Enriquez, R. F., McDonald, M. M., Zhang, L., During, M. J. et al. (2007). Novel role of Y1 receptors in the coordinated regulation of bone and energy homeostasis. *J. Biol. Chem.* 282, 19092-19102.

Feletou, M. and Levens, N. R. (2005). Neuropeptide Y2 receptors as drug targets for the central regulation of body weight. *Curr. Opin. Investig. Drugs* 6, 1002-1011.

Munoz, M. T. and Argente, J. (2002). Anorexia nervosa in female adolescents: endocrine and bone mineral density disturbances. *Eur. J. Endocrinol.* 147, 275-286.

Davenport, R. J. (2005). The skeleton goes to pot. *Sci. Aging Knowledge. Environ.* 2005, nf39.

Hinton, A., Bond, S. and Forgac, M. (2009). V-ATPase functions in normal and disease processes. *Pflugers Arch.* 457, 589-598.

Schaller, S., Henriksen, K., Sorensen, M. G. and Karsdal, M. A. (2005). The role of chloride channels in osteoclasts: ClC-7 as a target for osteoporosis treatment. *Drug News Perspect.* 18, 489-495.

Blair, H. C., Teitelbaum, S. L., Ghiselli, R. and Gluck, S. (1989). Osteoclastic bone resorption by a polarized vacuolar proton pump. *Science* 245, 855-857.

Holliday, L. S., Bubb, M. R., Jiang, J., Hurst, I. R. and Zuo, J. (2005). Interactions between vacuolar H+-ATPases and microfilaments in osteoclasts. *Journal of Bioenergetics and Biomembranes* 37, 419-423.

Toyomura, T., Murata, Y., Yamamoto, A., Oka, T., Sun-Wada, G. H., Wada, Y. and Futai, M. (2003). From Lysosomes to the Plasma Membrane: LOCALIZATION OF VACUOLAR TYPE H+-ATPase WITH THE a3 ISOFORM DURING OSTEOCLAST DIFFERENTIATION. *J. Biol. Chem.* 278, 22023-22030.

Li, Y. P., Chen, W., Liang, Y., Li, E. and Stashenko, P. (1999). Atp6i-deficient mice exhibit severe osteopetrosis due to loss of osteoclast-mediated extracellular acidification. *Nat. Genet.* 23, 447-451.

Sun-Wada, G. H., Toyomura, T., Murata, Y., Yamamoto, A., Futai, M. and Wada, Y. (2006). The a3 isoform of V-ATPase regulates insulin secretion from pancreatic beta-cells. *J. Cell Sci.* 119, 4531-4540.

Smith, A. N., Finberg, K. E., Wagner, C. A., Lifton, R. P., Devonald, M. A., Su, Y. and Karet, F. E. (2001). Molecular cloning and characterization of Atp6n1b: a novel fourth murine vacuolar H+-ATPase a-subunit gene. *J. Biol. Chem.* 276, 42382-42388.

Serrano, E. M., Ricofort, R. D., Zuo, J., Ochotny, N., Manolson, M. F. and Holliday, L. S. (2009). Regulation of vacuolar H(+)-ATPase in microglia by RANKL. *Biochem. Biophys. Res. Commun.* 389, 193-197.

Stover, E. H., Borthwick, K. J., Bavalia, C., Eady, N., Fritz, D. M., Rungroj, N., Giersch, A. B., Morton, C. C., Axon, P. R., Akil, I. et al. (2002). Novel ATP6V1B1 and ATP6V0A4 mutations in autosomal recessive distal renal tubular acidosis with new evidence for hearing loss. *J. Med. Genet.* 39, 796-803.

Moriyama, Y., Maeda, M. and Futai, M. (1992). The role of V-ATPase in neuronal and endocrine systems. *J. Exp. Biol.* 172, 171-178.

Neubert JK, Mannes AJ, Karai LJ, Jenkins AC, Zawatski L, Abu-Asab M, Iadarola MJ. (2008). Perineural resiniferatoxin selectively inhibits inflammatory hyperalgesia. Mol Pain. 2008 Jan 16;4:3.

Di, G. J., Boudkkazi, S., Mochida, S., Bialowas, A., Samari, N., Leveque, C., Youssouf, F., Brechet, A., Iborra, C., Maulet, Y. et al. (2010). V-ATPase membrane sector associates with synaptobrevin to modulate neurotransmitter release. *Neuron* 67, 268-279.

Hiesinger, P. R., Fayyazuddin, A., Mehta, S. Q., Rosenmund, T., Schulze, K. L., Zhai, R. G., Verstreken, P., Cao, Y., Zhou, Y., Kunz, J. et al. (2005). The v-ATPase V-0 subunit a1 is required for a late step in synaptic vesicle exocytosis in Drosophila. *Cell* 121, 607-620.

Cruciat, C. M., Ohkawara, B., Acebron, S. P., Karaulanov, E., Reinhard, C., Ingelfinger, D., Boutros, M. and Niehrs, C. (2010). Requirement of prorenin receptor and vacuolar H+-ATPase-mediated acidification for Wnt signaling. *Science* 327, 459-463.

Takahashi, K., Hiraishi, K., Hirose, T., Kato, I., Yamamoto, H., Shoji, I., Shibasaki, A., Kaneko, K., Satoh, F. and Totsune, K. (2010). Expression of (pro)renin receptor in the human brain and pituitary, and co-localisation with arginine vasopressin and oxytocin in the hypothalamus. *J. Neuroendocrinol.* 22, 453-459.

Nguyen, G. (2011). Renin and Prorenin Receptor in Hypertension: What's New? *Curr. Hypertens. Rep.* 13, 79-85.

Kasper, D., Planells-Cases, R., Fuhrmann, J. C., Scheel, O., Zeitz, O., Ruether, K., Schmitt, A., Poet, M., Steinfeld, R., Schweizer, M. et al. (2005). Loss of the chloride channel ClC-7 leads to lysosomal storage disease and neurodegeneration. *EMBO J.* 24, 1079-1091.

Kornak, U., Kasper, D., Bosl, M. R., Kaiser, E., Schweizer, M., Schulz, A., Friedrich, W., Delling, G. and Jentsch, T. J. (2001). Loss of the ClC-7 chloride channel leads to osteopetrosis in mice and man. *Cell* 104, 205-215.

Idris, A. I., Landao-Bassonga, E. and Ralston, S. H. (2010). The TRPV1 ion channel antagonist capsazepine inhibits osteoclast and osteoblast differentiation in vitro and ovariectomy induced bone loss in vivo. *Bone* 46, 1089-1099.

24

Clinical Application of Three-Dimensional Reverse Engineering Technology in Orthodontic Diagnosis

Bong-Kuen Cha
Gangneung-Wonju National University
Korea

1. Introduction

A three-dimensional (3D) surface scanning system was recently introduced in dental fields and has been used most extensively for example, for assessing morphological changes in maxillofacial surgery or in orthopedic treatment with a functional appliance. Another use for the 3D data acquisition in orthodontics is bending art system (BAS) or Invisalign® system introduced as a new treatment modality. However, research on the various clinical applications of 3D digital model is still in its early stage, as it has been used as a simple model analysis, a digitized data storage (Alcan *et al.*, 2009; Ayoub *et al.*, 2003; Birnbaum & Aaronson, 2008; Cha *et al.*, 2007; Choi et al., 2010; Costalos *et al.*, 2005; Dalstra & Melsen, 2009; Gracco *et al.*, 2007; Keating *et al.*, 2008; Krejci *et al.*, 1994; Leifert *et al.*, 2009; Macchi et al., 2006; Santoro *et al.*, 2003; Stevens *et al.*, 2006; Van der Linden, 1987).

This chapter is intended to investigate the possibility of the clinical application of 3D reverse engineering technology used in the analysis of orthodontic models and facial morphology.

The theme of this chapter is divided into seven parts:

1. The measuring accuracy and process of the 3D model scanning technique was evaluated in terms of linear, surface and volumetric parameters. The diverse clinical applications of model analysis, including measuring basal arch width, or sectional areas concerned will be presented.
2. Giving the evidences that the superimposition of the 3D digital maxillary model is clinically as reliable as cephalometric superimposition for assessing orthodontic tooth movements.
3. Presenting the clinical cases, using the superimposition technique for the 3D measuring of orthodontic tooth movement in maxilla.
4. Describing the clinical procedure for digital diagnostic setup.
5. Introducing a novel method concerning the volumetric assessment of tooth wear using 3D reverse engineering technology.
6. Presenting a quantitative 3D soft tissue facial analysis using a color coding system.
7. Presenting feasible methods of the integrating 3D digital model into a 3D facial image to visualize the anatomic position of the dentition.

1.1 Reliability of measurement and clinical application of 3D digital model

The accuracy and reproducibility of a 3D surface scanning device to record the surface detail of study models is well documented and evaluated with respect to linear, surface, and volumetric parameters in the literature (Alcan *et al.*, 2009; Cha *et al.*, 2007; Costalos *et al.*, 2005; Dalstra & Melsen, 2009; Eraso et al., 2007; Gracco et al., 2007; Horton et al., 2009; Keating *et al.*, 2008; Leifert *et al.*, 2009; Miller et al., 2003). We have taken a comparison study using 30 dental study models (Cha et al., 2007). Orthodontic linear measurements were recorded between landmarks, directly on the study models and indirectly on the 3D digital models by using the INUS dental scanning solution® (composed of Breuckmann's opto TOP scanner®, INUS Rapidform 2002®, Autoscan system®). The resolution of the Topometric & Photogrametric 3D scanner® after calibration is 8 μm and the reliability is 15 μm. This exceeds the accuracy required for orthodontic measurements such as the mesiodistal tooth width, arch length, and arch width. There were no significant differences between the measurements at the 1% level. The similar study (Keating et al., 2008) using another laser scanning device (Minolta VIVID® 900, non-contact 3D surface laser scanner, Konica Minolta Inc., Tokyo, Japan) also shows that the difference between measurements on the study and 3D digital models was 0.14 mm, and was not statistically significant. In conclusion, measurements carried out on 3D digital models are a valid and reliable alternative to those currently used in study models in orthodontic practice with the advantage of significantly reducing measurement time.

1.2 Some examples of research and clinical applications using 3D digital model

Tooth size, crowding or spacing, overjet, overbite, and Bolton analysis are typically measured by hand on study models. 3D digital model is valuable alternative to conventional study models and can be used to determine routine diagnostic value, such as the Bolton analysis, arch length discrepancy, sagittal or transverse symmetry (Cha et al., 2007; Santoro et al., 2003) (Fig. 1). Automatic identification system (the automatic recognition of tooth morphology) will be a suite of technologies, that enable and facilitate the accurate capture and rapid transmission of machine readable data, e.g. cusp tip or pit and fissure of certain teeth, to automated information systems, thereby enhancing the readiness of capabilities in support of their respective mission.

Furthermore it also held information, which could previously be gathered only by complicated laboratory procedure, as sawing or wax up etc. There are numerous clinical examples to illustrate how such information could be applied in the diagnostic or treatment evaluation in orthodontics (Fig. 2). In counterpoint to the two-dimensional analysis, it is possible with 3D digital model to determine further parameters, such as palatal volume before and after maxillary expansion (Fig. 3) or volume or surface square measure of the deep structure of the palate (Fig. 4).

3D digital model offers many advantages, including elimination of model breakage and storage problems, instant retrieval of models, ease of communication with patients and colleagues. A single set of 3D digital models typically requires 8 MByte of disc space. It means that the data of 5,000 patients can be stored on a 40 GByte drive. It enables the orthodontist to e-mail images if desired and is a convenient presentation tool (Cha *et al.*, 2007).

Disadvantages include lack of tactile input for the orthodontist and time needed to learn how to use the system (Santoro *et al.*, 2003). 3D digital models present several unique challenges compared with conventional study models. Because the 3D computer image is

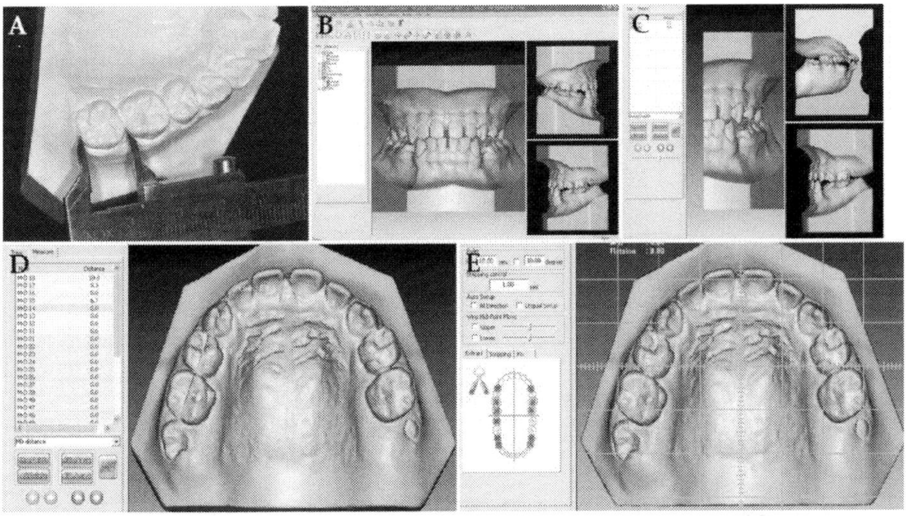

Fig. 1. **A**. Tooth size analysis: traditional manual method with sliding caliper. **B**. Gallery 3D digital model images in 3Txer software®(Orapix Co., Seoul, Korea). **C**. Selection of digital model for overbite and overjet measurements. Models can be rotated, which facilitates cross-sectioning at point of maximum overjet. **D**. Tooth size measurement tools (mesiodistal diameters) in 3Txer software®. E. Assessment of sagittal and transverse arch form symmetry in 3Txer software®.

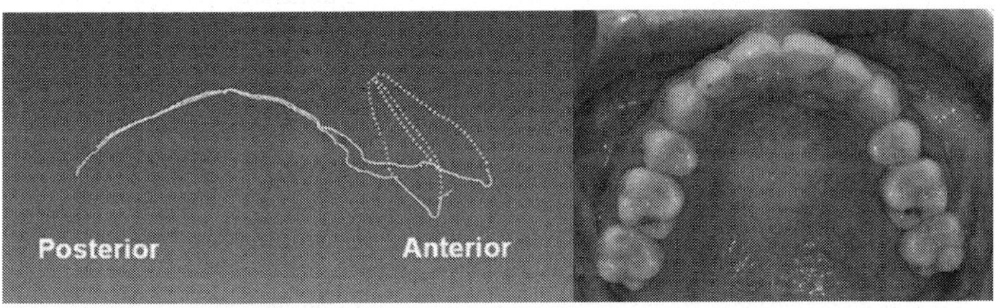

Fig. 2. Notice the change in palatal surface with gingival enlargement after retraction of anterior teeth. Enlarged soft tissue was denoted by the red arrow.

displayed on a 2D screen, the greatest challenge was observing crossbite. They will seem to have a positive overjet in the posterior segment when they really do not. Details for midlines, occlusal anatomy, and wear facets are not as clear on the 3D digital model (Stevens *et al.*, 2006).

Despite such limitations, 3D digital model provide a valuable source of information and continuous development of technology will suggest ways to overcome some of its shortcomings.

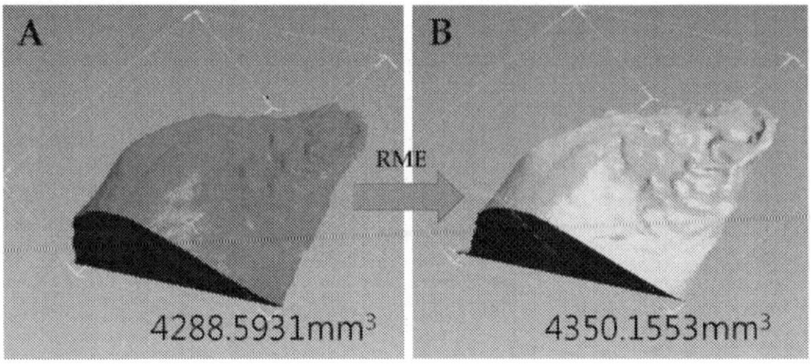

Fig. 3. Volumetric change of the palate before **A** and after **B** rapid maxillary expansion (volumetric change was about 61.6 mm^3).

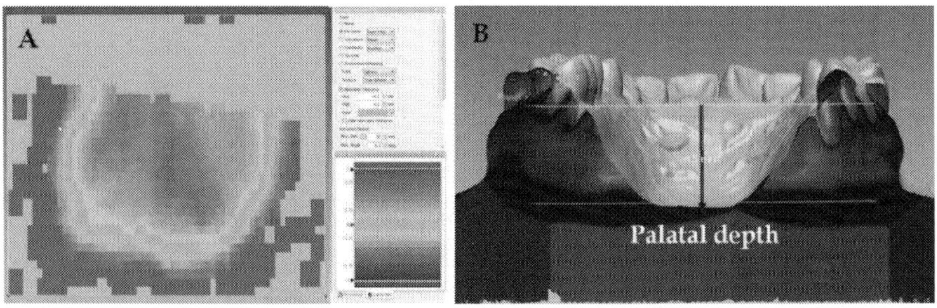

Fig. 4. **A**. Color contour analysis locating the deepest point that cannot be recognized accurately by manual method, light green means zero point, dark red area means deepest point of palate. **B.** Measuring accurate palatal depth from the arbitrary reference plane to the deepest point of mid-palatal suture located by using color contour analysis.

2. Evidences that the superimposition of the 3D digital maxillary model is clinically as reliable as cephalometric superimposition for assessing orthodontic tooth movement

Despite inherent errors, cephalometric superimpositions are currently the most widely used means for assessing sagittal and vertical tooth movement. However, there are some disadvantages and limitations of cephalometric radiographs and superimposition. Its drawbacks include difficulties in evaluating 3D tooth movement and identifying inherent landmarks. Further disadvantages are tracing errors, frequent radiation exposure, and high costs (Ghafari *et al.*, 1998).

We have performed a study, comparing 3D digital model superimposition with cephalometric superimposition (Cha *et al.*, 2007). The material was collected from initial and final maxillary study models and lateral cephalometric radiographs of 30 patients, who underwent orthodontic treatment with extraction of permanent teeth. The 3D superimposition was carried out using the surface-to-surface matching (best-fit method)

(Fig. 5). The antero-posterior movement of the maxillary first molar and central incisor was evaluated cephalometrically and on 3D digital models. The results revealed no statistical differences between the incisor and molar movements as assessed cephalometrically and by 3D model superimposition. These findings suggest that the 3D digital model superimposition technique used in this study is clinically as reliable as cephalometric superimposition for assessing orthodontic tooth movements.

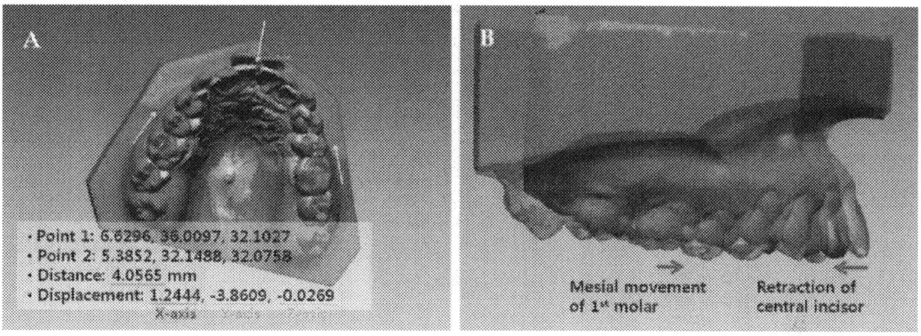

Fig. 5. Assessment of tooth movements on superimposed 3D digital models (red: before treatment, blue: after treatment). A. Occlusal view. B. Sagittal view.

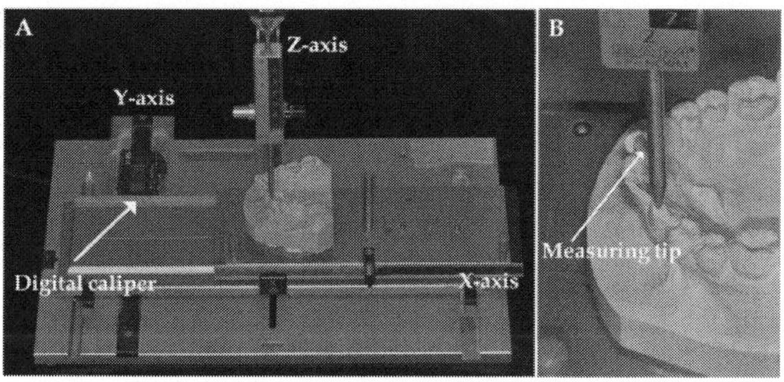

Fig. 6. Measurement of the study model with the Reference Measurement Instrument (RMI) **A**. Digital calipers for X-, Y-, and Z-axis. **B**. Measuring from the tip of the canine.

To evaluate the accuracy of the superimposition of 3D digital models using the palatal surface as a reference for measuring tooth movements, we have performed a comparison study of the correlation between the tooth movement of the setup model and that of the superimposition in its 3D digital model (Choi *et al.*, 2010). Teeth on the study model were randomly moved after sawing, subsequently scanned to produce another set of 3D digital models. 3D digital model were superimposed using the palatal area as reference via surface-to-surface matching and the changes in tooth movement were calculated. In the study models, the tooth movements were directly measured using the Reference Measurement Instrument (Fig. 6). The means of the anteroposterior (x-axis), transverse (y-axis), and vertical (z-axis) tooth movements of the study models and those of the digital models did not differ significantly, and very high correlations were found between the study models and the digital models.

Recently, Jang *et al.* (Jang *et al.*, 2009) superimposed serial models treated by premolar extraction by means of three miniscrews as registration landmarks (miniscrew-superimposition method) and compared with ruga-palate superimposition method. The displacement of the central incisors measured using the ruga-palate-superimposition method showed no significant difference with that measured using the miniscrew-superimposition method.

Moreover, with the superimposition method introduced here, it seems promising that, in the future, a simple mouse click will enable fast computer-assisted evaluation of 3D tooth movements (Choi *et al.*, 2010).

Despite promising possibilities of the applications, the validity of this method has not been examined in growing patients, who underwent orthopedic treatment, such as rapid maxillary expansion (RME) treatment or maxillary surgery. In addition, we must not overlook the fact, that we encounter difficulties when we try to superimpose the mandibular arch because of the lack of the stable registration area (Fig. 7). Further research on this field is needed to clarify the evidences for the stable area for the superimposition.

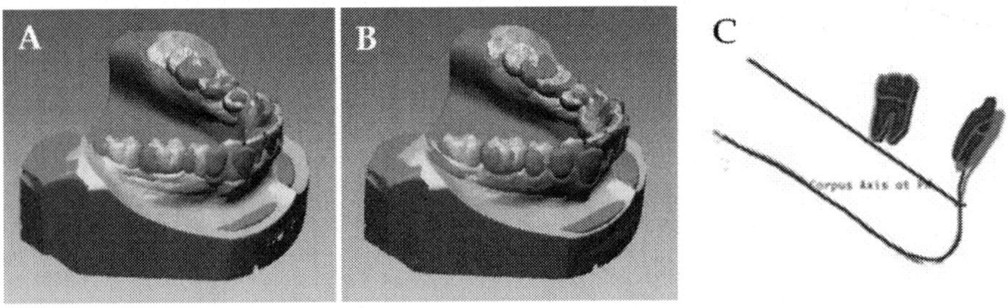

Fig. 7. Different results of mandibular superimposition due to the lack of stable registration area. Superimposition (**A)** shows no lingual movement of lower incisor. Note the tremendous lingual movement of lower incisor on superimposition (**B**) in same patient (red: before treatment, blue: after treatment). C. Superimposition on mandible in 2D cephalometrics shows lingual movement of lower incisor.

3. Presentation of clinical cases, using the superimposition technique for the 3D measurement of orthodontic tooth movement in maxilla

A 32-year-old Korean female presented with chief complaint of facial convexity. Cephalometric analysis showed a skeletal Class II relationship, significant obtuse mandibular plane angle, and retrognathic chin. After extraction of four premolars, pre-adjusted fixed appliances were bonded for initial leveling and alignment of both arches. An L-shaped mini-plate was adjusted to fit the contour of each cortical bone surface and was fixed with bone screws with the long arm exposed to the oral cavity, between upper first and second molars, for the intrusion of upper molars and retraction of upper dentition without any anchorage loss. After 30 months of orthodontic treatment, the patient showed a Class I occlusion with normal overbite, overjet and improved profile (Fig. 8).

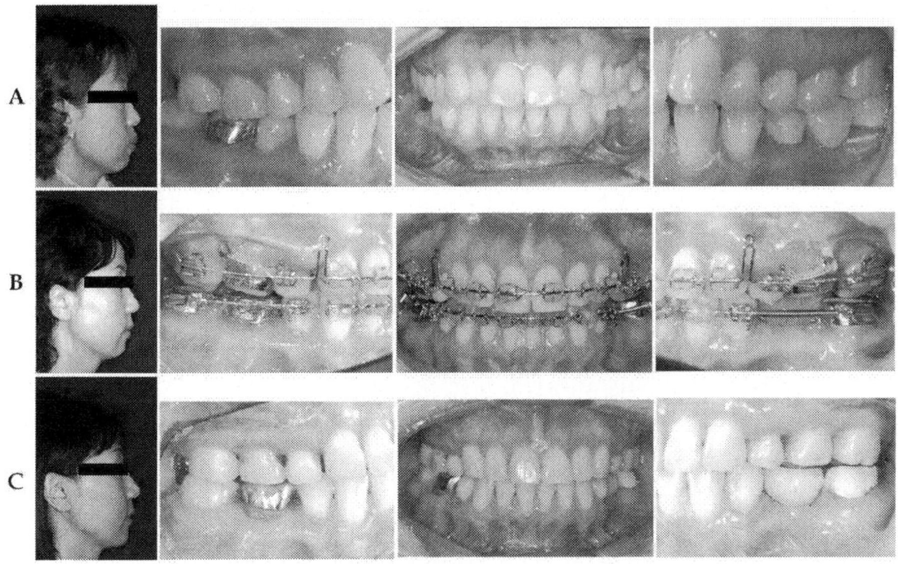

Fig. 8. A 32-year-old female with skeletal Class II relatiohship, hyperdivergent long-face pattern, and retrognathic chin. **A**. Pre-treatment. **B**. Contraction arch and miniplate for retraction of anterior teeth and intrusion of posterior teeth. **C**. Post-treatment.

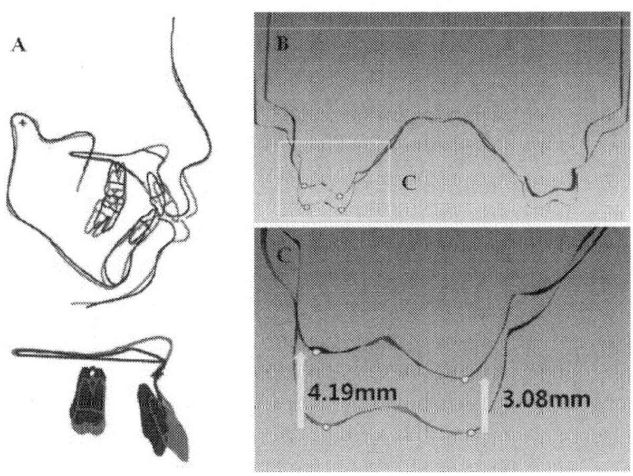

Fig. 9. **A**. Superimposition of pre-and post-treatment cephalometric tracings. Significant intrusion and distalization of upper molars were noted. (red: before treatment, blue: after treatment) **B**. Superimposition using 3D digital models. **C**. The amount of intrusion on the buccal and palatal cusp can be measured on the superimposed 3D digital models respectively. Note the different amount of intrusion between buccal and palatal cusp.

Superimposition of the pre- and post-treatment cephalometric radiography demonstrated significant intrusion of the upper posterior teeth. The entire upper dentition appeared to have been retracted. Fig. 9 shows, that in superimposed 3D digital model between before and after orthodontic treatment, the mesiobuccal cusp of upper right first molar was intruded 4.2 mm, on the other hand, palatal cusp as a functional cusp, was intruded only 3.1 mm. Such a result, it is impossible for us to get with the conventional cephalometric superimposition method.

A 10-year-old girl presented with a skeletal Class III malocclusion, a concave facial profile due to an anterior crossbite. Based on the cephalometric and clinical examinations, the patient was diagnosed as a functional Class III. The treatment plan for this patient included Class III activator (Fig. 10).

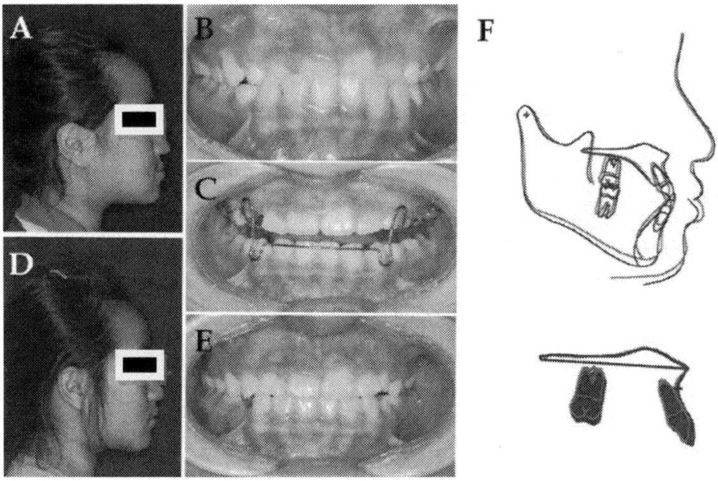

Fig. 10. A, B. Pre-treatment. Notice the anterior crossbite. C. Class III activator was used. D, E. Post-treatment. Notice normal overjet and overbite. F. Superimposition of pre-and post-treatment shows extrusion of upper molar and labioversion of upper incisors. (red: before treatment, blue: after treatment)

Post-treatment superimposed tracing revealed that anterior crossbite was corrected mainly by dentoalveolar movement and clockwise rotation of the mandible (Fig. 10). The maxillary incisors were flared and mandibular incisors were retruded and somehow extruded. However, correct measurement of the amount of tooth movement was not possible, because of inherent errors of the tracing and bisecting tracing of the cephalometrics.

The extrusion of upper molars exerts a downward vector of force on the mandible, causing the lower jaw to rotate downwards and backwards in a clockwise direction. Palatal cusp specially plays a more important role in this phenomenon rather than buccal cusp, which we are unable to measure separately in conventional superimposition of the 2D cephalometrics. Fig. 11 shows, that in superimposed 3D digital model between before and after orthodontic treatment, the mesiobuccal cusp of right upper first molar extruded 2.21 mm, on the other hand, mesiopalatal cusp as a functional cusp, extruded 1.30 mm. This different result might come from the change of the amount in the torque of the upper molars

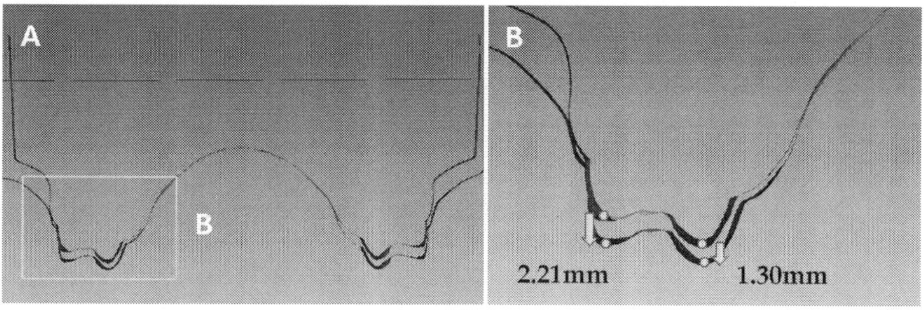

Fig. 11. **A, B** Different amount of the extrusion between mesiobuccal cusp and mesiopalatal cusp, which plays an important role as a functional cusp.

4. The clinical procedure for digital diagnostic setup and fabrication of indirect bonding tray

The diagnostic setup is a valuable aid in testing the effect of complex therapy, such as asymmetric extractions, space redistribution in the congenital missing cases. By replacing the teeth on the model in their desired position after suitable trimming, one can obtain an idea of the proportions between dental arch, apical area, occlusion and the degree to which the anterior teeth should be displaced sagittally (Fig. 12)(Van der Linden, 1987). The infusion of computer-aided design/computer-assisted machining (CAD/CAM Technology) enables now orthodontist or technicians to make virtual diagnostic setup, that provide not only diagnostic aids, but also simplify the laboratory procedure for precise indirect bonding (Fig. 13).

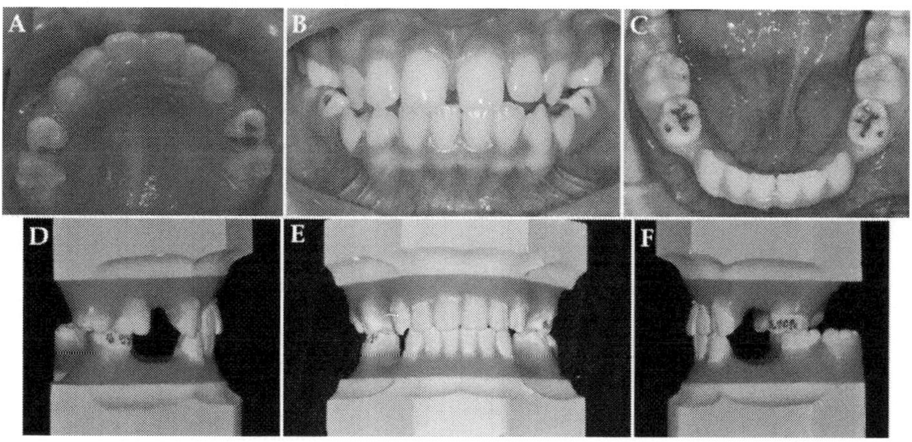

Fig. 12. **A~C**. This patient is Angle Class III with congenital missing teeth on #14, 15, 24, 25, 34, 35, 44, and 45. Treatment planning is prosthodontic treatment for #15, 25, 34, 35, 44, and 45 with full protraction of maxillary buccal teeth, as the lower anterior group remains unchanged. **D~F**. Traditional diagnostic set-up model.

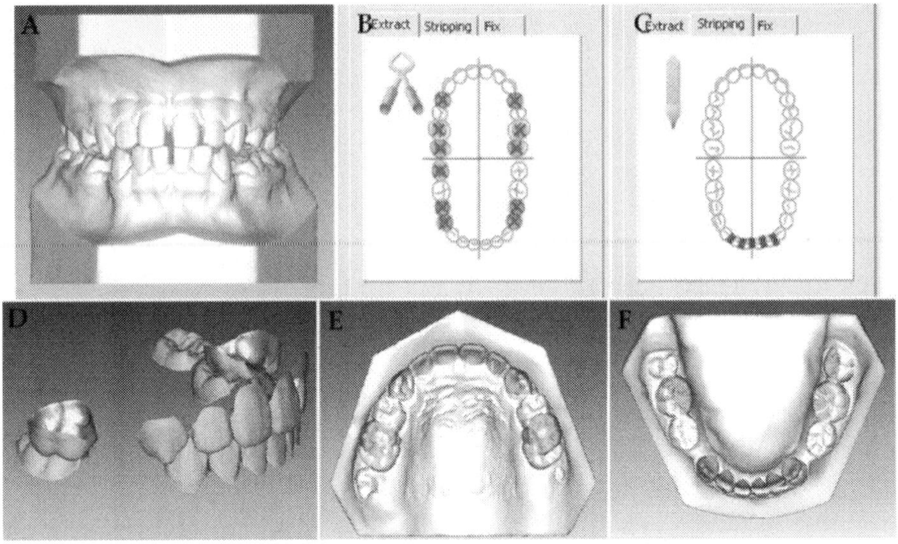

Fig. 13. 3D digital model in 3Txer software® (Orapix Co., Seoul, Korea). **A~C**. The program includes extractions or stripping functions, which can be planned in diagnostic set-up. In this case, we use "Extract" function. **D**. 3D virtual set-up in 3Txer software®. **E, F**. Superimpositions before and after set-up can visualize and quantify tooth movement in comparison to traditional set-up.

It is important in making the diagnostic setup to select correct arch form. For this purpose, we use an individualized template, which is able to give the precise arch form for each patient, provided by the 3Txer software® (Orapix Co., Seoul, Korea). These references are selected by the practitioner from a 3D virtual setup with virtual bracket positioning (Fig. 13).

Bracket positioning is an important factor for efficient orthodontic treatment. Traditionally, direct bonding of the bracket is used by most of the orthodontists. Advantages of direct bonding over the indirect procedure were summarized as follows (Zachrisson & Brobakken, 1978);

1. The bracket bases were fitted closer to the tooth surface.
2. It was easier to remove excess adhesive flash around the bracket bases.
3. The bonding adhesive constantly filled out the entire contact surface of the bracket.

As straight arch wire technique and lingual orthodontics were developed, because of the irregularity of lingual or labial tooth surface and the difficulty of access to some teeth, indirect bonding became very rapidly the technique of choice (Fillion, 2007).

Indirect bonding technique may be classified into two main categories; procedure with, or without setup of individual teeth. The difference between the two procedures is that while the purpose of the indirect bonding without setup is to reduce the possible positioning error often confronted in direct bonding, with setup is to realize the ideal straight arch wire technique that does not require arch wire bending. Fig. 14 shows typical procedure of indirect bonding without setup, using dual tray method.

A
C
B
D

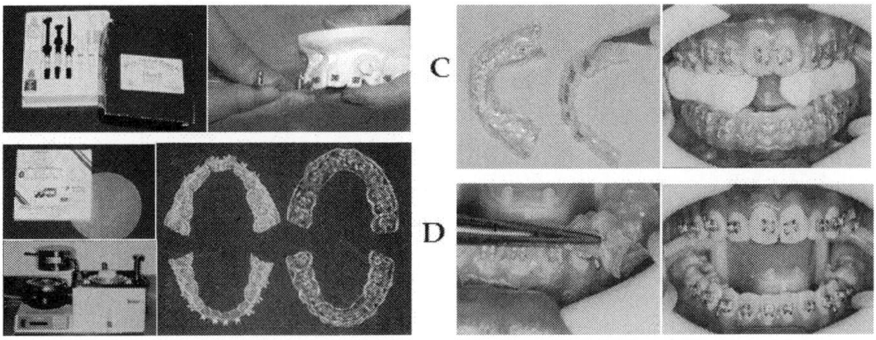

Fig. 14. Indirect bonding procedure. **A.** Apply double coat of liquid separator to dry stone models and positioning brackets using Phase II composite® on brackets' base. **B.** Fabricate two indirect transfer trays using 0.5 mm Copyplast material and 1.25 mm Biocryl material from Bioplast® company. **C.** Brackets' base is rinsed with acetone and the teeth are etched, rinsed, and dried. Excel composite® is added to brackets' base and the dual trays are applied. **D.** Removing transfer trays.

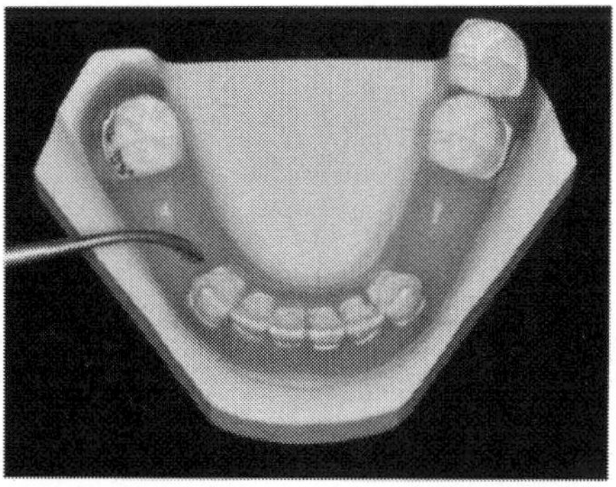

Fig. 15. The individual teeth are sawn out. Setting the separate block on the wax roll permits alternations in position.

In 1982, Myrberg and Warner (Myrberg & Warner, 1982) presented a technique, in which individual bracket placement indicators were made for each tooth based on the concept of a dental setup that suits the individual functional, occlusal, and esthetic requirements of each patient. Subsequent to this, numerous techniques have been developed based on indirect bonding from diagnostic setups (Hoffman, 1988). The traditional method of fabricating a diagnostic setup is to saw through the root areas, separate the teeth by hand, and affix them in their new positions with wax (Fig. 15). The technique is difficult to master and furthermore the laboratory procedure is tedious and time consuming for both the technician and orthodontist.

The rapid development of CAD/CAM technology enables not only bonding the brackets in preciously corrected position, but ensures that their individualized placements will produce the ideal occlusion incorporated in the virtual setup (Fillion, 2007).

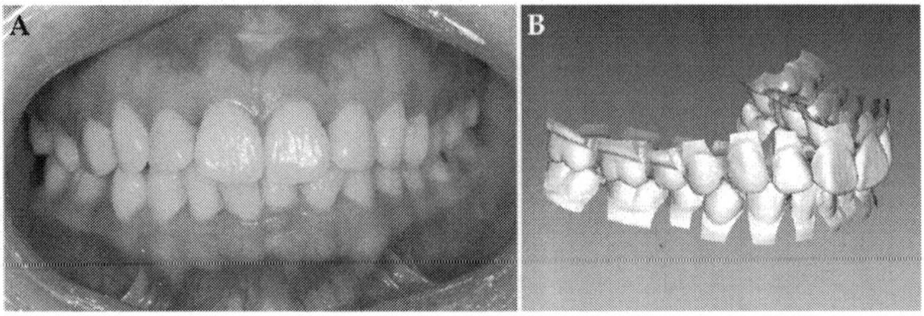

Fig. 16. **A**. This patient's chief complaint was anterior crowding. **B**. Visualization of the scanned model and establishing the geometrically independent tooth unit.

In the followings, an indirect bonding technique will be introduced and summarized based on a virtual setup from CAD/CAM transfer trays. For a more detailed discussion of this procedure, the reader can refer some publications (Fillion, 2007; 2010).

1. Dental arch should be segmented into individual dental units perceived as geometric units (Fig. 16).
2. Making the treatment plan, including extraction or non-extraction, stripping, final arch form. Such prescriptions are incorporated in 3Txer software®.
3. After setup, according to the selected prescription, upper and lower arch are manually adjusted to fit the final treatment result. (Fig. 17 C, D).
4. The virtual brackets are placed on the same horizontal plane and centered on each tooth. In this procedure, individual arch form (virtual arch) can be determined.(Fig. 17 E)
5. Virtual transfer trays are constructed. A rapid-prototype machine constructs in real time the transfer tray (Fig. 18 A).
6. Positioning the tray over the teeth and seating the tray (Fig. 18 B).

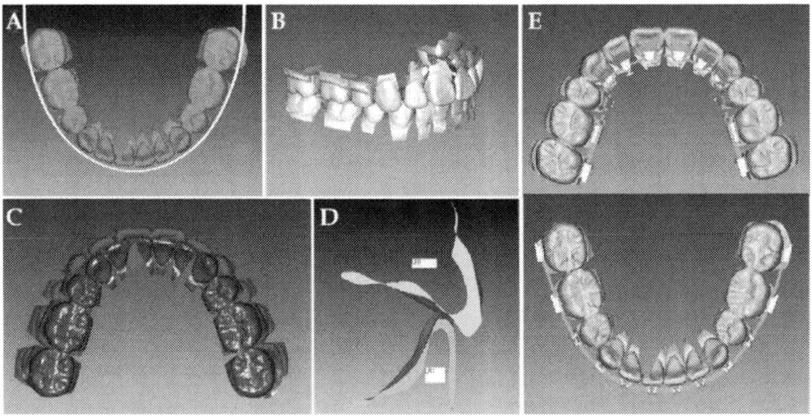

Fig. 17. **A**. Selection of the curve, on which the teeth will be positioned in construction of the set-up. **B**. Visualization of the set-up. **C, D**. Occlusion test: the red-colored zones represent the areas of contact. **E**. Precise positioning of the virtual brackets on the virtual set-up and placement of the ideal virtual arch wire.

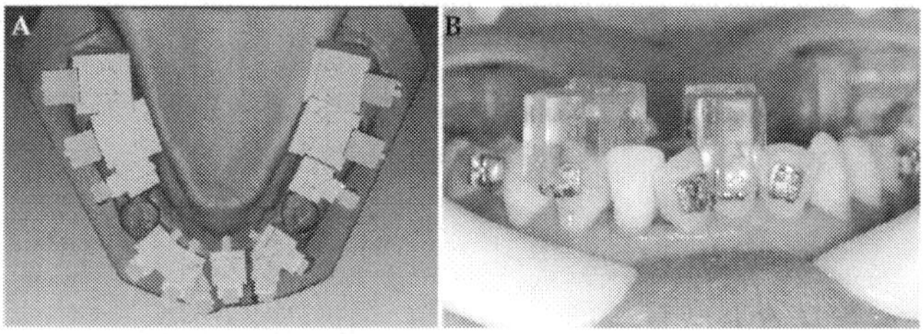

Fig. 18. **A**. Construction of the virtual transfer trays. **B**. Bonding of the brackets.

Material and equipment manufacturers continually introduce new and innovative products that further advance virtual technology. A fabrication procedure of virtual surgical splint procedure in virtual articulator has been also introduced, which spare the time consuming procedure of model surgery and surgical wafer fabrications (Song & Baek, 2009). Recently, a new imaging method, using computed tomography technology and laser scanning provides complete 3D views of the maxilla and the mandible, and the model setup with individual roots (Harrell *et al.*, 2002; Macchi *et al.*, 2006). The development of a 3D digital setup that displays individual crowns, roots and craniofacial structures will greatly help the clinician in diagnosis and treatment planning to determine various treatment options, monitor the changes after treatment over time, predict and display final treatment results, and measure treatment outcomes accurately (Macchi *et al.*, 2006).

Recently, Rangel and colleagues (Rangel *et a*l., 2008) reported the registration of digital models to 3D facial images. These multimodal images could improve our diagnosis and treatment planning processes and eventually will become the clinical standard, enhancing treatments provided by different specialties, including orthodontics, periodontics, prosthodontics, and restorative dentistry.

5. Introducing a novel method of the volumetric assessment of tooth wear using 3D reverse engineering technology

Tooth wear is defined as the non carious loss of tooth substance as a result of attrition, abrasion and erosion. Tooth attrition is regular and slow progressive loss of dental tissues as a consequence of tooth to tooth contact during mastication (Milicic *et al.*, 1987; Shafer *et al.*, 1983.) especially by parafunctions and unbalanced morphological occlusion.

Loss of occlusal surface of the tooth affects the vertical dimension and might induce deep bite (Ramjford & Ash, 1983). If there is attritional wear on the posterior teeth, they induce interference with completely seated TMJs and/or the anterior guidance (Dawson, 2007). High correlations among tooth wear, maximal bite force and the size of the gonial angle were reported (Kiliaridis *et al.*, 1995). Some previous studies reported the association between greater tooth wear and malocclusion (Carlsson *et al.*, 2003), although there were controversial opinions.

There are a few studies which investigated the relationship between tooth wear and orthodontic treatment (Kuijpers *et al.*, 2009). Until now there is no study focused on the tooth wear during orthodontic treatment, moreover no information about the quantity of tooth wear caused by orthodontic treatment. The main reason is probably due to the technical limit in quantifying the volumetric change of the tooth material. For that reason the most previous studies on tooth wear evaluated the tooth wear index only on study models. Recently, Cha *et*

al. (Cha et al., 2007) suggested the clinical method of the quantifying volumetric change due to tooth wear by using 3D digital model superimposition.
The followings will show you how to use the superimposition method of 3D digital models to quantify the amount of central incisor wear occurred during the orthodontic treatment (Fig. 19).
The maxillary and mandibular dental casts were taken before and after orthodontic treatment and scanned by a laser surface scanning system (KOD300®, Orapix co. LTD, Seoul, Korea) with the reliability of 50 ㎛. 3D virtual models of central incisors were reconstructed and imported to a 3D reverse modeling software (Rapidform XOR3®, INUS Technology, Seoul, Korea) (Fig 19. A, B). The 3D images of central incisor before and after orthodontic treatment were superimposed with best-fitting method. As reference area, the middle third of labial and lingual surface of central incisor were used, because these areas are considered to be rarely affected by attritional wear and the pathologic condition of gingival(Fig. 19 C)
To calculate the volume of central incisor, the 3 boundary planes were constructed on the 3D images of central incisor before treatment (Fig. 19 D, E). We compared the volume of the central incisors before and after treatment in relation with the boundary planes and we arrived at the conclusion that the second one was smaller (Fig. 19 F, G).
This technology can be applied into a quite diverse area in dentistry, e.g. quantity evaluation of teeth after prosthetic or conservative treatments.

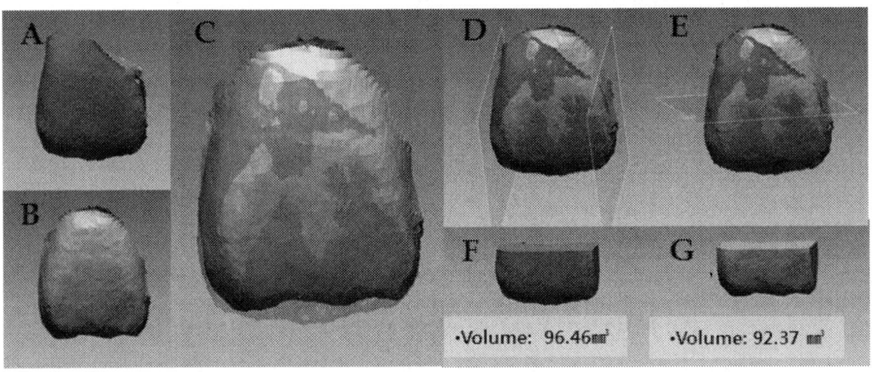

Fig. 19. Procedure for quantifying the amount of tooth wear. A. 3D digital model of maxillary incisor before orthodontic treatment (red). B. 3D digital model of the same tooth after orthodontic treatment (blue). C. Superimposition of A and B with best-fitting method using the middle third of labial and lingual surface as reference area. D, E. Mesial plane, distal plane, and gingival plane as boundary planes. F, G. 3D digital model before and after orthodontic treatment with the same boundary planes for volumetric calculation of tooth wear. The volume of tooth materials was reduced to about 4.09 mm³.

6. Presenting a quantitative 3D soft tissue facial analysis using a color coding system

Orthodontists have recognized that objective evaluation of facial morphology is important for the effective treatment planning and evaluation in reference to the growth change.

Traditionally, orthodontists have used radiographs to assess the soft tissue facial change, e.g. they measure 2D landmarks on the lateral cephalogram that arguably do not exist in a 3D body (Kau & Richmond, 2008). The problems in traditional cephalometrics also come from landmark identification of hard and soft tissues on x-rays because of the superimposition of several structures, which might be the major source of cephalometric errors. In the patient Fig. 20, it is showed that the facial contour angle was improved after orthognathic surgery but there is a limitation and difficulty to evaluate it at full extent three dimensionally.

Medical CT or Cone-beam CT (CBCT) can be an alternative, but possible overuse might lead to radiation exposure problems, together with financial burden. For the reason mentioned above, it should be stated that traditional longitudinal growth studies with radiation sources might present ethical and moral dilemmas. How to solve such an ethical dilemma? We think that the use of alternative surface imaging devices can be one step forward in handling such ethical dilemmas.

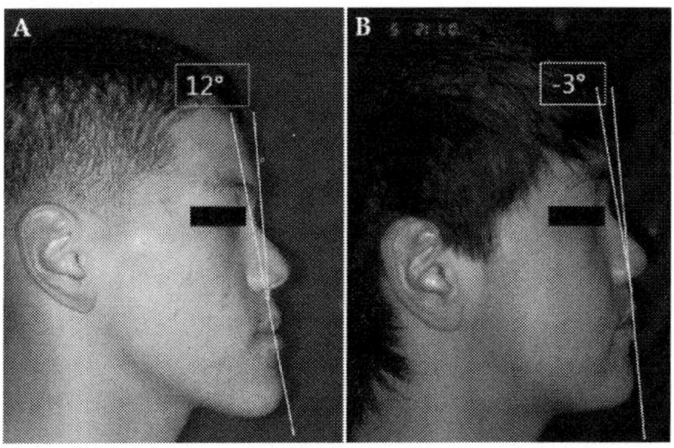

Fig. 20. **A**. Pre-treatment lateral view. **B**. Post-treatment lateral view. Note that although facial contour angle improved after surgery, there is a limitation to evaluate it at full extent.

With the advances in the technology, various devices, including laser scanners (Baik *et al.*, 2007), stereophotogrammetry (Ayoub *et al.*, 2003), and structured light systems (Weinberg *et al.*, 2004) have been used in acquiring the 3D images of the facial morphology. Among them, 3D laser scanner system or optical surface scanner is widely used because of its simple and rapid capture of the whole facial 3D image. It is quite likely that this system has a diverse possibility of clinical applications and researches (Baik *et al.*, 2007; Ismail & Moss, 2002; McCance *et al.*, 1997; McDonagh *et al.*, 2001; Moss, 2006; Moss *et al.*, 1995)

The laser scanning 3D technology allows to generate a high precision and can be used to calculate the morphological ground surface variations at different acquisition time intervals. The main advantages are that change due to growth or treatment of an individual can be monitored in three dimensions using this method, which is non-invasive and which can be repeated every few weeks (Moss, 2006; Moss *et al.*, 1995).

The registration program (Rapidform XOR3®, INUS technology, Seoul, Korea) enables superimposition of similar areas on two overlaid scans to demonstrate the surface differences in color coding system (Moss, 2006)(Fig. 22 E)

The purpose of 3D face registration is to align different 3D face data into a common coordinate system. So, registration is a crucial and indispensable step, as the accuracy of this step will greatly influence the performance of the whole face recognition system. The important step in the registration process is to determine which area will be used as a stable reference. The displacement, change in shape, or in size will be described relative to these structures. In the traditional 2D cephalometrics, the anterior cranial base e.g. Sella-Nasion is used for the superimpositions because of its relative stability after neural growth in brain. But locating 3D landmarks on complex curving structures is significantly more difficult (Miller et al., 2007; Morris et al., 1998; Moss et al., 1994).

Moss et al. (Moss *et al.*, 1994) combined five aforementioned anatomical landmarks (right and left endocanthion, right and left exocanthion and soft tissue Nasion) together with five constructed points projected onto the forehead. Hajeer et al. (Hajeer *et al.*, 2002) used seven superimposition points in the eye and nose area. Miller *et al.* (Miller et al., 2007) hold a view that the forehead area is stable area for superimposing 3D images. The superimposition points above were proved to be easy to locate and the landmarks well definable (Hoefert et al., 2010) (Fig. 21, Table 1).

There are, however, a number of problems that remain to be explored.

The forehead area with superimposition points 5, 6 and 7 in Fig. 21 and Table 1 were in an area, in which, according to the Bolton standards, 0.5 - 1.0 mm increase in Nasion-Sella line and a forward displacement of the frontal bone can be expected with normal growth in children between ages 4 and 5 (Hoefert et al., 2010). It means that the distance from sella turcica to foramen caecum does not increase after eruption of the first permanent molar and forehead can be used as a superimposing area.

However, this assumption is not supported by the mention that there was a correlation between frontal sinus pneumatization and the progression of skeletal maturity (Ruf & Pancherz, 1996). Another recent case reports by author (Cha *et al.*, 2011) provides the evidence that infraorbitale can be moved forward by maxillary protraction by using the surgical miniplate anchorage. These observations suggest further questions that must be reserved for a more extensive study.

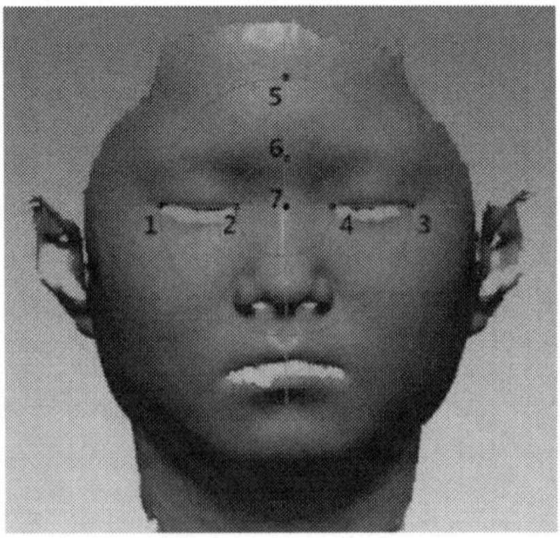

Fig. 21. Superimposition points (for explanation see Table 1).

Superimposition points	Description
Point 1	Right exocanthion
Point 2	Right endocanthion
Point 3	Left exocanthion
Point 4	Left endocanthion
Point 5	Intersection of forehead axis with the outer eye circle
Point 6	Intersection of forehead axis with the inner eye circle
Point 7	Middle of eye axis

Table 1. Superimposition points recommended by Hoefert *et al.* (Hoefert *et al.*, 2010).

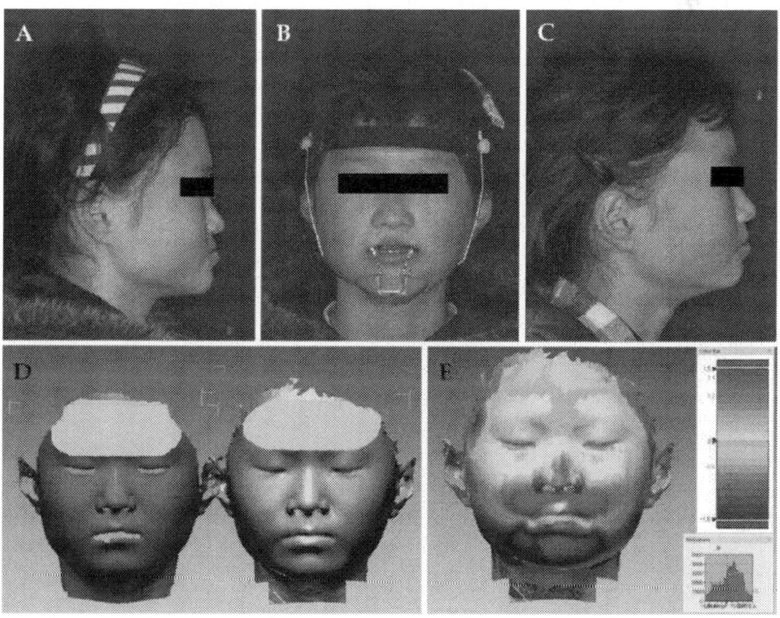

Fig. 22. 3D facial superimposition of the patient treated by maxillary protraction **A.** pre-treatment facial photo. **B.** Treatment by protraction headgear. **C.** Post-treatment facial photo. **D,E.** Superimposition of pre- and post-treatment 3D facial images using the forehead as reference area. According to the color-coding system, yellow/red color means forward movement, while blue color means backward movement.

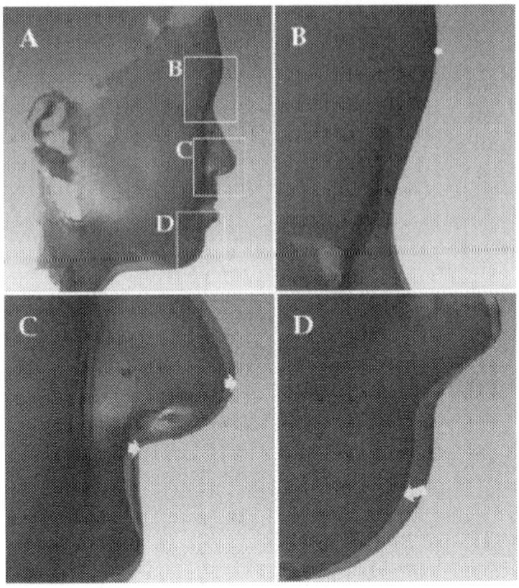

Fig. 23. **A**. Detailed sectional view of superimposition image in Fig. 22. **B**. Glabella was not changed. C. Nose tip and Subnasale was protruded by 0.6 mm and 1.2 mm, respectively. **D**. Pogonion was retruded in backward and downward direction by 2 mm.

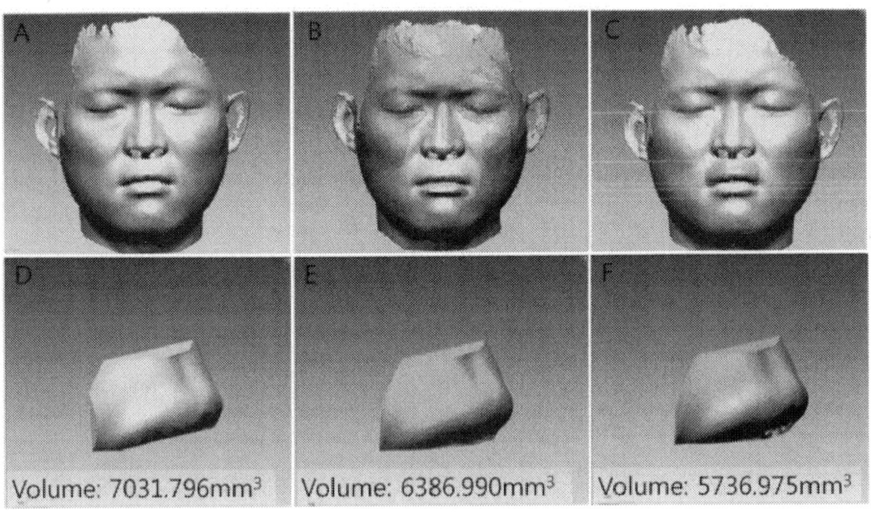

Fig. 24. Method for evaluating the volumetic change of the lip. **A~C.** 3D facial images were acquired and superimposition on forehead area was performed. To measure the volumetric change of the lip, boundary planes for the upper lip were constructed on the 3D facial images. **D~F.** The changes of lip volume before debonding (yellow), after debondig (green), and 6 months after debonding (blue).

Following is the example of the application of 3D facial registration for the evaluation of the change of facial morphology after orthopedic treatment. A patient who has a developing Class III malocclusion was monitored in order to assess the direction of growth and the rate of change after maxillary protraction therapy (Fig. 22 and 23).

There were no apparent changes to the central portion of the forehead and Glabella area (Fig. 23 B). There was general thickening of the lateral brow region, from 0.34 to 0.50 mm. The nose showed the positive change by 1.20 mm during the treatment (Fig. 23 C). There were visible but small positive changes in the cheek areas similar on both sides of the face. There was large and distinct forward and downward translation of the maxilla away from the forehead. There was elongation of the face leading to the downward projection of the soft-tissue chin (Fig. 23 D).

Another example (Fig. 24) represents the procedures for the evaluation of the quantitative change of lip volume between the final stage of the orthodontic treatment and after debonding procedure, to investigate the influence of bracket thickness for facial profile in 29 year-old male patients. The 3D facial images were imported into the Rapidform XOR3 software® (INUS technology, Seoul, Korea) and the superimposition method known as the best-fit was used on the reference area at the forehead, soft tissue glabella, including zygoma and nose.

To evaluate the volumetric change of the lip, 5 boundary planes were constructed on the 3D facial images. The volume in upper lip decreased 644.80 mm^3 immediately after debonding, and 650.01mm^3 more for the 6 month of retention period. The techniqueof the detailed volumetic measurement of soft tissue points to several promising applications for future research.

7. Presenting feasible methods of the integrating digital 3D model into a 3D facial image to visualize the anatomic position of the dentition

One area of high interest is the study of the integration of 3D digital model into a 3D facial image, which can be used as possible alternatives to 2D cephalometric superimposition. The 3D digital models of each dental arch are scanned independently and need to be related in space to represent the patient occlusion. Different methods have been developed for this purpose: visually assessing the study models' occlusion and matching their relative position in the virtual space; by scanning a wax bite, and registering the upper model to the upper side of the wax bite and the lower model to its lower side; by mounting the models in a bracket of known relative position, or by scanning the study models in occlusion and using that relative positional information to register the upper model to the lower one.

Rangel et al. (Rangel *et al.*, 2008) first introduced the procedure for the integration of 3D digital model in 3D facial image. Fig. 26 shows summarized procedures of digital model integration method.

For matching the 3D digital model to the 3D facial image, the anterior teeth were used as the registration surface.

1. To see the teeth on the 3D facial image, cheek retractors were used to pull the lips open, then a 3D facial image was made (Fig. 25 A and B).
2. A second 3D facial image was made from the patient at rest with the teeth in occlusion (Fig. 25 C).
3. 3D digital model is matched to the 3D facial image with the cheek retractors. To improve the accuracy of the registration, two step registration procedure were needed (Fig. 26 A~C).

4. Two 3D facial image at rest and with retractor were matched. Here as above, two step registration procedure were needed (Fig. 26 D~F).
5. Final 3D data set could be established (Fig. 27).

It seems technically possible to make a data set of a patient's face with the dentition positioned into this 3D picture. This procedure points to several promising applications for feature research about noncephalometric analysis or superimpositions.

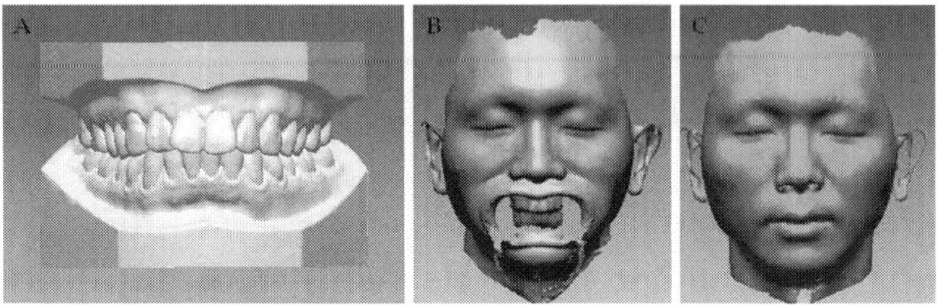

Fig. 25. **A.** 3D digital model. **B.** 3D facial image of the patient with cheek retractor. **C.** 3D facial image of the patient at rest position.

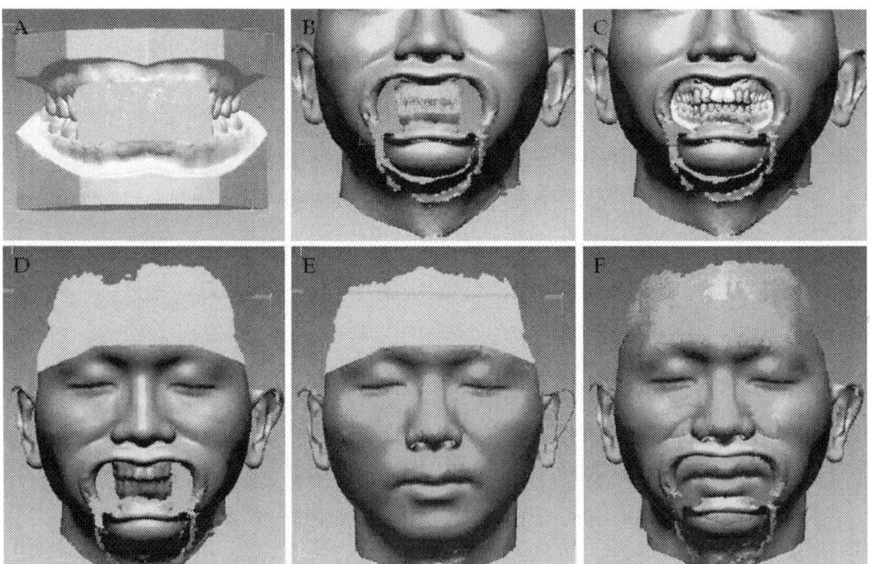

Fig. 26. Integration procedure of the 3D digital model into the 3D facial image. **A.** Region for surface registration is indicated on the 3D digital model(upper and lower anterior teeth were used). **B.** The same region in **A** is indicated on the 3D facial image with cheek retractor. **C.** Integration of 3D digital model and 3D facial image by using the registration area. **D, E.** Region for surface registration of two 3D facial images(forehead area was used). **F.** Superimposition of 3D facial images in **D** and **E.**

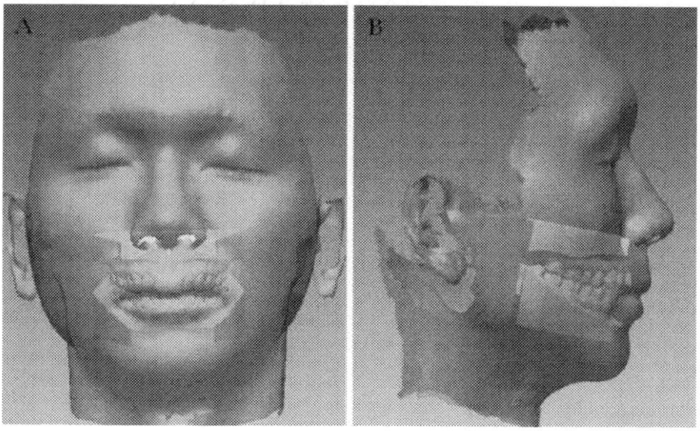

Fig. 27. Completed data set of the 3D digital model integrated into a 3D facial image. **A.** frontal view. **B.** profile view

8. Conclusion

In this chapter, we have reviewed the extent and limitation of the clinical application of 3D digital model and 3D facial image. The best-fit mathematical superimposition method of maxillary casts on the identical palatal vault is very accurate and allows for 3D evaluation of tooth movement. This technology can be also applied into a quite diverse area in dentistry, e.g. quantity evaluation of tooth material after conservative treatments or tooth wearing. The rapid development of CAD/CAM technology and the advances in 3D imaging of the face enable not only the virtual setup of the teeth but the results of treatment to be viewed from any perspective and to analyze the changes that have occurred by the treatment or growth.

9. References

Alcan, T.; Ceylanoglu, C. & Baysal, B. (2009). The relationship between digital model accuracy and time-dependent deformation of alginate impressions. *Angle Orthod*, Vol.79, No.1, pp. 30-36. ISSN 0003-3219

Ayoub, A.; Garrahy, A.; Hood, C.; White, J.; Bock, M.; Siebert, J.P.; Spencer, R. & Ray, A. (2003). Validation of a vision-based, three-dimensional facial imaging system. *Cleft Palate Craniofac J*, Vol.40, No.5, pp. 523-529. ISSN 1055-6656

Baik, H.S.; Jeon, J.M. & Lee, H.J. (2007). Facial soft-tissue analysis of Korean adults with normal occlusion using a 3-dimensional laser scanner. *Am J Orthod Dentofacial Orthop*, Vol.131, No.6, pp. 759-766. ISSN 1097-6752

Carlsson, G.E.; Egermark, I. & Magnusson, T. (2003). Predictors of bruxism, other oral parafunctions, and tooth wear over a 20-year follow-up period. *J Orofac Pain*, Vol.17, No.1, pp. 50-57. ISSN 1064-6655

Cha, B.K.; Choi, D.S.; Ngan, P.; Jost-Brinkmann, P.G.; Kim, S.M. & Jang, I.S. (2011). Maxillary protraction with miniplates providing skeletal anchorage in a growing Class III patient. *Am J Orthod Dentofacial Orthop*, Vol.139, No.1, pp. 99-112. ISSN 1097-6752

Cha, B.K.; Choi, J.I.; Jost-Brinkmann, P.G. & Jeong, Y.M. (2007). Applications of three-dimensionally scanned models in orthodontics. *Int J Comput Dent*, Vol.10, No.1, pp. 41-52. ISSN 1463-4201

Cha, B.K.; Lee, J.Y.; Jost-Brinkmann, P.G. & Yoshida, N. (2007). Analysis of tooth movement in extraction cases using three-dimensional reverse engineering technology. *Eur J Orthod*, Vol.29, No.4, pp. 325-331. ISSN 0141-5387

Choi, D.S.; Jeong, Y.M.; Jang, I.; Jost-Brinkmann, P.G. & Cha, B.K. (2010). Accuracy and reliability of palatal superimposition of three-dimensional digital models. *Angle Orthod*, Vol.80, No.4, pp. 497-503. ISSN 1945-7103

Costalos, P.A.; Sarraf, K.; Cangialosi, T.J. & Efstratiadis, S. (2005). Evaluation of the accuracy of digital model analysis for the American Board of Orthodontics objective grading system for dental casts. *Am J Orthod Dentofacial Orthop*, Vol.128, No.5, pp. 624-629. ISSN 0889-5406

Dalstra, M. & Melsen, B. (2009). From alginate impressions to digital virtual models: accuracy and reproducibility. *J Orthod*, Vol.36, No.1, pp. 36-41; discussion 14. ISSN 1465-3133

Dawson, P.E. (2007). *Functional occlusion: from TMJ to smile design*. Mosby. ISBN 978-0323033718, Philadelphia, USA

Eraso, F.E.; Parks, E.T.; Roberts, W.E.; Hohlt, W.F. & Ofner, S. (2007). Density value means in the evaluation of external apical root resorption: an in vitro study for early detection in orthodontic case simulations. *Dentomaxillofac Radiol*, Vol.36, No.3, pp. 130-137. ISSN 0250-832X

Fillion (2007). Computerized generated conception and fabrication of transfer trays for indirect bonding of lingual attachements: The Orapix system. *Rev Orthop Dento Facial*, Vol.41:1-15, pp. 1-15.

Ghafari, J.; Baumrind, S. & Efstratiadis, S.S. (1998). Misinterpreting growth and treatment outcome from serial cephalographs. *Clin Orthod Res*, Vol.1, No.2, pp. 102-106. ISSN 1397-5927

Gracco, A.; Buranello, M.; Cozzani, M. & Siciliani, G. (2007). Digital and plaster models: a comparison of measurements and times. *Prog Orthod*, Vol.8, No.2, pp. 252-259. ISSN 1723-7785

Hajeer, M.Y.; Ayoub, A.F.; Millett, D.T.; Bock, M. & Siebert, J.P. (2002). Three-dimensional imaging in orthognathic surgery: the clinical application of a new method. *Int J Adult Orthodon Orthognath Surg*, Vol.17, No.4, pp. 318-330. ISSN 0742-1931

Harrell, W.E., Jr.; Hatcher, D.C. & Bolt, R.L. (2002). In search of anatomic truth: 3-dimensional digital modeling and the future of orthodontics. *Am J Orthod Dentofacial Orthop*, Vol.122, No.3, pp. 325-330. ISSN 0889-5406

Hoefert, C.S.; Bacher, M.; Herberts, T.; Krimmel, M.; Reinert, S.; Hoefert, S. & Goz, G. (2010). Implementing a superimposition and measurement model for 3D sagittal analysis of therapy-induced changes in facial soft tissue: a pilot study. *J Orofac Orthop*, Vol.71, No.3, pp. 221-234. ISSN 1615-6714

Hoffman (1988). Indirect bonding with a diagnostic set-up. *J Clin Orthod*, Vol.8, pp. ISSN 509-511.

Horton, H.M.; Miller, J.R.; Gaillard, P.R. & Larson, B.E. (2009). Technique comparison for efficient orthodontic tooth measurements using digital models. *Angle Orthod*, Vol.80, No.2, pp. 254-261. ISSN 0003-3219

Ismail, S.F. & Moss, J.P. (2002). The three-dimensional effects of orthodontic treatment on the facial soft tissues--a preliminary study. *Br Dent J*, Vol.192, No.2, pp. 104-108. ISSN 0007-0610

Jang, I.; Tanaka, M.; Koga, Y.; Iijima, S.; Yozgatian, J.H.; Cha, B.K. & Yoshida, N. (2009). A novel method for the assessment of three-dimensional tooth movement during orthodontic treatment. *Angle Orthod*, Vol.79, No.3, pp. 447-453. ISSN 0003-3219

Kau, C.H. & Richmond, S. (2008). Three-dimensional analysis of facial morphology surface changes in untreated children from 12 to 14 years of age. *Am J Orthod Dentofacial Orthop*, Vol.134, No.6, pp. 751-760. ISSN 1097-6752

Keating, A.P.; Knox, J.; Bibb, R. & Zhurov, A.I. (2008). A comparison of plaster, digital and reconstructed study model accuracy. *J Orthod*, Vol.35, No.3, pp. 191-201; discussion 175. ISSN 1465-3125

Kiliaridis, S.; Johansson, A.; Haraldson, T.; Omar, R. & Carlsson, G.E. (1995). Craniofacial morphology, occlusal traits, and bite force in persons with advanced occlusal tooth wear. *Am J Orthod Dentofacial Orthop*, Vol.107, No.3, pp. 286-292. ISSN 0889-5406

Krejci, I.; Reich, T.; Bucher, W. & Lutz, F. (1994). [A new method for 3-dimensional wear measurement]. *Schweiz Monatsschr Zahnmed*, Vol.104, No.2, pp. 160-169. ISSN 1011-4203

Kuijpers, M.A.; Kiliaridis, S.; Renkema, A.; Bronkhorst, E.M. & Kuijpers-Jagtman, A.M. (2009). Anterior tooth wear and retention type until 5 years after orthodontic treatment. *Acta Odontol Scand*, Vol.67, No.3, pp. 176-181. ISSN 1502-3850 (Electronic)

Leifert, M.F.; Leifert, M.M.; Efstratiadis, S.S. & Cangialosi, T.J. (2009). Comparison of space analysis evaluations with digital models and plaster dental casts. *Am J Orthod Dentofacial Orthop*, Vol.136, No.1, pp. 16 e11-14; discussion 16. ISSN 1097-6752

Macchi, A.; Carrafiello, G.; Cacciafesta, V. & Norcini, A. (2006). Three-dimensional digital modeling and setup. *Am J Orthod Dentofacial Orthop*, Vol.129, No.5, pp. 605-610. ISSN 1097-6752

McCance, A.M.; Moss, J.P.; Fright, W.R.; Linney, A.D. & James, D.R. (1997). Three-dimensional analysis techniques--Part 2: Laser scanning: a quantitative three-dimensional soft-tissue analysis using a color-coding system. *Cleft Palate Craniofac J*, Vol.34, No.1, pp. 46-51. ISSN 1055-6656

McDonagh, S.; Moss, J.P.; Goodwin, P. & Lee, R.T. (2001). A prospective optical surface scanning and cephalometric assessment of the effect of functional appliances on the soft tissues. *Eur J Orthod*, Vol.23, No.2, pp. 115-126. ISSN 0141-5387

Milicic, A.; Gazi-Coklica, V. & Slaj, M. (1987). Dental attrition in preschool children. *Acta Stomatol Croat*, Vol.21, No.4, pp. 271-276. ISSN 0001-7019

Miller, L.; Morris, D.O. & Berry, E. (2007). Visualizing three-dimensional facial soft tissue changes following orthognathic surgery. *Eur J Orthod*, Vol.29, No.1, pp. 14-20. ISSN 0141-5387

Miller, R.J.; Kuo, E. & Choi, W. (2003). Validation of Align Technology's Treat III digital model superimposition tool and its case application. *Orthod Craniofac Res*, Vol.6 Suppl 1, pp. 143-149. ISSN 1601-6335

Morris, D.O.; Illing, H.M. & Lee, R.T. (1998). A prospective evaluation of Bass, Bionator and Twin Block appliances. Part II--The soft tissues. *Eur J Orthod*, Vol.20, No.6, pp. 663-684. ISSN 0141-5387

Moss, J.P. (2006). The use of three-dimensional imaging in orthodontics. *Eur J Orthod*, Vol.28, No.5, pp. 416-425. ISSN 0141-5387

Moss, J.P.; Linney, A.D. & Lowey, M.N. (1995). The use of three-dimensional techniques in facial esthetics. *Semin Orthod*, Vol.1, No.2, pp. 94-104. ISSN 1073-8746

Moss, J.P.; McCance, A.M.; Fright, W.R.; Linney, A.D. & James, D.R. (1994). A three-dimensional soft tissue analysis of fifteen patients with Class II, Division 1 malocclusions after bimaxillary surgery. *Am J Orthod Dentofacial Orthop*, Vol.105, No.5, pp. 430-437. ISSN 0889-5406

Myrberg, N.E. & Warner, C.F. (1982). Indirect bonding technique. *J Clin Orthod*, Vol.16, No.4, pp. 269-272. ISSN 0022-3875

Nagasaka, S.; Fujimura, T. & Segoshi, K. (2003). Development of a non-radiographic cephalometric system. *Eur J Orthod*, Vol.25, No.1, pp. 77-85. ISSN 0141-5387

Orapix (2010). *3Txer 3D virtual treatment planner.* Orapix www.orapix.com.

Ramjford, S.P. & Ash, M.M. (1983). *Occlusion,* W.B.Saunders, ISBN 978-0721655918, Philadelphia, USA

Rangel, F.A.; Maal, T.J.; Berge, S.J.; van Vlijmen, O.J.; Plooij, J.M.; Schutyser, F. & Kuijpers-Jagtman, A.M. (2008). Integration of digital dental casts in 3-dimensional facial photographs. *Am J Orthod Dentofacial Orthop*, Vol.134, No.6, pp. 820-826. ISSN 1097-6752

Ruf, S. & Pancherz, H. (1996). Frontal sinus development as an indicator for somatic maturity at puberty? *Am J Orthod Dentofacial Orthop*, Vol.110, No.5, pp. 476-482. ISSN 0889-5406

Santoro, M.; Galkin, S.; Teredesai, M.; Nicolay, O.F. & Cangialosi, T.J. (2003). Comparison of measurements made on digital and plaster models. *American journal of orthodontics and dentofacial orthopedics*, Vol.124, No.1, pp. 101-105. ISSN 0889-5406

Song, K.G. & Baek, S.H. (2009). Comparison of the accuracy of the three-dimensional virtual method and the conventional manual method for model surgery and intermediate wafer fabrication. *Oral Surg Oral Med Oral Pathol Oral Radiol Endod*, Vol.107, No.1, pp. 13-21. ISSN 1528-395X

Stevens, D.R.; Flores-Mir, C.; Nebbe, B.; Raboud, D.W.; Heo, G. & Major, P.W. (2006). Validity, reliability, and reproducibility of plaster vs digital study models: comparison of peer assessment rating and Bolton analysis and their constituent measurements. *American journal of orthodontics and dentofacial orthopedics*, Vol.129, No.6, pp. 794-803. ISSN 0889-5406

Weinberg, S.M.; Scott, N.M.; Neiswanger, K.; Brandon, C.A. & Marazita, M.L. (2004). Digital three-dimensional photogrammetry: evaluation of anthropometric precision and accuracy using a Genex 3D camera system. *Cleft Palate Craniofac J*, Vol.41, No.5, pp. 507-518. ISSN 1055-6656

Zachrisson, B.U. & Brobakken, B.O. (1978). Clinical comparison of direct versus indirect bonding with different bracket types and adhesives. *Am J Orthod*, Vol.74, No.1, pp. 62-78. ISSN 0002-9416

25

Recent Advances in the Genetics of Orthodontics

Yoko Tomoyasu, Tetsutaro Yamaguchi and Koutaro Maki
Department of Orthodontics, School of Dentistry, Showa University
Japan

1. Introduction

Consideration of genetic factors is an essential element of diagnosis that underlies orofacial traits. In particular, orthodontic clinicians may have an interest in craniofacial growth and tooth movement. These parts of the diagnostic process are important to understand the cause of the problem before attempting treatment. In this chapter, we present our studies on the genetic causes of external apical root resorption and mandibular morphology, and review related studies.

2. External apical root resorption (EARR)

External apical root resorption (EARR) is a common outcome following orthodontic treatment. The factors associated with this phenomenon are genetic background, the length of treatment, the magnitude of the orthodontic forces, the type of orthodontic movement, trauma and others (Brin & Bollen, 2011). Abnormal root shape is also a significant risk factor in root resorption (Kjaer, 1995). Allergy and asthma may also be high-risk factors for the development of excessive root resorption during orthodontic tooth movement (Nishioka et al., 2006).

Interleukin 1 beta IL-1B, a potent bone-resorptive cytokine, is a key component of the complex signaling pathways leading to root resorption. The proinflammatory cytokine IL-1 is a key mediator of the inflammatory response and regulates the proliferation of fibroblasts in the gingival and periodontal ligaments. The level of IL-1B notably increases in the human gingival crevicular fluid during orthodontic treatment (Uematsu et al., 1996). The levels of IL-1 correlate with individual differences in the amount of tooth translation (Iwasaki et al., 2001) and are thought to play a role in susceptibility to EARR (Davidovitch, 1991). Moreover, *IL-1B*-knockout mice demonstrate significantly greater root resorption than wild-type controls when undergoing experimental orthodontic treatments (Viecilli et al., 2009).

A C-to-T single nucleotide polymorphism (SNP) in *IL-1B*, rs1143634, may be causally associated with susceptibility to EARR. The TT genotype of this polymorphism has been associated with a 4-fold increase in IL-1B production (Pociot et al., 1992; di Giovine et al., 1995). Al-Qawasmi et al. (2003) reported an association of this polymorphism with the risk of EARR in the Caucasian population. Subjects homozygous for the C allele had a 5.6-fold

(95% confidence interval, 1.9–21.2) increased risk of EARR greater than 2 mm compared with those not homozygous for the C allele.

2.1 EARR and the Il-1B gene in the Japanese

Differences in tooth shape are used to characterize race and to provide an indication of racial affinity between human populations. For example, there are differences in the approximal root topography of teeth in the Chinese population compared with other populations (Ong & Neo, 1990). Sameshima & Sinclair (2001) reported that Asian patients experienced significantly less root resorption than Caucasian or Hispanic patients. We examined the association between a single polymorphism (rs1143634) in *IL-1B* and root resorption in 54 Japanese subjects (Tomoyasu et al., 2009a). Lateral cephalograms and panoramic radiographs were obtained from 54 Japanese subjects comprising 18 men and 36 women. The roots of three types of teeth were measured on pretreatment and posttreatment lateral cephalometric and panoramic radiographs. The roots of the maxillary and mandibular central incisors were measured from the pretreatment and posttreatment cephalometric radiographs. The mesial and distal roots of the left and right sides were measured on the panoramic radiographs. We amplified DNA by polymerase chain reaction, and genotyped the SNP by DNA sequencing. We found no significant difference between the genotype frequencies of the *IL-1B* SNP rs1143634 and the amount of root resorption in the Japanese population (Tables 1, 2).

	Maxillary incisor (mm)				Mandibular incisor (mm)			
	n	Mean	S.D.	P	n	Mean	S.D.	P
CC	45	2.1	2	0.29	48	1.7	1.5	0.86
CT	6	2.9	1.3		6	1.7	1.8	
	Mandibular mesial incisor (mm)				Mandibular incisor (mm)			
	n	Mean	S.D.	P	n	Mean	S.D.	P
CC	46	0.5	1.4	0.39	46	0.5	0.7	0.27
CT	6	0.7	1		6	1.2	1.6	

Table 1. The relationship between the *IL-1B* SNP rs1143634 and the amount of root resorption of the maxillary incisor, mandibular incisor, mandibular mesial molar, and mandibular distal molar in Japanese subjects. No statistical significance of the differences between the *IL-1B* genotype and the amount of root resorption was found.

	Unaffected groups (<2.0mm)		Affected groups (≥2.0mm)		
IL-1B marker	CC	CT	CC	CT	P
Maxillary central incisor	22	2	23	4	0.47
Mandibular central incisor	31	3	17	3	0.48
Mandibular first molar, mesial root	45	5	1	1	0.08
Mandibular first molar, distal root	44	5	2	1	0.22

Table 2. Relationship between the unaffected and affected groups by genotype. Subjects were classified as unaffected (<2.0 mm) or affected (≥2.0 mm), according to the amount of root resorption. No statistical significance of the differences between the *IL-1B* genotype and the classification of root resorption was determined.

2.2 Accuracy of EARR measurements

In our study, we failed to replicate in the Japanese population the previously reported association between the *IL-1B* polymorphism and EARR. In our study, we used lateral cephalograms to measure the amount of root resorption. In the study by Al-Qawasmi et al. (2003), lateral cephalograms and panoramic radiographs were used to measure EARR. However, the intraoral radiograph is more useful for measuring the amount of root resorption than the panoramic radiograph or lateral cephalogram. McFadden et al. (1989) indicated that errors in measurement using electronic calipers on lateral cephalometric films were approximately 2.5 times more frequent than the errors using periapical radiographs. Sameshima & Asgarifar (2001) suggested that the use of panoramic radiographs to measure root resorption might overestimate the amount of root loss by 20% or more, and that they are not as precise or reliable as intraoral radiographs (Bastos Lages et al., 2009).

To solve this problem, Bastos Lages et al. (2009) used periapical radiographs to determine the presence and severity of EARR to reduce the bias related to the diagnosis of EARR by other types of radiographs. In this report, the positive association was replicated in the Brazilian population.

They described that errors will certainly continue to occur until an accurate three-dimensional imaging system is available, because the accuracy of periapical x-rays for EARR measurements is unlikely that any inconsistencies in evaluating root resorption by this method in our study seriously biased the estimates of EARR.

2.3 Ethnic differences in the frequency of the *IL-1B* polymorphism

It is well known that differences in SNP frequencies among human populations are ethnicity-dependent (Wang et al., 2008). Ethnic factors are also considered to be a major variable in evaluating predisposition to EARR (Sameshima & Sinclair, 2001).

We characterized the ethnic variation at the *IL-1B* locus by examining the allele frequencies of the *IL-1B* polymorphism among individuals with different ethnic backgrounds. DNA samples from 24 Han Chinese, 24 African Americans, 24 European Americans, and 24 Hispanics were obtained, but no craniofacial measurements taken, and were used as reference populations for the allele frequencies of the *IL-1B* SNP.

There were marked differences in the frequency of the T allele of rs1143634 among the various ethnic populations (Table 3). The highest frequency (29.2%) was observed in the European Caucasians. The African American and Hispanic populations carried the T allele at frequencies of 10.4% and 14.7%, respectively. In contrast, the Japanese and Han Chinese populations carried the T allele at the markedly lower frequencies of 5.6% and 2.5%, respectively.

	Japanese	Han Chinese	African American	European Caucasian	Hispanic
n	54	24	24	24	24
C	94.4%	97.5%	89.6%	70.8%	85.3%
T	5.6%	2.5%	10.4%	29.2%	14.7%

Table 3. Allele distribution of the *IL-1B* SNP rs1143634 among different ethnicities.

The marked allelic diversity between different ethnic groups at this locus may explain our failure to identify any association between rs1143634 and EARR in the Japanese. We observed that Asian populations have a higher frequency of the C allele than other ethnic groups. In our data, only six Japanese subjects had a T allele. The failure to detect an association between the rs1143634 and root resorption in the Japanese may be due to the study being underpowered to detect a polymorphism that occurs at a relatively low frequency. In contrast, in the populations in which positive associations with EARR were identified, namely Caucasians and Brazilians, the T allele occurs at a higher frequency (Caucaisans: C; 70.8%, T; 29.2%, Tomoyasu et al., 2009a) (Brazilians: C; 43.4%, T; 56.6%, Bastos Lages et al., 2009), respectively. Further studies evaluating the genetic determinants of root resorption susceptibility are required.

3. Mandibular morphology and the growth hormone receptor gene

Craniofacial morphology has a strong genetic component but it is also influenced by environmental factors, making it a complex trait to study. Growth hormone (GH) is a craniofacial morphological determinant; it plays a major role in the growth and development of the craniofacial complex by directly and indirectly modulating the size and the angular relationships of the craniofacial structures (Ramirez-Yanez et al., 2005). Children with deficient or excess GH have been reported to develop unique craniofacial configurations (Pirinen et al., 1994). Disproportionate growth of the cranial base structures and jaws results in facial retrognathia, which entails a proportionately smaller posterior than anterior facial height in persons of short stature with GH deficiency (Kjelberg et al., 2000). GH therapy for children with short stature or Turner syndrome results in characteristic patterns of craniofacial growth (Van Erum et al., 1988; Simmons, 1999). Responses to systemic GH therapy are time- and site-dependent in the craniofacial region, and are associated with an increase in cartilage growth, particularly within the mandibular ramus (Van Erum et al., 1988; Simmons, 1999). Children who receive long-term GH replacement therapy show exaggerated growth of the craniofacial skeleton, especially with respect to the height of the mandibular ramus (Funatsu et al., 2006; Forsberg et al., 2002). A comparison of children with Turner syndrome who received recombinant human GH treatment and a large cross-sectional control group showed a statistically significant increase in ramus growth associated with mandibular ramus height, but not with mandibular body length, maxillary length, or anterior cranial base length (Rongen-Westerlaken et al., 1993).

Growth hormone receptors (GHRs) have been shown by molecular genetic analysis to be present in the mandibular condyle (Lewinson et al., 1994). Analysis of the *Ghr* knockout mouse has revealed that the GH→GHR→insulin-like growth factor 1 system is important in postnatal growth and that GHR plays a role in maintaining proportional skeletal growth (Sjogren et al., 2000). In *Ghr* knockout mice, the height of the mandibular ramus is significantly reduced (Ramirez-Yanez et al., 2005), and disproportionate skeletal growth is reflected by decreased femur:crown-rump and femur:tibia ratios (Sjogren et al., 2000). There are diverse mutations and polymorphisms in the *GHR* gene in humans. Reports have shown a relationship between *GHR* and idiopathic short stature (Goddard et al., 1995) and Laron syndrome (growth hormone insensitivity syndrome), which is marked by a characteristic facial appearance. Interestingly, patients with GHR deficiency showed significantly decreased vertical facial growth (Schaefer et al., 1994). Therefore, GHR is suggested to have site-, area-, or region-specific effects (Hartsfield, 2005).

3.1 Relationship between the *GHR* gene and mandibular morphology in the Japanese

We quantitatively evaluated the relationship between craniofacial morphology and the P561T variant in exon 10 of the *GHR* gene in the non-syndromic Japanese population (Yamaguchi et al., 2001). DNA and cephalograms were obtained from 50 Japanese men and 50 Japanese women. To analyze craniofacial morphology, measurements were made on tracings of lateral cephalograms under standardized conditions. We measured cranial base length (nasion-sella; N–S), maxillary length (point A-pterygomaxillary fissure; A'-PTM'), overall mandibular length (gnathion-condylion; Gn–Co), mandibular corpus length (pogonion-gonion; Pog'-Go), and mandibular ramus height (condylion-gonion; Co-Go) (Figure 1). Body height was also measured. We identified a significant association of the polymorphic GHR gene (P561T, rs6184) with mandibular ramus height (P = 0.0181) (Table 4).

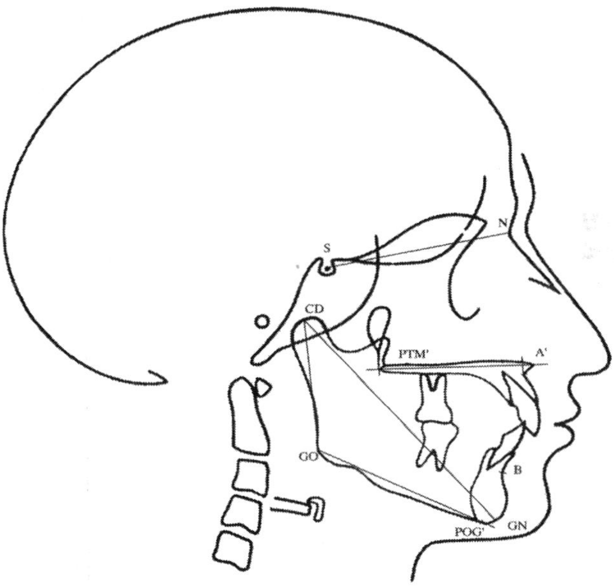

Fig. 1. Cephalometric reference points and lines used to assess the relationship between *GHR* gene variants. N–S, cranial base length; A'–PTM', maxillary length; Co–Go, mandibular ramus length; Pog'–Go; mandibular corpus length; Gn–Co, overall mandibular length.

	P561T	n	Body Height (cm)	N-S (mm)	A'-PTM' (mm)	Gn-Co (mm)
Subjects	CC	86	165.2±7.8	71.0±3.6	50.9±3.3	126.3±9.5
(100)	CA	14	163.4±10.5	70.0±4.6	50.4±3.7	122.3±9.6
	P		0.32	0.6	0.47	0.12
Men	CC	44	171.0±5.5	72.6±3.6	52.1±3.1	131.6±7.0
(50)	CA	6	173.7±6.5	72.6±5.1	53.0±3.5	131.4±7.4
	P		0.4	0.55	0.53	0.98
Women	CC	42	159.2±4.6	69.3±2.7	49.6±3.0	120.7±8.6
(50)	CA	8	155.6±3.9	68.1±3.3	48.4±2.5	115.5±3.1
	P		0.38	0.32	0.26	0.06

	P561T	n	Pog'-Go(mm)	Co-Go(mm)	Height/Co-Go
Subjects	CC	86	81.2±6.0	63.5±6.9	2.7±0.2
(100)	CA	14	79.3±7.2	58.9±6.1	2.9±0.3
	P		0.32	.018*	.013*
Men	CC	44	84.3±4.7	68.5±4.4	2.5±0.2
(50)	CA	6	86.3±3.7	64.9±2.1	2.7±0.1
	P		0.37	.021*	.015*
Women	CC	42	78.0±5.6	58.3±4.9	2.8±0.3
(50)	CA	8	74.2±3.7	54.4±3.5	2.9±0.3
	P		0.07	.025*	.028*

Table 4. The relationship between *GHR* gene variants and linear measurements in 50 men and 50 women. *P < 0.05.

To confirm these findings, we extended our previous study, genotyping approximately 1.7-times more non-syndromic Japanese individuals than analyzed in a previous report. Genomic DNA and lateral cephalograms were obtained from 167 Japanese subjects comprising 50 men and 117 women. The male subjects were the same as those we reported previously. We genotyped these individuals for five SNPs in the coding region of GHR (exon 10): C422F (rs6182, GG and GT genotype), S473S (rs6176, CC and CT genotype), P477T (rs6183, CC and CA genotype), I526L (rs6180, AA, AC and CC genotype), and P561T (rs6184, CC and CA genotype). We identified a significant relationship between the P56IT and C422F genotypes with mandibular ramus height in the Japanese population (P < 0.05; Table 5). These two polymorphisms are in linkage disequilibrium (Tomoyasu et al., 2009b).

			Body height (cm)			N-S (mm)		
		n	Mean	S.D.	P	Mean	S.D.	P
C422F	GG	135	161.6	7.9	0.16	69.7	3.4	0.66
	GT	16	164.6	10.2		69.3	4.4	
S473S	CC	137	161.9	8.4	0.95	69.6	3.5	0.32
	CT	11	161.1	6.1		70.5	2.8	
P477T	CC	146	161.6	8.3	0.47	69.6	3.5	0.58
	CA	4	163.8	9.1		69.5	4.8	
I526L	AA	77	162.7	8.8	0.47	69.5	3.5	0.56
	AC	44	161	7.9		70.2	4	
	CC	32	161.4	6.9		69.4	2.6	
P561T	CC	135	161.6	7.9	0.16	69.7	3.4	0.66
	CA	16	164.6	10.2		69.3	4.4	

			A′-PTM′ (mm)			Gn-Co (mm)		
		n	Mean	S.D.	P	Mean	S.D.	P
C422F	GG	135	50	4.8	0.95	122.9	9.3	0.63
	GT	16	49.9	3.1		121.7	8.5	
S473S	CC	137	49.9	4.8	0.71	122.9	9.2	0.89
	CT	11	49.8	2.1		123	9.7	
P477T	CC	146	49.9	4.7	0.54	122.7	9.1	0.15
	CA	4	51.3	3.5		130.5	11.4	
I526L	AA	77	50.1	3.2	0.06	124.2	9.7	0.19
	AC	44	50.7	3.1		121.6	8.7	
	CC	32	48.1	7.9		121.4	7.7	
P561T	CC	135	50	4.8	0.95	122.9	9.3	0.63
	CA	16	49.9	3.1		121.7	8.5	

			Pog′-Go (mm)			Co-Go (mm)		
		n	Mean	S.D.	P	Mean	S.D.	P
C422F	GG	135	79.5	5.6	0.78	61.6	6.5	0.02*
	GT	16	79.9	7.2		57.9	6.1	
S473S	CC	137	79.9	5.9	0.31	61.5	6.5	0.54
	CT	11	78.5	6.4		60.9	5.6	
P477T	CC	146	79.8	6	0.23	61.3	6.4	0.17
	CA	4	83.3	5.7		65.6	4.5	
I526L	AA	77	80.1	5.8	0.82	62.4	6.7	0.13
	AC	44	79.6	5.5		61.1	6.8	
	CC	32	79.5	6.8		59.7	5.4	
P561T	CC	135	79.5	5.6	0.78	61.6	6.5	0.02*
	CA	16	79.9	7.2		57.9	6.1	

Table 5. Relationship between 5 SNPs in the GHR and 6 linear measurements of body height and craniofacial morphology in 167 Japanese subjects. *P < 0.05.

	n	Body height(cm) Mean	S.D.	P	N-S (mm) Mean	S.D.	P
d3/fl-GHR							
fl/fl	92	171.2	7.2	0.24	75.3	3.8	0.92
fl/d3	24	169.7	6.3		75.6	3.8	
d3/d3	9	173.7	3.9		75.4	4.4	
C422F/P561T							
GG/CC	124	170.6	7.1	0.49	75.2	3.8	0.7
GT/CA	24	169.6	6.7		75.2	3.7	
S473S							
CC	145						
CT	3						
P477T							
CC	145						
CA	3						
I526L							
AA	62	171.5	7.2	0.19	75.8	3.7	0.24
AC	61	170	7.2		74.8	3.3	
CC	24	169	6.3		75.1	4.5	

	n	A'-PTM'(mm) Mean	S.D.	P	Gn-Co (mm) Mean	S.D.	P
d3/fl-GHR							
fl/fl	92	52	3.2	0.79	139.6	8.3	0.21
fl/d3	24	52.2	3.4		137.8	6.9	
d3/d3	9	51.3	2.5		142.7	10.4	
C422F/P561T							
GG/CC	124	52.1	3.3	0.32	138.7	8	0.38
GT/CA	24	51.3	2.9		137.7	8.6	
S473S							
CC	145						
CT	3						
P477T							
CC	145						
CA	3						
I526L							
AA	62	52.6	3.2	0.24	139.1	8.7	0.71
AC	61	51.7	3.2		137.9	7.8	
CC	24	51.7	3.7		139.2	7.9	

	n	Pog'-Go(mm) Mean	S.D.	P	Co-Go(mm) Mean	S.D.	P
d3/fl-GHR							
fl/fl	92	84.8	5.5	0.12	72	7.6	0.59
fl/d3	24	82.8	5.2		70.7	6.3	
d3/d3	9	84.5	4.5		72.5	6.6	
C422F/P561T							
GG/CC	124	83.9	5.5	0.77	71.9	7.1	0.02*
GT/CA	24	84.2	5.3		68.5	5.5	
S473S							
CC	145						
CT	3						
P477T							
CC	145						
CA	3						
I526L							
AA	62	84.3	5.7	0.82	72	7.6	0.68
AC	61	83.5	5.3		71.2	6.5	
CC	24	84.2	84.2		71.1	7.4	

Table 6. The relationship between six SNPs in GHR and six linear measurements of body height and craniofacial morphology in 159 Korean subjects. $*P < 0.05$.

3.2 Relationship between the *GHR* gene and mandibular morphology in Asian populations

Following our report of an association between an exon 10 SNP in the *GHR* gene and mandibular ramus height in the Japanese (Yamaguchi et al., 2001), Zhou et al. (2005) reported the association of another exon 10 *GHR* polymorphism, I526L, with mandibular height in 95 Han Chinese subjects. We did not replicate this finding in 167 Japanese subjects (Tomoyasu et al., 2009b).

We also evaluated the association of *GHR* polymorphisms with mandibular ramus height in the Korean population (Kang et al., 2009). Genomic DNA samples and lateral cephalograms were obtained from 159 Korean subjects, comprising 100 men and 59 women. We tested the five aforementioned exon 10 SNPs plus a common polymorphism *d3/fl-GHR* that results in genomic deletion of exon 3 (Urbanek et al., 1992; Pantel et al., 2000). Two common isoforms of GHR, one full-length (fl-GHR) and the other lacking the extracellular domain encoded by exon 3 (d3-GHR), are associated with differences in responsiveness to GH. Children carrying at least one *d3-GHR* allele show a 1.7- to 2-fold greater response to GH than do *fl-GHR/fl-GHR* homozygotes (Dos-Santos et al., 2004). This common polymorphism has also been associated with the degree of height increase in response to GH therapy in French children of short stature who were born small for gestational age or with idiopathic short stature (Dos-Santos et al., 2004), as well as in German Turner syndrome patients (Binder et al., 2006), and Brazilian GH-deficient children (Jorge et al., 2006).

Table 6 shows the frequencies of the six *GHR* genotypes and the relationships between these genotypes and six linear measurements of body height and craniofacial morphology in 159 Korean subjects. Heterozygosity for S473S and P477T (genotypes CT and CA, respectively) was found in only three subjects. Therefore, statistical analysis was not performed for S473S or P477T. Genotype-specific association analysis revealed that mandibular ramus height only was significantly correlated with the P561T (a C-to-A transversion) and C422F (a G-to-T transversion) variants (P = 0.024). The *d3/fl-GHR* polymorphism was not associated with any measurement. These data replicated our findings in the Japanese population, but were different from the findings reported for the Han Chinese population.

We confirmed an association between polymorphisms P561T and C422F and mandibular ramus height. Individuals with the genotype CC for polymorphism P561T and the genotype GG for polymorphism C422F had a significantly greater mandibular height than those with genotypes CA and GT, respectively.

3.3 Ethnic differences in the *GHR* SNP allele frequencies

A clue to understanding ethnic differences in the association between the *GHR* locus and mandibular ramus height might be gained by determining the allelic frequencies of the five SNPs among 24 Han Chinese, 24 African Americans, 24 European Americans, and 24 Hispanics. we examined the allelic frequencies of the five SNPs among 24 Han Chinese, 24 African Americans, 24 European Americans, and 24 Hispanics. We found that the allele frequencies vary considerably (Table 7).

The reason for the difference between Japanese/Koreans and Chinese remains unclear; however, we did find widely discordant allele frequencies in the *GHR* exon 10 SNPs between some of the different ethnic groups. Indeed, the association of *GHR* is different depending on ethnicity in other cases, such as Laron syndrome (Hopp et al., 1996; Shevah et al., 2004) and idiopathic short stature (Blum et al., 2006; Hujeirat et al., 2006; Bonioli et al.,

2005; Sjoberg et al., 2001; Sanchez et al., 1998; Johnston et al., 2000). These differences might imply the need for independent studies on the association of *GHR* with craniofacial morphology in each ethnic group. The mandibular size of Japanese people appears to be slightly smaller than that of European-Americans (Miyajima et al., 1996) or Caucasians (Ishii et al., 2001; Ishii et al., 2002; Ishizuka et al., 1989).

		Japanese (n=167)	Han Chinese (n=24)	African American (n=24)	European American (n=24)	Hispanic (n=24)
C422F	G	94.1%	79.4%	100.0%	100.0%	100.0%
	T	5.9%	20.6%	0.0%	0.0%	0.0%
S473S	C	96.3%	97.3%	100.0%	97.5%	100.0%
	T	3.7%	2.6%	0.0%	2.5%	0.0%
P477T	C	98.7%	100.0%	100.0%	100.0%	100.0%
	A	1.3%	0.0%	0.0%	0.0%	0.0%
I526L	A	46.7%	38.2%	64.3%	58.3%	62.4%
	C	53.3%	61.8%	35.6%	41.6%	37.5%
P561T	C	94.7%	80.0%	100.0%	100.0%	100.0%
	A	5.2%	19.9%	0.0%	0.0%	0.0%

Table 7. Allele distribution of 5 SNPs in exon10 of the GHR

On average, the allele frequencies for populations from different continents differ by 16–19%, and for populations within a continent, such as Koreans and Japanese, they differ by 5–10% (Miller et al., 2005). These differences may be sufficiently large, even among the closely related Korean, Japanese, and Chinese populations, to cause substructural problems for case-control genetic studies of complex traits. Indeed, our findings in the Japanese and Korean populations were not replicated in the Han Chinese. A haplotype-based study based on HapMap data is required to assess the differences among Asian populations, and a larger-scale study with the ethnicities kept distinct is required to obtain a conclusive result (Roeder et al., 2006; Ambrosius et al., 2004; Schork et al., 2002; Longmate et al., 2001). Our work emphasizes the importance of close matching of ethnic groups, especially when measuring craniofacial morphology, which is known to vary by ethnicity (Miyajima et al., 1996; Ishii et al., 2001; Ishii et al., 2002; Ioi et al., 2007).

Growth hormone insensitivity syndrome of genetic origin has been linked to many different mutations of *GHR*, and is associated with a wide range of severities of clinical and biochemical phenotypes. Mandibular growth is also influenced by multiple factors, among which heterozygous *GHR* mutations appear to play a more or less important role, depending on the kind of mutation and on the overall genetic make-up of the individual. Although there is continuing interest in the functional importance of the P56IT and C422F variants, their precise roles remain unknown. The availability of an environmental factor (*i.e.*, orthopedic treatment) has made it possible to initiate therapeutic trials on children with short ramus height. Sasaki et al. (2007) reported a Japanese patient with ectodermal dysplasia, and proposed that the P561T variant could be a genetic marker for mandibular growth. Sasaki et al. (2009) reported that a difference in mandibular growth between P561T heterozygous and wild-type individuals could be demonstrated by cephalometric measurements during childhood. A heterozygous P561T mutation may affect mandibular growth during early childhood, as it is hypothesized to function as an inhibitory factor in the process of mandibular growth. *GHR* is considered a possible genetic marker for mandibular ramus height (Sasaki et al., 2007). This genetic factor might be considered along with other factors associated with mandibular growth when planning treatment to influence mandibular height, such as Herbst appliances, functional appliances, headgear, and facemask therapy.

3.4 Mandibular prognathism

We previously reported a genome-wide linkage analysis with 90 mandibular prognathism sib-pairs from an Asian population, and identified three significantly linked chromosomal loci: 1p36, 6q25, and 19p13.2 (Yamaguchi et al., 2005). These do not include the *GHR* locus on chromosome 5. We did not find any *GHR* gene SNPs that were associated with mandibular corpus length or overall mandibular length; there was also no identified association in the Chinese population (Zhou et al., 2005).

Recently, there have been four reports describing mandibular prognathism-related genes or loci. Jang et al. (2010) reported that polymorphisms in matrilin-1 could be used as a marker for genetic susceptibility to mandibular prognathism. Xue et al. (2010) reported an association between genetic polymorphisms in the erythrocyte membrane protein band 4.1 gene and mandibular prognathism. Li et al. (2010, 2011) reported a novel suggestive linkage locus for mandibular prognathism in two Chinese pedigrees. The linked region, around SNP rs875864 on chromosome 4, contains candidate genes include *EVC* and *EVC2* (Li et al., 2010), and that on chromosome 4 between rs1468507 and rs7141857 contains candidate genes including transforming growth factor, beta 3 and latent transforming growth factor beta binding protein (Li et al., 2011). Further studies will be needed to find the rare variants causing mandibular prognathism.

3.5 Conclusion

While various environmental factors contribute to morphogenesis of the mandible, genetic factors play a substantial role (Chang et al., 2006). However, there are very few reports that have examined the correlation between craniofacial morphology and genotype. Our studies have succeeded in elucidating susceptibility locus-related non-syndromic craniofacial morphology. We have also found marked diversities in the allelic frequencies of GH receptor polymorphisms within a multi-ethnic study population, which might partly explain the differing craniofacial morphologies among different ethnicities. Recent advances in clinical genetics have increased our knowledge of the genetic impact on craniofacial phenotypes. Identifying the genetic susceptibility for specific craniofacial phenotypes would enable more effective diagnosis and treatment for patients while they were still growing.

4. Acknowledgments

We are deeply grateful to the study participants. We also thank our collaborators, Ituro Inoue (National Institute of Genetics), Atsushi Tajima (Tokushima University), Ryosuke Kimura (University of the Ryukyus), Soo Byung Park (Pusan National University), Miyuki Watanabe (Showa University), Masaaki Yamaguchi (Showa University), and Yoshinobu Shibasaki (Showa University). The protocols used in our studies were approved by the relevant Ethics Committees, and all patients gave their written informed consent to participate in the study before samples were taken. The dbSNP numbers are taken from the dbSNP database at the National Center for Biotechnology Information. (http://www.ncbi.nlm.nih.gov/SNP/)

5. References

Al-Qawasmi, RA.; Hartsfield, JK Jr.; Everett, ET.; Flury, L.; Liu, L.; Foroud, TM. et al. (2003). Genetic predisposition to external apical root resorption. *Am J Orthod Dentofacial Orthop,* Vol. 123, No. 3, pp. 242-252, ISSN 0889-5406

Ambrosius, WT.; Lange, EM. & Langefeld, CD. (2004). Power for genetic association studies with random allele frequencies and genotype distributions. *Am J Hum Genet,* Vol. 74, No. 4, pp. 683-693, ISSN 0002-9297

Bastos Lages, EM.; Drummond, AF.; Pretti, H.; Costa, FO.; Lages, EJ.; Gontijo, AI. et al. (2009). Association of functional gene polymorphism IL-1beta in patients with external apical root resorption. *Am J Orthod Dentofacial Orthop,* Vol. 136, No. 4, pp. 542-546, ISSN 1097-6752

Binder, G.; Baur, F.; Schweizer, R. & Ranke, MB. (2006). The d3-growth hormone receptor polymorphism is associated with increased responsiveness to GH in Turner syndrome and short SGA children. *J Clin Endocrinol Metab,* Vol. 91, No. 2, pp. 659–664, ISSN 0021-972X

Blum, WF.; Machinis, K.; Shavrikova, EP.; Keller, A.; Stobbe, H.; Pfaeffle, RW. et al. (2006). The growth response to growth hormone (GH) treatment in children with isolated GH deficiency is independent of the presence of the exon 3-minus isoform of the GH receptor. J Clin Endocrinol Metab, Vol. 91, No. 10, pp. 4171-4174, ISSN 0021-972X

Bonioli, E.; Taro, M.; Rosa, CL.; Citana, A.; Bertorelli, R.; Morcaldi, G. et al. (2005). Heterozygous mutations of growth hormone receptor gene in children with idiopathic short stature. *Growth Horm IGF Res,* Vol. 15, No. 6, pp. 405-410, ISSN 1096-6374

Brin, I.; Bollen, AM. (2011). External apical root resorption in patients treated by serial extractions followed by mechanotherapy. *Am J Orthod Dentofacial Orthop,* Vol. 139, No. 2, pp. e129-134, ISSN 1097-6752

Chang, HP.; Tseng, YC. & Chang, HF. (2006). Treatment of mandibular prognathism. *J Formos Med Assoc,* Vol. 105, No. 10, pp. 781-790, ISSN 0929-6646

Davidovitch Z. (1991). Tooth movement. *Crit Rev Bio Med,* Vol. 2, No. 4, pp. 411-450, ISSN 1045-4411

di Giovine, FS.; Cork, MJ.; Crane, A.; Mee, JB. & Duff, GW. (1995). Novel genetic association of an IL-1B gene variation a +3953 with IL-1B protein production and psoriasis. *Cytokine,* Vol. 7, No. 6, pp. 606, ISSN 1043-4666

Dos-Santos, C.; Essioux, L.; Teinturier, C.; Tauber, M.; Goffin, V. & Bougneres, P. (2004). A common polymorphism of the growth hormone receptor is associated with increased responsiveness to growth hormone. *Nat Genet,* Vol. 36, No. 7, pp. 720-724, ISSN 1061-4036

Forsberg, CM.; Krekmanova, L. & Dahllof, G. (2002). The effect of growth hormone therapy on mandibular and cranial base development in children treated with total body irradiation. *Eur J Orthod,* Vol. 24, No. 3, pp. 285–292, ISSN 0141-5387

Funatsu, M.; Sato, K. & Mitani, H. (2006). Effects of growth hormone on craniofacial growth. *Angle Orthod,* Vol. 76, No. 6, pp. 970–977, ISSN 0003-3219

Goddard, AD.; Covello, R.; Luoh, SM.; Clackson, T.; Attie, KM.; Gesundheit, N. et al. (1995). Mutations of the growth hormone receptor in children with idiopathic short stature. The Growth Hormone Insensitivity Study Group. *N Engl J Med,* Vol. 333, No. 17, pp. 1093-1098, ISSN 0028-4793

Hartsfield, JK. (2005). Genetics and Orthodontics, In: *Orthodontics: Current Principles & Techniques, 4th ed.,* Graber, TM.; Vanarsdall, RL. & Vig, KWL, pp. 101-115, Mosey, ISBN 0323026214, St. Louis

Hopp, M.; Rosenbloom, AL.; Griffiths, J.; Kgwete, S. & Vaccarello, MA. (1996). Growth hormone receptor deficiency (Laron syndrome) in black African siblings. *S Afr Med J,* Vol. 86, No. 3, pp. 268-270, ISSN 0256-9574

Hujeirat, Y.; Hess, O.; Shalev, S. & Tenenbaum-Rakover, Y. (2006). Growth hormone receptor sequence changes do not play a role in determining height in children with idiopathic short stature. *Horm Res,* Vol. 65, No. 4, pp. 210-216, ISSN 0301-0163

Ioi, H.; Nakata, S.; Nakasima, A. & Counts, AL. (2007). Comparison of cephalometric norms between Japanese and Caucasian adults in anteroom-posterior and vertical dimension. *Eur J Orthod,* Vol. 29, No. 5, pp. 493–499, ISSN 0141-5387

Ishii, N.; Deguchi, T. & Hunt, NP. (2001). Craniofacial morphology of Japanese girls with Class II division 1 malocclusion. *J Orthod,* Vol. 28, No. 3, pp. 211-215, ISSN 1465-3125

Ishii, N.; Deguchi, T. & Hunt, NP. (2002). Morphological differences in the craniofacial structure between Japanese and Caucasian girls with Class II Division 1 malocclusions. *Eur J Orthod,* Vol. 24, No. 1, pp. 61-67, ISSN 0141-5387

Ishizuka, K.; Yamazaki, T.; Inoue, K.; Kouchi, K.; Ou, B. & Namura, S. (1989). A morphological study of the cranial base and dentofacial structure of Japanese with Angle Class II, div. 1 malocclusion--as compared with American white with Angle Class II, div. 1 malocclusion. *Nippon Kyosei Shika Gakkai Zasshi,* Vol. 48, No. 1, pp. 1-6, ISSN 0021-454X

Iwasaki, LR.; Haack, JE.; Nickel, JC.; Reinhardt, RA. & Petro, TM. (2001). Human interleukin-1 beta and interleukin-1 receptor antagonist secretion and velocity of tooth movement. *Arch Oral Biol,* Vol. 46, No. 2, pp. 185-189, ISSN 0003-9969

Jang, JY.; Park, EK.; Ryoo, HM.; Shin, HI.; Kim, TH.; Jang, JS. et al. (2010). Polymorphisms in the Matrilin-1 gene and risk of mandibular prognathism in Koreans. *J Dent Res,* Vol. 89, No. 11, pp. 1203-1207, ISSN 1544-0591

Johnston, LB.; Pashankar, F.; Camacho-Hubner, C.; Savage, MO. & Clark, AJ. (2000). Analysis of the intracellular signalling domain of the human growth hormone receptor in children with idiopathic short stature. *Clin Endocrinol,* Vol. 52, No. 4, pp. 463-469, ISSN 0300-0664

Jorge, AA.; Marchisotti, FG.; Montenegro, LR.; Carvalho, LR.; Mendonca, BB. & Arnhold, IJ. (2006). Growth hormone (GH) pharmacogenetics: influence of GH receptor exon 3 retention or deletion on first-year growth response and final height in patients with severe GH deficiency. *J Clin Endocrinol Metab,* Vol. 91, No. 2, pp. 1076–1080, ISSN 0021-972X

Kang, EH.; Yamaguchi, T.; Tajima, A.; Nakajima, T.; Tomoyasu, Y.; Watanabe, M. et al. (2009). Association of the growth hormone receptor gene polymorphisms with mandibular height in a Korean population. *Arch Oral Biol,* Vol. 54, No. 6, pp. 556-562, ISSN 1879-1506

Kjaer I. (1995). Morphological characteristics of dentitions developing excessive root resorption during orthodontics treatment. *Eur J Orthod,* Vol. 17, No. 1, pp. 25-34, ISSN 0141-5387

Kjelberg, H.; Beiring, M. & Wikland, KA. (2000). Craniofacial morphology, dental occlusion, tooth eruption, and dental maturity in boys of short stature with or without growth hormone deficiency. *Eur J Oral Sci,* Vol. 108, No. 5, pp. 359–367, ISSN 0909-8836

Li, Q.; Zhang, F.; Li, X. & Chen, F. (2010). Genome scan for locus involved in mandibular prognathism in pedigrees from China. *PLoS One,* Vol. 10, No. 5, pp. e12678, ISSN 1932-6203

Li, Q.; Li, X.; Zhang, F. & Chen, F. (2011). The identification of a novel locus for mandibular prognathism in the Han Chinese population. J Dent Res, Vol. 90, No. 1, pp. 53-57, ISSN 1544-0591

Lewinson, D.; Bialik, GM. & Hochberg, Z. (1994) Differential effects of hypothyroidism on the cartilage and the osteogenic process in the mandibular condyle: recovery by growth hormone and thyroxine. *Endocrinology,* Vol. 135, No. 4, pp. 1504–1510, ISSN 0013-7227

Longmate, JA. (2001). Complexity and power in case-control association studies. *Am J Hum Genet,* Vol. 68, No. 5, pp. 1229-1237, ISSN 0002-9297

McFadden, WM.; Engstrom, C.; Engstrom, H. & Anholm, JM. (1989). A study of the relationship between incisor intrusion and root shortening. *Am J Orthod Dentofacial Orthop,* Vol. 96, No. 5, pp. 390–396, ISSN 0889-5406

Miller, RD.; Phillips, MS.; Jo, I.; Donaldson, MA.; Studebaker, JF. & Addleman, N. et al. (2005). The SNP Consortium Allele Frequency Project. High-density single-nucleotide polymorphism maps of the human genome. *Genomics,* Vol. 86, No. 2, pp. 117–126, ISSN 0888-7543

Miyajima, K.; McNamara, JA Jr.; Kimura, T.; Murata, S. & Iizuka, T. (1996). Craniofacial structure of Japanese and European-American adults with normal occlusions and well-balanced faces. *Am J Orthod Dentofacial Orthop,* Vol. 110, No. 4, pp. 431-438, ISSN 0889-5406

Nishioka, M.; Ioi, H.; Nakata, S.; Nakasima, A. & Counts, A. (2006). Root resorption and immune system factors in the Japanese. *Angle Orthod,* Vol. 76, No. 1, pp. 103-108, ISSN 0003-3219

Ong, G. & Neo, J. (1990). A survey of approximal root concavities in an ethnic Chinese population. *Arch Oral Biol,* Vol. 35, No. 11, pp. 925-928, ISSN 0003-9969

Pantel, J.; Machinis, K.; Sobrier, ML.; Duquesnoy, P.; Goosens, M. & Amselem, S. (2000). Species-specific alternative splice mimicry atthe growth hormone receptor locus revealed by the lineage of retroelements during primate evolution. *J Biol Chem,* Vol. 275, No. 25, pp. 18664–18669, ISSN 0021-9258

Pirinen, S.; Majurin, A.; Lenko, HL. & Koski K. (1994). Craniofacial features in patients with deficient and excessive growth hormone. *J Craniofac Genet Dev Biol,* Vol. 14, No. 3, pp. 144-152, ISSN 0270-4145

Pociot, F.; Mølvig, J.; Wogensen, L.; Worsaae, H. & Nerup, J. (1992). A TaqI polymorphism in the human interleukin-1 beta (IL-1 beta) gene correlates with IL-1 beta secretion in vitro. *Eur J Clin Invest,* Vol. 22, No. 6, pp. 396-402, ISSN 0014-2972

Ramirez-Yanez, GO.; Smid, JR.; Young, WG. & Waters, MJ. (2005). Influence of growth hormone on the craniofacial complex of transgenic mice. *Eur J Orthod,* Vol. 27, No. 5, pp. 494-500, ISSN 0141-5387

Roeder, K.; Bacanu, SA.; Wasserman, L. & Devlin, B. (2006). Using linkage genome scans to improve power of association in genome scans. *Am J Hum Genet,* Vol. 78, No. 2, pp. 243-252, ISSN 0002-9297

Rongen-Westerlaken, C.; Vd Born, E.; Prahl-Andersen, B.; Von Teunenbroek, A.; Manesse, P.; Otten, BJ. et al. (1993). Effect of growth hormone treatment on craniofacial growth in Turner's syndrome. *Act Paediatric,* Vol. 82, No. 4, pp. 364–368, ISSN 0803-5253

Sameshima, G.T. & Asgarifar, KO. (2001). Assessment of root resorption and root shape: periapical vs panoramic films, *Angle Orthod,* Vol. 71, No. 3, pp. 185–189, ISSN 0003-3219

Sameshima, GT. & Sinclair, PM. (2001). Predicting and preventing root resorption: Part I. Diagnostic factors. *Am J Orthod Dentofacial Orthop,* Vol. 119, No. 5, pp. 505-510, ISSN 0889-5406

Sanchez, JE.; Perera, E.; Baumbach, L. & Cleveland, WW. (1998). Growth hormone receptor mutations in children with idiopathic short stature. *J Clin Endocrinol Metab,* Vol. 83, No. 11, pp. 4079-4083, ISSN 0021-972X

Sasaki, Y.; Kaida, C.; Saitoh, I.; Fujiwara, T. & Nonaka, K. (2007). Craniofacial growth and functional change in oligodontia with ectodermal dysplasia: a case report. *J Oral Rehabil,* Vol. 34, No. 3, pp. 228-235, ISSN 0305-182X

Sasaki, Y.; Satoh, K.; Hayasaki, H.; Fukumoto, S.; Fujiwara, T. & Nonaka, K. (2009). The P561T polymorphism of the growth hormone receptor gene has an inhibitory effect on mandibular growth in young children. *Eur J Orthod,* Vol. 31, No. 5, pp. 536-541, ISSN 1460-2210

Schaefer, GB.; Rosenbloom, AL.; Guevara-Aguirre, J.; Campbell, EA.; Ullrich, F.; Patil, K. et al. (1994). Facial morphometry of Ecuadorian patients with growth hormone receptor deficiency/Laron syndrome. *J Med Genet,* Vol. 31, No. 8, pp. 635-639, ISSN 0022-2593

Schork, NJ. (2002). Power calculations for genetic association studies using estimated probability distributions. *Am J Hum Genet,* Vol. 70, No. 6, pp. 1480-1489, ISSN 0002-9297

Shevah, O.; Rubinstein, M. & Laron, Z. (2004). Molecular defects of the growth hormone receptor gene, including a new mutation, in Laron syndrome patients in Israel: relationship between defects and ethnic groups. *Isr Med Assoc J,* Vol. 6, No. 10, pp. 630-633, ISSN 1565-1088

Simmons, KE. (1999). Growth hormone and craniofacial changes: preliminary data from studies in Turner's syndrome. *Pediatrics,* Vol. 104, No. 4, pp. 1021-1024, ISSN 0031-4005

Sjoberg, M.; Salazar, T.; Espinosa, C.; Dagnino, A.; Avila, A.; Eggers, M. et al. (2001). Study of GH sensitivity in chilean patients with idiopathic short stature. *J Clin Endocrinol Metab,* Vol. 86, No. 9, PP. 4375-4381, ISSN 0021-972X

Sjogren, K.; Bohlooly, YM.; Olsson, B.; Coschigano, K.; Tornell, J.; Mohan, S. et al. (2000). Disproportional skeletal growth and markedly decreased bone mineral content in growth hormone receptor -/- mice. Biochem Biophys Res Commun, Vol. 267, No. 2, pp. 603-608, ISSN 0006-291X

Tomoyasu Y.; Yamaguchi T.; Tajima A.; Nakajima T.; Inoue I. & Maki K. (2009a). External apical root resorption and interleukin-1B gene polymorphism in Japanese population. *Orthod Waves,* Vol. 68, No. 4, pp. 152-157, ISSN 1344-0241

Tomoyasu, Y.; Yamaguchi, T.; Tajima, A.; Nakajima, T.; Inoue, I. & Maki K. (2009b). Further evidence for an association between mandibular height and the growth hormone receptor gene in a Japanese population. *Am J Orthod Dentofacial Orthop,* Vol. 136, No. 4, pp. 536-541, ISSN 1097-6752

Uematsu, S.; Mogi, M. & Deguchi, T. (1996). Interleukin (IL)-1 beta, IL-6, tumor necrosis factor-alpha, epidermal growth factor, and beta 2-microglobulin levels are elevated in gingival crevicular fluid during human orthodontic tooth movement. *J Dent Res,* Vol. 75, No. 1, pp. 562-567, ISSN 0022-0345

Urbanek, M.; MacLeod, JN.; Cooke, NE. & Liebhaber SA. (1992). Expression of a human growth hormone (hGH) receptor isoform is predicted by tissue-specific alternative splicing of exon 3 of the hGH receptor gene transcript. *Mol Endocrinol,* Vol. 6, No. 2, pp. 279–287, ISSN 0888-8809

Van Erum, R.; Mulier, G.; Carels, C. & de Zegher, F. (1988). Craniofacial growth and dental maturation in short children born small for gestational age: effect of growth hormone treatment. Own observations and review of the literature. *Horm Res,* Vol. 50, No. 3, pp. 141-146, ISSN 0301-0163

Viecilli, RF.; Katona, TR.; Chen, J.; Hartsfield, JK Jr. & Roberts, WE. (2009). Orthodontic mechanotransduction and the role of the P2X7 receptor. *Am J Orthod Dentofacial Orthop,* Vol. 135, No. 6, pp. 694e1–16, ISSN 1097-6752

Wang, XD.; Deng, XY.; Chen, J.; Li, JL.; Chen, X.; Zhao, LZ. et al. (2008). Single nucleotide polymorphisms of the pregnane x receptor gene in Han Chinese and a comparison with other ethnic populations. *Pharmacology,* Vol. 81, No. 4, pp. 350-354, ISSN 1423-0313

Xue, F.; Wong, R. & Rabie, AB. (2010). Identification of SNP markers on 1p36 and association analysis of EPB41 with mandibular prognathism in a Chinese population. *Arch Oral Biol,* Vol. 55, No. 11, pp. 867-872, ISSN 1879-1506

Yamaguchi, T.; Maki, K. & Shibasaki, Y. (2001). Growth hormone receptor gene variant and mandibular height in the normal Japanese population. *Am J Orthod Dentofacial Orthop,* Vol. 119, No. 6, pp. 650-653, ISSN 0889-5406

Yamaguchi, T.; Park, SB.; Narita, A.; Maki, K. & Inoue I. (2005). Genome-wide linkage analysis of mandibular prognathism in Korean and Japanese patients. *J Dent Res,* Vol. 84, No. 3, pp. 255-259, ISSN 0022-0345

Zhou, J.; Lu, Y.; Gao, XH.; Chen, YC.; Lu, JJ.; Bai, YX. et al. (2005). The growth hormone receptor gene is associated with mandibular height in a Chinese population. *J Dent Res,* Vol. 84, No. 11, pp. 1052-1056, ISSN 0022-0345